Essentials of Pain Medicine

Essentials of Pain Medicine

Editor: Eva Fitzgerald

FOSTER ACADEMICS
www.fosteracademics.com

www.fosteracademics.com

FOSTER ACADEMICS

Cataloging-in-Publication Data

Essentials of pain medicine / edited by Eva Fitzgerald.
p. cm.
Includes bibliographical references and index.
ISBN 978-1-63242-837-0
1. Pain medicine. 2. Pain--Treatment. 3. Medicine. 4. Pharmacology. I. Fitzgerald, Eva.
RB127 .E87 2019
617.9--dc23

Foster Academics,
118-35 Queens Blvd., Suite 400,
Forest Hills, NY 11375, USA

ISBN 978-1-63242-837-0 (Hardback)

Printed and bound in China.

Contents

Preface

Pain medicine is the branch of medicine dealing with the management of pain for improving the quality of life of patients suffering from pain. When a pathology is resistant to treatment and pain persists, and when the underlying cause of pain can not be understood, the task of pain medicine is to relieve suffering. An important goal of pain management is to address pain in such a way that it is effective and causes as little side effects as possible. NSAIDs, opioids, muscle relaxants, antiepileptic and anti-inflammatory drugs, cannabinoids, antidepressants, anticonvulsants, etc. are medications that are prescribed for mild, acute, severe and chronic pain. For the treatment of chronic pain, whether due to malignant or benign processes, a three-step Analgesic Ladder recommends the kind of prescription for mild, moderate and severe pain and the way to increase analgesia. This book presents the complex subject of pain medicine in the most comprehensible language. From theories to research to practical applications, case studies related to all contemporary topics of relevance to this field have been included in this book. With state-of-the-art inputs by acclaimed experts of this field, this book targets students and professionals.

This book is a comprehensive compilation of works of different researchers from varied parts of the world. It includes valuable experiences of the researchers with the sole objective of providing the readers (learners) with a proper knowledge of the concerned field. This book will be beneficial in evoking inspiration and enhancing the knowledge of the interested readers.

In the end, I would like to extend my heartiest thanks to the authors who worked with great determination on their chapters. I also appreciate the publisher's support in the course of the book. I would also like to deeply acknowledge my family who stood by me as a source of inspiration during the project.

Editor

1

Psychiatric Disorders in Complex Regional Pain Syndrome (CRPS): The Role of the Consultation-Liaison Psychiatrist

Michael Brinkers,[1] Paulina Rumpelt,[2] Anke Lux,[3] Moritz Kretzschmar,[1] and Giselher Pfau[1]

[1]Department of Anaesthesiology and Intensive Care Medicine, Otto-von-Guericke-University Magdeburg, Magdeburg, Germany
[2]Department of Diagnostic and Interventional Radiology, Oberlausitz-Kliniken, Bautzen, Germany
[3]Department for Biometrics and Medical Informatics, Otto-von-Guericke-University Magdeburg, Magdeburg, Germany

Correspondence should be addressed to Moritz Kretzschmar; moritz.kretzschmar@med.ovgu.de

Academic Editor: Federica Galli

Background. Complex regional pain syndrome (CRPS) is a multifactorial disorder with complex aetiology and pathogenesis. At the outpatient pain clinic of Magdeburg University Hospital, all patients, without exception, are subject to permanent psychiatric care delivered by a consultation-liaison psychiatrist. In CRPS, psychological stabilization and treatment of the neuropathic aspects are equally important. The aim of this single-center retrospective study was to determine mental/psychiatric defects impairing pain processing at the time of investigation and show the effects of treating mental disorders and neuropathic pain with the same psychotropic drugs. *Method.* On admission, the consultation-liaison psychiatrist examined the mental state of every patient in a semistructured interview according to AMDP (working group for methods and documentation in psychiatry). Due to the model of the Department of Anaesthesiology, we are able to compare the group of CRPS patients with all other outpatients treated for pain. *Results.* The medical treatment of psychiatric dysfunction leads to an analgesic effect. Only every second CRPS patient had an additional psychiatric diagnosis, and 15.6% were diagnosed with depressive mood disorders and show a higher prevalence of depressive symptoms than the general population and exceed the mean for all patients treated in our pain clinic. *Conclusions.* In neuropathies, treatment of the neuropathic pain has a modulating effect on mental disorders. As CRPS patients are frequently affected by depressions, and owing to the connection between depression and suicidal tendencies, patients should be seen by a consultation-liaison psychiatrist, and nonpsychiatrists should pay special attention to this patient group.

1. Introduction

The complex regional pain syndrome (CRPS) can be divided into two groups:

(i) CRPS I, formerly known as reflex sympathetic dystrophy (RSD)—here, no nerve lesions can be identified.

(ii) CRPS II (formerly known as causalgia). The symptoms of this syndrome include evidence of a nerve lesion [1].

As CRPS belongs to the neuropathic diseases, the patients were subject to drug therapy, with special attention paid to the administration of anticonvulsant and antidepressant drugs. Wertli et al. [2] performed a meta-analysis and concluded that anticonvulsant and antidepressant drugs had no satisfying effect. By contrast, psychiatric drugs are indicated in the case of psychiatric alterations, such as agitation, anxiety, or depressive moods. CRPS in association with psychiatric disorders has only been investigated in limited studies, as the patients rarely undergo a routine and thorough psychological-psychiatric examination [3]. Rommel et al. recommend a psychological cotreatment of the patients. On the one hand, psychiatric alterations, mainly depression and anxiety, are registered in this way. On the other hand, these comorbidities should be treated with psychotherapy and/or medication. However, the question of whether psychological factors should be regarded as risk factors for CRPS is a highly controversial issue [4–6].

The care by a consultation-liaison (CL) psychiatrist is a permanent feature of the Department of Anaesthesiology, where the CL psychiatrist is employed full time since 2001. All patients, without exception, undergo psychological evaluation. In this way, it is possible to obtain an overview of the group of CRPS patients and relate them to the entire group of outpatients treated for pain.

This retrospective study describes the neuropathic and psychiatric aspects of CRPS patients and their treatment.

2. Patients and Methods

2.1. Patients. For this retrospective study, we collected data from CRPS patients examined at the Department of Anaesthesiology (Medical Faculty of Otto-von-Guericke University) between January 1, 2001, and June 30, 2014. Data were analysed after consultation with the Ethics Committee of Otto-von-Guericke University and in strict compliance with data protection by pseudonymization. The correctness of the referral diagnosis of CRPS for outpatient treatment was checked and confirmed at our clinic according to the clinical data and criteria published by Stanton-Hicks et al. [1], Jänig and Stanton-Hicks [7] and, after adoption by the IASP in 2010, according to the Budapest criteria [8]. A comparison of the criteria before and after 2010 is displayed in Table 1.

One of the central issues of the patients' medical history is pain quality and pain severity. The Visual Analogue Scale (VAS) is a 10 cm scale that measures the severity of pain. The scale has different descriptors at each end on a horizontal line (VAS 0 is no pain, and 10 is the worst pain). In addition to the current pain level (current VAS), the patients are interviewed for their maximum (maximum VAS), minimum (minimum VAS), and target VAS ("Which pain level would you accept if we say that we cannot reach VAS 0?").

To complete the medical history, the CL psychiatrist questioned the patients in a semistructured interview according to AMDP to get an overview of their psychic state. To evaluate and classify the findings, a comparison was made with the entire group of pain outpatients with corresponding somatic and psychiatric diagnoses for the period 2001–June 2014.

2.2. Assessment and Questionnaires

2.2.1. AMDP (Working Group for Methods and Documentation in Psychiatry). The AMDP System is a Manual for the Assessment and Documentation of Psychopathology. The AMDP is an addition to a small number of instruments that have been created and tested in an international setting [10].

2.2.2. SCL-90-R. The SCL-90-R assesses psychological distress in terms of nine primary symptom dimensions and three summary scores termed global scores. SCL-90-R test was applied to all patients involved in this study. Somatization (SOM), Obsessive-Compulsive (O-C), Anxiety (ANX), Hostility (HOS), Phobic Anxiety (PHOB), Paranoid Ideation (PAR), and Psychoticism (PSY) subscales of SCL-90-R test were performed, and general assessment of SCL-90-R test was performed by the means of Global Severity Index (GSI). Its score is found by the average of the ratings of all items (range 0–4). GSI results indicate general assessment of SCL-90-R questionnaire.

2.3. Statistical Analysis. Statistical analysis was conducted with IBM SPSS version 24 (Armonk, NY, USA).

At first, descriptive analyses were carried out. The associations between qualitative variables were investigated by contingency table analyses using Pearson's chi-square test. The Mann–Whitney test was applied for comparison between quantitative variables (VAS). Wilcoxon's paired test was used to ascertain differences in quantitative data (VAS) between the time of the last consultation and the time of admission. This was done separately for the different groups to be investigated (CRPS I/CRPS II, F-diagnosis yes/no).

In all statistical tests, an error probability of α of 0.05 was assumed (all p values < 0.05 are considered significant).

3. Results

3.1. Demographic Data. Since the consequent registration of patients with somatic and psychiatric diagnoses at the Department of Anaesthesiology of Magdeburg Medical Faculty began in 2001, 64 CRPS patients (18 males and 46 females) have been treated (effective date: June 30, 2014). From the time of admission onwards, patients' age ranged from 19 to 89 years, with a mean (±standard deviation) of 49.6 ± 13.1 years. It must be pointed out that 47 patients developed CRPS after surgery. The demographic data are presented in Table 2.

A questionnaire was used to obtain an overview of all treatments applied for each patient to date and current medication was noted. These were as follows:

(1) Medical treatment ($n = 59$)

(2) Physical therapy with remedial gymnastics ($n = 48$), lymphatic drainage ($n = 12$), occupational therapy ($n = 8$), manual treatment ($n = 7$), electrotherapy ($n = 8$), and transcutaneous electrical nerve stimulation ($n = 13$)

(3) Psychotherapy ($n = 8$) and autogenic training ($n = 6$)

(4) Invasive treatments with intra-articular injection of corticosteroids ($n = 14$), local anaesthesia ($n = 3$), stellate ganglion block ($n = 2$), spinal cord stimulation ($n = 2$), and intravenous therapy with NMDA receptor antagonist ($n = 1$)

(5) Alternative medicine with acupuncture ($n = 7$)

An overview of administered substance classes after optimization and stepwise adaptation of the therapy is presented in Table 3. The staff of our department substantially increased the administration of low-potency opioids and psychotropic drugs such as anticonvulsants and antidepressants.

Clinical examination and electrophysiological studies performed in all the patients revealed CRPS II in 21 patients

TABLE 1: IASP criteria for the diagnosis of CRPS before and after 2010.

IASP diagnostic criteria for complex regional pain syndrome (CRPS)* up to 2010 [9]	IASP diagnostic criteria for complex regional pain syndrome (CRPS) after 2010 [8]
(1) The presence of an initiating noxious event, or a cause of immobilization†	(1) Continuing pain, which is disproportionate to any inciting event
(2) Continuing pain, allodynia, or hyperalgesia in which the pain is disproportionate to any known inciting event	(2) Must report at least one symptom in three of the four following categories: Sensory: reports of hyperalgesia and/or allodynia Vasomotor: reports of temperature asymmetry and/or skin color changes and/or skin color asymmetry. Sudomotor/edema: reports of edema and/or sweating changes and/or sweating asymmetry. Motor/trophic: reports of decreased range of motion and/or motor dysfunction (weakness, tremor, dystonia) and/or trophic changes (hair, nails, skin)
(3) Evidence at some time of edema, changes in skin blood flow, or abnormal sudomotor activity in the region of pain (can be sign or symptom)	(3) Must display at least one sign# at the time of evaluation in two or more of the following categories: Sensory: evidence of hyperalgesia (to pinprick) and/or allodynia (to light touch and/or deep somatic pressure and/or joint movement) Vasomotor: evidence of temperature asymmetry and/or skin color changes and/or asymmetry. Sudomotor/edema: evidence of edema and/or sweating changes and/or sweating asymmetry. Motor/trophic: evidence of decreased range of motion and/or motor dysfunction (weakness, tremor, dystonia) and/or trophic changes (hair, nails, skin)
(4) This diagnosis is excluded by the existence of other conditions that would otherwise account for the degree of pain and dysfunction	(4) There is no other diagnosis that better explains the signs and symptoms

*If seen without "major nerve damage," diagnose CRPS I; if seen in the presence of "major nerve damage," diagnose CRPS II. #A sign is counted only if it is observed at the time of diagnosis. †Not required for diagnosis; 5–10% of patients will not have this.

TABLE 2: Demographic data with mean value (±SD); median (range).

Male/female	18/46
Age at onset of pain	49.6 years (±13.1 years)
Age at last consultation	53.6 years (±12.8 years)
Time period between onset of pain and outpatient admission	1.6 years (±2.5); 0.5 years (immediately,13.3 years)
Time period between diagnosis and outpatient presentation	0.4 years (±1.0); 0.02 years (immediately, 7.5 years)
Treatment period	2.4 years (±3.6); 0.6 years (one consultation up to 15 years)
Number of consultations	23 (±37); 9 (1,190 consultations)
Upper/lower extremities	56/8
CRPS type I/type II	43/21
Number of patients with surgery before onset of CRPS	47

The VAS value of all 64 patients was 5.0 ± 2.5. Value at the end of therapy: 3.6 ± 2.1 ($p = 0.226$).

and CRPS I in 43 patients. Neuropathic complaints (burning, stabbing, cutting, tingling, shooting, and electrifying sensations) were mentioned by 60 of the 64 patients.

3.2. SCL-90-R. Altogether, the GSI data of 47 patients (73.4%) were compared. For 17 patients, no data were available. GSI had a mean value of 53.8 ± 8.4 (median 55.0, range from 33 to 70). Thirty-seven patients (78.3%) had GSI scores ≤ 60 (no increased mental stress), whereas 10 patients (21.3%) had GSI scores > 60. These patients showed increased values (total values > 61) for anxiety (scale 5: 65.0 ± 3.6) and depression (scale 4: 70.0 ± 4.6).

3.3. CRPS Patients with Psychiatric Diagnosis. Twenty-eight of 64 CRPS patients received a psychiatric diagnosis. For 36 patients (56.3%), the psychiatric findings were unremarkable. Seven of 28 patients with psychiatric diagnosis received a double diagnosis (25.0%), one patient a triple diagnosis (3.6%), and one patient a quadruple diagnosis (3.6%). The diagnoses are presented in Table 4.

Table 3: Overview of drug therapy distribution of drugs before outpatient admission and after adaptation of medication.

Drugs	Before admission (n)	At present or at end of therapy (n)
Low-potency opioids	24	40
High-potency opioids	6	11
NSAID	45	5
Anticonvulsant drugs	10	30*
Antidepressant drugs	6	39**
Neuroleptics	0	2
Glucocorticoids	4	0
Calcitonin	3	1

*Gabapentin, $n = 15$; pregabalin, $n = 9$; **amitriptyline, $n = 20$; mirtazapine, $n = 7$; venlafaxine, $n = 6$.

3.3.1. Psychiatric Diagnoses—A Comparison between CRPS Patients and the Common Patient Cohort of the Department of Anaesthesiology. The psychiatric examinations of all the patients treated at the Department of Anaesthesiology ($n = 2439$) gave the following picture:

(1) The psychological findings of 805 patients (33%) were unremarkable.

(2) 1634 patients (67%) had at least one psychiatric diagnosis.

(3) 866 (35.5%) of the patients had two, 173 (7.1%) had three, 10 (0.4%) had four, and two patients (0.1%) had five psychiatric diagnoses at the same time.

(4) Depression (F3) was diagnosed in 15.5% ($n = 378$).

(5) 207 (8.5%) of the patients abused pain killers or other substances.

(6) 636 patients (26.1%) were affected by a neurotic spectrum disorder (F4 = conversion disorder, anxiety disorder, somatoform disorder, adjustment disorder, and hypochondriasis).

The CRPS patients and all the other pain outpatients of our department were compared for the frequency of psychiatric diagnoses. This comparison revealed that CRPS patients were less frequently affected by organic defects including symptomatic psychiatric disorders (F0), as well as by neurotic stress and somatoform disorders. No anxiety disorders were noted. They also more frequently suffered from personality and behavioral disorders (F6) without any psychopathological findings ($p < 0.001$). These differences especially apply to female patients ($p = 0.005$).

Psychiatric findings classified as F3 and F4 (mood and adjustment disorders) of patients with somatic pain diagnoses (different somatic pain groups according to Klinger et al. [11]) in our pain clinic are presented in Table 5.

CRPS patients had the lowest proportion of psychiatric disorders and come after the group of patients with tumour pain. However, as far as the F3 depressions are concerned, their proportion is higher than the mean of the entire group of pain patients.

3.4. Reduction in Pain Severity

3.4.1. Pain Severity in CRPS I and CRPS II Patients. On admission, CRPS patients with nerve lesions had a significantly higher VAS level than those without (VAS 5.6 ± 2.5 versus VAS 4.1 ± 2.5, $p = 0.037$). At the end of the medication switch, CRPS patients with nerve lesions reached a VAS pain level of 4.25 ± 2.2 and those without nerve lesions reached a VAS level of 3.39 ± 2.2 (Figure 1).

3.4.2. Pain Severity in CRPS Patients with Psychiatric Diagnosis. There were significant differences in patients with psychiatric diagnosis on admission. The VAS data at presentation were as follows (psychiatric diagnosis yes/no):

VAS current: 5.63/3.97 ($p = 0.031$)

VAS minimum: 4.0/2.63 ($p = 0.015$)

VAS target: 3.08/2.03 ($p = 0.008$)

Here, the CRPS patients with psychiatric diagnosis showed significantly higher VAS values. No differences were found for VAS maximum (8.07/7.89; $p = 0.658$) and VAS end (4.08/3.39; $p = 0.228$).

Furthermore, patients with a psychiatric diagnosis showed significantly decreased VAS values at the end of therapy/record date ($p = 0.02$) when compared to the baseline values (Figure 2).

4. Discussion

Consensus has been reached in the literature that CRPS is a serious disease characterized by a heterogeneous expression and a course that is difficult to predict. The reason for this lies in numerous influences, including psychological factors [12]. Therefore, it is necessary to search for factors that either favour the development of or are caused by CRPS, thus complicating the course. Therefore, early diagnosis is the best prerequisite for a good prognosis [13].

Although this retrospective study focused on psychological aspects, a multimodal approach to pain therapy was adhered to in all patients. This included physical therapy and lymphatic drainage when indicated.

This study did not concentrate on remarkable life events or coping strategies [12, 14], but rather placed emphasis on psychological factors and psychiatric diagnoses.

The majority of authors assume that in CRPS patients, psychological disorders and changes in the patients' behavior are to a greater extent a consequence of the pain rather than the cause [15]. Other study groups report that psychiatric disorders had already been diagnosed before CRPS occurs [16, 17].

Table 4: Psychiatric diagnoses of ICD-10 for CRPS patients.

Diagnostic group	Commentary	Number of patients
F0	*Organic, including symptomatic, mental disorders*	*Total 3*
F07	Organic personality disorder	3
F1	*Mental and behavioral disorders due to psychoactive substance use*	*Total 6*
F10	Mental and behavioral disorders due to use of alcohol	3
F13.1	Harmful use of sedatives or hypnotics	1
F17.2	Dependence syndrome due to use of tobacco	2
F2	*Schizophrenia, schizotypal, and delusional disorders*	*Total 2*
F24	Induced delusional disorder	1
F25.2	Schizoaffective disorder, mixed type	1
F3	*Mood (affective) disorders*	*Total 10*
F32.0	Mild depressive episode	1
F32.1	Moderate depressive episode	3
F34.0	Cyclothymia	2
F34.1	Dysthymia	4
F4	*Neurotic, stress-related, and somatoform disorders*	*Total 11*
F42.1	Predominantly compulsive acts (obsessional rituals)	1
F43.2	Adjustment disorders	6
F44	Dissociative (conversion) disorders	2
F45.0	Somatization disorder	1
F45.4	Persistent somatoform pain disorder	1
F6	*Disorders of adult personality and behavior*	*Total 7*
F60.4	Histrionic personality disorder	1
F60.7	Dependent personality disorder	1
F60.8	Other specific personality disorders	2
F60.9	Personality disorder, unspecified	1
F62.8	Chronic pain personality syndrome	1
F66.0	Sexual maturation disorder	1
F9	*Behavioral and emotional disorders with onset usually occurring in childhood and adolescence*	*Total 1*
F95.1	Chronic motor or vocal tic disorder	1

Table 5: Percentage of mood disorders (F3) and neurotic spectrum disorders (F4) in different somatic pain groups according to Klinger, arranged in ascending order for F3.

Diagnosis	*n*	F3 (%)	F4 (%)	Total percentage of F-diagnoses (%)
Vascular pain in limbs	18	5.6	16.7	61.1
Neuropathia totally	276	7.2	15.9	55.8
Cancer pain	148	9.5	7.4	39.2
Chest pain	43	11.6	34.9	62.8
Muscle-joint pain	456	13.4	27.2	65.6
Chronic low back pain with radiculopathia	87	14.9	19.5	64.4
CRPS	*64*	*15.6*	*17.2*	*43.8*
Abdominal pain	88	15.9	36.4	81.8
Chronic low back pain without radiculopathia	905	16.9	31.4	71.7
Headache and facial pain	185	20.0	22.7	62.2
Fibromyalgia and panalgesia	171	25.7	31.6	86.5
Cenesthesia	62	25.8	16.1	72.6

Numerous case reports characterize CRPS patients as anxious, strained, irritated, emotionally labile, or depressive [18–20]. The description of these patients focused on either personal traits or psychological factors, such as depression or anxiety [21–24], which are presumed to occur more frequently in CRPS patients. This corresponds to the personal traits mentioned above. Anxiety, in particular, is associated with higher risk of developing CRPS after fractures [25]. According to Rommel et al. [3], increased anxiety is a factor that increases pain [25]. In our study though, the questionnaire SCL-90-R revealed that only a small patient cohort was affected by anxiety.

Psychiatric disorders, such as depressive mood disorders or anxiety disorders, have only rarely been investigated. Two study groups have tried to ascertain the proportion of psychiatric disorders in CRPS by using SCID for DSM-III

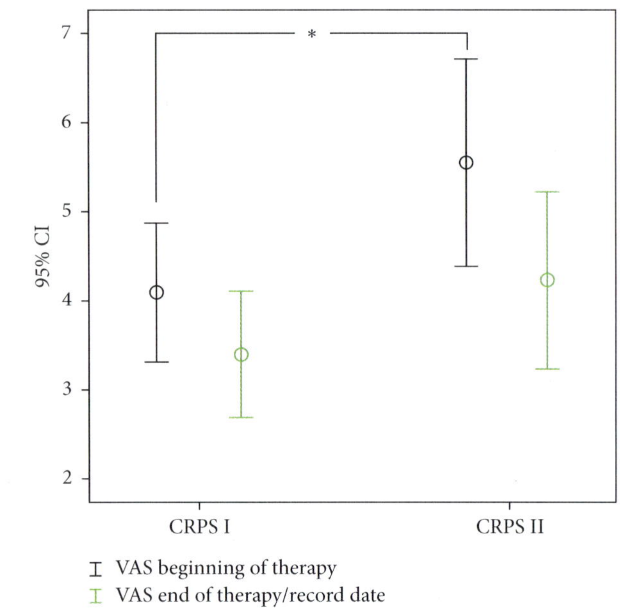

Figure 1: The course of average VAS between CRPS types I and II. Time point 1: beginning of therapy; time point 2: end of medication switch/record date; *significant difference between CRPS type I and type II at the beginning of therapy.

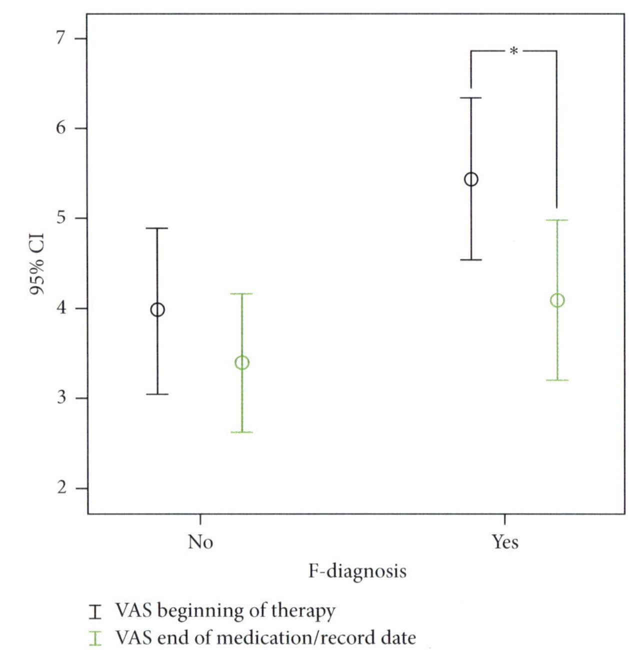

Figure 2: The course of average VAS between CRPS patient with or without F-diagnosis. Time point 1: beginning of therapy; time point 2: end of medication switch/record date; *significant difference to beginning of therapy.

and DSM-IV (Structured Clinical Interview for Diagnostic and Statistical Manual of Mental Disorders). In 1998, Monti et al. [13] compared pain diseases with a neuropathic component. They compared 25 patients with CRPS I and 25 patients with chronic back pain following a herniated disk using a structured clinical interview according to SCID for DSM-III. 20% and 24% of the patient groups fulfilled the criteria for a major depression (i.e., F3 depression). Of the nondepressed patients, 60% and 64% showed no sign of a personality disorder. Thus, no significant differences were noted.

In their most recent systematically performed psychiatric investigation performed in 2001, Rommel et al. [3] concentrated on the recognition of psychiatric disorders in CRPS. That study included 40 patients interviewed according to SCID for DSM-IV. The interview for that study was performed by an experienced psychologist. Thirty-seven of 40 patients were evaluated. Eight patients (22%) were found to be psychologically normal in the preliminary finding and at the time of examination. Rommel et al. registered adjustment disorders in twelve of the 37 patients and major depressions (F32.1) in five patients and summarized these deficiencies as psychiatric disorders occurring after CRPS. Due to the fact that depression episodes occurred in six patients before CRPS, in five patients after CRPS, and in seven patients in the further course, it has to be presumed that cyclothymic courses with interim inconspicuous stages ($6/37 = 16.2\%$) were responsible. Furthermore, these patients constituted a minority compared to those affected by adjustment disorders (6 versus 12). The majority of patients showed signs of anxiety before onset of CRPS.

In our study, we registered a depression rate of 15.6%, which is similar to the percentage reported by Rommel et al. When compared to the entire group, anxiety disorders were not diagnosed.

In our department, both an anaesthesiologist and a permanently present CL psychiatrist take care of all the pain patients. This means that psychological findings are available for all patients (100%). Compared to the entire patient cohort of the Department of Anaesthesiology, the proportion of psychiatric disorders in CRPS patients is lower. A specific comparison with back pain and muscle-joint pain revealed that the proportion was considerably lower.

According to Feliu and Edwards [26], specific predisposing factors of the psychological or psychiatric kind which trigger or intensify CRPS do not exist for CRPS patients, nor can these factors be found in other patients with chronic pain.

However, compared to the common population, the CRPS patients of our study show

(1) a higher prevalence (15.6%) for depression. The TACOS study in Germany (Transitions in Alcohol Consumption and Smoking) interviewed 4075 persons by telephone and found that 11.5% of the questioned participants were affected by major depression [27],

(2) a higher prevalence for depression compared to the majority of somatic patients of the entire group,

(3) that concerning depression, our data are similar to those of Rommel et al. [3].

Rommel et al. concluded that depressive mood disorders constitute a factor that promotes disease and intensifies pain.

In our study, pain was more intense in patients with psychiatric disorders. Other studies also confirm that psychiatric disorders intensify pain in CRPS patients [28].

In general, patients with neuropathic pain have a lower incidence of depression than patients with other forms of physical pain. In our study population, 7.2% had a F3 diagnosis, while 15.9% of CRPS patients showed a F3 diagnosis (Table 5). Smith et al. found lower suicidal tendencies in patients with neuropathic pain compared to stomach pain and explain this by the concept that neuropathic pain has a physical and anatomic correlate [29].

In a publication from our study group, we could show that neuropathic pain has an incidence of 8.2% for F3 depression as opposed to lower back pain (14.0%) and muscle-joint pain (15.0%) in a population of 485 outpatients assessed over a consecutive 6-month period [30].

Maier et al. found in a general population a prevalence of 4.5% for F3 depression [31], whereas Elisei et al. located them at 17% [32].

Different therapies have been recommended for the treatment of CRPS. A large number of studies have investigated the analgesic effects of different therapy forms [33]. However, success can be achieved only by combination of different therapies and early diagnosis [34]. Another aspect needs to be added: Our study is the first to emphasize the bipolar efficacy spectrum of analgetically effective psychiatric drugs. As CRPS patients have comorbidity with F3 depression, these patients should be treated with dual active psychotropic drugs, that is, serotonin-noradrenaline reuptake inhibitors (SNRIs) as opposed to selective serotonin reuptake inhibitors (SSRIs) [30]. In the treatment of depression and pain, SNRIs have a direct analgetic influence on pain and the pain is reduced indirectly by increasing the threshold for neuralgia. Therefore, the treatment with dual active psychotropic drugs could have facilitated the reduction in VAS pain scores we found.

Due to the association between depression and suicidal tendencies among pain patients [35–37], surveillance by nonpsychiatrists [38, 39] and increased psychological care [40] are recommended in current literature.

4.1. Limitations of the Study. This study only compared the psychiatric diagnoses of CRPS patients with those of other chronic pain patients in an outpatient clinic of a university hospital. It was not the aim of this study to perform an expansive psychological assessment or to systematically determine radical and stressing life events and their timely assignment to the disease process.

Also, the diagnostic criteria of CRPS were revised and adopted by the IASP in 2010. The Budapest Criteria have a sensitivity nearly identical to that for the IASP criteria, but with substantially improved specificity, and furthermore lead to improved diagnostic consistency between clinicians [8].

5. Conclusions

CRPS is a syndrome that offers an extremely variable picture. Emphasis is placed on two psychiatric factors (anxiety and depression). Some authors assign a repeatedly noted anxiety to a type of personality, whereas others regard this as a clue to anxiety disorders and their differential diagnoses [41]. In our retrospective study, increased anxiety was noted only in a small number of patients.

The depressions were assigned to affective disorders (F3) in two publications based on SCID for DSM-III [13] and, respectively, on SCID for DSM-IV [3]. Chronic pain patients in general and CRPS patients in particular are affected by a larger number of depressions compared to the normal population.

However, as the number of cases is very small, this conclusion should be regarded with caution. But those data are confirmed by current investigations and by comparison with all disease courses evaluated by the Department of Anaesthesiology to date. As depressions may lead to a higher rate of suicidality in CRPS patients [35, 37], psychological and psychiatric treatment is recommended as early as possible.

Acknowledgments

This work was funded by Institutional Resources of the Department of Anaesthesiology and Intensive Care Medicine, Otto-von-Guericke-University Magdeburg.

References

[1] M. Stanton-Hicks, W. Janig, S. Hassenbusch, J. D. Haddox, R. Boas, and P. Wilson, "Reflex sympathetic dystrophy: changing concepts and taxonomy," *Pain*, vol. 63, no. 1, pp. 127–133, 1995.

[2] M. M. Wertli, A. G. Kessels, R. S. Perez, L. M. Bachmann, and F. Brunner, "Rational pain management in complex regional pain syndrome 1 (CRPS 1)—a network meta-analysis," *Pain Medicine*, vol. 15, no. 9, pp. 1575–1589, 2014.

[3] O. Rommel, A. Willweber-Strumpf, P. Wagner, D. Surall, J.-P. Malin, and M. Zenz, "Psychological abnormalities in patients with complex regional pain syndrome (CRPS)," *Der Schmerz*, vol. 19, no. 4, pp. 272–284, 2005.

[4] A. Beerthuizen, D. L. Stronks, F. J. Huygen, J. Passchier, J. Klein, and A. V. Spijker, "The association between psychological factors and the development of complex regional pain syndrome type 1 (CRPS1)—a prospective multicenter study," *European Journal of Pain*, vol. 15, no. 9, pp. 971–975, 2011.

[5] A. Beerthuizen, A. van't Spijker, F. J. Huygen, J. Klein, and R. De Wit, "Is there an association between psychological factors and the Complex Regional Pain Syndrome type 1 (CRPS1) in adults? A systematic review," *Pain*, vol. 145, no. 1, pp. 52–59, 2009.

[6] R. S. Perez, W. W. Zuurmond, P. D. Bezemer et al., "The treatment of complex regional pain syndrome type I with free radical scavengers: a randomized controlled study," *Pain*, vol. 102, no. 3, pp. 297–307, 2003.

[7] W. Jänig and M. Stanton-Hicks, *Reflex Sympathetic Dystrophy—A Reappraisal:* 6, IASP Press, Seattle, WC, USA, 1996.
[8] R. N. Harden, S. Bruehl, R. S. Perez et al., "Validation of proposed diagnostic criteria (the "budapest criteria") for complex regional pain syndrome," *Pain*, vol. 150, no. 2, pp. 268–274, 2010.
[9] H. Merskey and N. Bogduk, "Classification of chronic pain. Descriptions of chronic pain syndromes and definitions of pain terms. Prepared by the International association for the study of pain, subcommittee on taxonomy," *Pain Supplement*, vol. 3, pp. S1–S226, 1986.
[10] W. Guy and T. A. Ban, *The AMDP-System: Manual for the Assessment and Documentation of Psychopathology*, Springer, Berlin, Heidelberg, Germany, 1982.
[11] R. Klinger, H. Denecke, B. Glier et al., "Quality control in the therapy of chronic pain. Results obtained by a task force of the German section of the international association for the study of pain on psychological assessment of chronic pain. XI. assessment and multiaxial classification of pain," *Der Schmerz*, vol. 11, no. 6, pp. 378–385, 1997.
[12] C. Maihofner, "Complex regional pain syndrome: a current review," *Der Schmerz*, vol. 28, no. 3, pp. 319–336, 2014.
[13] D. A. Monti, C. L. Herring, R. J. Schwartzman, and M. Marchese, "Personality assessment of patients with complex regional pain syndrome type I," *Clinical Journal of Pain*, vol. 14, no. 4, pp. 295–302, 1998.
[14] J. H. Geertzen, H. De Bruijn, A. T. De Bruijn-Kofman, and J. H. Arendzen, "Reflex sympathetic dystrophy: early treatment and psychological aspects," *Archives of Physical Medicine and Rehabilitation*, vol. 75, no. 4, pp. 442–446, 1994.
[15] R. J. Schwartzman and T. L. McLellan, "Reflex sympathetic dystrophy. A review," *Archives of Neurology*, vol. 44, no. 5, pp. 555–561, 1987.
[16] M. D. Chard, "Diagnosis and management of algodystrophy," *Annals of the Rheumatic Diseases*, vol. 50, no. 10, pp. 727–730, 1991.
[17] J. M. Gybels and W. H. Sweet, "Neurosurgical treatment of persistent pain. Physiological and pathological mechanisms of human pain," *Pain and Headache*, vol. 11, pp. 1–402, 1989.
[18] M. Buhring, "Reflex dystrophy following so-called whiplash injury of the cervical spine," *Zeitschrift fur Orthopadie und ihre Grenzgebiete*, vol. 122, no. 3, pp. 281–286, 1984.
[19] M. E. Lynch, "Psychological aspects of reflex sympathetic dystrophy: a review of the adult and paediatric literature," *Pain*, vol. 49, no. 3, pp. 337–347, 1992.
[20] H. J. Pollack, R. Neumann, and E. Pollack, "Sudeck's disease and the psyche," *Beitrage zur Orthopadie und Traumatologie*, vol. 27, no. 8, pp. 463–468, 1980.
[21] D. J. Bean, M. H. Johnson, W. Heiss-Dunlop, A. C. Lee, and R. R. Kydd, "Do psychological factors influence recovery from complex regional pain syndrome type 1? A prospective study," *Pain*, vol. 156, no. 11, pp. 2310–2318, 2015.
[22] S. Bruehl and C. R. Carlson, "Predisposing psychological factors in the development of reflex sympathetic dystrophy. A review of the empirical evidence," *Clinical Journal of Pain*, vol. 8, no. 4, pp. 287–299, 1992.
[23] J. A. Lohnberg and E. M. Altmaier, "A review of psychosocial factors in complex regional pain syndrome," *Journal of Clinical Psychology in Medical Settings*, vol. 20, no. 2, pp. 247–254, 2013.
[24] G. Pendon, A. Salas, M. Garcia, and D. Pereira, "Complex regional pain syndrome type 1: analysis of 108 patients," *Reumatología Clínica*, vol. 13, no. 2, pp. 73–77, 2017.
[25] B. Dilek, B. Yemez, R. Kizil et al., "Anxious personality is a risk factor for developing complex regional pain syndrome type I," *Rheumatology International*, vol. 32, no. 4, pp. 915–920, 2012.
[26] M. H. Feliu and C. L. Edwards, "Psychologic factors in the development of complex regional pain syndrome: history, myth, and evidence," *Clinical Journal of Pain*, vol. 26, no. 3, pp. 258–263, 2010.
[27] C. Meyer, H. J. Rumpf, U. Hapke et al., "Lifetime prevalence of mental disorders in general adult population. Results of TACOS study," *Der Nervenarzt*, vol. 71, no. 7, pp. 535–542, 2000.
[28] A. Vouilloz, O. Deriaz, G. Rivier, C. Gobelet, and F. Luthi, "Biopsychosocial complexity is correlated with psychiatric comorbidity but not with perceived pain in complex regional pain syndrome type 1 (algodystrophy) of the knee," *Joint Bone Spine*, vol. 78, no. 2, pp. 194–199, 2011.
[29] M. T. Smith, R. R. Edwards, R. C. Robinson, and R. H. Dworkin, "Suicidal ideation, plans, and attempts in chronic pain patients: factors associated with increased risk," *Pain*, vol. 111, no. 1, pp. 201–208, 2004.
[30] M. Brinkers, G. Pfau, and C. Schneemilch, "Aspects of liaison psychiatry care of patients in a university pain clinic," *Der Schmerz*, vol. 32, no. 2, pp. 115–120, 2018.
[31] C. Maier, R. Baron, T. R. Tolle et al., "Quantitative sensory testing in the German Research Network on Neuropathic Pain (DFNS): somatosensory abnormalities in 1236 patients with different neuropathic pain syndromes," *Pain*, vol. 150, no. 3, pp. 439–450, 2010.
[32] S. Elisei, L. Pauselli, P. M. Balducci et al., "Mood disorders in general hospital inpatients: one year data from a psychiatric consultation-liaison service," *Psychiatria Danubina*, vol. 25, no. 2, pp. S268–S271, 2013.
[33] N. S. Atalay, O. Ercidogan, N. Akkaya, and F. Sahin, "Prednisolone in complex regional pain syndrome," *Pain Physician*, vol. 17, no. 2, pp. 179–185, 2014.
[34] R. Albazaz, Y. T. Wong, and S. Homer-Vanniasinkam, "Complex regional pain syndrome: a review," *Annals of Vascular Surgery*, vol. 22, no. 2, pp. 297–306, 2008.
[35] B. J. Fisher, J. A. Haythornthwaite, L. J. Heinberg, M. Clark, and J. Reed, "Suicidal intent in patients with chronic pain," *Pain*, vol. 89, no. 2, pp. 199–206, 2001.
[36] I. Jimenez-Rodriguez, J. M. Garcia-Leiva, B. M. Jimenez-Rodriguez, E. Condés-Moreno, F. Rico-Villademoros, and E. Calandre, "Suicidal ideation and the risk of suicide in patients with fibromyalgia: a comparison with non-pain controls and patients suffering from low-back pain," *Neuropsychiatric Disease and Treatment*, vol. 10, pp. 625–630, 2014.
[37] J. Sharp and B. Keefe, "Psychiatry in chronic pain: a review and update," *Current Psychiatry Reports*, vol. 7, no. 3, pp. 213–219, 2005.
[38] M. A. Ilgen, F. Kleinberg, R. V. Ignacio et al., "Noncancer pain conditions and risk of suicide," *JAMA Psychiatry*, vol. 70, no. 7, pp. 692–697, 2013.
[39] L. Sanna, A. L. Stuart, J. A. Pasco et al., "Suicidal ideation and physical illness: does the link lie with depression?," *Journal of Affective Disorders*, vol. 152–154, pp. 422–426, 2014.
[40] J. W. Gilbert, G. R. Wheeler, B. B. Storey et al., "Suicidality in chronic noncancer pain patients," *International Journal of Neuroscience*, vol. 119, no. 10, pp. 1968–1979, 2009.
[41] S. M. Stahl and S. Soefje, "Panic attacks and panic disorder: the great neurologic imposters," *Seminars in Neurology*, vol. 15, no. 2, pp. 126–132, 1995.

2

Effectiveness of Sequential Viscosupplementation in Temporomandibular Joint Internal Derangements and Symptomatology

Roberta Maria Drumond Furtado Bossi Fonseca,[1] Eduardo Januzzi,[2] Luciano Ambrosio Ferreira,[3,4] Eduardo Grossmann,[5] Antonio Carlos Pires Carvalho,[3] Pedro Gonçalves de Oliveira,[6] Érica Leandro Marciano Vieira,[7] Antônio Lúcio Teixeira,[7,8] and Camila Megale Almeida-Leite[1,9]

[1]*Programa de Pós-Graduação em Patologia, Faculdade de Medicina, Universidade Federal de Minas Gerais (UFMG), Belo Horizonte, MG, Brazil*
[2]*Faculdade Ciodonto, Sete Lagoas, MG, Brazil*
[3]*Departamento de Radiologia, Faculdade de Medicina, Universidade Federal do Rio de Janeiro, Rio de Janeiro, RJ, Brazil*
[4]*9 Hospital Maternidade Therezinha de Jesus-HMTJ/JF, Suprema-Faculdade de Ciências Médicas e da Saúde, Juiz de Fora, Brazil*
[5]*Departamento de Ciências Morfológicas, Instituto de Ciências Básicas da Saúde, Universidade Federal do Rio Grande do Sul, Porto Alegre, RS, Brazil*
[6]*Faculdade de Farmácia, Universidade Anhembi Morumbi, São Paulo, SP, Brazil*
[7]*Departamento de Clínica Médica, Faculdade de Medicina, UFMG, Belo Horizonte, MG, Brazil*
[8]*Department of Psychiatry and Behavioral Sciences, The University of Texas, Houston, TX, USA*
[9]*Departamento de Morfologia, Instituto de Ciências Biológicas, UFMG, Belo Horizonte, MG, Brazil*

Correspondence should be addressed to Camila Megale Almeida-Leite; camila@icb.ufmg.br

Academic Editor: Fabiana Ballanti

Viscosupplementation is a minimally invasive technique that replaces synovial fluid by intra-articular injection of hyaluronic acid (HA). Although effective in some joints, there is not conclusive evidence regarding temporomandibular disorders. This case series described the efficacy of a viscosupplementation protocol in intra-articular temporomandibular disorders. Ten patients with a diagnosis of disc displacement and/or osteoarthritis by Research Diagnostic Criteria for Temporomandibular Disorders (RDC/TMD) were submitted to four monthly injections of low or medium molecular weight HA. Pain, mandibular function, image analysis by tomography and magnetic resonance, and quality of life were assessed at baseline and follow-ups (1 and 6 months). Pain, jaw range-of-motion, mandibular function, and quality of life improved at follow-up evaluations. Osteoarthritis changes decreased, and 20% of patients improved mandibular head excursion after treatment. Resolution of effusion and improvement in disc morphology were observed for most patients. This viscosupplementation protocol reduced pain and symptoms associated with internal derangement of temporomandibular joint, improved quality of life, and showed benefits from both low and medium molecular weight HA in alternate cycles.

1. Introduction

Temporomandibular disorders (TMDs) are a heterogeneous group of disorders involving the temporomandibular joint (TMJ), the masticatory muscles, and associated structures [1–3]. TMD affect 5 to 12% of population [4], and their management causes high costs to public health [5]. The most common signs and symptoms include pain, TMJ sounds, and limitation of mandibular movement, which can compromise daily activities and quality of life [2, 6].

According to American Academy of Orofacial Pain (AAOP), diagnosis and classification of TMD are divided into two major groups: muscle and joint disorders, with their respective subdivisions [3]. Among intra-articular TMD, disc displacement with or without reduction and degenerative joint disorders (osteoarthrosis and osteoarthritis) are the most frequent alterations. They are associated to changes in quantity and quality of synovial fluid (SF) [3, 7].

Viscosupplementation (VS) is a minimally invasive technique that involves replacement of synovial fluid by intra-articular injection of hyaluronic acid (HA) which restores its concentration and molecular weight in joint cavity [8]. HA is an important component of synovial fluid and is produced by type B synoviocytes. These molecules are involved by a large amount of water and provide suitable viscosity and elasticity for synovial fluid [9]. Studies about the effects of exogenous HA with different molecular weights have been performed. It has been suggested that high molecular weight HA is important in lubrication and protection of joint structures due to its improvement of highly hydrated and rheological environment [10, 11]. In contrast, low molecular weight HA induces its endogen production by type B synoviocytes restoring natural properties of synovial fluid [12, 13].

VS has been proven to be effective for knee and other large joints [14], and it can stimulate de novo synthesis of HA and inhibits release of inflammatory mediators by synoviocytes [8], such as cytokines and metalloproteinases that have been associated with osteoarthritis, mediating pain, and tissue damage [15–18].

Regarding TMD, there is not conclusive evidence [19–21]. Several studies have shown that VS can improve lubrication and biomechanical properties of TMJ and eliminate or reduce joint-related pain [22–26], but different concentrations and molecular weights of HA, varied number of intra-articular injections, and treatment cycles made it difficult to establish an effective approach [19–21]. Recent systematic reviews have shown that HA intra-articular injections in TMJ can be beneficial in improving pain and symptoms of TMDs and in regulating inflammatory mediators better than placebo, but they highlight that further clinical research is necessary to establish its effectiveness, mainly in comparison to corticosteroid [19–21]. Moreover, these works emphasize that an adequate protocol with number of injections, appropriate molecular weight of HA, minimum effective dose, and long-term side effects should be addressed [19–21].

Based upon clinical use of VS in joint disorders, including TMD, and the need of an efficient protocol for treatment, we describe a case series of four monthly injections of low and medium molecular weight HA in superior TMJ compartment and analyze TMJ dysfunction and quality of life through validated instruments and TMJ image analysis.

2. Materials and Methods

This study was approved by the Ethics Committee of Universidade Federal de Minas Gerais, Belo Horizonte, Brazil (CAAE-24911314.3.0000.5149) and registered in Brazilian Registry of Clinical Trials (RBR-6759yz). All procedures were performed in accordance with the ethical standards of institutional and/or national research committee and with the principles stated in the 1964 Helsinki Declaration and its later amendments. All patients provided written informed consent before inclusion in the study and received free and unconditional treatment.

Ten consecutive patients fulfilling the following inclusion criteria were selected from university orofacial pain division or from a private orofacial pain clinic: age between 18 and 70, diagnosis of disc displacement with or without reduction, and/or osteoarthritis according to the Research Diagnostic Criteria for Temporomandibular Disorders (RDC/TMD Axis I). Patients with rheumatologic diseases, neuropathic pain, or history of previous TMJ surgery, trauma, or fractures were excluded. No other treatment for TMD (physical therapy, jaw exercises, heat pack to the jaw, and muscle relaxants) was allowed during the study period, and anamnesis before each session was performed to control it.

2.1. Viscosupplementation. All ten selected patients underwent a cycle of four injections (1 per month) of 1 mL of HA in upper joint compartment of both joints as previously described [7]. Low MW HA (500–730 kDa, Polireumin®) was used in months 1 and 3 and medium MW HA (1,000–2,000 kDa, Osteonil Mini®) was injected in months 2 and 4. All injection procedures were conducted by the same physician. Baseline evaluation and two follow-up assessments (1 month and 6 months) were performed after the end of the treatment.

2.2. Clinical Evaluation. Clinical evaluations were performed by the same experienced operator after training and calibration by RDC/TMD examination protocol [27]. The following parameters were assessed at the time of diagnosis (baseline) and at each appointment during treatment (data not shown) and follow-ups (1 and 6 months after treatment): (1) pain intensity by 0–10 numeric rating scale (NRS) (0 = no pain and 10 = worst possible pain) [28]; (2) pain quality by multidimensional McGill Pain Questionnaire (MPQ), which characterizes emotional and sensory aspects of pain with scores ranging from 1 to 78 [29]; (3) pain-related impact of life by Manchester Orofacial Pain Disability Scale (MOPDS-Brazil), a 26-item Likert scale questionnaire with scores ranging from 0 to 52 [30]; (4) jaw range-of-motion by interincisal distance; (5) severity of craniomandibular dysfunction by Clinical Dysfunction Index Craniomandibular (IDCCM), ranging from 0 to 5 [31]; (6) functional limitation by Mandibular Function Impairment Questionnaire (MFIQ), a 17-item Likert scale questionnaire with final score ranging from 0 to 5 [32]; (7) quality of life by Oral Health Impact Profile (OHIP- 49) with values from 0 to 280 [33].

2.3. Image Analysis. The patients' left and right joints were examined by cone-beam computerized tomography (CBCT) and by magnetic resonance imaging (MRI) at baseline and at final follow-up (6 months after treatment). Images were interpreted by a blind experienced radiologist and all available slices were evaluated. In CBCT, osteoarthritic (OA) changes were defined according to Ahmad et al. [34] by the presence of sclerosis (loss of convex aspect in the articular surface), osteophyte (reactive bone spirits), erosion (cortical rupture), and subchondral cyst (pseudocyst infiltrated in the subcortical region). All parameters were analyzed in sagittal and coronal views of 1 mm interval through Radiocef Studio 2 software as previously described [34]. The distance of the outmost points of detected alterations were compared between baseline and final follow-up images in the same tomographic slice. Position of mandibular head in relation to temporal bone was assessed by visual inspection of the CBCT scan slides and categorized as normal mobility, hypomobility or hypermobility. In MRI, posterior band disc joint position in sagittal and coronal views was evaluated as previously described [18], and methods of image analysis for MRI was similar of CBCT. Presence of reduction, adhesion, and effusion (inflammatory signals) was also analyzed. In addition, morphology of disc was classified as previously described [35].

2.4. Statistical Analysis. Statistical analysis was performed using MINITAB® software version 17. For clinical data, within-patient differences among baseline and follow-up values were assessed by paired t-tests for comparing mean change or Wilcoxon signed rank test for comparing median change. Osteoarthritic changes between baseline and final follow-up (6 months) were evaluated by paired t-test for comparing mean change (erosion) or by Wilcoxon signed rank test for comparing median change (sclerosis, osteophyte, and flattening). P values of 0.05 or less were considered significant. All graphs were created by GraphPad Prism 5.0 software.

3. Results

Demographic characteristics (age, gender, race/ethnicity, marital status, and scholarity) of sample are shown in Table 1.

3.1. Clinical Evaluation. At baseline, 50% of patients ($n = 5$ patients) had myofascial pain according to RDC/TMD Axis I Group I (muscle disorders) (Table 2). In RDC/TMD Axis I Group II disorders (disc displacement), 90% ($n = 9$ patients) were diagnosed with disc displacement with reduction (ADDR). Whereas, in RDC/TMD Axis I Group III (other joint conditions), 10% ($n = 1$ patient) had arthralgia at rest and mandibular function and 20% ($n = 2$ patients) had osteoarthosis/osteoarthritis diagnosis.

One and 6 months after treatment, there was a significant change in patient diagnosis according to the RDC/TMD Axis I Group I, that is, no patient was diagnosed with myofascial pain. No changes were observed in RDC/TMD Axis I Group II, except for one patient. In RDC/TMD Axis I Group III, the patient with arthralgia became symptomless and one of the patients formerly diagnosed with osteoarthritis was diagnosed with osteoarthrosis.

Mouth opening without pain improved at 1 month after treatment in comparison to baseline (Figure 1(a)). Craniomandibular dysfunction showed significant improvement 1 and 6 months after treatment (Figure (1b)). Pain intensity was significantly decreased at 1 and 6 months (Figure 1(c)), as well as McGill pain scores (Figure 1(d)).

Moreover, orofacial pain disability was improved at 1 and 6 months follow-up evaluations (Figure 2(a)) and better mandibular function was detected 6 months after treatment (Figure 2(b)). Quality of life reported by patients showed improvement at both follow-up evaluations in comparison to baseline (Figure 2(c)).

3.2. Image Analysis. At baseline, both TMJs of all patients were examined by CBCT and MRI. Osteoarthritic changes evaluation by CBCT showed significant decrease in presence of osteophyte, flattening, sclerosis, and erosion of mandibular head at 6 months after treatment (Table 3). Hypoplasia and hyperplasia of mandibular head, deviation in form, subcortical cysts, generalized sclerosis, loose joint body or bone ankylosis were not found at baseline or 6 months follow-up. In addition, CBCT has shown that 20% of patients (2 patients) have improved standard excursion of mandibular head in both joints after treatment.

Soft tissue evaluation by MRI before and 6 months after treatment showed the following: (1) all patients had disc displacement with reduction before and after treatment; (2) all patients had alterations in disc position in at least one of the views (sagittal and/or coronal) after treatment; (3) one patient showed remission of right disc adhesion after treatment; (4) all patients (4 joints) who had effusion signal before treatment evolved to resolution of effusion 6 months after treatment (Table 4). Regarding disc shape, all patients showed stabilization or improvement in disc morphology of both joints, except for one patient.

4. Discussion

In this case series, we evaluated the effectiveness of a protocol of four injections of low and medium MW HA on pain, mandibular function, signs of intra-articular disease by image analysis, and quality of life in ten patients with TMD.

After treatment, disc displacement diagnosis by MRI or RDC/TMD was not changed, except for one patient, which was expected since TMJ discs cannot be replaced by minimal invasive technique [36]. Disc position in coronal view was altered in 5 joints after treatment, and this may be due to better lubrication and recovery of mandibular dynamics obtained by VS. Joint sound is the clinical sign that RDC/TMD utilizes for disc displacement diagnosis, but disc position can only be determined by MRI analysis [27]. Since VS improves joint lubrication and biomechanics, joint sound may not be present even when disc is displaced. This might be the case for the patient that had a change in clinical diagnosis by RDC/TMD, although image analysis did not change.

Table 1: Demographic characteristics of patients.

Patient	Age	Gender	Race/ethnicity	Marital status	Education
1	35	F	Other or unstated	Never married	High school or less
2	47	F	Other or unstated	Married	High school or less
3	34	M	Other or unstated	Married	High school or less
4	66	F	White	Married	High school or less
5	20	F	White	Never married	Undergraduate degree
6	30	F	Other or unstated	Married	High school or less
7	19	F	White	Never married	Undergraduate degree
8	27	F	Other or unstated	Never married	Postgraduate degree
9	43	F	Other or unstated	Divorced	High school or less
10	37	F	White	Never married	Postgraduate degree

M: male; F: female.

Table 2: RDC/TMD diagnosis at baseline and follow-ups (1 and 6 months).

Patient		Research diagnostic criteria Axis I Group I	Group II Right	Group II Left	Group III Right	Group III Left
1	Baseline	MPWLO	ADDR	ADDR	—	—
	Follow-up (1 month)	—	ADDR	ADDR	—	—
	Follow-up (6 months)	—	ADDR	ADDR	—	—
2	Baseline	—	ADDR	ADDR	—	—
	Follow-up (1 month)	—	ADDR	ADDR	—	—
	Follow-up (6 months)	—	ADDR	ADDR	—	—
3	Baseline	—	ADDR	ADDR	—	—
	Follow-up (1 month)	—	—	—	—	—
	Follow-up (6 months)	—	—	—	—	—
4	Baseline	—	ADDR	ADDR	—	—
	Follow-up (1 month)	—	ADDR	ADDR	—	—
	Follow-up (6 months)	—	ADDR	ADDR	—	—
5	Baseline	MP	ADDR	ADDR	Arthralgia	Arthralgia
	Follow-up (1 month)	—	ADDR	ADDR	—	—
	Follow-up (6 months)	—	ADDR	ADDR	—	—
6	Baseline	MP	ADDR	ADDR	Osteoarthritis	Osteoarthritis
	Follow-up (1 month)	—	ADDR	ADDR	Osteoarthritis	Osteoarthrosis
	Follow-up (6 months)	—	ADDR	ADDR	Osteoarthritis	Osteoarthrosis
7	Baseline	MP	ADDR	ADDR	—	—
	Follow-up (1 month)	—	ADDR	ADDR	—	—
	Follow-up (6 months)	—	ADDR	ADDR	—	—
8	Baseline	—	ADDR	ADDR	—	—
	Follow-up (1 month)	—	ADDR	ADDR	—	—
	Follow-up (6 months)	—	ADDR	ADDR	—	—
9	Baseline	—	—	—	Osteoarthrosis	Osteoarthritis
	Follow-up (1 month)	—	—	—	Osteoarthrosis	Osteoarthritis
	Follow-up (6 months)	*	*	*	*	*
10	Baseline	MPWLO	ADDR	ADDR	—	—
	Follow-up (1 month)	—	ADDR	ADDR	—	—
	Follow-up (6 months)	*	*	*	*	*

RDC/TMD Axis I Group I (muscle disorders): MP = myofascial pain, MPWLO = myofascial pain with limited opening; Group II (disc displacement): ADDR = disc displacement with reduction; Group III (other joint conditions). *Patient did not attend final follow-up.

All patients initially diagnosed with muscle pain (myofascial), joint pain (arthralgia), or limited mouth opening have improved pain and function and those diagnoses were not observed at follow-ups. Pain relief was observed by a significant reduction of pain intensity and scores measured by NRS, McGill, and MOPDS. This may be attributed to different mechanisms regarding TMJ, such as anti-inflammatory effects of HA injection with consequent decrease of metalloproteinases and proinflammatory mediators in synovial fluid, as well as improvement of joint biomechanics [10–13]. In this work, measurement of synovial fluid inflammatory mediators was not performed to

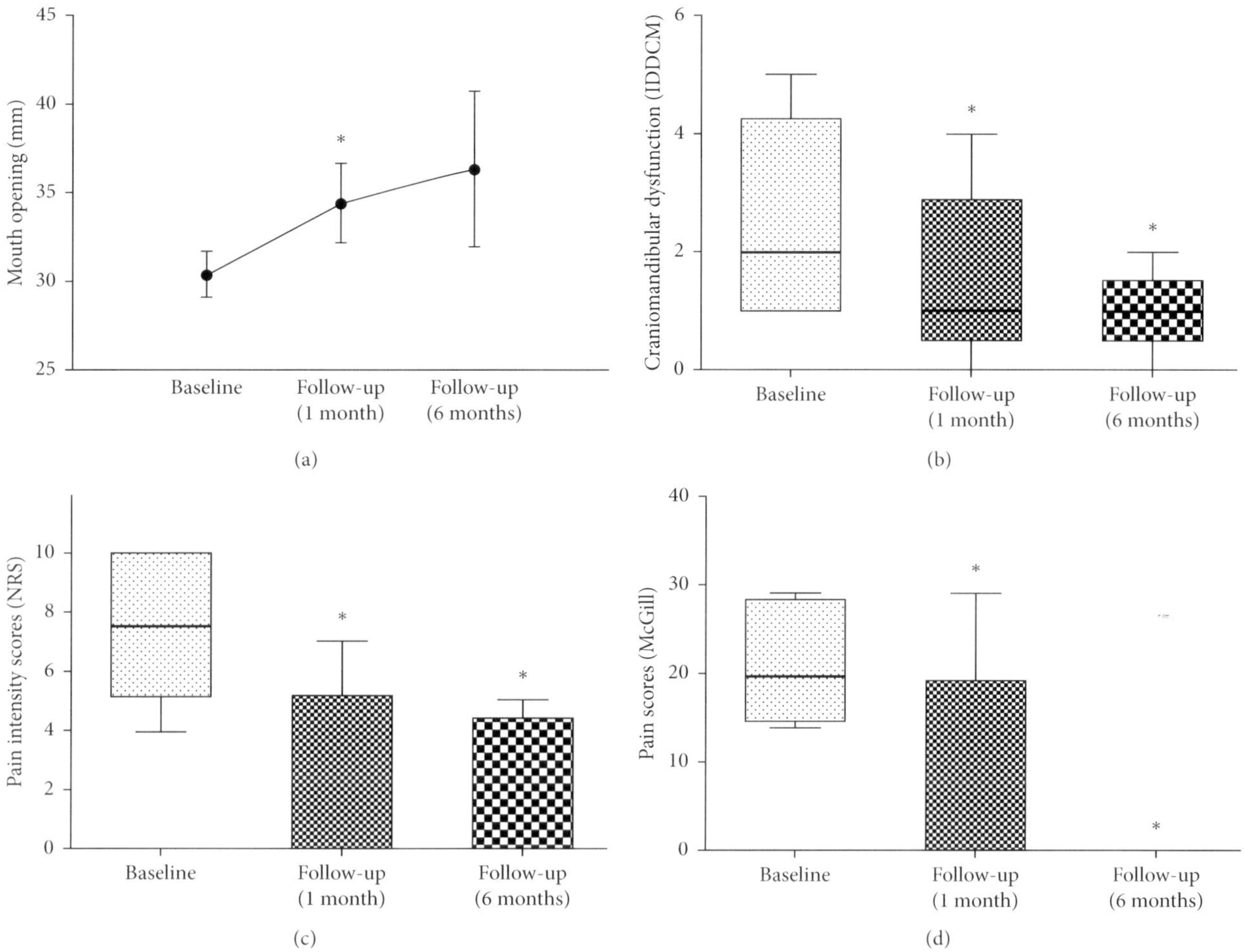

Figure 1: (a) Improvement on mouth opening without pain (measured in mm) at 1 and 6 months after treatment. This parameter was analyzed only on patients who showed limited mouth opening at baseline. Bars represent standard deviation (SD). Student's *t*-test; $^*p = 0.039$; $n = 5$ patients (1-month follow-up) and 3 patients (6-month follow-up). (b) Decrease in scores of craniomandibular dysfunction (IDDCM-Helkimo Index) at 1 and 6 months after treatment. Box and whisker show quartiles, the band inside the box is the median, and the ends of the whiskers represent minimum and maximum values. Wilcoxon signed rank test; $^*p = 0.034$ (1-month follow-up) and $^*p = 0.038$ (6-month follow-up); $n = 10$ patients (1-month follow-up) and 8 patients (6-month follow-up). (c) Decrease in NRS pain intensity at 1 and 6 months after treatment. This parameter was analyzed only on patients who showed pain at baseline. Box and whisker show quartiles, the band inside the box is the median, and the ends of the whiskers represent minimum and maximum values. Wilcoxon signed rank test; $^*p = 0.018$ (1-month follow-up) and $^*p = 0.05$ (6-month follow-up); $n = 6$ patients (1-month follow-up) and 4 patients (6-month follow-up). (d) Decrease in McGill pain scores at 1 and 6 months after treatment. This parameter was analyzed only on patients who showed pain at baseline. Box and whisker show quartiles, the band inside the box is the median, and the ends of the whiskers represent minimum and maximum values. Wilcoxon signed rank test; $^*p = 0.042$ (1-month follow-up) and $^*p = 0.05$ (6-month follow-up); $n = 6$ patients (1-month follow-up) and 4 patients (6-month follow-up)

avoid invasive technique of TMJ, which could create bias in treatment outcome. Moreover, masticatory muscles promote jaw movements and their functionality is related to structural and functional integrity of TMJ [2]. Hence, relief or improvement of joint symptoms, as well as restoration of biomechanics by VS protocol, may be associated with better function of adjacent muscles and pain relief. Moreover, diminished peripheral inputs by restored TMJ may lead to improvement of central sensitization and muscle pain [37].

VS protocol tested here showed significant improvement in mouth opening amplitude both in clinical and radiologic evaluations. This outcome in clinical examination has also been shown in other studies of VS but with different protocols [7, 8, 24, 25] and may be due to restoration of joint lubrication. Moreover, VS was able to improve medial disc position, shown by MRI, which may have contributed to better mandible movements, TMJ biomechanics, and quality of life.

Less severe dysfunction was observed after treatment. Evaluation of mandible function by MFIQ has also shown improvement. More importantly, patients' evaluation of quality of life has improved. Other studies have also shown beneficial outcomes of VS by mouth opening, pain intensity, and subjective parameters such as satisfaction with treatment [7, 24, 25]. However, to our knowledge, objective evaluation of TMJ dysfunction, mandible function, and quality of life through validated instruments is first described here.

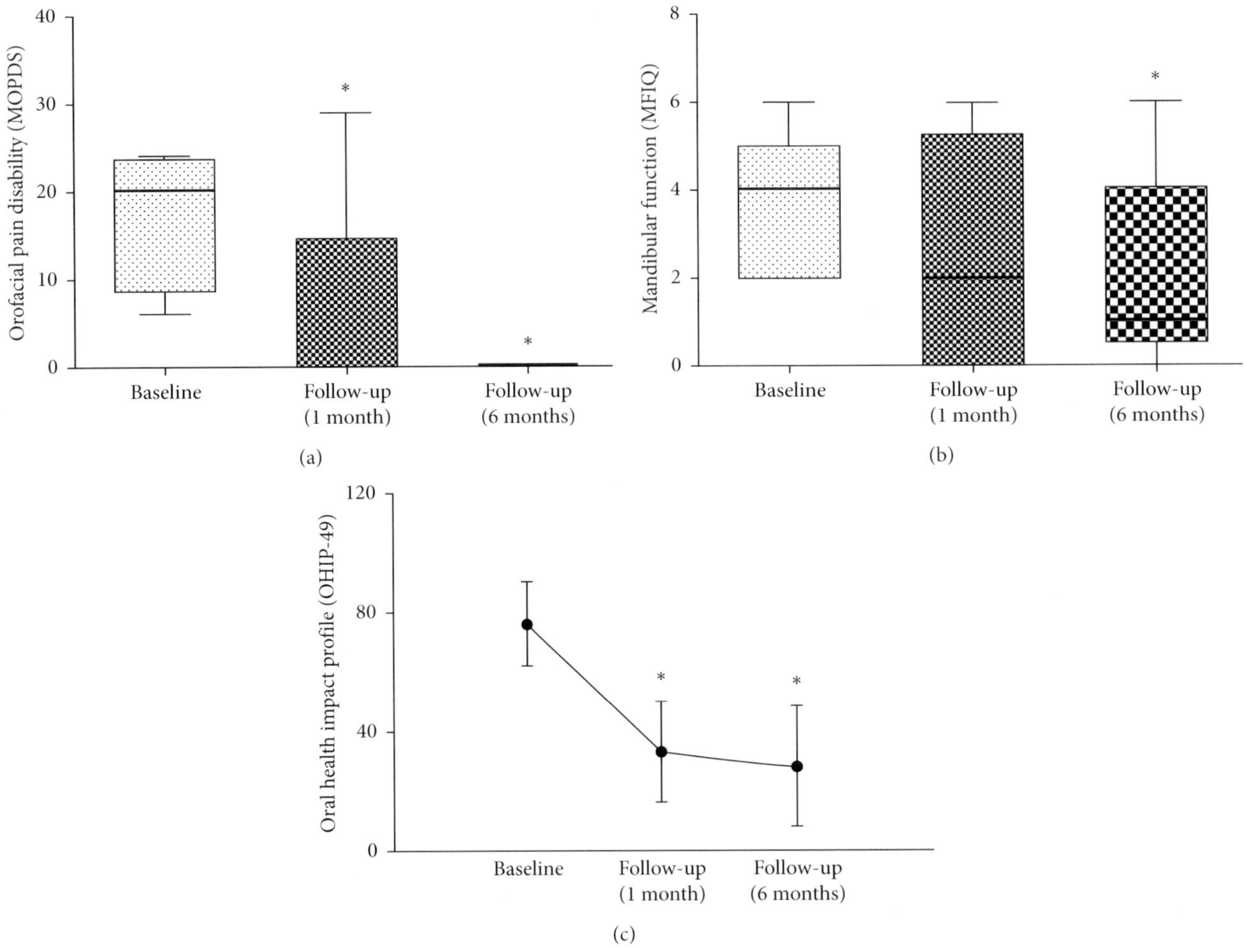

FIGURE 2: (a) Improvement on orofacial pain disability at 1 and 6 months after treatment. This parameter was analyzed only on patients who showed pain at baseline. Box and whisker show quartiles, the band inside the box is the median, and the ends of the whiskers represent minimum and maximum values. Wilcoxon signed rank test; $^{*}p = 0.042$ (1-month follow-up) and $^{*}p = 0.05$ (6-month follow-up); $n = 6$ patients (1-month follow-up) and 4 patients (6-month follow-up). (b) Improvement on mandibular function MFIQ at 6 months after treatment. Box and whisker show quartiles, the band inside the box is the median, and the ends of the whiskers represent minimum and maximum values. Wilcoxon signed rank test; $p < 0.05$ (1-month follow-up) and, $^{*}p = 0.038$ (6-month follow-up); $n = 10$ patients (1-month follow-up) and 8 patients (6-month follow-up). (c) Decrease of impact on quality of life (OHIP-49) at 1 and 6 months. Bars represent standard deviation (SD). Student's t-test; $^{*}p = 0.029$ (1-month follow-up) and $^{*}p = 0.035$ (6-month follow-up); $n = 10$ patients (1-month follow-up) and 8 patients (6-month follow-up).

It is important to highlight that pain relief as well as improvement in mouth opening, mandibular function, and quality of life may also be a result of observed remission of myofascial pain itself. As mentioned, masticatory muscles and TMJ are structurally functionally related [2]. Moreover, reduction on pain could be also attributed to a better consciousness of mandibular function or to a placebo effect as a consequence of being under of examination and treatment for TMD. However, this hypothesis cannot be tested or excluded at this time.

Only a few studies have used image analysis to evaluate TMD treatment efficacy [18, 26]. In this work, image analysis revealed positive effects of established therapeutics in shape and function of hard and soft tissues of TMJ. VS improvement of biomechanics and lubrication seems to stabilize disc shape and avoid greater deformities, which is relevant for the course of the disease [34]. Moreover, effusion signals were not observed after treatment and our VS protocol showed effectiveness in recovery of joint inflammation and OA degenerative changes. VS beneficial effects such as reduction of joint friction, improvement of rheological environment [10, 11], and induction of endogen production of HA [12, 13] may lead to anatomical rearrangement and can justify CBCT and MRI tissue remodeling observed here.

Among studies that have shown efficacy of VS in TMD, different methods have been described and, as a result, there is an effort of researchers and clinicians to establish an effective protocol for treatment of TMD, as already established for other joints [7, 12, 24, 38]. The present study shows a new protocol of four injections of low and medium MW HA in TMJ with relevant clinical effectiveness on pain, jaw range of motion, dysfunction degree, and quality of life. Furthermore, it is important to emphasize that VS as a single intra-articular treatment is less aggressive than other techniques such as arthrocentesis [7, 24], associated or not with VS, with safety and economic advantages.

Table 3: CBCT evaluation of osteoarthritis changes at baseline and at final (6 months) follow-up.

Patient		Osteoarthritis changes of TMJ (mm)							
		Sclerosis		Erosion		Osteophyte		Flattening	
		Right joint	Left joint	Right joint	Left joint	Right joint	Left joint	Right joint	Left joint
2	Baseline	2.370	1.270	1.410	0.420	1.580	0.000	4.510	0.000
	Final	1.020	1.220	0.410	0.290	1.040	0.000	3.130	0.000
3	Baseline	1.210	1.630	0.000	0.000	0.590	0.000	4.950	4.620
	Final	1.060	0.870	0.000	0.000	0.510	0.000	2.220	2.160
4	Baseline	1.800	1.400	0.000	0.000	0.000	0.000	4.070	2.910
	Final	1.280	1.100	0.000	0.000	0.000	0.000	2.000	2.470
5	Baseline	2.470	1.960	1.080	0.730	1.870	1.190	5.570	4.560
	Final	1.550	1.950	0.850	0.350	1.300	0.850	2.520	2.220
6	Baseline	1.610	1.520	0.730	0.000	2.230	0.000	6.380	3.480
	Final	1.560	1.030	0.420	0.000	1.110	0.000	2.410	3.190
7	Baseline	1.020	1.090	0.000	0.550	1.240	1.220	3.250	3.620
	Final	0.920	0.770	0.000	0.190	1.030	0.770	1.650	3.300
8	Baseline	0.880	0.680	0.000	0.000	0.430	0.430	0.460	4.140
	Final	0.690	1.630	0.000	0.000	0.000	0.410	2.220	4.110
Baseline	Mean or median	1.460		0.340		0.510		4.105	
	SD	—		0.470		—		—	
	25%	1.120		—		0.000		3.300	
	75%	1.750		—		1.230		4.600	
Final	Mean or median	1.140		0.170		0.460		2.440	
	SD	—		0.250		—		—	
	25%	0.940		—		0.000		2.220	
	75%	1.550		—		0.980		3.170	
P value	Paired *t*-test			0.022*					
	Wilcoxon test	0.041*				0.00*		0.027*	

Media and standard deviation (SD) are shown for erosion (parametric data). Median, 25th percentile (25%), and 75th percentile (75%) are shown for other parameteres (nonparametric data); *p* values of 0.05 or less were considered significant.

Table 4: MRI evaluation of TMJ disc position and adhesion at baseline and at final (6 months) follow-up.

Patient		TMJ soft tissues evaluation							
		Right joint				Left joint			
		Sagittal plane*	Coronal plane*	Adhesion	Reduction	Sagittal plane*	Coronal plane*	Adhesion	Reduction
2	Baseline	AI	S	No	Yes	A	Lateral	No	Yes
	Final	AI	S	No	Yes	A	S	No	Yes
3	Baseline	S	Medial	Yes	Yes	S	S	No	Yes
	Final	A	S	No	Yes	A	S	No	Yes
4	Baseline	A	S	No	Yes	AI	S	No	No
	Final	A	S	No	Yes	S	S	No	Yes
5	Baseline	A	S	No	No	AI	Lateral	No	No
	Final	A	S	No	Yes	A	S	No	Yes
6	Baseline	A	Lateral	No	Yes	A	S	No	Yes
	Final	A	S	No	Yes	AI	S	No	Yes
7	Baseline	A	S	No	Yes	S	S	No	Yes
	Final	S	S	No	Yes	S	Lateral	No	Yes
8	Baseline	A	Lateral	No	Yes	A	S	No	Yes
	Final	A	S	No	No	A	S	No	Yes

*Position of disc posterior band to functional surface of the mandibular head in sagittal and coronal planes: S: superior; A: anterior; AI: anteroinferior. Two patients did not attend final follow-up and 1 could not be submitted to CBCT or MRI because of pregnancy.

The use of HA of different MW in alternated monthly injections is a new perspective of VS in TMD and allows association of biomechanical properties of high MW AH and biological effects of lower MW AH. Hence, this protocol of treatment is able to promote fast and sustained effects, as suggested by results.

The literature describes different time intervals between applications [24, 38]. We believe that 1-month interval may allow HA acting inside joint for longer periods, which favor the effects of the next injection and the treatment itself. In addition, treatment cycle with monthly injections may be more tolerated by patients and offer some economic benefits, as it postpones a new cycle. Improvement of pain, mandibular function, and quality of life are in accordance to this finding, and relief of TMD signs and symptoms offered by VS may have restored local and systemic functions.

Although we show promising results regarding the described protocol for TMJ VS, we are aware of the limitations of this work. We believe its greater contribution may be the description of a new perspective to be tested in a well-controlled clinical trial in future research studies. Our small number of patients and the study design as an open label noncontrolled trial does not allow inference of VS positive effects to all TMD patients. However, case series is a descriptive work that illustrates novel features in clinical practice, its sample represents common clinical population, and generates new research questions [39]. Hence, this study aimed at sharing a description of some well succeeded cases of sequential VS in TMJ internal derangements. Moreover, case series usually describes 5 to 7 cases [40], and our sample is in accordance to this type of work, even with loss of 2 patients at final follow-up.

VS protocol shown here reduced pain and symptoms associated with internal derangement of TMJ and improved quality of life of TMD patients. Randomized clinical trials of this treatment protocol should deserve attention in future researches.

Acknowledgments

R. M. Fonseca received an MSc scholarship from Coordenação de Aperfeiçoamento de Pessoal de Nível Superior (CAPES/Brazil). C. M. Almeida-Leite was funded by Conselho Nacional de Desenvolvimento Científico e Tecnológico (CNPq) (Grant 459228/2014-5). A. L. Teixeira was supported by CNPq and Fundação de Amparo à Pesquisa de Minas Gerais (FAPEMIG). This study appreciates TRB Pharma (Brazil) for donation of hyaluronic acid for viscosupplementation (Polireumin and Osteonil Mini), Radioscan (Brazil) for cone-beam computerized tomography examination, and Hermes Pardini (Brazil) for magnetic resonance imaging.

References

[1] C. McNeill, "Management of temporomandibular disorders: concepts and controversies," *Journal of Prosthetic Dentistry*, vol. 77, no. 5, pp. 510–522, 1997.

[2] S. J. Scrivani, D. A. Keith, and L. B. Kaban, "Temporomandibular disorders," *New England Journal of Medicine*, vol. 359, no. 25, pp. 2693–2705, 2008.

[3] R. De Leeuw and G. D. Klasser, *Orofacial Pain: Guidelines for Assessment, Diagnosis and Management*, Quintessence Publ. Co, Chicago, IL, USA, 5th edition, 2008.

[4] National Institute of Dental and Craniofacial Research, November 2015, http://www.nidcr.nih.gov/DataStatistics/FindDataByTopic/FacialPain/PrevalenceTMJD.htm.

[5] E. Schiffman, R. Ohrbach, E. Truelove et al., "Diagnostic criteria for temporomandibular disorders (DC/TMD) for clinical and research applications: recommendations of the International RDC/TMD Consortium Network and Orofacial Pain Special Interest Group," *Journal of Oral and Facial Pain and Headache*, vol. 28, no. 1, pp. 6–27, 2014.

[6] N. Mobilio, I. Casetta, E. Cesnik, and S. Catapano, "Prevalence of self-reported symptoms related to temporomandibular disorders in an Italian population," *Journal of Oral Rehabilitation*, vol. 38, no. 12, pp. 884–890, 2011.

[7] L. Guarda-Nardini, S. Masiero, and G. Marioni, "Conservative treatment of temporomandibular joint osteoarthrosis: intra-articular injection of sodium hyaluronate," *Journal of Oral Rehabilitation*, vol. 32, no. 10, pp. 729–734, 2005.

[8] R. Thein, B. Haviv, A. Kidron, and S. Bronak, "Intra-articular injection of hyaluronic acid following arthroscopic partial meniscectomy of the knee," *Orthopedics*, vol. 33, no. 10, p. 724, 2010.

[9] H. Hempfling, "Intra-articular hyaluronic acid after knee arthroscopy: a two-year study," *Knee Surgery, Sports Traumatology, Arthroscopy*, vol. 15, no. 5, pp. 537–546, 2007.

[10] C. Alpaslan, A. Bilgihan, G. H. Alpaslan, B. Güner, M. Ozgür Yis, and D. Erbaş, "Effect of arthrocentesis and sodium hyaluronate injection on nitrite, nitrate, and thiobarbituric acid-reactive substance levels in the synovial fluid," *Oral Surgery, Oral Medicine, Oral Pathology, Oral Radiology, and Endodontology*, vol. 89, no. 6, pp. 686–690, 2000.

[11] G. Alpaslan and C. Alpaslan, "Efficacy Of TMJ arthrocentesis with and without injection of sodium hyaluronate," *International Journal of Oral and Maxillofacial Surgery*, vol. 26, pp. 613–618, 1997.

[12] P. Ghosh and D. Guidolin, "Potential mechanism of action intra articular hyaluronan therapy in osteoarthritis are the effects molecular weigtht depedent?," *Seminars in Arthritis and Rheumatism*, vol. 32, no. 1, pp. 10–37, 2002.

[13] L. Wei, H. Xiong, B. Li et al., "Change of HA molecular size and boundary lubrication in synovial fluid of patients with temporomandibular disorders," *Journal of Oral Rehabilitation*, vol. 37, no. 4, pp. 271–277, 2010.

[14] T. E. Clegg, D. Caborn, and C. Mauffrey, "Viscosupplementation with hyaluronic acid in the treatment for cartilage lesions: a review of current evidence and future directions," *European Journal of Orthopaedic Surgery and Traumatology: Orthopédie Traumatologie*, vol. 23, no. 2, pp. 119–124, 2013.

[15] D. C. Bauer, D. J. Hunter, S. B Abramson et al., "Classification of osteoarthritis biomarkers: a proposed approach," *Osteoarthritis and Cartilage*, vol. 14, no. 8, pp. 723–727, 2006.

[16] E. B. Dam, M. Loog, C. Christiansen et al., "Identification of progressors in osteoarthritis by combining biochemical and MRI-based markers," *Arthritis Research and Therapy*, vol. 11, no. 8, p. R115, 2009.

[17] J. C. Rousseau and P. D. Delmas, "Biological markers in osteoarthritis," *Nature Clinical Practice Rheumatology*, vol. 3, no. 6, pp. 346–356, 2007.

[18] L. H. Cevidanes, D. Walker, J. Schilling et al., "3D osteoarthritic changes in TMJ condylar morphology correlates with specific systemic and local biomarkers of disease," *Osteoarthritis and Cartilage*, vol. 22, no. 10, pp. 1657–1667, 2014.

[19] M. C. Goiato, E. V. da Silva, R. A. de Medeiros, K. H. Túrcio, and D. M. Dos Santos, "Are intra-articular injections of hyaluronic acid effective for the treatment of temporomandibular disorders? a systematic review," *International Journal of Oral and Maxillofacial Surgery*, vol. 45, no. 12, pp. 1531–1537, 2016.

[20] V. Iturriaga, T. Bornhardt, C. Manterola, and P. Brebi, "Effect of hyaluronic acid on the regulation of inflammatory mediators in osteoarthritis of the temporomandibular joint: a systematic review," *International Journal of Oral and Maxillofacial Surgery*, vol. 46, no. 5, pp. 590–595, 2017.

[21] M. A. Moldez, V. R. Camones, G. E. Ramos, M. Padilla, and R. Enciso, "Effectiveness of intra-articular injections of sodium hyaluronate or corticosteroids for intracapsular temporomandibular disorders: a systematic review and meta-analysis," *Journal of Oral and Facial Pain and Headache*, vol. 32, no. 1, pp. 53–66, 2018.

[22] M. C. Reid, "Viscosupplementation for osteoarthritis: a primer for primary care physicians," *Advances in Therapy*, vol. 30, no. 11, pp. 967–986, 2013.

[23] J. Escoda-Francolí, E. Vázquez-Delgado, and C. Gay-Escoda, "Scientific evidence on the usefulness of intraarticular hyaluronic acid injection in the management of temporomandibular dysfunction," *Medicina Oral, Patología Oral y Cirugía Bucal*, vol. 15, no. 4, pp. 644–648, 2010.

[24] D. Manfredini, F. Piccotti, and L. Guarda-Nardini, "Hyaluronic acid in the treatment of TMJ disorders: a systematic review of the literature," *Cranio*, vol. 28, no. 3, pp. 166–176, 2010.

[25] L. Guarda-Nardini, A. Rossi, R. Arboretti, S. Bonnini, E. Stellini, and D. Manfredini, "Single- or multiple-session viscosupplementation protocols for temporomandibular joint degenerative disorders: a randomized clinical trial," *Journal of Oral Rehabilitation*, vol. 42, no. 7, pp. 521–528, 2015.

[26] C. Li, X. Long, M. Deng, J. Li, H. Cai, and Q. Meng, "Osteoarthritic changes after superior and inferior joint space injection of hyaluronic acid for the treatment of temporomandibular joint osteoarthritis with anterior disc displacement without reduction: a cone-beam computed tomographic evaluation," *Journal of Oral and Maxillofacial Surgery*, vol. 73, no. 2, pp. 232–244, 2015.

[27] S. Dworkin and L. LeResche, "Research diagnostic criteria for temporomandibular disorders: review, criteria, examinations, and specifications, critique," *Journal of Craniomandibular Disorders: Facial and Oral Pain*, vol. 6, no. 4, pp. 301–355, 1992.

[28] J. T. Farrar, J. P. Young Jr., L. LaMoreaux, J. L. Werth, and R. M. Poole, "Clinical importance of changes in chronic pain intensity measured on an 11-point numerical pain rating scale," *Pain*, vol. 94, no. 2, pp. 149–158, 2001.

[29] R. Melzack, "The McGill Pain Questionnaire: major properties and scoring methods," *Pain*, vol. 1, no. 3, pp. 277–299, 1975.

[30] V. R. Aggarwal, M. Lunt, J. M. Zakrzewska, G. J. Macfarlane, and T. V. Macfarlane, "Development and validation of the Manchester orofacial pain disability scale," *Community Dentistry and Oral Epidemiology*, vol. 33, no. 2, pp. 141–149, 2005.

[31] M. Helkimo, "Studies on function and dysfunction of the masticatory system. 3. Analyses of anamnestic and clinical recordings of dysfunction with the aid of indices," *Svensk Tandlakare Tidskrift*, vol. 67, pp. 165–181, 1974.

[32] B. Stegenga, L. G. de Bont, R. de Leeuw, and G. Boering, "Assessment of mandibular function impairment associated with temporomandibular joint osteoarthrosis and internal derangement," *Journal of Orofacial Pain*, vol. 7, no. 2, pp. 183–195, 1993.

[33] G. D. Slade and A. J. Spencer, "Development and evaluation of the oral health impact profile," *Community Dental Health*, vol. 11, no. 1, pp. 3–11, 1994.

[34] M. Ahmad, L. Hollender, Q. Anderson et al., "Research diagnostic criteria for temporomandibular disorders (RDC/TMD): development of image analysis criteria and examiner reliability for image analysis," *Oral Surgery, Oral Medicine, Oral Pathology, Oral Radiology, and Endodontology*, vol. 107, no. 6, pp. 844–860, 2009.

[35] S. Murakami, A. Takahashi, H. Nishiyama, M. Fujishita, and H. Fuchihata, "Magnetic resonance evaluation of the temporomandibular joint disc position and configuration," *Dento Maxillo Facial Radiology*, vol. 22, no. 4, pp. 205–207, 1993.

[36] J. R. Gonçalves, D. S. Cassano, L. Rezende, and L. M. Wolford, "Disc repositioning: does it really work?," *Oral and Maxillofacial Surgery Clinics of North America*, vol. 27, no. 1, pp. 85–107, 2015.

[37] M. H. Ossipov, G. O. Dussor, and F. Porreca, "Central modulation of pain," *Journal of Clinical Investigation*, vol. 120, no. 11, pp. 3779–3787, 2010.

[38] D. Manfredini, S. Bonnini, R. Arboretti, and L. Guarda-Nardini, "Temporomandibular joint osteoarthritis: an open label trial of 76 patients treated with arthrocentesis plus hyaluronic acid injections," *International Journal of Oral and Maxillofacial Surgery*, vol. 38, no. 8, pp. 827–834, 2009.

[39] B. Kooistra, B. Dijkman, T. A. Einhorn, and M. Bhandari, "How to design a good case series," *Journal of Bone and Joint Surgery-Americanm*, vol. 91, no. 3, pp. 21–26, 2009.

[40] F. M. Abu-Zidan, A. K. Abbas, and A. F. Hefny, "Clinical "case series": a concept analysis," *African Health Sciences*, vol. 12, no. 4, pp. 557–562, 2012.

3

Incidence of Delirium in Critically Ill Cancer Patients

Luis A. Sánchez-Hurtado,[1,2] Nancy Hernández-Sánchez,[3] Mario Del Moral-Armengol,[2] Humberto Guevara-García,[1] Francisco J. García-Guillén,[1] Ángel Herrera-Gómez,[1] and Silvio A. Ñamendys-Silva[1,4,5]

[1]*Department of Critical Care Medicine, Instituto Nacional de Cancerología, Mexico City, Mexico*
[2]*Department of Critical Care Medicine, Hospital Especialidades Centro Médico Nacional La Raza, Mexican Institute of Social Security, Mexico City, Mexico*
[3]*Department of Critical Care Medicine, UMAE Hospital de Traumatologia "Dr. Victor de la Fuente Narvaez", Mexican Institute of Social Security, Mexico City, Mexico*
[4]*Department of Critical Care Medicine, Instituto Nacional de Ciencias Médicas y Nutrición Salvador Zubirán, Mexico City, Mexico*
[5]*Department of Critical Care Medicine, Medica Sur Clinic & Foundation, Mexico City, Mexico*

Correspondence should be addressed to Silvio A. Ñamendys-Silva; snamendys@incan.edu.mx

Academic Editor: Bruno Gagnon

Objective. The aim of this study was to estimate the incidence of delirium and its risk factors among critically ill cancer patients in an intensive care unit (ICU). *Materials and Methods.* This is a prospective cohort study. The Confusion Assessment Method for the Intensive Care Unit (CAM-ICU) was measured daily at morning to diagnose delirium by a physician. Delirium was diagnosed when the daily was positive during a patient's ICU stay. All patients were followed until they were discharged from the ICU. Using logistic regression, we estimated potential risk factors for developing delirium. The primary outcome was the development of ICU delirium. *Results.* There were 109 patients included in the study. Patients had a mean age of 48.6 ± 18.07 years, and the main reason for admission to the ICU was septic shock (40.4%). The incidence of delirium was 22.9%. The mortality among all subjects was 15.6%; the mortality rate in patients who developed delirium was 12%. The only variable that had an association with the development of delirium in the ICU was the days of use of mechanical ventilation (OR: 1.06; CI 95%: 0.99–1.13; $p = 0.07$). *Conclusion.* Delirium is a frequent condition in critically ill cancer patients admitted to the ICU. The duration in days of mechanical ventilation is potential risk factors for developing delirium during an ICU stay. Delirium was not associated with a higher rate of mortality in this group of patients.

1. Introduction

Delirium is an acute brain dysfunction, characterized by an acute change or fluctuation in mental status, inattention, disorganized thinking, or an alteration in level of consciousness [1–4]. A delirium assessment is a necessary routine task within an intensive care unit (ICU) because the presence of delirium is associated with morbidity, mortality, prolonged ICU hospitalization, increased time on a ventilator, and overall greater healthcare costs [5–7]. Delirium has long-term consequences, such as prolonged cognitive impairment, impaired activities of daily living, and decreased quality of life in survivors of a critical illness [8, 9]. Multiple risk factors for delirium, classified as predisposing and precipitating risk factors, include age, presence of a previous illness, high severity of acute illness, and therapeutic options such as mechanical ventilation, sedation, emergency surgery, and metabolic disorders, among others [5, 10].

The prevalence of delirium in the ICU setting has been reported to range from 20 to 40%; when mechanical ventilation is used, this rate increases to 60–80%. This wide range can be explained by a number of characteristics including illness severity and the instrument used. In specialized ICUs, the prevalence may be higher [2, 5]. Older critically ill patients may have a rate of more than 80% [9].

In oncological patients, delirium is the most common neuropsychiatric complication and has the same consequences as in critically ill patients without cancer [11, 12]. The reported incidence rate varies widely, from 10 to 85%, depending on the stage of cancer [12, 13]. However, when oncological patients are critically ill, there is very minimal information about the frequency of delirium. The vast majority of information on this topic has come from hospitalized or palliative oncological patients [13]. In this context, the aim of the current study was to describe the incidence of delirium and identify risk factors for its development among critically ill cancer patients who are hospitalized in an ICU.

2. Materials and Methods

2.1. Patient Population and Characteristics. A prospective, observational cohort study was conducted at the ICU of Instituto Nacional de Cancerologia located in Mexico City. We included all consecutive patients admitted to the ICU during the period between December 2015 and May 2016. The medical surgical ICU has nine beds exclusively for oncology patients. This study was approved by the institutional review board, and the need for informed consent was waived. Demographic and clinical data were collected using a paper form. The following information was collected: age, gender, ICU admission diagnosis, medical or surgical disorder, type of tumor (leukemia, lymphoma, or solid tumor), oncological disease status (recent diagnosis, active disease, complete remission, and others), disease stage (localized, metastatic, and others), type of treatment offered (chemotherapy, radiotherapy, or surgical), performance status [14] and the Karnofsky performance status scale [15], comorbidities, use of mechanical ventilation, diagnosis of acute renal failure, use and type of sedation, analgesic, steroids, antibiotics, and transfusion requirements. We calculated the Sequential Organ Failure Assessment (SOFA) [16] and the Mexican Sequential Organ Failure Assessment (MEXSOFA) score for evaluation of organic failures [17]. We measured the presence and severity of pain with the Numerical Rating for Pain Scale (NRP) or Behavioral Pain Scale (BPS), depending on the use of mechanical ventilation [18]. We recorded length of time before admission to the ICU (days), length of stay in the ICU stays (days), and subsequent hospital stay.

2.2. Delirium Assessment. The primary outcome was the development of ICU delirium, defined as a positive assessment for delirium during a patient's ICU stay. A delirium was diagnosed when the Confusion Assessment Method for the Intensive Care Unit (CAM-ICU) [1]. All the evaluations were performed by the same intensivist physician previously trained to perform the CAM-ICU measurement [1]. The patients were screened at the time of admission and each day in the morning (10:00–11:00 AM). According to the original description of CAM-ICU, presence of delirium, it was defined by changes in the next aspects: acute change or fluctuating course of mental state, inattention, altered level of consciousness, and disorganized thinking. The CAM-ICU aspect of the presence of acute changes or fluctuating course of mental state in the past 24 hours, through oscillation of the consciousness level according to the Richmond Agitation-Sedation Scale (RASS), all patients with RASS ≥ 3 (movement or ocular opening to the verbal call but without visual contact) were considered eligible for the evaluation of the presence of delirium. This evaluation can be performed in sedated patients and patients with no sedation, as well as in those submitted to mechanical ventilation. We do not perform the CAM-ICU if a patient is unconscious, comatose, or under deep sedation (i.e., RASS −4 or −5).

2.3. Statistical Analysis. Statistical analyses were performed using the Statistical Package for Social Sciences program (SPSS version 20.0, Chicago, IL). The Kolmogorov–Smirnov test was used to evaluate the distribution of variables. Continuous variables are reported as the mean ± SD or median (25–75% interquartile range (IQR)). Nominal variables are presented as percentages. Differences between groups were assessed using the chi-square test, Fisher's exact test, Student's t-test, or Mann–Whitney U test, as appropriate. Univariate and multivariate logistic regression analyses were used to identify factors associated with delirium. Variables with p values ≤ 0.200 in the univariate analysis or those considered clinically relevant (age, SOFA score, type of neoplasm and extension, comorbidities, and acute kidney injury) were entered into the multivariate analysis. In the multivariate model, $p < 0.050$ was used to denote statistically significant association between each variable and delirium. Results are presented as odds ratios (ORs) and their associated 95% confidence intervals (CIs). The area under the receiver operating characteristic curve was used to assess the discrimination of the model. Goodness of fit (Hosmer–Lemeshow) was calculated to assess the relevance of the logistic regression model (calibration), where p values > 0.05 indicate good model fit.

3. Results

During the period of study data collection, 109 patients were hospitalized in the ICU, and all were included in the analysis. The mean age was 49.25 ± 18.23 years old, and 62 (56.9%) were women. A total of 52 (47%) patients presented one or more comorbidities, and arterial hypertension and diabetes mellitus occurred most frequently. The main reason for ICU admission was septic shock ($n = 44$, 40.4%), hypovolemic shock ($n = 25$, 22.9%), and acute respiratory failure ($n = 12$, 11%). In terms of the type of solid tumor, the principal organs affected were the colon ($n = 15$, 13.8%), cervical uterus ($n = 13$, 11.9%), esophagus ($n = 7$, 6.4%), and ovaries ($n = 7$, 6.4%). The demographic characteristics of the patients based on the presence of delirium are present in Table 1.

Table 1: Demographic and clinical data of patients.

	With delirium	Without delirium	p
Number of patients, n (%)	25 (22.9)	84 (77.1)	
Age (years), median ± standard deviation (SD)	55.4 ± 17.55	47.42 ± 18.13	$0.050^{\$}$
Sex, n (%)			
Women	16 (64)	46 (54.8)	0.410^{*}
Comorbidities, n (%)	11 (44)	41 (48.8)	0.670^{*}
Arterial hypertension	4 (16)	14 (16.7)	0.930^{+}
Diabetes mellitus	4 (16)	12 (14.3)	0.760^{+}
Heart failure	6 (24)	22 (26.2)	0.830^{*}
Type of patient, n (%)			
Medical condition	12 (48)	34 (40.5)	0.500^{+}
Surgical condition	13 (52)	50 (59.5)	
Place before admission to ICU, n (%)			
Emergency room	0	2 (2.4)	
Ward	15 (60)	42 (50)	
Operating room	10 (40)	40 (47.6)	
Reason for admission to ICU, n (%)			
Septic shock	11 (44)	33 (39.3)	0.670^{*}
Hypovolemic shock	2 (8)	23 (27.4)	0.060°
Acute respiratory failure	5 (20)	7 (8.3)	0.100^{*}
Postsurgical care	1 (4)	6 (7.14)	0.999°
Postcardiac arrest care	3 (12)	3 (3.57)	0.130^{*}
Type of malignancies, n (%)			
Solid tumor	14 (56)	61 (72.6)	0.110^{*}
Hematologic neoplasm	11 (44)	23 (27.4)	
Status of oncological disease, n (%)			
Recent diagnosis	10 (40)	38 (33.3)	
Active disease	9 (36)	49 (58.3)	0.540^{*}
Complete remission	6 (24)	7 (8.3)	
Extension of neoplasm, n (%)			
Local or regional	17 (15.6)	72 (66)	0.040^{*}
Metastatic	8 (7.3)	12 (11)	
Treatment for cancer, n (%)			
Surgical treatment	13 (52)	42 (50)	0.860^{*}
Chemotherapy	9 (36)	46 (54.8)	0.100^{*}
Radiotherapy	6 (24)	1 (1.2)	0.410^{+}
Karnofsky score	80 (65–95)	80 (70–90)	0.780°
ECOG	1 (0.5–2.5)	1 (1–2)	0.770°
SOFA score at admission to ICU	7 (5–10.5)	7 (3.5–10)	0.450°
MEXSOFA score at admission to ICU	8 (6–11)	8 (4–11)	0.420°
Mortality in the ICU, n (%)	3 (12)	14 (16.7)	0.750^{+}

ICU: intensive care unit; SOFA: Sequential Organ Failure Assessment score, MEXSOFA: Mexican Sequential Organ Failure Assessment score; IQR: interquartile range; $^{\$}$Student's t; *chi-squared; $^{+}$Fisher's exact; $^{\circ}$Mann–Whitney U.

The incidence of delirium was 22.9% ($n = 25$), and patients spent a median of 3 days (IQR: 1.5–7.5) in the ICU before the delirium onset. The most frequently observed subtype of delirium was mixed 44% ($n = 11$), hypoactive delirium 24% ($n = 6$), and hyperactive delirium 28% ($n = 7$). The mortality among all subjects was 15.6% ($n = 17$), and in patients who developed delirium, mortality was 12% ($n = 3$).

After reviewing the potential risk factors and clinical characteristics under investigation in the current study, we found several significant differences between patients with delirium and those without delirium; more specifically, patients with delirium were found to be on mechanical ventilation for a greater number of day, were older in age, and their cancer had metastasized (Tables 1 and 2). These characteristics, as well as other characteristic deemed clinically relevant, were included in univariate and multivariate logistic regression models; results of the analyses indicate that mechanical ventilation for a greater number of day is associated with the development of delirium in the ICU (Table 3).

4. Discussion

Delirium is a frequent complication in patients hospitalized or admitted to the ICU. This study found that in patients admitted to a mixed oncology ICU, the incidence of delirium was 22.9%. The time in days of use of mechanical ventilation was the only characteristic associated with the development of delirium at the ICU when adjusted for another variable. Moreover, in the current sample of patients, there was no difference in mortality rate when delirium was present or absent.

Table 2: Risk factors for development of delirium.

	With delirium	Without delirium	p
Alcoholism, n (%)	3 (12)	15 (17.9)	0.760^{+}
Smoking, n (%)	4 (16)	18 (21.4)	0.770^{+}
Acute kidney injury at time of admission to the ICU, n (%)	16 (64)	37 (44)	0.080*
Mechanical ventilation at admission to the ICU, n (%)	19 (76)	54 (64.3)	0.270^{+}
Time with mechanical ventilation (days), median (IQR)	8 (4–11)	2 (1–10)	0.010^{+}
Use of sedative in the ICU, n (%)	17 (68)	50 (59.5)	0.44*
Use of benzodiazepines, n (%)	9 (36)	31 (36.9)	0.930°
Use of mixed sedation, n (%)	3 (12)	2 (2.4)	0.080^{+}
Analgesic with opioids, n (%)	22 (88)	73 (87)	0.999*
Numerical Rating for Pain Scale	2.5 (0.5–4.5)	2.5 (0–5)	0.860°
Behavioral Pain Scale	3 (3–3)	3 (3–3)	0.930°
Use of steroids in the ICU, n (%)	8 (32)	23 (27.4)	0.650*
Use of vasopressor in the ICU, n (%)	18 (72)	57 (67.9)	0.690*
Transfusion during stay in the ICU, n (%)	10 (40)	41 (48.8)	0.490*
Use of antibiotic in the ICU, n (%)	25 (100)	78 (92.9)	0.330*
Time before admission to the ICU (days), median (IQR)	4 (1–9.5)	2 (1–13.5)	0.510°
Time in the ICU (days), median (IQR)	7 (2-5-13)	2 (1–6.75)	0.007°

ICU: intensive care unit; IQR: interquartile range; *chi-squared; $^{+}$Fisher's exact; $^{\circ}$ Mann–Whitney U.

Table 3: Risk factors for delirium in oncological critical ill patients, univariate and multivariate analysis.

	Univariate			Multivariate		
	OR	CI 95%	p	OR	CI 95%	p
Time with mechanical ventilation (days)	**1.06**	**0.99–1.13**	**0.070**	**1.06**	**0.99–1.13**	**0.070**
Time in the ICU (days)	1.07	1.01–1.14	0.020			
Hematologic neoplasm	2.08	0.82–5.25	0.040			
Metastasis	2.83	0.99–7.98	0.040			
Age (years)	1.03	0.99–1.05	0.050			
Hypovolemic shock	0.23	0.05–1.05	0.060			
Use mixed sedation	5.59	0.88–35.56	0.070			
Acute kidney injury at admission to the ICU	2.26	0.89–5.68	0.080			
Chemotherapy	0.46	0.18–1.17	0.100			
Acute respiratory failure	2.75	0.79–9.58	0.110			
Postcardiac arrest care	3.68	0.69–19.52	0.130			
Use of mechanical ventilation	1.76	0.63–4.88	0.270			
MEXSOFA score at admission to the ICU	1.05	0.93–1.18	0.410			
SOFA score at admission to the ICU	1.04	0.93–1.18	0.440			
Use of sedative in the ICU	1.44	0.56–3.72	0.440			
Postsurgical care	0.54	0.06–4.72	0.580			
Septic shock	1.21	0.49–2.99	0.670			
Analgesics with opioids	0.91	0.23–3.53	0.880			
Use of benzodiazepines	0.96	0.38–2.43	0.930			

ICU: intensive care unit; SOFA: Sequential Organ Failure Assessment score; MEXSOFA: Mexican Sequential Organ Failure Assessment score; CI: confidence interval; Hosmer–Lemeshow χ^2 =9.24, p = 0.240; auROC: 0.69 (CI 95% 0.57–0.82), p = 0.0100.

Previously reported estimates of delirium incidence in critically ill patients ranged from 10 to 80%; this wide range depends on a factor such as the type of acute condition requiring ICU admission, with the highest incidence rates found in older patients and those who are in the postoperative period [6, 18, 19]. Prior researchers have theorized that the wide range of reported delirium incidence rates were a result of different methods for diagnosing delirium, as well as the clinical conditions. The results of our study, which was conducted in an oncological ICU, are similar to other non-oncological populations; moreover, this study also found lower rates of delirium than in studies with oncological patients on mechanical ventilation [5, 19].

There are a number of different risk factors for developing delirium in the ICU, including patients' age, severity of illness, use of sedatives, use of mechanical ventilation, preexisting conditions, and other factors [6]. In our study, several of these risk factors were frequently observed in patients with delirium, although there was not a significant statistical association; however, any of them showed a statistical association in patients with delirium.

The use of mechanical ventilation is a fully identified risk factor for the development of delirium, and the duration in days of this therapeutic strategy and support has also shown association [20, 21] as authors have shown in the same way as has been observed in our results, where it was the only variable with a weak association with development of delirium, despite the evident difference in the duration of the days of mechanical ventilation between subjects with delirium and those who did not develop it.

Oncological patients with hematological or solid neoplasm frequently present with many predisposing risk factors for delirium, including frailty, comorbidities, polypharmacy, and malnutrition; however, a limitation of the current study is that we did not measure these variables as potential confounders variables [12, 22].

Several studies have shown the consistent relationship between delirium and mortality in oncological and non-oncological patients, in both the ICU and a general hospital setting [5, 19]; however, in our study, we found a low overall rate of mortality, and there were no differences in the mortality rates of patients with and without delirium. Patients typically have a lower mortality rate when they spend less time on mechanical ventilation, spend less time in the ICU, and have a high proportion of solid tumor [23], which may explain the current findings. Our study found a lower patient mortality rate compared to other studies with critically ill cancer patients, despite similar patient organ failure in our study and previous studies, as measured by the SOFA score. Patients included in our study had better performance status, which may explain the difference in research finding [19].

This study has important limitations. First, the study was conducted in a single cancer center and has a small sample size. These limitations may affect the external validity of our results, limiting their utility in other ICU environments. Second, we did not consider the metastasis site (when it was present in patients), which may have been a potential confounding variable.

5. Conclusion

Delirium is a frequent condition in critically ill cancer patients admitted to the ICU. The duration in days of mechanical ventilation is a potential risk factor for developing delirium during an ICU stay. Delirium was not associated with a higher rate of mortality in this group of patients.

References

[1] E. Ely, R. Margolin, J. Francis et al., "Evaluation of delirium in critically ill patients: validation of the Confusion Assessment Method for the intensive Care Unit (CAM-ICU)," *Critical Care Medicine*, vol. 29, no. 7, pp. 1370–1379, 2001.

[2] T. Girard, P. Pandharipande, and E. Ely, "Delirium in the intensive care unit," *Critical Care: The Official Journal of the Critical Care Forum*, vol. 12, no. 3, p. s3, 2008.

[3] A. Morandi, P. Pandharipande, M. Trabucchi et al., "Understanding international differences in terminology for delirium and other types of acute brain dysfunction in critically ill patients," *Intensive Care Medicine*, vol. 34, no. 10, pp. 1097–1915, 2008.

[4] P. Pandaripande, W. Ely, R. Arora et al., "The intensive care delirium research agenda: a multinational, interprofessional perspective," *Intensive Care Medicine*, vol. 43, no. 9, pp. 1329–1339, 2017.

[5] J. Salluh, M. Soares, J. Teles et al., "Delirium epidemiology in critical care (DECCA): an international study," *Critical Care: The Official Journal of the Critical Care Forum*, vol. 14, no. 6, p. R210, 2010.

[6] J. Salluh, T. Sharshar, and J. Kress, "Does this patient have delirium?," *Intensive Care Medicine*, vol. 43, no. 5, pp. 693–695, 2017.

[7] P. Pandharipande, J. Jackson, and W. Ely, "Delirium: acute cognitive dysfunction in the critically ill," *Current Opinion in Critical Care*, vol. 11, pp. 360–368, 2005.

[8] J. Devlin, J. Fong, G. Frase, and R. Riker, "Delirium assessment in the critically ill," *Intensive Care Medicine*, vol. 33, no. 6, pp. 929–940, 2007.

[9] R. Cavallazzi, M. Saad, and P. Marik, "Delirium in the ICU: an overview," *Annals of Intensive Care*, vol. 2, no. 1, p. 49, 2012.

[10] I. Zaal, J. Devlin, L. Peelen, and A. Slooter, "A systematic review of risk factors for delirium in the ICU," *Critical Care Medicine*, vol. 43, no. 1, pp. 40–47, 2015.

[11] A. Caraceni and F. Simonetti, "Palliating delirium in patient with cancer," *Lancet Oncology*, vol. 10, no. 2, pp. 164–172, 2009.

[12] W. Breitbat and Y. Alici, "Evidence-based treatment of delirium in patients with cancer," *Journal of Clinical Oncology*, vol. 30, no. 11, pp. 1206–1214, 2012.

[13] C. Danes-Farriols, C. Landa-Teran, A. Ruiz-Ripoll, and J. Planas-Domingo, "Prevalence of delirium in patients with advanced cancer admitted to a palliative unit," *Medicina Paliativa*, vol. 23, no. 4, pp. 165–171, 2016.

[14] M. Oken, R. Creech, D. Tormey et al., "Toxicity and response criteria of the cooperative oncology group," *American Journal of Clinical Oncology*, vol. 5, no. 6, pp. 649–655, 1982.

[15] C. Schag, R. Heinrich, and P. Ganz, "Karnofsky performance status revisited: Reliability, validity, and guidelines," *Journal of Clinical Oncology*, vol. 2, no. 3, pp. 187–193, 1984.

[16] J. Vincent, R. Moreno, J. Takala et al., "The SOFA (Sepsis-related Organ Failure Assessment) score to describe organ dysfunction/failure. On behalf of the Working Group on Sepsis-Related Problems of the European Society of Intensive Care Medicine," *Intensive Care Medicine*, vol. 22, no. 7, pp. 707–710, 1996.

[17] S. Namendys, M. Silva, G. Vásquez et al., "Application of a modified sequential organ failure assessment score to critically ill patients," *Brazilian Journal of Medical and Biological Research*, vol. 46, no. 2, pp. 186–193, 2013.

[18] E. Bilge, M. Kaya, G. Senel, and S. Ünver, "The incidence of delirium at postoperative intensive care unit in adults patients," *Turkish Journal of Anesthesia and Reanimation*, vol. 43, no. 4, pp. 232–239, 2015.

[19] S. Mori, J. R. T. Takeda, F. S. A. Carrara, C. R. Cohrs, S. S. V. Zanei, and I. Y. Whitaker, "Incidence and factors related to delirium in an intensive care unit," *Revista da Escola de Enfermagem da USP*, vol. 50, no. 4, pp. 585–591, 2016.

[20] C. Bullock, S. Richards, J. Winchester, T. Jackson, and C. Small, "Delirium in critically military patients following trauma: a cohort analysis," *Journal of the Intensive Care Society*, vol. 17, no. 1, pp. 12–18, 2016.

[21] M. van den Boogaard, L. Schoonhoven, J. van der Hoeven, T. van Achterberg, and P. Pickkers, "Incidence and short-term consequences of delirium in critically patients: a prospective

observational cohort study," *International Journal of Nursing Studies*, vol. 49, no. 7, pp. 775–783, 2012.
[22] N. Sarhill, D. Walsh, K. A. Nelson, S. LeGrand, and M. P. Davis, "Assessment of delirium in advanced cancer: the use of the beside confusion scale," *American Journal of Hospice and Palliative Care*, vol. 18, no. 5, pp. 335–341, 2001.
[23] I. Almeida, M. Soares, F. Bozza et al., "The impact of acute brain dysfunction in the outcome of mechanical ventilated cancer patients," *PLoS One*, vol. 9, no. 1, Article ID e85332, 2014.

4

Chemical Composition and Antioxidant, Analgesic, and Anti-Inflammatory Effects of Methanolic Extract of *Euphorbia retusa* in Mice

Jazia Sdayria,[1,2] Ilhem Rjeibi,[1] Anouar Feriani,[1] Sana Ncib,[3] Wided Bouguerra,[3] Najla Hfaiedh,[1] Abdelfattah Elfeki,[2] and Mohamed Salah Allagui[2]

[1]*Research Unit of Macromolecular Biochemistry and Genetic, Faculty of Sciences of Gafsa, University of Gafsa, 2112 Gafsa, Tunisia*
[2]*Laboratory of Animal Ecophysiology, Faculty of Science of Sfax, University of Sfax, 3018 Sfax, Tunisia*
[3]*Common Services Unit for Research, Faculty of Sciences of Gafsa, University of Gafsa, 2112 Gafsa, Tunisia*

Correspondence should be addressed to Ilhem Rjeibi; rjeibii@yahoo.fr

Academic Editor: Shinya Kasai

Plants provide an alternative source to manage different human disorders due to various metabolites. The aim of this study is to investigate the phytochemical constituents of the methanolic extracts of *Euphorbia retusa* and to evaluate their antioxidant, anti-inflammatory, and analgesic activities. The phytochemical results obtained by HPLC and by chemical assay reactions have revealed the richness of the methanolic extract of *E. retusa* in active compounds, in particular polyphenols, flavonoids, and tannins. The methanolic extract shows significant antioxidant activities *in vitro*, in the DPPH and the FRAP assays. The antinociceptive activity was evaluated using acetic acid and hot-plate models of pain in mice. The anti-inflammatory activity was evaluated by carrageenan-induced paw edema. Oral pretreatment with the methanolic extract of *E. retusa* (200 mg/kg) exhibited a significant inhibition of pain induced either by acetic acid or by the heating plate and in a manner comparable to the standard drug paracetamol. *E. retusa* significantly reduced paw edema starting from the 3rd hour after carrageenan administration by increasing the activity of antioxidant enzymes (SOD, CAT, and GPx) in liver and paw tissues and decreasing the levels of MDA. These results may confirm the interesting potential of this plant as a treatment of various inflammatory and pain diseases.

1. Introduction

Inflammatory reaction is one of the most important defense mechanisms against tissue injury caused by physical and chemical agents, noxious stimuli, heat, antigen-antibody reaction, and microbial effect. Inflammatory response occurs in two distinct phases: an acute and a chronic. The acute phase is a preliminary crisis absolutely necessary for the healing processes characterized by local vasodilatation, increased capillary permeability, and the release of inflammatory mediators like histamine, serotonin, and prostaglandins. The chronic phase is the result of failure to eliminate acute inflammation, an autoimmune response to a self-antigen characterized by infiltration of leukocytes and phagocytic cells [1]. Chronic inflammation can last for several months and even years and can eventually cause several diseases such as rheumatoid arthritis, atherosclerosis, asthma, heart disease, ulcerative colitis, and some cancers. Therefore, inflammation must be well regulated in these early stages.

Several studies have demonstrated that the main mechanisms involved in the inflammatory reaction are closely associated with the generation of free radicals and the creation of oxidative stress. In fact, during the inflammation process, several reactive oxygen species (ROS) including nonradical hydrogen peroxide (H_2O_2), singlet oxygen ($^1O_2$), nitric oxide (NO), superoxide ($O2^{\cdot-}$), hydroxyl ($HO^{\cdot}$), and peroxyl (ROO–) radicals are overexpressed by neutrophils and macrophages and play an important role in the host defense mechanism [2]. Besides their defensive effects, this overproduction leads to tissue injury by damaging macromolecules and lipid peroxidation of membranes [3]. In addition, ROS propagate inflammation by stimulating the release of cytokines, such as interleukin-1, tumour necrosis factor-alpha (TNF-α), and interferon-gamma (IFN-γ). Thus, free radicals are important mediators that provoke or sustain inflammatory processes, and consequently, cells and tissues require antioxidant enzymes, including superoxide dismutase, catalase, and glutathione peroxidase to neutralize and decompose these reactive oxygen species [2, 4].

Currently, nonsteroidal anti-inflammatory drugs (NSAIDs) are widely prescribed because of their efficacy in the management of pain, inflammation, and rheumatic disorders. However, their long-term therapeutic use is often associated with adverse effects such as gastrointestinal ulcers and renal insufficiency [5]. For these reasons, the use of medicinal plants has become the new strategy of several studies to develop and introduce new drugs with greater safety and efficiency. Indeed, medicinal plants contain a large number of bioactive molecules of multiple interests not only in traditional medicine but also in the food and pharmaceutical industry. These molecules include alkaloids, phenolic acids, tannins, and flavonoids which possess interesting biological activities like anti-inflammatory, anticarcinogenic, antimicrobial, and antioxidant.

Euphorbia is the largest genus of the family Euphorbiaceae and comprises about 1000 species. Many researchers have shown that *Euphorbia* species possess antitumoral activity [6], antimicrobial activity [7], inhibition of HIV-1 viral infection [8], and antihyperglycemic and hypolipidemic activities [9]. *Euphorbia retusa* locally called "lebina" is an annual herb abundantly found throughout the Mediterranean area. It is characterized by long alternate blue-green leaves which contain toxic and skin-irritant milky latex very rich in tetracyclic triterpene compounds [10]. This herb has been used in traditional medicine as a cure for warts, trichiasis, and venomous bites [11]. However, to our knowledge, *E. retusa* is less studied than the other species of their family. There is some scientific work that has reported the isolation of many compounds including flavonol glycosides [12] and triterpenoids and fatty acids from the aerial part of this plant [13]. Diterpenoids and triterpenoids were also isolated from the roots [13]. For biological properties, only a recent study conducted by Abdallah [14] has demonstrated the antimicrobial activity of this plant. Therefore, the present study is aimed at determining the phytochemical composition of the methanolic extract of *E. retusa* using standard analytical methods followed by exploring their potential antioxidant, antinociceptive, and anti-inflammatory activities by *in vivo* and *in vitro* models.

2. Materials and Methods

2.1. Chemicals and Reagents. The chemicals and reagents used in this work such as Folin–Ciocalteu reagent, 2,2-diphenyl-1-picrylhydrazyl (DPPH), ascorbic acid, gallic acid, vanillic acid, rutin, epicatechin, coumaric acid, catechin, 2,6-di-tert-butyl-4-hydroxy-carboxylic acid (BHT), sodium carbonate, aluminum chloride ($AlCl_3$), sodium nitrate ($NaNO_2$), sodium carbonate (Na_2CO_3), sodium hydroxide (NaOH), and hydrogen peroxide (H_2O_2) were purchased from Sigma-Aldrich Chemical (St. Louis, MO). HPLC-grade solvent methanol, acetonitrile, and acetic acid were purchased from Carlo Erba Reactif-CDS. Carrageenan was also obtained from Sigma-Aldrich Chemical (St. Louis, MO).

2.2. Plant Material. The leaves of *Euphorbia retusa* were collected from the Gafsa region in the southwest of Tunisia (34°22′59″N latitude and 8°09′00″E longitude) during November 2015. The plant leaves were washed and dried in shade for up to two weeks. The dried leaves were crushed, using an electric grinder, into fine powders and stored at room temperature in a dry place.

2.3. Extraction Procedure. The dried powder leaves of *E. retusa* were extracted by the maceration method. 50 mL of methanol was added to 5g of leaves and was left to stand under agitation for 24 h. Subsequently, the solution was filtered using a filter paper. The methanol extract was evaporated under reduced pressure at room temperature, and the obtained residue was preserved at 4°C for further analysis.

2.4. Determination of Total Polyphenol Contents. The total polyphenol content of the methanol extract was carried out according to the Folin–Ciocalteu method [15]. This method consists of mixing 0.25 mL of the extract (1 mg/mL) with 1.25 mL of the Folin–Ciocalteu reagent (diluted 10 times with distilled water). After 5 min, 1 mL of sodium carbonate solution (7.5%) was added, and the mixture was incubated at 45°C for 2 hours. The absorbance of the solution obtained was measured at 765 nm using a spectrophotometer (Shimadzu UV-190). A calibration curve was prepared in parallel under the same operating conditions using gallic acid as positive control. The phenol contents were expressed in terms of milligrams of the gallic acid equivalent (GAE) per gram of the extract (mg·GAE/g extract).

2.5. Determination of Flavonoid Contents. The flavonoid content was determined according to the aluminum chloride colorimetric method of Djeridane et al. [16]. Briefly, 0.5 mL of the extract (1 mg/mL) was mixed with 0.15 mL of 5% sodium nitrite. After 5 min, 0.15 mL of 10% $AlCl_3$ solution was added to the mixture, followed by the addition of 1 mL of 1.0 M·NaOH after one min, and diluted with 1.2 mL of distilled water. The standard solution of quercetin (0–400 μg/mL) was prepared in the same conditions. The absorbance of the extract and standard solutions was read at 430 nm using a spectrophotometer (Shimadzu UV-190). The total flavonoid content was determined from the calibration curve and expressed as milligrams of the quercetin equivalent (QE) per gram of the extract (mg·QE/g extract).

2.6. Condensed Tannin Contents. The Broadhurst and Jones method [17] modified by Heimler et al. [18] was used for the determination of the condensed tannin content. 400 μL of the extract (1 mg/mL) or standard solution (1 mg/mL) was mixed with 3 mL of 4% vanillin initially dissolved in methanol and 1.5 mL of concentrated sulfuric acid. The mixture was incubated for 15 min, and the absorbance was taken at 430 nm using a spectrophotometer (Shimadzu UV-190). Catechin solution was used as a reference, and the content of condensed tannins was expressed as mg of the catechin equivalent/mg of the extract.

2.7. Identification of the Phenolic Compounds and Flavonoids by HPLC. For the identification of the phenolic compounds and flavonoids present in the plant extract, a Varian ProStar HPLC system equipped with a reverse C18 column (Varian; 150 nm × 4.6 mm, particle size 5 μm), a ternary pump (ProStar 230), and a diode barrier detector (ProStar 330) was used. The chromatographic analyses were a gradient elution consisting of two solvents: solvent A (100% methanol) and solvent B (0.05% acetic acid aqueous solution). The gradient conditions were 35% A and 65% B at $t = 1$ min, 50% A and 50% B at $t = 30$ min, and 90% A and 10% B at $t = 40$ min. The flow rate was 1 mL/min, and the injection volume was 20 μL at 25°C. The identification was carried out at 280 nm for phenolic acids and at 365 nm for flavonoids using gallic acid, epicatechin, coumaric acid, apigenin, and naringenin as standard phenolic acids and rutin, quercetin, and kaempferol as standard flavonoids and based on comparison with retention times and coinjection.

2.8. Antioxidant Activity

2.8.1. DPPH Radical Scavenging Activity Assay. The capacity to scavenge the free radical 2,2-diphenyl-1-picrylhydrazyl (DPPH) was estimated according to the method of Yang et al. [19]. Briefly, 1 mL of the methanol extract at different concentrations (0.05 to 0.4 mg/mL) was mixed with 1 mL of 50 mm DPPH ethanolic solution. The mixtures were kept in the dark for 30 min, and the absorbance was measured at 517 nm using Shimadzu UV-190. Butylhydroxytoluene (BHT) used as positive control was prepared under the same conditions. Each test was performed in triplicate. The DPPH radical scavenging activity (RSA) was calculated as follows:

$$\text{RSA}\ (\%) = \frac{\text{absorbance of DPPH} - \text{absorbance of the sample}}{\text{absorbance of DPPH}} \times 100. \tag{1}$$

2.8.2. Ferric-Reducing Antioxidant Power Assay. The ability of the extract to reduce the ferric ion (Fe^{3+}) present in the $K_3[Fe(CN)6]$ complex to ferrous ion (Fe^{2+}) was evaluated by the method described by Oyaizu [20]. Briefly, 2.5 mL of the plant extract at different concentrations (0–300 μg/mL), 2.5 mL of sodium phosphate buffer (0.2 M, pH 6.6), and 2.5 mL of potassium ferricyanide (1% w/v in distilled water) were combined in a test tube and incubated in a water bath at 50°C for 20 min. Following this, 2.5 mL of trichloroacetic acid solution (10%, w/v) was added, and the mixture was centrifuged at 3000 rpm for 10 min. Finally, a 2.5 mL aliquot of the supernatant was mixed with 2.5 mL of distilled water and 0.5 mL of a 0.1% (w/v) solution of ferric chloride ($FeCl_3$). The manipulation was carried out in triplicate. The absorbance was read spectrophotometrically at 700 nm. Ascorbic acid was used as a standard antioxidant, and the results were presented as the change in absorbance as a function of concentration; increased absorbance of the reaction mixture indicates greater reducing power.

2.9. Pharmacological Activities In Vivo

2.9.1. Animals. Swiss albino mice weighing 20–30 g were obtained from the Central Pharmacy of Tunisia, Tunis, Tunisia. The animals were housed in a spacious indoor cage and were kept in the animal room under controlled conditions (12 h light-dark cycle; temperature 22 ± 2°C; relative humidity 60 ± 5%) with free access to food pellets (SNA, Sfax, Tunisia) and tap water ad libitum. Before two weeks of the experiment, the animals were divided into normal control groups and test groups pretreated with the methanolic extract of *E. retusa*, paracetamol, and indomethacin of six animals per group. The experiments on laboratory animals were carried out according to Guide for the Care and Use of laboratory Animals approved by the Animal Ethics Committee.

2.9.2. Acute Toxicity. For evaluating the acute toxicity, mice were divided into different groups and treated with increasing oral doses of the *E. retusa* methanolic extract (100–200–400–600–800–1000 mg/kg) in distilled water. After administration of the extracts, the animals were kept under regular observation for 48 h for any mortality or behavioral changes.

2.9.3. Analgesic Activity

(1) Hot-Plate Test. This test was carried out according to the method described by Turner [21]. It is based upon induction of thermal stimulus by putting the mice in a glass beaker setting on the surface of the hot plate thermostatically controlled at 55°C. Reaction time, measured in seconds, was recorded when the animals licked their forepaws and jumped. The increase in reaction time indicates analgesic activity. For this test, 3 groups of 6 mice each were used. Group 1 (control group) received 1 mL distilled water, group 2 (*E. retusa* group) was pretreated orally (p.o.) with the *E. retusa* methanol extract (200 mg/kg), and group 3 (positive control group) was pretreated with paracetamol (100 mg/kg, p.o.). *E. retusa* extract

and paracetamol were administered with free access to an aqueous solution of both for two weeks.

(2) Writhing Test. The analgesic effect of the plant extract was assessed by the acetic acid abdominal constriction test according to the method described by Sawadogo et al. [22]. The animals were selected and divided into three groups of six mice each. Group 1 served as a normal control and was given 1 mL distilled water. Group 2 was pretreated orally (p.o.) with the *E. retusa* methanol extract at 200 mg/kg. Group 3 was pretreated with standard paracetamol at 100 mg/kg, p.o. After 15 days of pretreatment, all mice were intraperitoneally injected with 10 mL of 1% acetic acid. The number of abdominal writhings for each mouse was recorded during 30 min. Analgesic activity was expressed as a percentage of pain inhibition which was calculated according to the following formula:

$$\%\ \text{inhibition} = \frac{((\text{number of writhes})\ \text{control} - (\text{number of writhes})\ \text{treated})}{(\text{number of writhes})\ \text{control}} \times 100. \tag{2}$$

2.9.4. Anti-Inflammatory Activity. The anti-inflammatory activity of *E. retusa* was evaluated using the carrageenan-induced mice paw edema model [23]. Inflammation was induced by the injection of 1% carrageenan in physiological water (0.9% NaCl) at a dose of 100 μL into the subplantar region of the right hind paw of the mice. Four groups of six mice per group were used for the study: an untreated negative control group receiving a physiological solution by subplantar injection, an untreated positive control group injected with carrageenan (Carr), a reference group pretreated orally with indomethacin (10 mg/kg, p.o.) and injected with carrageenan (Carr + Indo), and the fourth group pretreated orally with the *Euphorbia* methanol extract (200 mg/kg, p.o.) and injected with carrageenan (Carr + Eu). The evolution of the volume of edema was followed by the measurement of the paw diameter of each mouse before and at 1, 2, 3, 4, 5, and 6 h after induction of inflammation using a manual calliper. For each group, the percentages of inflammation and inhibition of edema were calculated by the following formulas:

$$\begin{aligned} \%\ \text{inflammation} &= \frac{(VT - \text{V0})}{\text{V0}} \times 100, \\ \%\ \text{inhibition} &= \frac{((VT - \text{V0})\ \text{control} - (VT - \text{V0})\ \text{treated group})}{(VT - \text{V0})\ \text{control}} \times 100, \end{aligned} \tag{3}$$

where VT is the paw size obtained at various times, while V0 is the paw size obtained before any treatment.

At the end of the experiment, the animals were sacrificed and the right hind paw tissue and liver were dissected, rinsed in ice-cold normal saline, and homogenized in ice-cold phosphate buffer (pH 7.4). Then, the homogenate was centrifuged at 3000 × g for 10 min. The supernatant was collected and kept at −20°C in a refrigerator for MDA and the antioxidant enzymes (CAT, SOD, and GPx) activity assays.

(1) Determination of Tissue Lipid Peroxidation. The concentration of malondialdehyde (MDA), an indicator of lipid peroxidation, was evaluated by the thiobarbituric acid-reacting substances (TBARS) method [24]. This method is based on the fact that peroxidation of most membrane systems leads to the release of small amounts of MDA which react with thiobarbituric acid (TBA) in the acidic high temperature and form a red-complex TBARS. The absorbance of TBARS was determined at 532 nm. Lipid peroxidation was expressed as nmoles of TBARS.

(2) Determination of Antioxidant Enzyme Activity. The biochemical parameters were analyzed to check the protective activity of the methanolic extract of *E. retusa* by the following methods: total superoxide dismutase (SOD) activity was evaluated by measuring its ability to inhibit the photoreduction of nitroblue tetrazolium (NBT) [25].The photoreduction of NBT was mediated by superoxide anions generated by the xanthine/xanthine oxidase system and monitored at 550 nm. One unit of SOD is defined as the amount of enzymes required to inhibit the rate of NBT reduction by 50%. Total catalase (CAT) activity estimation was determined by measuring the hydrogen peroxide dissipation at 240 nm, using the method of Aebi [26]. Glutathione-peroxidase (GPX) activity was measured by detecting the oxidating state of NADPH at 340 nm according to the method used by Flohe and Gunzler [27]. The protein concentration of the tissue was determined by the method of Bradford [28], using bovine serum albumin as a standard.

2.10. Statistical Analysis. Results in this study were presented as the mean ± standard deviation (SD) and as the percentage. All analyses were statistically evaluated by ANOVA and using Student's t-test. $p \leq 0.05$ was considered significant.

3. Results

3.1. Total Phenolic, Flavanoid, and Condensed Tannin Content. The total polyphenolic content of the leaf extracts

Table 1: The phytochemical composition and antioxidant capacity of the methanolic extract of *Euphorbia retusa*.

	Phytochemical composition			Antioxidant activity	
	Total phenolics (mg·GAE/g·DW)[a]	Total flavonoids (mg·QE/g·DW)[b]	Condensed tannins (mg·QE/g·DW)[c]	DPPH (EC_{50}, mg/ml)	FRAP (EC_{50}, mg/ml)
Euphorbia retusa	280.21 ± 0.085	20.50 ± 0.107	41.39 ± 0.198	131.23 ± 7.47	104.05 ± 12.82
Vitamin C	—	—	—	76.88 ± 16.88	48.46 ± 7.72

[a]Total phenolic content as the gallic acid equivalent. [b]Total flavonoid content as the quercetin equivalent. [c]Condensed tannin as the quercetin equivalent. Values are expressed as mean ± standard deviation (n = 3).

was approximately 280.21 ± 0.085 mg of gallic acid/g of plant extracts. The total flavonoid content was estimated to be equivalent to 20.50 ± 0.107 mg of quercetin/g of plant extracts. Besides, the condensed tannin content of the leaf extracts of *E. retusa* expressed in mg of the catechin equivalents/g of plant extracts was 41.39 ± 0.198 mg/g (Table 1).

3.2. HPLC Analysis. The HPLC analysis of the *E. retusa* methanol extract revealed the presence of phenolic acids and flavonoids. The HPLC elution profile recorded at 280 nm showed 5 phenolic acids: gallic acid, epicatechin, coumaric acid, apigenin, and naringenin (Figure 1(a)) with concentrations of 1111.41 μg/mL, 198.52 μg/mL, 147.73 μg/mL, 7.89 μg/mL, and 6.13 μg/mL, respectively (Table 2), while the HPLC elution profile of flavonoids (Figure 1(b); Table 2) recorded at 360 nm identified 3 compounds: rutin, quercetin, and kaempferol, with concentrations of 50.74 μg/mL, 6.78 μg/mL, and 14.42 μg/mL.

3.3. Antioxidant Capacity

3.3.1. DPPH Radical Scavenging Activity. The evolution of the antiradical activity of the extract of *Euphorbia, in vitro*, against the DPPH radical was dose-dependent (Figure 2). Indeed, as the concentration of the extract increases, the anti-DPPH activity also increases until a maximum concentration (0.4 mg/mL) was reached. The antioxidant capacity was determined from IC_{50}, which corresponds to the concentration necessary to reduce 50% of the DPPH radical. The extract of *E. retusa* presents IC_{50} with 130 mg/mL which means low activity compared to BHT used as a positive control (40 mg/mL) (Table 1)

3.3.2. Ferric-Reducing Antioxidant Assay (FRAP). The antioxidant capacity of the extract was also measured by the FRAP method. As shown in Figure 3, the reducing power of the extract was dependent on the extract concentration compared to the ascorbic acid standard. The activity increased with the increasing concentration of the extract. The reducing power of the *Euphorbia* extract at 300 mg/mL was found to be 0.61 ± 0.12 of the absorbance unit. This activity appeared important but significantly lower than that of ascorbic acid (0.87 ± 0.059) ($p < 0.05$). The effective concentration EC_{50} was 246.66 μg/ml ± 100.16 and 130.71 μg/mL ± 91.21 in *E. retusa* and ascorbic acid, respectively.

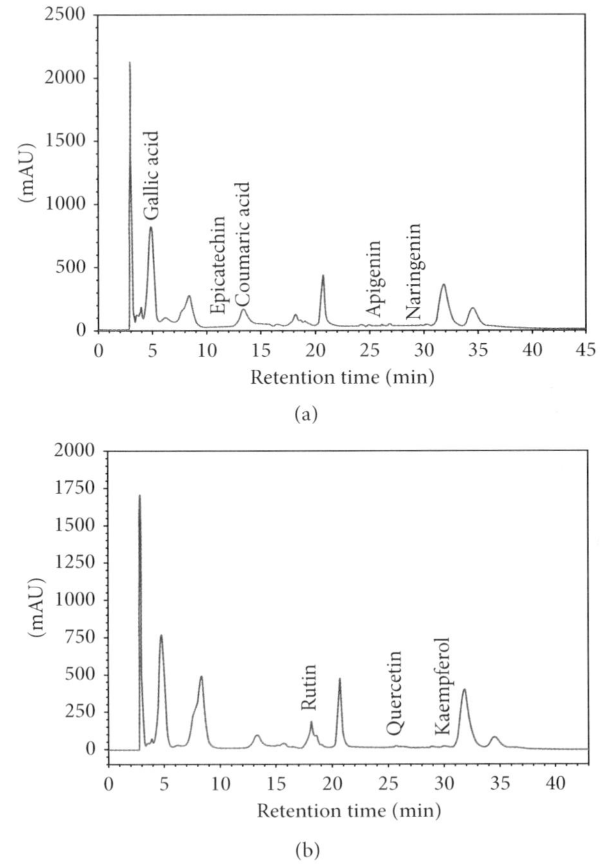

Figure 1: HPLC/DAD chromatogram of the methanol extract of *Euphorbia retusa*. (a) HPLC profile of phenolic acids at 280 nm; (b) HPLC profile of flavonoids at 360 nm.

3.4. Pharmacological Activities In Vivo

3.4.1. Acute Toxicity. The acute toxicity of *E. retusa* was conducted for evaluating their safety at different doses. *E. retusa* did not generate any behavioral changes, and no death was observed with the maximum dose of 1000 mg/kg BW. In this study, a dose of 200 mg/kg BW was chosen to investigate the antioxidant, analgesic, and anti-inflammatory activities of the methanolic extract of *E. retusa* in experimental animals.

3.4.2. Writhing Test. Table 3 shows acetic acid-induced writhing responses in mice. The methanolic extract of *E. retusa* (200 mg/kg) and paracetamol (100 mg/kg) significantly reduced the number of abdominal writhings elicited

Table 2: Composition of flavonoids and phenolic acids of the methanol extract of *Euphorbia retusa*.

	Compounds	Concentration (μg/mL)
Phenolic acids	Gallic acid	1111.41
	Epicatechin	198.52
	Coumaric acid	147.73
	Apigenin	7.89
	Naringenin	6.13
Flavonoids	Rutin	50.74
	Quercetin	6.78
	Kaempferol	14.42

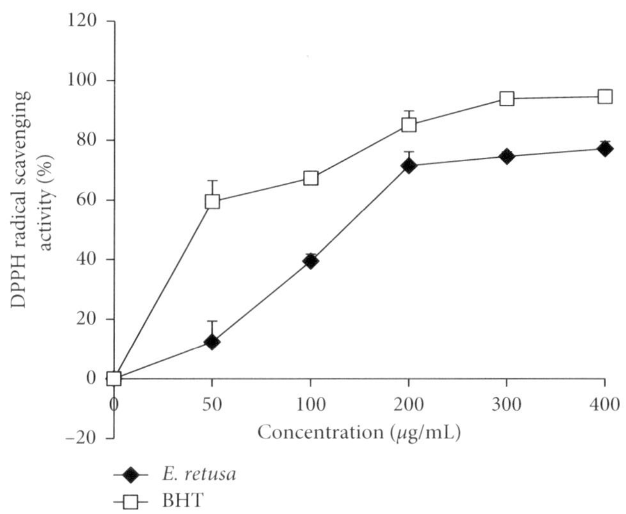

Figure 2: The antiradical activity of *Euphorbia retusa* against the radical DPPH. Values are represented as mean ± standard deviation ($n = 3$).

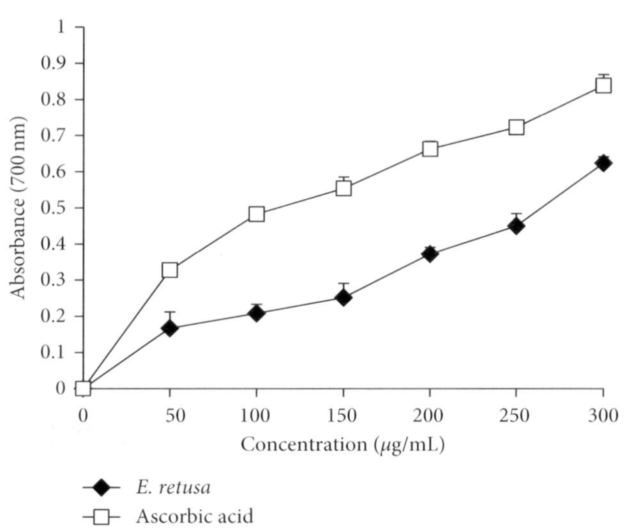

Figure 3: The reducing power of *Euphorbia retusa* and ascorbic acid by the FRAP assay. Values are expressed as mean ± standard deviation ($n = 3$).

by acetic acid when compared to the control group, indicating their analgesic activities. The percentages of inhibition of the pain were 55% for the extract of *Euphorbia* and 70% for the paracetamol.

Table 3: Effect of the methanolic extract of *Euphorbia retusa* on the abdominal contortions induced by acetic acid in mice.

Group	Dose (mg/kg)	Number of writhes	Inhibition (%)
C (distilled water)	1 mL/kg	20.16 ± 8.97	—
Euphorbia retusa	200 mg/kg	9 ± 9.52**	55.37
Paracetamol	100 mg/kg	6 ± 4.56***	70.24

The values are expressed as mean ± SEM ($n = 6$). *** $p < 0.001$ and ** $p < 0.01$ as compared to the control.

Table 4: Effect of the methanolic extract of *Euphorbia retusa* on thermal nociception induced by a hot plate in mice paws.

Group	Dose (mg/kg)	Reaction time (s)	Inhibition (%)
C (NaCl)	10 mL/kg	31.85 ± 14.45	—
Euphorbia retusa	200 mg/kg	151 ± 27.69***	78.90
Paracetamol	100 mg/kg	127.5 ± 34.06***	75.01

The values are expressed as mean ± SEM ($n = 6$). *** $p < 0.001$ as compared to the control.

3.4.3. Hot-Plate Test. The results obtained from the hot-plate test are presented in Table 4. The oral pretreatment of mice with the *E. retusa* methanol extract caused a significant ($p < 0.001$) increase of the latency time of reaction in comparison with the control group. The reference drug significantly inhibited the hot-plate-induced pain compared to the control group. The inhibition rates of hot-plate-induced pain by *E. retusa* compared with the positive control were 78.90% and 75.01%, respectively.

3.4.4. Anti-Inflammatory Activity. The development of edema in control and treated groups for 6h is represented in Figure 4. The percentage of inflammation in the group (Carr) was increased progressively, and in a highly significant ($p < 0.001$) way over time, it was increased from 65% at the first hour to 120% at the 6th hour. However, this percentage of inflammation was decreased over time and in a comparable manner in the groups pretreated with indomethacin or the methanolic extract of *Euphorbia*; in fact, it was decreased from 57% at the 2nd hour to 32% after 6 hours in the group pretreated with the extract of the plant (Carr + Eu). This is well confirmed in Figure 4(a) that presents the paws of the different groups of mice taken after the completion of the experiment.

As seen in Figure 4(c), the extract of *E. retusa* shows significant inhibition of edema in the 2nd, 3rd, 4th, 5th, and 6th hour after injection of Carr. However, this inhibition was more important than that of mice receiving Indo, used as positive controls indicating anti-inflammatory activities of *Euphorbia*.

(1) Effects of the E. retusa Extract on the MDA Level. The evolution of dermal lipid peroxidation is illustrated in Figure 5. In the Carr group, we noted a highly significant increase ($p < 0.001$) of the MDA level compared to the control group. However, the pretreatment of mice with the methanolic extract of *E. retusa* and indomethacin significantly decreased the MDA levels in paw tissue.

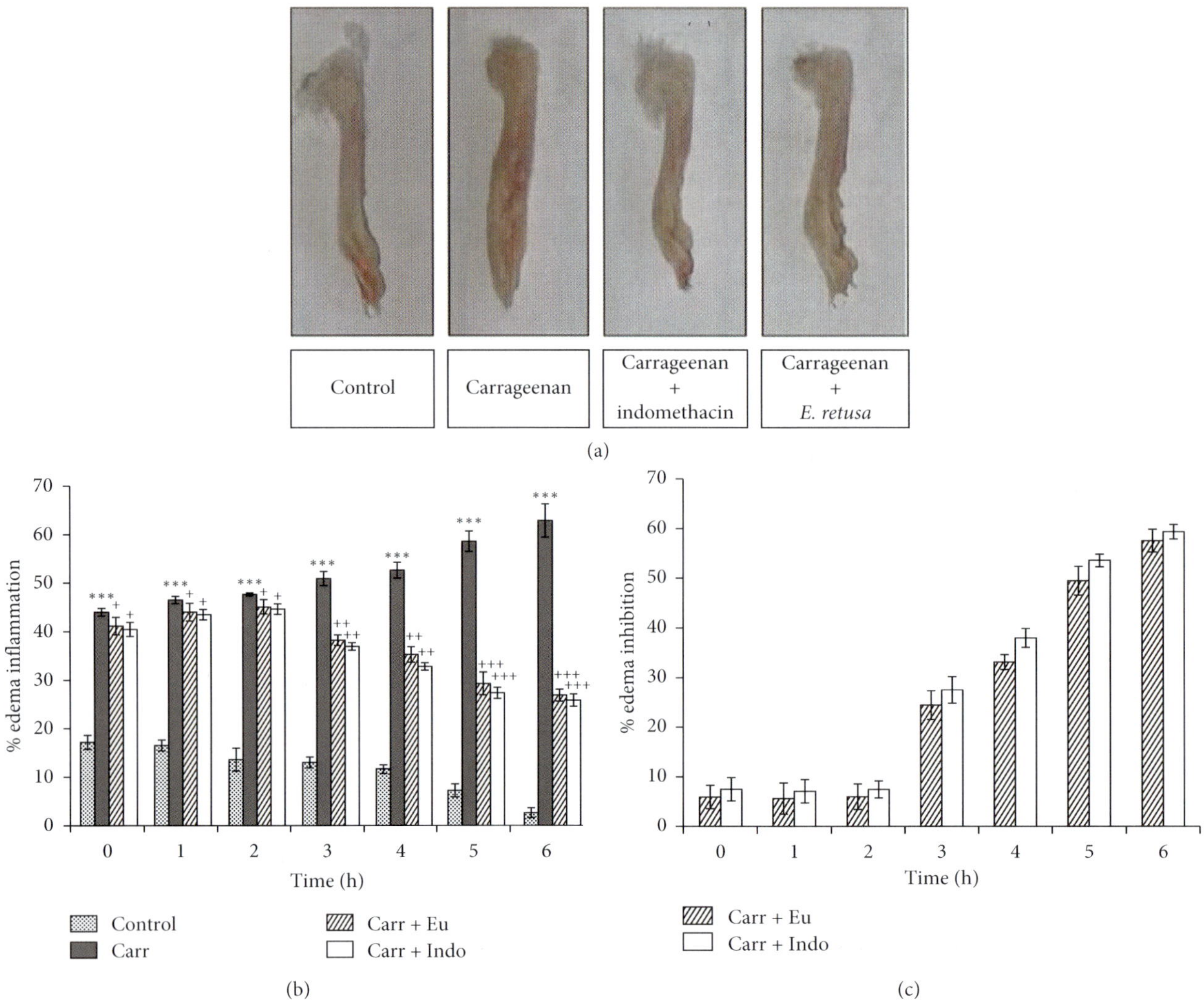

FIGURE 4: (a) The paw of mice treated with carrageenan and/or indomethacin or the methanolic extract of *Euphorbia retusa*. (b) Percentage inflammation of the paws of mice induced by local injection of carrageenan and/or indomethacin or the methanolic extract of *Euphorbia retusa*. Control: normal mice injected with isotonic saline solution (NaCl) 0.9%; Carr: mice injected with carrageenan 1%; Carr + Indo: mice pretreated with indomethacin and injected with carrageenan; Carr + Eu: mice pretreated with the methanolic extract of *E. retusa* and injected with carrageenan. (c) Percent inhibition of paw edema in mice pretreated with the *Euphorbia retusa* extract and indomethacin, induced after local injection of carrageenan. Values are represented as mean ± SD ($n = 6$) in each group. $^{*}p < 0.05$, $^{**}p < 0.01$, and $^{***}p < 0.001$. $^{*}p$: compared with the control; ^{+}p: compared with carrageenan.

(2) Effects of the E. retusa Extract on the Activities of Antioxidant Enzymes. The changes of the activities of antioxidant enzymes in liver and paw tissues of all treated groups were assessed. The results presented in Table 5 show that carrageenan administration significantly decreased SOD, CAT, and GPx activities in liver and paw tissues in comparison with the control group ($p < 0.001$). However, a significant restoration in these enzymatic antioxidant activities was observed in the group pretreated with *E. retusa* (200 mg/kg), as well as with 10 mg/kg indomethacin.

4. Discussion

Nowadays, phytotherapy, based on scientific works, is becoming an important alternative pathway in the world to find effective natural medicines without any adverse effects. The objective of the present work is to study the phytochemical properties of the methanolic extract of *E. retusa* and to evaluate its antioxidant, analgesic, and anti-inflammatory activities. The phytochemical investigation of the methanolic extract of *E. retusa* revealed significant levels of polyphenols, tannins, and flavonoids. The HPLC analysis has provided more precise information on the chemical nature of the bioactive compounds present in the methanolic extract of *E. retusa*. Among the polyphenols, gallic acid, epicatechin, coumaric acid, apigenin, and naringenin and among the flavonoids, rutin, quercetin, and kaempferol were identified. Several studies have indicated that these phytochemical compounds are responsible for the antioxidant and anti-inflammatory properties of multiple medicinal plants [29, 30].

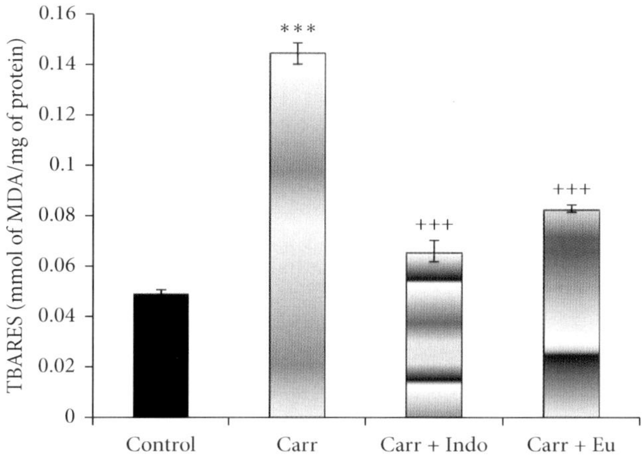

FIGURE 5: Effects of *Euphorbia retusa* and indomethacin on MDA concentrations in paw edema. The values are expressed as mean ± SEM ($n = 4$; $^{***}p < 0.001$ compared with the control group; $^{+++}p < 0.01$ compared with the carrageenan-treated group).

The antioxidant activity of the *E. retusa* methanol extract was evaluated *in vitro* by using the DPPH and FRAP tests. In methanol, DPPH occurs as a free radical of purple color that becomes weak after acquiring the proton of the antioxidant. Thus, measuring the reduction of the color intensity of the methanolic DPPH solution can be used to evaluate the ability of antioxidants to give the proton. The methanol extract exhibited good scavenging ability which may be due to donation of an electron or hydrogen to stabilize DPPH free radicals. In addition, in the present study, the *E. retusa* extract showed a powerful antioxidant activity on the FRAP assay which measures the ability to reduce the ferricyanide complex of Fe^{3+} to the ferrous (Fe^{2+}) form through donating a hydrogen atom. Antioxidant potential of a plant extract might be due to its richness in polyphenols and flavonoids. These bioactive compounds are known by their redox properties and chemical structure, which might play an important role in chelating transition metals and scavenging free radicals [31].

Thermal stimulation by the hot plate and chemical irritation by acetic acid are the two analgesic testing methods employed with the objective of identifying possible peripheral and central effects of the *E. retusa* methanol extract. The acetic acid writhing test was used to study the peripheral analgesic effect of a substance. The methanol extract of *E. retusa* significantly reduced the number of writhings caused by the injection of acetic acid. The injection of acetic acid induces a response characterized by the contraction of the abdominal muscles, an extension of the forearms, and lengthening of the body. These symptoms are believed to be related to the release of endogenous mediators of pain such as serotonin, histamine, bradykinin, and prostaglandins. These chemical mediators stimulate peripheral nociceptive neurons and induce dilatation of arterioles and venules with contraction and separation of endothelial cells, resulting in increased vascular permeability [32]. The writhing test is a typical model to study the inflammatory pain. However, this test is very sensitive because the abdominal writhing response can be suppressed by muscle relaxants and nonsteroidal anti-inflammatory drugs (NSAIDs), such as aspirin, diclofenac, and indomethacin, which could lead to misinterpretation of the results. Therefore, it was considered that the use of other additional pain models is necessary. The hot-plate test was used to evaluate the central analgesic activity by measuring the reaction time of the perception of pain. The heat stimulation sensitizes peripheral nerve endings, and the impulses generated propagate to the brain via the spinal cord. Hence, this test is primarily used to evaluate the ability of a substance to inhibit pain of central origin. In our study, we found that *E. retusa* possess antinociceptive activity against chemically and thermally induced nociception. The mechanism of analgesic activity of *E. retusa* could be due to their bioactive substances that raised the pain threshold by depressing pain receptors centrally in the brain [33]. This antinociceptive activity may be related to the reduction in the liberation of the inflammatory mediators or to the blockage of receptors resulting in the peripheral antinociceptive effect [34]. The richness of our extract in phenolic compounds, mainly gallic acid, and flavonoids can justify this activity. These compounds are known by their anti-inflammatory activity because of their influence on the metabolism of arachidonic acid and the release of histamine; they inhibit the production of prostaglandin and the expression of cyclooxygenase [35]. Flavonoids also act on the expression of adhesion molecules and proinflammatory cytokines by various mechanisms including inhibition of transcription of the nuclear factor by inhibiting kinases involved in signal transduction [36].

In the present study, the anti-inflammatory activity of the methanolic extract of *E. retusa* was evaluated using the carrageenan-induced paw edema model. The molecular and cellular mechanism of the Carr-induced inflammation is well characterized and is widely used to study the inflammatory process of the skin, as well as to identify anti-inflammatory agents that may be useful in the treatment of local exogenous inflammatory disorders [37]. Carrageenan can induce local inflammation biphasic. The early phase (1-2 h) is related to the excessive production of chemical mediators such as histamine, serotonin, and bradykinin, while the delayed phase (3-6h) is linked to the production of prostaglandins, leukotrienes, and free radicals that contribute to the increase of vascular permeability, which facilitates the infiltration of neutrophils and accumulation of plasma fluid into the interstitial space which leads to edema [38]. The degree of paw swelling is a good index in assessing the anti-inflammatory activity. Our results revealed that the methanolic extract of *E. retusa* significantly inhibited the edema formation in both the first and second phases and in a manner similar to the indomethacin. The anti-inflammatory activity of *E. retusa* in the first phase could be due to the possible suppression of histamine signaling by the mast cell stabilizing effect [39] and direct inhibition of histamine H1 receptor and histidine decarboxylase gene transcriptions [40]. The anti-inflammatory activity of *E. retusa* increases in the second phase and reaches its maximum at 6 hours. This could be explained by the possible inhibition of the release and/or synthesis of cyclooxygenase (COX-2) or lipoxygenase products by the *E. retusa* extract.

Table 5: Effect of carrageenan on antioxidant enzyme activities in liver and paw tissues of mice.

	Liver			Paw		
	SOD	CAT	GPx	SOD	CAT	GPx
Control	12.83 ± 2.67	1.94 ± 0.20	77.40 ± 4.63	20.08 ± 1.04	0.14 ± 0.01	70.32 ± 3.73
Carr	$6.48 \pm 0.28^{***}$	$0.53 \pm 0.18^{**}$	$22.54 \pm 4.92^{***}$	$8.66 \pm 0.93^{***}$	$0.04 \pm 0.01^{**}$	$12.23 \pm 3.32^{***}$
Carr + Indo	$12.19 \pm 0.35^{+++}$	$1.45 \pm 0.24^{+}$	$54.74 \pm 4.66^{+++}$	$17.90 \pm 1.23^{+++}$	$0.12 \pm 0.01^{+}$	$44.75 \pm 2.95^{+++}$
Carr + Eu	$10.60 \pm 0.52^{+++}$	$0.89 \pm 0.24^{+}$	$45.35 \pm 1.91^{+++}$	$16.79 \pm 1.06^{+++}$	$0.10 \pm 0.01^{+}$	$26.73 \pm 3.08^{+++}$

CAT: μmol of H_2O_2 destroyed/min/mg of protein; SOD: U/mg protein; GPx: μmol of NADPH oxidized/min/mg of protein. Values are expressed as mean ± SD of six mice in each group. Carr group versus control group: $^{**}p < 0.01$ and $^{***}p < 0.001$. Carr + Indo or Carr + Eu group versus Carr group: $^{+}p < 0.05$, $^{++}p < 0.01$, and $^{+++}p < 0.001$. Carr: carrageenan; Indo: Indomethacin; Eu: *Euphorbia retusa*.

Indeed, the cyclooxygenase is an important enzyme that allows conversion of arachidonic acid to prostaglandins, under stimulation by various proinflammatory cytokines including bacterial lipopolysaccharide (LPS), TNF-α, IL-1β, IL-6, and interferon-γ, in the second inflammatory phase of the carrageenan-induced edema model [2]. Indomethacin (standard drug) also exhibited strong anti-inflammatory potential after 3, 4, and 5 h of carrageenan injection to mice. Nonsteroidal anti-inflammatory drugs (NSAIDs), such as indomethacin, target the cyclooxygenase enzyme, thereby inhibiting the formation of the paw edema [41]. Furthermore, the higher anti-inflammatory activity of the *E. retusa* extract seems to be closely correlated with its richness in polyphenolic constituents. In fact, flavonoids such as rutin, quercetin, and kaempferol, identified by HPLC in the methanolic extract of *E. retusa*, have been known in several previous studies as potent inhibitors of proinflammatory cytokines and cyclooxygenase [42]. These bioactif compounds can inhibit lysosomal enzyme secretion and arachidonic acid release from membranes by inhibiting lipoxygenase, cyclooxygenase, and phospholipase A2. From the cyclooxygenase pathway, arachidonic acid inhibition by inflamed cells could reduce endoperoxides, prostaglandins, prostacyclin, and thromboxanes, while from the lipoxygenase pathway, it could reduce hydroperoxy and hydroxyeicosatetraenoic acids and leukotrienes [43]. Then, anti-inflammatory activities of polyphenols have been well documented. In addition, several researches have reported that some polyphenols inhibit arachidonic acid peroxidation and possess cyclooxygenase inhibitory or stimulatory effects [44, 45].

The inflammatory response is also associated with the neutrophil infiltration and production of the reactive free radical species derived from them. In fact, inflammation induces excessive production of reactive oxygen species (ROS) involved in the genesis of oxidative stress, which generates oxidative imbalance [46]. Against oxidative stress condition, defense systems produce antioxidant enzymes, such as SOD, CAT, and GPx [47]. In the present work, we found that the carrageenan injection generates a highly significant decrease in the activities of SOD, CAT, and GPx in the untreated group at the tissue compared with the control group ($p < 0.001$). We assume that this reduction in activities may be related to the high use of the produced antioxidant enzymes that act as scavengers of free radicals generated during the inflammatory process. Hence, the oral pretreatment with *E. retusa* significantly increases the activity of enzymatic antioxidants (SOD, CAT, and GPx) compared with the carrageenan group. The anti-inflammatory effect exhibited by this plant might be related to its antioxidant properties [48]. During inflammatory processes, the ROS have been proposed to mediate cell damage via a number of independent mechanisms including the inactivation of antioxidant enzymes. Lipid oxidation serves as a marker of cellular damage *in vivo*. MDA production is due to free radical attack on the plasma membrane. Thus, the inflammatory effect would result in the accumulation of MDA. Enhancing the levels of glutathione and SOD then reduces the MDA production [49]. Therefore, endogenous glutathione plays an important role against carrageenan-induced local inflammation [50, 51]. In the present study, SOD, CAT, and GPx activities increased in the paw and liver tissues following the pretreatment with *E. retusa* and were coupled to the significant decrease in MDA. The antioxidant effects of *E. retusa* observed in our study *in vitro* and *in vivo* may be related to their richness in polyphenolic compounds. Among these compounds, gallic acids and flavonoids are capable of inhibiting the oxidants released by leukocytes and other phagocytes by increasing enzymatic antioxidants in tissues [52, 53]. These natural compounds, endowed with interesting antioxidant activities, could prevent multiple kinds of inflammations strongly linked to an excess of free radicals.

5. Conclusion

In conclusion, this work reveals the antioxidant, antinociceptive, and anti-inflammatory effects *in vitro* and *in vivo* of *E. retusa*. These effects seem to be related to their richness in polyphenolic compounds which inhibit the production of several inflammatory mediators such as MDA and COX-2 in the edema paw and increase the activities of SOD, CAT, and GPx in the liver. Thus, these bioactive compounds show an antinociceptive activity in both peripheral and central levels. Therefore, with these pharmacological properties, *E. retusa* can be considered an effective agent for the treatment of pain and inflammation.

Acknowledgments

The authors greatly appreciate the technical support provided by the Unit of Common Services, Faculty of Sciences Gafsa, Tunisia.

References

[1] M. Harsh, *Inflammation and Healing, Textbook of Pathology*, Jaypee Brothers Medical Publishers Ltd., New Delhi, India, 5th edition, 2005.

[2] J. S. Deng, C. S. Chi, S. S. Huang, P. H. Shie, T. H. Lin, and G. J. Huang, "Antioxidant, analgesic, anti-inflammatory activities of the ethanolic extracts of *Taxillus liquidambaricola*," *Journal of Ethnopharmacology*, vol. 137, no. 3, pp. 1161–1171, 2011.

[3] S. L. Aitken, E. L. Karcher, and P. Rezamand, "Evaluation of antioxidant and proinflammatory gene expression in bovine mammary tissue during the periparturient period," *Journal of Dairy Science*, vol. 92, no. 2, pp. 589–598, 2009.

[4] F. Conforti, S. Sosa, M. Marrelli et al., "The protective ability of Mediterranean dietary plants against the oxidative damage: the role of radical oxygen species in inflammation and the polyphenol, flavonoid and sterol contents," *Food Chemistry*, vol. 112, no. 3, pp. 587–594, 2009.

[5] J. L. Wallace and L. Vong, "NSAID-induced gastrointestinal damage and the design of GI-sparing NSAIDs," *Current Opinion Investigational Drugs*, vol. 9, no. 11, pp. 1151–1156, 2008.

[6] N. Duarte, N. Gyemant, P. M. Abreu, J. Molnar, and M. J. U. Ferreira, "New macrocylic lathyrane diterpenes, from *Euphorbia lagascae*, as inhibitors of multidrug resistance of tumor cells," *Planta Medica*, vol. 72, no. 2, pp. 162–168, 2006.

[7] S. Murugan, R. Anand, P. Uma-Devi, N. Vidhya, and K. A. Rajesh, "Efficacy of *Euphorbia milli* and *Euphorbia pulcherrima* on aflatoxin producing fungi (*Aspergillus flavus* and *Aspergillus parasiticus*)," *African Journal of Biotechnology*, vol. 6, pp. 718-719, 2007.

[8] M. Hezareh, "Prostratin as a new therapeutic agent targeting HIV viral reservoirs," *Drug News and Perspectives*, vol. 18, no. 8, pp. 496–450, 2005.

[9] T. Shamim, M. Ahmad, and M. Mukhtar, "Antihyperglycemic effects of methanolic extract of *Euphorbia* prostrate on alloxan induced diabetic rabbits," *European Scientific Journal*, vol. 10, no. 10, 2014.

[10] L. A. G. Refahy, "Study on flavonoids and triterpenoids content of some Euphorbiaceae plants," *Journal of Life Sciences*, vol. 5, pp. 100–107, 2011.

[11] J. Bellakhdar, *La Pharmacope´e Marocaine Traditionnelle*, Ibis Press, Paris, France, 1997.

[12] N. A. M. Salah, "Flavonol glycosides of *Euphorbia retusa* and *E. sanctae-catharinae*," *Phytochemistry*, vol. 24, no. 2, pp. 371-372, 1985.

[13] H. Haba, C. Lavaud, A. M. Abdulmagid, and M. Benkhaled, "Diterpenoids and triterpenoids from *Euphorbia retusa*," *Journal of Naturals Products*, vol. 72, no. 7, pp. 1258–1264, 2009.

[14] M. E. Abdallah, "Antimicrobial properties and phytochemical constituents of the methanol extracts of *Euphorbia retusa* Forssk. and *Euphorbia terracina* L. from Saudi Arabia," *South Asian Journal of Experimental Biology*, vol. 4, pp. 48–53, 2014.

[15] V. L. Singleton and J. A. Rossi, "Colorimetry of total phenolics with phosphomolybdic-phosphotungstic acid reagents," *American Journal of Enology and Viticulture*, vol. 16, pp. 144–153, 1965.

[16] A. Djeridane, M. Yousfi, B. Nadjemi, D. Boutassouna, P. Stocker, and N. Vidal, "Antioxidant activity of some Algerian medicinal plants extracts containing phenolic compounds," *Food Chemistry*, vol. 97, no. 4, pp. 654–660, 2006.

[17] R. B. Broadhurst and W. T. Jones, "Analysis of condensed tannins using acidified vanillin," *Journal of Science of Food and Agriculture*, vol. 29, no. 9, pp. 788–794, 1978.

[18] D. Heimler, P. Vignolini, M. G. Dini, F. Vincieri, and A. Rmani, "Antiradical activity and polyphenol composition of local Brassicaceae edible varieties," *Food Chemistry*, vol. 99, no. 3, pp. 464–469, 2006.

[19] J. Yang, J. Guo, and J. Yuan, "In vitro antioxidant properties of rutin," *LWT-Food Science of Technology*, vol. 41, no. 6, pp. 1060–1066, 2008.

[20] M. Oyaizu, "Studies on products of browning reactions: antioxidative activities of products of browning reaction prepared from glucosamine," *Japanese Journal of Nutrition*, vol. 44, no. 6, pp. 307–315, 1986.

[21] R. A. Turner, "Analgesics," in *Screening Methods in Pharmacology*, R.A. Turner and P. Hebban, Eds., p. 100, Academic Press, New York, NY, USA, 1965.

[22] W. R. Sawadogo, R. Boly, and M. Lompo, "Anti-inflammatory, analgesic and antipyretic activities of *Dicliptera verticillata*," *International Journal of Pharmacology*, vol. 2, no. 4, pp. 435–438, 2006.

[23] C. A. Winter, E. A. Risley, and G. W. Nuss, "Carrageenan-induced edema in hind paw of the rat as an assay for anti-iflammatory drugs," *Proceeding of the Society for Experimental Biology and Medicine*, vol. 111, no. 3, pp. 544–547, 1962.

[24] H. H. Draper and M. Hadley, "Malondialdehyde determination as index of lipid peroxidation," *Methods in Enzymology*, vol. 186, pp. 421–431, 1990.

[25] Y. Sun, L. W. Oberley, and Y. Li, "A simple method for clinical assay of superoxide dismutase," *Clinical Chemistry*, vol. 34, no. 3, pp. 497–500, 1988.

[26] H. Aebi, "Catalase *in vitro*," *Methods in Enzymology*, vol. 105, pp. 121–126, 1984.

[27] L. Flohe and W. A. Gunzler, "Assays of glutathione peroxidase," *Methods in Enzymology*, vol. 105, pp. 114–121, 1984.

[28] M. M. Bradford, "A rapid and sensitive method for the quantitation of microgram quantities of protein utilizing the principle of protein-dye binding," *Analytical of Biochemistry*, vol. 72, no. 1-2, pp. 248–254, 1976.

[29] O. A. Fawole, A. R. Ndhlala, S. O. Amoo, J. F. Finnie, and J. Van Staden, "Antiinflammatory and phytochemical properties of twelve medicinal plants used for treating gastro-intestinal ailments in South Africa," *Journal of Ethnopharmacology*, vol. 123, no. 2, pp. 237–243, 2009.

[30] G. Costa, V. Francisco, M. C. Lopes, M. T. Cruz, and M. T. Batista, "Intracellular signaling pathways modulated by phenolic compounds: application for new anti-inflammatory drugs discovery," *Current Medicinal Chemistry*, vol. 19, no. 18, pp. 2876–2900, 2012.

[31] A. A. Mohamed, A. A. Khalil, and H. E. S. El-Beltagi, "Antioxidant and antimicrobial properties of kaff maryam (*Anastatica hierochuntica*) and doum palm (*Hyphaene thebaica*)," *Grasas Aceites*, vol. 61, no. 1, pp. 67–75, 2010.

[32] C. O. Okoli, P. A. Akah, S. V. Nwafor, A. I. Anisiobi, I. N. Ibegbunam, and O. Erojikwe, "Antiinflammatory activity of hexane leaf extract of *Aspilia africana* C.D. Adams," *Journal of Ethnopharmacology*, vol. 109, no. 2, pp. 219–225, 2007.

[33] S. P. Gawade, "Acetic acid induced painful endogenous infliction in writhing test on mice," *Journal of Pharmacology and Pharmacotherapeutics*, vol. 3, no. 4, p. 348, 2012.
[34] N. M. Gomes, C. M. Rezende, S. P. Fontes, M. E. Matheus, M. A. C. Pinto, and P. D. Fernandes, "Characterization of the antinociceptive and anti-inflammatory activities of fractions obtained from *Copaifera multijuga* Hayne," *Journal of Ethnopharmacology*, vol. 128, no. 1, pp. 177–183, 2010.
[35] K. Madden, L. Flowers, R. Salani et al., "Proteomics-based approach to elucidate the mechanism of antitumor effect of curcumin in cervical cancer," *Prostaglandins, Leukotrienes and Essential Fatty Acids*, vol. 80, no. 1, pp. 9–18, 2009.
[36] J. Gonzalez-Gallego, S. Sanchez-Campos, and M. J. Tunon, "Anti-inflammatory properties of dietary flavonoids," *Nutrición hospitalaria*, vol. 22, no. 3, pp. 287–293, 2007.
[37] P. P. Kumar and G. Kuttan, "*Vernonia cinerea* L. scavenges free radicals and regulates nitric oxide and proinflammatory cytokines profile in carrageenan induced paw edema model," *Immunopharmacology and Immunotoxicology*, vol. 31, no. 1, pp. 94–102, 2009.
[38] E. Hvattum and D. Ekeberg, "Study of the collision induced radical cleavage of flavonoid glycosides using negative electrospray ionization tandem quadrupole mass spectrometry," *Journal of Mass Spectrometry*, vol. 38, no. 1, pp. 43–49, 2003.
[39] S. Shashidhara, A. V. Bhandarkar, and M. Deepak, "Comparative evaluation of successive extracts of leaf and stem bark of *Albizia lebbeck* for mast cell stabilization activity," *Fitoterapia*, vol. 79, no. 4, pp. 301-302, 2008.
[40] I. M. Nurul, H. Mizuguchi, M. Shahriar et al., "*Albizia lebbeck* suppresses histamine signalling by the inhibition of hisamine H1 receptor and histidine decarboxylase gene transcriptions," *International Immunopharmacolgy*, vol. 11, no. 11, pp. 1766–1772, 2011.
[41] S. Khan, M. H. Mehmood, A. N. Akbar Ali, F. S. Ahmed, A. Dar, and A.-H. Gilani, "Studies on anti-inflammatory and analgesic activities of betel nut in rodents," *Journal of Ethnopharmacolgy*, vol. 135, no. 3, pp. 654–661, 2011.
[42] M. Sermaani, "Evaluation of phytochemical and antibacterial activity of *Pedalium murex* Linn," *Root International Research Journal of Pharmacy*, vol. 2, pp. 131–134, 2011.
[43] A. Tjølsen and K. Hole, "Animal models of analgesia," in *The Pharmacology of Pain*, A. Dickenson and J. Besson, Eds., vol. 130, pp. 1–20, Springer, Berlin, Germany, 1997.
[44] V. Viji and A. Helen, "Inhibition of lipoxygenases and cyclooxygenase-2 enzymes by extracts isolated from *Bacopa monnieri* (L.) Wettst.," *Journal of Ethnopharmacology*, vol. 118, no. 2, pp. 305–311, 2008.
[45] W. Jing, C. Xinyi, H. Li, L. Li, L. Hongfei, and L. Wei, "Effects of tea polyphenols on the expression of NF-kB, COX-2 and surviving in Lewis lung carcinoma xenografts in C57Bl/6 mice," *Chinese Journal of Lung Cancer*, vol. 15, pp. 271–276, 2012.
[46] S. Vircheva, G. Nenkova, and A. Georgieva, "Effects of desipramine on the antioxidant status in rat tissues at carrageenan-induced paw inflammation," *Cell Biochemistry and Function*, vol. 30, no. 1, pp. 18–23, 2012.
[47] L. Petrov, E. Tzvetanova, and A. Pavlova, "In-vivo effects of nociceptin and its structural analogue [Orn9] nociceptin on the antioxidant status of rat blood and liver after carrageenan-induced paw inflammation," *Central European Journal of Medicine*, vol. 5, no. 1, pp. 123–131, 2010.
[48] L. Bignotto, J. Rocha, B. Sepodes et al., "Anti-inflammatory effect of lycopene on carrageenan-induced paw oedema and hepatic ischaemia-reperfusion in the rat," *British Journal of Nutrition*, vol. 102, no. 1, pp. 126–133, 2009.
[49] P. C. Hsieh, Y. L. Ho, G. J. Huang et al., "Hepatoprotective effect of the aqueous extract of *Flemingia macrophylla* on carbon tetrachloride-induced acute hepatotoxicity in rats through anti-oxidative activities," *American Journal of Chinese Medicine*, vol. 39, no. 2, pp. 349–365, 2011.
[50] S. Cuzzocrea, G. Costantino, B. Zingarelli, E. Mazzon, A. Micali, and A. P. Caputi, "The protective role of endogenous glutathione in carrageenan induced pleurisy in the rat," *European Journal of Pharmacology*, vol. 372, no. 2, pp. 187–197, 1999.
[51] Z. R. Lai, W. H. Peng, Y. L. Ho et al., "Analgesic and anti-inflammatory activities of the methanol extract of *Kalanchoe gracilis* (L.) DC stem in mice," *American Journal of Chinese Medicine*, vol. 38, no. 3, pp. 529–546, 2010.
[52] M. H. Huang, S. S. Huang, B. S. Wang et al., "Antioxidant and anti-inflammatory properties of *Cardiospermum halicacabum* and its reference compounds ex vivo and in vivo," *Journal of Ethnopharmacology*, vol. 133, no. 2, pp. 743–750, 2011a.
[53] S. S. Huang, C. S. Chiu, H. J. Chen et al., "Antinociceptive activities and the mechanisms of anti-inflammation of asiatic acid in mice," *Evidence Based Complementary and Alternative Medicine*, vol. 2011, Article ID 895857, 10 pages, 2011.

5

Psychological Factors Associated with Phantom Limb Pain

Xaver Fuchs,[1,2] **Herta Flor**,[2,3] **and Robin Bekrater-Bodmann**[2]

[1] *Biopsychology and Cognitive Neuroscience, Faculty of Psychology and Sports Science, Bielefeld University, Bielefeld, Germany*
[2] *Department of Cognitive and Clinical Neuroscience, Central Institute of Mental Health, Medical Faculty Mannheim, Heidelberg University, Mannheim, Germany*
[3] *Center for Neuroplasticity and Pain (CNAP), SMI®, Department of Health Science and Technology, Aalborg University, Aalborg, Denmark*

Correspondence should be addressed to Xaver Fuchs; xaver.fuchs@uni-bielefeld.de

Academic Editor: Edita Navratilova

Phantom limb pain (PLP) is a common phenomenon occurring after the amputation of a limb and can be accompanied by serious suffering. Psychological factors have been shown to play an important role in other types of chronic pain, where they are pivotal in the acquisition and maintenance of pain symptoms. For PLP, however, the interaction between pain and psychological variables is less well documented. In this review, we summarize research on the role of emotional, motivational, cognitive, and perceptual factors in PLP. The reported findings indicate that emotional factors modulate PLP but might be less important compared to other types of chronic pain. Additional factors such as the amount of disability and adjustment to the amputation appear to also play a role. Bidirectional relationships between stress and PLP have been shown quite consistently, and the potential of stress and tension reduction in PLP treatment could be further exploited. Little is known about the role of cognitive variables such as attention or expectation. Catastrophizing seems to aggravate PLP and could be targeted in treatment. Body perception is altered in PLP and poses a potential target for novel mechanistic treatments. More research on psychological factors and their interactions in PLP is needed.

1. Introduction

The amputation of a limb represents a serious disruption of body integrity and is associated with a number of negative consequences, particularly disability and postamputation pain. Although severe chronic residual limb pain is rare (occurring in less than 10% of the amputees), the majority of amputees (above two-thirds) report at least mild residual limb pain [1]. As a consequence of changes in the posture and strain of the remaining body parts, secondary pain is reported by a high proportion of the amputees, with high rates (more than 20% each) of pain in the remaining limbs, the shoulders, and the neck or the upper back [2, 3]. Almost all amputees also report about ongoing awareness of a phantom limb, with 60–80% complaining about phantom limb pain (PLP), that is, a painful sensation perceived in the amputated limb and thus located outside the physical borders of the body [4–6]. PLP usually begins early after an amputation (e.g., [7]), and in most amputees, PLP becomes chronic with a large variability in intensity, frequency, and quality [6, 8]. PLP leads to personal suffering [9], reduced quality of life [10], and impairs sleep [6]. PLP is still a challenge for pain research and treatment.

Neuroplastic changes occurring in the brain after an amputation have been a major focus in PLP research for the last two decades (for reviews, see [11, 12]). In contrast, less research has focused on psychological factors, and although they play an important role in other types of chronic pain, for example, chronic musculoskeletal pain (e.g., [13–15]), their role in PLP remains less well studied and less well understood (e.g., [16]). Furthermore, review articles directly addressing psychological factors in PLP are rare. Sherman et al. [17] and Hill [18] reviewed and critically discussed evidence from earlier studies and showed that PLP cannot be related to unresolved grief due to limb loss, denial, psychosomatic manifestations, pathological misinterpretation of somatic sensations, or personality disorders (e.g., [19–21]). The proposed relationship between personality factors and PLP could not be substantiated ([17]; for a discussion, see [18]).

Since the reviews cited above [17, 18] have been published two and three decades ago, respectively, the present work focuses and summarizes the research on the role of psychological variables from the late 90s to the present. We further focus on emotional factors, motivational aspects such as stress and stress coping, cognitive factors, and the role of body perception in the development and maintenance of chronic PLP and its potential for treatment approaches.

2. Emotional Factors

Much research on emotional processing in chronic pain has focused on comorbid anxiety and depression, which have a high prevalence in chronic pain (cf. [22–24]). For example, a health survey in a representative German sample [25] found an interview-based [26] prevalence of 8.1% for chronic pain disorder. Compared to the healthy population, the 12-month prevalence for anxiety disorders was significantly elevated in both male (33% versus 7%, odds ratio = 5.65) and female (37% versus 20%, odds ratio = 2.69) chronic pain patients. Mood disorders were also significantly more prevalent in chronic pain patients compared to pain-free participants (men: 30% versus 7%, odds ratio = 5.48; women: 30% versus 15%, odds ratio = 2.69). In line with the role of anxiety and mood disturbances (especially depression) in chronic pain, similar relationships can also be expected for chronic PLP. In the following sections, we will summarize findings on the role of depression and anxiety in PLP and will show that it is important to take specific characteristics of the sample into account, especially whether the sample consisted of amputees in early or later stages after amputation and whether concomitant pain was present.

2.1. Depression and Anxiety in Early-Stage Amputees. Especially in early stages after amputation, comorbidity rates of mental disorders in amputees can be related to factors other than PLP. Factors like chronic diseases leading to the amputation, traumatization, secondary pain, disability caused by the amputation, and adaptation to the new situation can give rise to anxiety and depression independently of PLP. The modulation of pain by emotional factors may therefore be different in early and late stage amputees. For example, Shukla et al. [27] reported high rates of depression (about 50%) and anxiety (above 35%) in amputees in the postoperative phase, regardless of PLP. In contrast, in samples that were more heterogeneous in age, time since amputation, or the cause of amputation, prevalence rates for depression and anxiety were lower than the rates reported by Shukla et al. [27] for recently amputated participants. For example, a prevalence of 19% was reported for depressive symptoms [28] and of 24% for both depression and anxiety symptoms [29]. In these studies, the association of depression and anxiety with PLP (which is most prevalent shortly after amputation [1]) has not been specifically investigated. Consequently, recent amputations should be seen as a special case, and in fact, there is evidence that depression in the postamputation phase is more strongly related to concerns about disability than PLP [28, 30, 31]. However, a different relationship has been observed for preamputation anxiety. Raichle et al. [32] investigated the relationship between overall anxiety levels prior to lower limb amputation and PLP and found that they were positively related particularly with PLP intensity (up to five days after amputation), even when postoperative analgesic medication was controlled for. The analysis of the interplay between emotional states and PLP can be better determined in later stages, when disability and adaptation to the new situation are no longer dominating topics. However, even in later stages, PLP is frequently related to disability and it is important to consider both disability- and pain-related issues.

2.2. Depression in Later Stages after Amputation. As already stated, symptoms of depression are common in the acute phase after an amputation. However, several studies showed that the rates of depressive symptoms decline during the following years. Horgan and MacLachlan [33] published a review on psychosocial adjustments following lower limb amputations and concluded that depression in the first years after amputation is most strongly associated with disability and that, by two years after amputation, depression rates have dropped to a level comparable to those of healthy people. However, even at later stages, it is important to distinguish between disability, somatic symptoms, pain, and depression. Whyte and Niven [31] used the Beck Depression Inventory (BDI [34]) to assess depressive symptoms in a sample of amputees with PLP in the chronic stage. They observed a significant positive correlation of PLP and BDI scores; however, they found that this correlation was mainly driven by PLP being correlated with items of the BDI that assess performance or somatic symptoms that are often seen in chronic pain. The problem that the BDI (and possibly other depression scales as well) tends to overestimate depression in samples with physical diseases and chronic pain has been pointed out before [35]. This highlights that the diagnostic instrument needs to be taken into account in the interpretation of studies on amputees and that psychopathology might be overestimated due to somatic symptoms associated with amputations. Desmond and MacLachlan [36] used the Hospital Anxiety and Depression Scale (HADS [37]) to screen for anxiety and depression and the Impact of Event Scale [38] to assess the severity of posttraumatic stress. They tested a sample comprising exclusively older male amputees (N = 582) with long-standing traumatic amputation (at least 10 years). Importantly, the HADS specifically excludes items concerning intrusions or physical symptoms of depression to avoid confounding when assessing groups with somatic disorders. In this homogeneous sample, the authors found elevated scores for depression, anxiety, and posttraumatic stress. In the amputee sample, values potentially indicating clinically relevant depression were observed three times more often than expected for the normal population. This study also found differential associations between psychological distress and postamputation pain: amputees showed higher values in depressive symptoms, avoidance, and intrusions if they suffered from either residual limb pain or residual limb pain *and* PLP but not if they suffered from PLP alone, indicating that chronic PLP might be different from other postamputation pain in terms of psychological distress. However, it is not entirely clear which factors caused the differences between the subgroups. The authors assumed that residual limb pain more strongly conflicts with prosthesis use so that their results might have been associated with activity restriction-induced negative affect [39]. Desmond and MacLachlan's [36] results suggest that PLP and depression are—if at all—only weakly associated if residual limb pain is accounted for. However, their sample consisted of former military service members who were mostly male, at younger age when serving, and suffered from traumatic limb loss in the line of duty with no preceding pain or diseases, and thus, these findings should not be generalized to other populations. Another study [40] reported the results of a survey that used a stratified sample of 914 amputees, which might provide more general norms. To assess depressive symptoms, the authors used the Center for Epidemiological Studies Depression Scale [41], which is also better suited for assessing depression in populations with chronic health problems. Pain bothersomeness was assessed individually for PLP, residual limb pain, and back pain. There was a significant correlation between pain bothersomeness and depressive symptoms within each of the groups. Depressive symptoms were almost three times more likely to be present in subjects who were extremely bothered by PLP than in subjects reporting not to be bothered. However, this association was even stronger in residual limb pain and back pain. Another study [42] compared depression and anxiety between PLP patients and other patients suffering from nonphantom neuropathic pain caused by trauma or surgery. Like another study mentioned above [36], this study used the HADS. This study found that amputees with PLP showed fewer symptoms of both depression and anxiety compared to patients with other types of neuropathic pain; however, residual limb pain was not accounted for. Fuchs et al. [43] reported on affective distress and pain-related interference as assessed by the West Haven-Yale Multidimensional Pain Inventory [44], a questionnaire assessing different dimensions of pain-related burden, in large samples of patients with chronic back pain and musculoskeletal pain compared to three amputee groups with (a) none but PLP, (b) non but residual limb pain, and (c) both PLP and residual limb pain. In line with the results from other studies [36, 40, 42], persons with either PLP or residual limb pain showed less affective distress and pain interference compared to chronic back pain or musculoskeletal pain patients. Concurrent PLP and residual limb pain was associated with higher burden compared to the groups that reported only one type of postamputation pain. However, even the amputees suffering from both pain types always showed less-intense burden than patients with chronic back pain or musculoskeletal pain. In a longitudinal study, Castillo et al. [45] assessed depression and pain in subjects with lower limb trauma at 3, 6, 12, and 24 months after injury. Pain predicted depression, but depression did not predict pain. It is important to note, however, that not all subjects in this study were amputees and that the study also did not make a distinction between PLP and other types of limb trauma-associated pain.

Taken together, these studies suggest that the association between pain and depression might be weaker in PLP than in other chronic pain conditions, including residual limb pain. In addition to a differentiation between specific pain types in amputees, it is important to consider the diagnostic tools and the composition of study samples.

2.3. Anxiety in Later Stages after Amputation. Anxiety is assumed to be both an etiological and a maintaining factor of chronic pain, especially as it is associated with avoidance of activity and perceived disability [46]. Similar to depression, anxiety symptoms are common in an early stage after amputation [27, 29], and anxiety levels decline in the first years after amputation [29, 33]. However, anxiety does not appear to be exclusively related to PLP shortly after amputation. Horgan and MacLachlan [33] stated that anxiety in acute amputees mainly relates to changes in body image, altered social role and social discomfort, and adaptation to a new identity. The preoccupation of amputees with topics relating to identity and social functioning (rather than pain) was also found in a qualitative study that explored amputees' experiences using a semistandardized interview [47]. Similar to what has been observed for depression, Whyte and Niven [31] also found that, in an early phase after amputation, anxiety was mainly correlated with somatic symptoms (e.g., insomnia) but not necessarily with pain.

There are only few studies on the association of anxiety and PLP after the immediate consequences of an amputation have subsided. The study by Desmond and MacLachlan [36] showed that compared to pain-free amputees, anxiety levels were higher in long-term amputees with chronic PLP or residual limb pain. However, those levels were still within the range of the healthy population. In their longitudinal study, Castillo et al. [45] showed that, in a late, chronic phase of pain following lower-extremity trauma, subsequent pain was predicted by anxiety but not by depression. However, as mentioned above, this study included amputees and nonamputees and did not differentiate between PLP and other types of pain.

3. The Role of Stress and Tension in PLP

Stress is thought to play a key role in the development and maintenance of chronic pain. As outlined in the diathesis-stress model of chronic pain [46, 48], various dysfunctional affective, cognitive, and behavioral responses mediate the relationship between stressors and pain symptoms in chronic pain patients. It has been proposed that similar to other types of chronic pain, stress can trigger pain episodes in PLP [24, 49]. Although some studies can be found, which will be discussed in the following paragraphs, there is generally less research on the role of stress in PLP compared to more common types of chronic pain (e.g., chronic back pain or headache [24]).

Sherman and colleagues conducted several studies on this topic and proposed that there are complex interactions between the central nervous system, sympathetic arousal, and characteristics of the residual limb [50]. For example, Sherman and Bruno [51] showed that the temperature of the residual limb compared to the intact limb is decreased in amputees with PLP, which has been related to decreased near-surface blood flow. The authors further showed a significant relationship between the extent of temperature differences and PLP quality such as burning, tingling, and throbbing. Discharges of peripheral input can be mediated by autonomic nervous system activity which could explain why situational (external) stressors and internal states (e.g., tension and anxiety) interact and trigger PLP episodes. In fact, Sherman et al. [52] demonstrated that there is a close temporal relationship between PLP and involuntary contractions of residual limb muscles: muscle activity bursts, which were recorded using surface electromyographic signals, preceded the experience of PLP. Involuntary contractions of residual limb muscles have been directly related to anxiety, tension, and stress [53]. This relationship is also supported by studies using relaxation-focused interventions to reduce PLP: In a review, Sherman [54] suggested that most treatments for PLP show success rates of 30% or below that might be merely due to placebo effects; only treatments reducing tension showed better effects and can be considered as successful treatments. Preliminary beneficial effects have also been shown for biofeedback. In a case study, total and enduring relief of PLP and an increasing temperature of the residual limb were observed following a residual limb EMG and temperature biofeedback training [55]. In another study, improvements in pain of at least 30% were observed in 6 out of 7 patients after six sessions of residual limb temperature biofeedback training [56]. However, this study lacked a control group, and better controlled studies on biofeedback in PLP are needed to evaluate its effectiveness.

Angrilli and Köster [57] experimentally investigated the effect of stress induction on amputees with and without PLP. Stress was induced in the amputees by means of three different induction methods: (a) having them deliver a free speech about memories of the amputation, (b) applying a cold pressor pain test, and (c) performing a mental arithmetic task. As measures of sympathetic stress responses, the authors recorded the heart rate and blood pressure levels. Amputees with PLP showed stronger psychophysiological stress reactions compared to amputees without PLP only in the free-speech task. This study thus suggests that amputees with PLP show enhanced stress responses, at least when the stressors are autobiographic and specific (e.g., reminders of their pain or amputation), similar to findings in chronic musculoskeletal pain patients [58]. Moreover, the results support the hypothesis that distressing pain memories (see below) play a role in PLP [59–61]. Heightened stress reactivity in amputees with PLP has also been demonstrated on a cortical level. Using electroencephalography, Larbig et al. [62] showed that PLP patients display increased cortical activity when presented with verbal pain-associated material.

The studies described above support the notion that PLP relates to both peripheral and central arousal and that PLP episodes might be influenced by emotional distress. Katz [63] proposed a model explaining the close connection between cognitive and affective processes and PLP. In amputees, the threshold for somatic sensations in the phantom limb might be lowered due to the loss of inhibitory control. The underlying mechanisms are proposed to be identical to those when healthy participants experience somatic sensations while affectively aroused. The reduced threshold for sympathetic activation might allow even events of much lower salience to trigger somatic sensations in the phantom limb, which further indicates that brain regions involved in cognitive and affective processes might contribute to a sympathetic-efferent/somatic-afferent cycle of activity. Interestingly, sympathetic arousal might also play a role in other chronic pain conditions and might further be related to maladaptive plasticity in the brain. For example, in patients suffering from complex regional pain syndrome (CRPS), sympathetic blocks have been shown to restore the organization in the primary somatosensory cortex [64]. CRPS is a condition characterized by ongoing pain perceived in upper or lower extremities, which shares similarities with PLP, as in terms of neuroplastic changes in the sensorimotor cortex [65, 66]. However, up to now, the contribution of sympathetic arousal to PLP remains largely unexplored.

How do these laboratory findings on the interaction between stress, peripheral or central arousal, and PLP relate to more naturalistic contexts and to daily life stressors? Giummarra et al. [67] developed a structured questionnaire on specific triggers of PLP episodes and investigated their frequency of occurrence in a sample of 264 amputees. Although behavioral triggers (e.g., trying to use the phantom) and stimulation of the residual limb (e.g., movement, touch, or pressure) were the most common trigger categories (50% and 37%, resp.), emotional triggers such as emotional distress, exhaustion, or thinking of the missing limb were still reported by 23% of the amputees. Moreover, 20% reported influences of the weather and another 11% reported about referred sensations originating from the intact limb. These results support the notion that PLP episodes often follow emotional distress and that residual limb activity interacts with PLP experience [52, 57]. However, these data are based on cross-sectional and subjective reports and may therefore be prone to memory biases or express implicit theories rather than actual events. Instead of using cross-sectional questionnaire data, Arena et al. [68] conducted a longitudinal study employing pain and stress diaries. Twenty-seven male amputees with PLP completed the diaries four times a day for six months. The authors performed a cross-lagged correlation analysis to detect relationships between stress and PLP over time. A significant relationship between stress and PLP was found in 74% of the amputees. The authors observed that, (a) in 63% of the sample, stress and pain covaried simultaneously, (b) in 44%, a change in pain preceded a change in stress, and (c) in

37%, a change in stress preceded a change in pain. This study thus supports the interpretation that even on the level of daily life stressors, there is a bidirectional relationship between PLP and stress. Taken together, findings from the laboratory and naturalistic observations are well in line with each other and support the role of stress in PLP.

Another reference to altered stress processing in PLP comes from studies investigating the importance of traumatization due to limb loss and initiated the developments of novel treatments of PLP [69]. Preliminary data indicate that a trauma-focused psychological treatment, aiming at traumatic amputation-related memories, successfully reduced PLP [70], probably due to the improvement of regulation of sympathetic arousal [71]. Consequently, an eye movement desensitization and reprocessing treatment, which has been applied in the treatment of posttraumatic stress disorder, showed promising effects in reducing PLP-associated suffering [72], although the specificity of this intervention needs to be clarified.

4. Cognitive Factors

Pain experience can be modulated by cognitive factors such as attention, memory, expectations, beliefs, appraisals, and (cognitive) coping strategies [24, 73, 74]. For many of these factors, little is known about how they specifically modulate PLP [18]. Although we do not know how attentional processes modulate PLP, some indirect indications exist. For example, hypnosis alters attentional processes and can be efficient in modulating both acute and chronic pain (for reviews, see [75, 76]). A reduction of PLP by hypnotherapy has been shown in a case study [77], although more studies are needed. Placebo effects, which are partly based on expectation [78], can also be used to alleviate neuropathic pain [79] and might potentially be effective in PLP although this has not been tested. Finally, the literature shows detrimental effects of catastrophizing on PLP, which are probably also mediated via attentional and expectation processes [80]. In the following sections, we will review relevant findings on memory, coping styles, and catastrophizing and their importance for PLP.

4.1. Memory for Pain. Several theories of chronic pain suggest that both declarative and nondeclarative memory processes contribute to the development and maintenance of chronic pain via neuroplastic changes in the nervous system [81–83]. One example for this process is central sensitization, referring to a hyperexcitability of the central nervous system and associated lowered pain thresholds [84]. In different groups with chronic pain, structural and functional reorganization within pain-processing brain areas has been shown, which might represent a neural correlate of pain memory [81, 85, 86].

For amputees in particular, memory processes have been discussed for both nonpainful phantom sensations and PLP. Katz and Melzack [61] and Katz [87] proposed a crucial role of *somatosensory memories* for both PLP and nonpainful phantom phenomena (e.g., phantom limb awareness or phantom sensations). Anderson-Barnes et al. [88] suggested that phantom sensations could be explained by *proprioceptive memories* and that they might become associated with pain perceived before the amputation by means of learning mechanisms. Due to tumor, vascular disease, or injury, an amputation is often preceded by pain in the affected limb. Katz and Melzack [61] suggested that pain prior to the amputation is encoded and can later be triggered, for example, by peripheral input stemming from the residual limb. This triggered preamputation pain is then experienced as PLP. Maladaptive plasticity that is positively correlated with PLP [65] can be seen as neural underpinning of pain memory in amputees. These processes might be more severe if chronic pain has already been present prior to amputation [81, 85, 86], potentially influencing the formation of a pain memory. The theory of a relationship between preamputation pain (that leaves behind a memory trace) and PLP is supported by retrospective reports that have shown similarities between memories referring to somatosensory perceptions in the affected limb in the phase before amputation and later phantom sensations [60, 61]. For example, in the study by Katz and Melzack [61], almost 60% of the amputees who reported having had pain before the amputation also reported that similar pain qualities continued or recurred later on in the phantom limb. However, reports about preamputation pain that were gathered retrospectively might be prone to memory bias. Prospective studies, on the contrary, give more valid information on the relationship between preamputation pain and PLP and showed that PLP during the first six months, but not long-term PLP, was predicted by pain before amputation [89, 90].

Finally, in line with the observation that chronic pain patients often complain about forgetfulness, impairments of both working memory and long-term memory have been discussed for chronic pain (for reviews, see [91–93]). Although empirical studies have used various methods and have found heterogeneous results when testing memory performance, reviews and meta-analyses indicate that chronic pain patients show poorer performance on memory tests [91–93]. In a recent review, Mazza et al. [91] have argued that poor performance in working and long-term memory tests of chronic pain patients might be related to impaired encoding and/or retrieval processes. In addition, this study also indicated a memory bias towards selectively remembering pain-related events. Whether processes of working memory or long-term memory are also associated with PLP has not yet been systematically studied.

4.2. Coping Strategies. The general term *pain coping* describes functional or dysfunctional styles to deal with pain after it has been attended to and interpreted (appraised) as being a threat [94, 95]. Pain coping can be divided into cognitive and behavioral strategies and also includes catastrophizing, which will be discussed in detail in the following section. Cognitive coping strategies comprise, for example, distraction from a sensation or reinterpretation of pain [96]. Examples for behavioral coping strategies are increasing or decreasing social or physical activity or seeking social or medical support [94, 96]. Hill [96] systematically described coping styles in amputees with PLP by having sixty male PLP patients complete the Coping Strategies Questionnaire [95]. Using principal component analysis, she found that the factor structure in PLP patients resembled the one originally discovered by Rosenstiel and Keefe [95] in a sample of chronic back pain patients. In the study by Hill [96], three main components were found—cognitive coping, helplessness, and pain denial—which explained about 20% of the variance in both PLP and psychological distress. In addition, most of the variance in these variables was accounted for by catastrophizing, representing a core facet of the helplessness factor. The author concluded that the repertoire of PLP sufferers contains only a limited amount of coping strategies that actually help to alleviate distress and pain and that successful coping rather means *not* to catastrophize. In a later study by Hill et al. [97], catastrophizing explained 26% of the variance in PLP, whereas other strategies only explained 3%. Interestingly, although male and female amputees do not differ in respect of PLP prevalence when the cause of amputation is controlled for, females report greater levels of pain interference [98]. This sex effect might contribute to differences in reported strategies to cope with PLP, with women showing significantly higher degrees of catastrophizing than males [98].

The conclusion that PLP patients use rather few coping strategies was confirmed by another study applying a different methodological approach. Whyte and Niven [99] had 89 amputees collect diary entries assessing PLP and coping strategies once per hour for one week. Instead of using standardized questions, coping strategies were captured using a free format. Analyses revealed that the amputees used a limited number of strategies that could be classified into distraction, relaxation, seeking support, exercise, manipulation of the residual limb, and drug or alcohol use. Importantly, none of the reported strategies was shown to be effective in reducing PLP. This study thus confirms that PLP sufferers tend to use less effective coping strategies.

4.3. Catastrophizing. Pain catastrophizing is a maladaptive cognitive coping style that is characterized by an exaggerated, negative orientation towards pain and anticipation of negative outcomes. There is evidence that catastrophizing predicts chronic pain and associated impairment [94, 100, 101]. Several studies found that catastrophizing was significantly positively correlated with the magnitude of PLP in amputees [80, 96, 97, 102–105]. Jensen et al. [103] found that between one and six months after amputation, the change in PLP and depressive symptoms could be predicted by catastrophizing and lack of social support and overtly solicitous responses from family members. In a later study [102], these results were replicated for a period of 12 and 24 months after amputation. Surprisingly, in these studies, more intense catastrophizing was associated with an *improvement* of PLP and depression symptomatology six and 24 months after amputation. These results, at first glance, seem contradictory; however, they might be explained by regression to the mean artefacts, caused by the strong correlation between PLP, depression, and catastrophizing at the first time point in the studies, and thus, there was little room left for the patients to further aggravate at the second time point. Hence, the lagged relationships in these two studies do not necessarily indicate that catastrophizing predicts improvement of PLP. Rather, the results highlight the importance of taking the initial magnitude of pain into account. Another longitudinal study supporting the aggravating effect of catastrophizing on PLP was performed by Richardson et al. [104]. These authors found that catastrophizing before the amputation significantly predicted PLP six months after the amputation, whereas pain before the amputation was only weakly related to later PLP.

Relationships between catastrophizing and PLP have been investigated in two studies by Vase et al. [80, 105]. In the first study [105], catastrophizing accounted for 35% of the variance in PLP after statistically controlling for depression and anxiety. In addition, catastrophizing correlated positively with wind-up-like pain, elicited by pinprick stimulation applied to the residual limb. Wind-up is a dynamical pain phenomenon which is usually assessed by repetitive application of moderately painful stimuli of equal intensity. Due to temporal summation processes, stimuli are perceived as increasingly painful. However, strong enhancement in perceived pain in this paradigm indicates exaggerated summation or sensitization processes, which have previously been reported for chronic pain patients [106, 107]. Vase et al. [105] suggested that catastrophizing and wind-up might interact and contribute to PLP. In the second study [80], the authors used electroencephalographic recordings of cortical responses to noxious and nonnoxious stimuli presented at the amputees' affected and nonaffected limbs. For stimuli presented on the affected side, there was a significant correlation between catastrophizing and the power at the N/P135 dipole, suggesting an origin of cortical activity in the area of the secondary somatosensory cortex. The authors concluded that this finding might be explained by the fact that catastrophizing implies hypervigilant attention to noxious and nonnoxious stimuli. Another study showed that catastrophizing is not only related to PLP but also to disability as it predicted physical and psychosocial disability in amputees [108].

5. Changes in Body Perception and Their Relationship to PLP

The changes in physical integrity after amputation are accompanied by alterations in cortical body representation and body perception. Moseley et al. [109] introduced the body matrix concept, describing a widely distributed frontoparietal brain network involved in processing a combined representation of body and space for maintaining homeostatic control and enabling protective behavior. Amputation-induced changes in this network and their behavioral and perceptual consequences have been repeatedly studied in the past (e.g., [110–113]).

Previous studies have shown that brain changes in amputees with PLP compared to amputees without PLP are pronounced and that PLP intensity is positively correlated with shifts in sensorimotor body representation (e.g., [65, 114]). These reorganization processes appear to be mirrored in altered body perception. For example, reorganization in the primary sensory cortex is not only correlated with PLP but also with the experience of a telescopic distortion (e.g., [115]), that is, the perception that the phantom limb shortens or, in extreme cases, retracts into the residual limb over time. Other cognitive alterations were observed for functions involving spatial transformations of body parts that appear to involve posterior and superior parietal regions and intraparietal regions (cf. [116]). Thus, amputees with PLP perform worse when they have to mentally rotate their limbs (e.g., [117]), and a negative association between performance in mental limb rotation and the frequency of PLP has been shown [118]. This suggests that phantom sensations in general [119] and PLP in particular are associated with impairments in the body schema, describing a flexible central representation of body posture that is needed for action. Since mental rotation of body parts involves motor imagery processes [120], and since the associated neural mechanisms are different in amputees with PLP compared to amputees without PLP [121], these results highlight the impaired mentalization of motor execution specifically for painful phantom limbs. Consequently, it has been suggested that the central body representation itself should be a target of therapeutic approaches [122], and thus, novel treatments aim at normalizing the underlying processes [123–130]. Interestingly, the amputees' body perception might be important for the effectiveness of these treatments [6, 127].

The PLP-specific alterations in body representation also have consequences for higher-order emotional and cognitive processes. In a nationwide study, Bekrater-Bodmann et al. [4] surveyed a large cohort of amputees for the presence of residual limb pain and PLP and additionally for their body-related dream content. Specifically, they assessed the proportion with which the amputees dreamed of themselves as being impaired (i.e., amputated) versus having an intact (i.e., nonamputated) body. The majority of amputees recalled their body appearance in dreams as intact, even decades after the amputation. PLP correlated positively with the recall of an impaired body in dreams, indicating that suffering in the awake state influences body representation in dreams. This relationship was rather unspecific because for residual limb pain, the same relationship was found. However, although dream content is rather difficult to interpret, these results suggest that the impaired physical body has a higher salience in postamputation pain sufferers than in pain-free amputees. In line with this notion, there is new evidence that PLP is related to implicit attitudes towards amputated bodies in general. By using an Implicit Association Test, Macauda et al. [131] showed that amputees implicitly prefer intact bodies. In fact, amputees did not differ from a nonamputated control group. Interestingly, PLP intensity was significantly and positively correlated with the preference for intact bodies. It remains open how these findings are related to those from an earlier study [132] in which amputees were instructed to draw their body images and in which amputees suffering from PLP drew their bodies as intact more often than amputees without PLP. To which extent this is mediated by emotional factors remains to be determined. Prospective studies need to carefully consider and examine the complex interplay between PLP, body-related higher-order cognitions, and emotional processing.

6. Summary and Conclusions

In this review article, we summarized and discussed the research on emotional factors, stress, cognition, and body perception in PLP. Most research on emotional factors focused on depression and anxiety. Rates of depression and anxiety are high in early stages after amputation; however, both conditions are probably not (or only weakly) associated with the occurrence of PLP but rather with problems related to the adaption to the new situation. In later stages, depression and anxiety might contribute to PLP, but these associations appear to be weaker than in other types of chronic pain. Up to now, it remains an open question why depression and anxiety might be less relevant in PLP than in other chronic pain states. One reason, which has already been suggested by Desmond and MacLachlan [36], might be that PLP less strongly interferes with everyday activity—and compared to residual limb pain even with prosthesis use—than other chronic pain syndromes. Another reason might be that, in the case of chronic back pain, emotional and cognitive variables might play a more important etiological role. For example, the fear-avoidance model of chronic pain [14] states that fear and avoidance of movement are acquired through a fear-conditioning process that might favor chronicity. Over time, avoidance of movement leads to disability and recurrent pain, which strengthens the learned association and leads to a vicious circle consisting of pain, disability, and fear. The model therefore suggests that fear conditionability might be a risk factor for chronic pain that is acquired in such a way. That chronic back pain patients show enhanced fear conditioning has been shown in several studies (e.g., [133]). The role of anxiety and negative affect in the acquisition of movement-related fear has also been shown experimentally [134, 135]. Another series of neuroimaging studies further suggest that emotional learning processes predict the transition from the acute phase to the chronic phase in back pain (for a review, see [136]). Whether these conditioning and emotional learning mechanisms are also important in PLP needs to be addressed in future studies.

Concerning stress, we showed that research, on the whole, suggests that there are bidirectional relationships between stress and PLP, probably due to interactions of the central and peripheral nervous systems. The bidirectional relationships between stress and PLP have been demonstrated both in experimental studies and more naturalistic settings. Given the relatively clear picture that can be drawn from this line of research, the utility of altering central and peripheral stress responses in clinical interventions should be explored. More recent studies also suggest that therapeutic interventions used in traumatization can be useful to treat PLP.

Little is known about the role of cognitive factors such as attention/distraction or expectation, which are commonly discussed as mediators of the pain experience. Memory is a well-represented topic in the PLP literature. However, it has not been clearly delineated which declarative and nondeclarative components are relevant and how they relate to neuroplasticity. Research on the role of catastrophizing in PLP shows that this coping style is positively associated with PLP presence, and longitudinal studies further indicate that catastrophizing aggravates PLP. Apart from avoiding catastrophizing, little is known about effective coping with PLP. Finally, we briefly discussed the role of body representation and body perception in PLP on which there have been many studies in the recent years and which are often perceived as the most promising targets for treating PLP (for reviews, see [137–140]). We also found evidence that cortical body representations might interact with psychological variables, but that until now, only few studies have focused on connections between these topics.

Compared to other types of pain, there has been little research on the role of psychological variables in PLP. whether psychological variables are less important for PLP or whether they have merely been neglected needs to be determined in future studies that take emotional, motivational, perceptual, and cognitive variables into account.

References

[1] L. Nikolajsen, "Phantom limb," in *Wall and Melzack's Textbook of Pain*, S. B. McMahon, P. D. Wall, and R. Melzack, Eds., Elsevier, Saunders, Philadelphia, PA, USA, 2013.

[2] M. A. Hanley, D. M. Ehde, M. Jensen, J. Czerniecki, D. G. Smith, and L. R. Robinson, "Chronic pain associated with upper-limb loss," *American Journal of Physical Medicine and Rehabilitation*, vol. 88, no. 9, pp. 742–779, 2009.

[3] K. Ostlie, R. J. Franklin, O. H. Skjeldal, A. Skrondal, and P. Magnus, "Musculoskeletal pain and overuse syndromes in adult acquired major upper-limb amputees," *Archives of Physical Medicine and Rehabilitation*, vol. 92, no. 12, pp. 1967–1973, 2011.

[4] R. Bekrater-Bodmann, M. Schredl, M. Diers et al., "Post-amputation pain is associated with the recall of an impaired body representation in dreams—results from a nation-wide survey on limb amputees," *PLoS One*, vol. 10, no. 3, Article ID e0119552, 2015.

[5] P. L. Ephraim, S. T. Wegener, E. J. MacKenzie, T. R. Dillingham, and L. E. Pezzin, "Phantom pain, residual limb pain, and back pain in amputees: results of a national survey," *Archives of Physical Medicine and Rehabilitation*, vol. 86, no. 10, pp. 1910–1919, 2005.

[6] U. Kern, V. Busch, M. Rockland, M. Kohl, and F. Birklein, "Prävalenz und risikofaktoren von phantomschmerzen und phantomwahrnehmungen in Deutschland [prevalence and risk factors of phantom limb pain and phantom limb sensations in Germany. A nationwide field survey]," *Der Schmerz*, vol. 23, no. 5, pp. 479–488, 2009.

[7] T. S. Jensen, B. Krebs, J. Nielsen, and P. Rasmussen, "Phantom limb, phantom pain and stump pain in amputees during the first 6 months following limb amputation," *Pain*, vol. 17, no. 3, pp. 243–256, 1983.

[8] D. M. Desmond and M. MacLachlan, "Prevalence and characteristics of phantom limb pain and residual limb pain in the long term after upper limb amputation," *International Journal of Rehabilitation Research*, vol. 33, no. 3, pp. 279–282, 2010.

[9] J. C. Bosmans, T. P. B. M. Suurmeijer, M. Hulsink, C. P. van der Schans, J. H. B. Geertzen, and P. U. Dijkstra, "Amputation, phantom pain and subjective well-being: a qualitative study," *International Journal of Rehabilitation Research*, vol. 30, no. 1, pp. 1–8, 2007.

[10] C. P. van der Schans, J. H. B. Geertzen, T. Schoppen, and P. U. Dijkstra, "Phantom pain and health-related quality of life in lower limb amputees," *Journal of Pain and Symptom Management*, vol. 24, no. 4, pp. 429–436, 2002.

[11] H. Flor, L. Nikolajsen, and T. S. Jensen, "Phantom limb pain: a case of maladaptive CNS plasticity?," *Nature Reviews Neuroscience*, vol. 7, no. 11, pp. 873–881, 2006.

[12] C. R. Jutzeler, A. Curt, and J. L. K. Kramer, "Relationship between chronic pain and brain reorganization after deafferentation: a systematic review of functional MRI findings," *NeuroImage: Clinical*, vol. 9, pp. 599–606, 2015.

[13] T. Pincus and S. Morley, "Cognitive-processing bias in chronic pain: a review and integration," *Psychological Bulletin*, vol. 127, no. 5, pp. 599–617, 2001.

[14] J. W. S. Vlaeyen and S. J. Linton, "Fear-avoidance and its consequences in chronic musculoskeletal pain: a state of the art," *Pain*, vol. 85, no. 3, pp. 317–332, 2000.

[15] M. C. Bushnell, M. Čeko, and L. A. Low, "Cognitive and emotional control of pain and its disruption in chronic pain," *Nature Reviews Neuroscience*, vol. 14, no. 7, pp. 502–511, 2013.

[16] J. Foell, R. Bekrater-Bodmann, H. Flor, and J. Cole, "Phantom limb pain after lower limb trauma origins and treatments," *International Journal of Lower Extremity Wounds*, vol. 10, no. 4, pp. 224–235, 2011.

[17] R. A. Sherman, C. J. Sherman, and G. M. Bruno, "Psychological factors influencing chronic phantom limb pain: an analysis of the literature," *Pain*, vol. 28, no. 3, pp. 285–295, 1987.

[18] A. Hill, "Phantom limb pain: a review of the literature on attributes and potential mechanisms," *Journal of Pain and Symptom Management*, vol. 17, no. 2, pp. 125–142, 1999.

[19] C. M. Parkes, "Factors determining the persistence of phantom pain in the amputee," *Journal of Psychosomatic Research*, vol. 17, no. 2, pp. 97–108, 1973.

[20] C. M. Parkes, "Psycho-social transitions: comparison between reactions to loss of a limb and loss of a spouse," *British Journal of Psychiatry*, vol. 127, no. 3, pp. 204–210, 1975.

[21] S. H. Frazier and L. C. Kolb, "Psychiatric aspects of pain and the phantom limb," *Orthopedic Clinics of North America*, vol. 1, pp. 481–495, 1970.

[22] D. A. Fishbain, R. Cutler, H. L. Rosomoff, and R. S. Rosomoff, "Chronic pain-associated depression: antecedent or consequence of chronic pain? A review," *Clinical Journal of Pain*, vol. 13, no. 2, pp. 116–137, 1997.

[23] R. J. Gatchel, Y. B. Peng, M. L. Peters, P. N. Fuchs, and D. C. Turk, "The biopsychosocial approach to chronic pain: scientific advances and future directions," *Psychological Bulletin*, vol. 133, no. 4, pp. 581–624, 2007.

[24] H. Flor and D. C. Turk, *Chronic Pain: An Integrated Biobehavioral Approach 1 Pap/Cdr Edition*, IASP Press, Seattle, WA, USA, 2011.

[25] C. Fröhlich, F. Jacobi, and H. U. Wittchen, "DSM-IV pain disorder in the general population," *European Archives of Psychiatry and Clinical Neuroscience*, vol. 256, no. 3, pp. 187–196, 2006.

[26] American Psychiatric Association, and American Psychiatric Association, *Diagnostic and Statistical Manual of Mental Disorders: DSM-IV-TR, Text Revision*, American Psychiatric Association, Washington, DC, USA, 4th edition, 2000.

[27] G. D. Shukla, S. C. Sahu, R. P. Tripathi, and D. K. Gupta, "A psychiatric study of amputees," *British Journal of Psychiatry*, vol. 141, no. 1, pp. 50–53, 1982.

[28] C. P. Mall, J. K. Trivedi, U. S. Mishra et al., "Psychiatric sequelae of amputation: I immediate effects," *Indian Journal of Psychiatry*, vol. 39, pp. 313–317, 1997.

[29] R. Singh, D. Ripley, B. Pentland et al., "Depression and anxiety symptoms after lower limb amputation: the rise and fall," *Clinical Rehabilitation*, vol. 23, no. 3, pp. 281–286, 2009.

[30] J. K. Trivedi, C. P. Mall, U. S. Mishra et al., "Psychiatric sequelae of amputation: II long term effects," *Indian Journal of Psychiatry*, vol. 39, pp. 318–323, 1997.

[31] A. S. Whyte and C. A. Niven, "Psychological distress in amputees with phantom limb pain," *Journal of Pain and Symptom Management*, vol. 22, no. 5, pp. 938–946, 2001.

[32] K. A. Raichle, T. L. Osborne, M. P. Jensen, D. M. Ehde, D. G. Smith, and L. R. Robinson, "Preoperative state anxiety, acute postoperative pain, and analgesic use in persons undergoing lower limb amputation," *Clinical Journal of Pain*, vol. 31, no. 8, pp. 699–706, 2015.

[33] O. Horgan and M. MacLachlan, "Psychosocial adjustment to lower-limb amputation: a review," *Disability and Rehabilitation*, vol. 26, no. 14-15, pp. 837–850, 2004.

[34] A. T. Beck and R. A. Steer, "Internal consistencies of the original and revised Beck Depression Inventory," *Journal of Clinical Psychology*, vol. 40, no. 6, pp. 1365–1367, 1984.

[35] J. R. Peck, T. W. Smith, J. R. Ward, and R. Milano, "Disability and depression in rheumatoid arthritis. A multi-trait, multi-method investigation," *Arthritis and Rheumatism*, vol. 32, no. 9, pp. 1100–1106, 1989.

[36] D. M. Desmond and M. MacLachlan, "Affective distress and amputation-related pain among older men with long-term, traumatic limb amputations," *Journal of Pain and Symptom Management*, vol. 31, no. 4, pp. 362–368, 2006.

[37] A. S. Zigmond and R. P. Snaith, "The hospital anxiety and depression scale," *Acta Psychiatrica Scandinavica*, vol. 67, no. 6, pp. 361–370, 1983.

[38] N. J. Zilberg, D. S. Weiss, and M. J. Horowitz, "Impact of event scale: a cross-validation study and some empirical evidence supporting a conceptual model of stress response syndromes," *Journal of Consulting and Clinical Psychology*, vol. 50, no. 3, pp. 407–414, 1982.

[39] H. M. Marshall, M. P. Jensen, D. M. Ehde, and K. M. Campbell, "Pain site and impairment in individuals with amputation pain," *Archives of Physical Medicine and Rehabilitation*, vol. 83, no. 8, pp. 1116–1119, 2002.

[40] B. D. Darnall, P. Ephraim, S. T. Wegener et al., "Depressive symptoms and mental health service utilization among persons with limb loss: results of a national survey," *Archives of Physical Medicine and Rehabilitation*, vol. 86, no. 4, pp. 650–658, 2005.

[41] L. S. Radloff, "The CES-D scale: a self-report depression scale for research in the general population," *Applied Psychological Measurement*, vol. 1, no. 3, pp. 385–401, 1977.

[42] H. Kazemi, S. Ghassemi, S. M. Fereshtehnejad, A. Amini, P. H. Kolivand, and T. Doroudi, "Anxiety and depression in patients with amputated limbs suffering from phantom pain: a comparative study with non-phantom chronic pain," *International Journal of Preventive Medicine*, vol. 4, pp. 218–225, 2013.

[43] X. Fuchs, R. Bekrater-Bodmann, and H. Flor, "Phantom pain: the role of maladaptive plasticity and emotional and cognitive variables," in *Pain, Emotion and Cognition*, G. Pickering and S. Gibson, Eds., pp. 189–207, Springer International Publishing, Berlin, Germany, 2015, Available at: http://link.springer.com/chapter/10.1007/978-3-319-12033-1_12.

[44] H. Flor, T. E. Rudy, N. Birbaumer, B. Streit, and M. M. Schugens, "Zur anwendbarkeit des west haven-yale multidimensional pain inventory im deutschen Sprachraum," *Der Schmerz*, vol. 4, no. 2, pp. 82–87, 1990.

[45] R. C. Castillo, S. T. Wegener, S. E. Heins, J. A. Haythornthwaite, E. J. MacKenzie, and M. J. Bosse, "Longitudinal relationships between anxiety, depression, and pain: results from a two-year cohort study of lower extremity trauma patients," *Pain*, vol. 154, no. 12, pp. 2860–2866, 2013.

[46] D. C. Turk, "A diathesis-stress model of chronic pain and disability following traumatic injury," *Pain Research and Management*, vol. 7, no. 1, pp. 9–19, 2002.

[47] H. Senra, R. A. Oliveira, I. Leal, and C. Vieira, "Beyond the body image: a qualitative study on how adults experience lower limb amputation," *Clinical Rehabilitation*, vol. 26, no. 2, pp. 180–191, 2012.

[48] H. Flor, N. Birbaumer, and D. C. Turk, "The psychobiology of chronic pain," *Advances in Behaviour Research and Therapy*, vol. 12, no. 2, pp. 47–84, 1990.

[49] R. A. Sherman, J. G. Arena, C. J. Sherman, and J. L. Ernst, "The mystery of phantom pain: growing evidence for psychophysiological mechanisms," *Biofeedback and Self-Regulation*, vol. 14, no. 4, pp. 267–280, 1989.

[50] R. A. Sherman, *Phantom Pain*, Springer, Boston, MA, USA, 1997, http://link.springer.com/10.1007/978-1-4757-6169-6.

[51] R. A. Sherman and G. M. Bruno, "Concurrent variation of burning phantom limb and stump pain with near surface blood flow in the stump," *Orthopedics*, vol. 10, pp. 1395–1402, 1987.

[52] R. A. Sherman, V. D. Griffin, C. B. Evans, and A. S. Grana, "Temporal relationships between changes in phantom limb pain intensity and changes in surface electromyogram of the residual limb," *International Journal of Psychophysiology*, vol. 13, no. 1, pp. 71–77, 1992.

[53] R. A. Sherman, N. Gall, and J. Gormly, "Treatment of phantom limb pain with muscular relaxation training to disrupt the pain-anxiety-tension cycle," *Pain*, vol. 6, no. 1, pp. 47–55, 1979.

[54] R. A. Sherman, "Published treatments of phantom limb pain," *American Journal of Physical Medicine*, vol. 59, pp. 232–244, 1980.

[55] G. Belleggia and N. Birbaumer, "Treatment of phantom limb pain with combined EMG and thermal biofeedback: a case report," *Applied Psychophysiology and Biofeedback*, vol. 26, no. 2, pp. 141–146, 2001.

[56] R. N. Harden, T. T. Houle, S. Green et al., "Biofeedback in the treatment of phantom limb pain: a time-series analysis," *Applied Psychophysiology and Biofeedback*, vol. 30, no. 1, pp. 83–93, 2005.

[57] A. Angrilli and U. Köster, "Psychophysiological stress responses in amputees with and without phantom limb pain," *Physiology and Behavior*, vol. 68, no. 5, pp. 699–706, 2000.

[58] H. Flor, D. C. Turk, and N. Birbaumer, "Assessment of stress-related psychophysiological reactions in chronic back pain

patients," *Journal of Consulting and Clinical Psychology*, vol. 53, no. 3, pp. 354–364, 1985.

[59] H. Flor, "Phantom-limb pain: characteristics, causes, and treatment," *Lancet Neurology*, vol. 1, no. 3, pp. 182–189, 2002.

[60] M. J. Giummarra, N. Georgiou-Karistianis, M. E. R. Nicholls, S. J. Gibson, M. Chou, and J. L. Bradshaw, "Maladaptive plasticity: imprinting of past experiences onto phantom limb schemata," *Clinical Journal of Pain*, vol. 27, no. 8, pp. 691–698, 2011.

[61] J. Katz and R. Melzack, "Pain 'memories' in phantom limbs: review and clinical observations," *Pain*, vol. 43, no. 3, pp. 319–336, 1990.

[62] W. Larbig, P. Montoya, H. Flor, H. Bilow, S. Weller, and N. Birbaumer, "Evidence for a change in neural processing in phantom limb pain patients," *Pain*, vol. 67, no. 2, pp. 275–283, 1996.

[63] J. Katz, "Phantom limb experience in children and adults: cognitive and affective contributions," *Canadian Journal of Behavioural Science*, vol. 25, no. 3, pp. 335–354, 1993.

[64] P. Stude, E. K. Enax-Krumova, M. Lenz et al., "Local anesthetic sympathectomy restores fMRI cortical maps in CRPS I after upper extremity stellate blockade: a prospective case study," *Pain Physician*, vol. 17, no. 5, pp. E637–E644, 2014.

[65] H. Flor, T. Elbert, S. Knecht et al., "Phantom-limb pain as a perceptual correlate of cortical reorganization following arm amputation," *Nature*, vol. 375, no. 6531, pp. 482–484, 1995.

[66] C. Maihöfner, H. O. Handwerker, B. Neundörfer, and F. Birklein, "Patterns of cortical reorganization in complex regional pain syndrome," *Neurology*, vol. 61, no. 12, pp. 1707–1715, 2003.

[67] M. J. Giummarra, N. Georgiou-Karistianisl, M. E. R. Nichollsl, S. J. Gibsonl, M. Choul, and J. L. Bradshawl, "The menacing phantom: what pulls the trigger?," *European Journal of Pain*, vol. 15, no. 7, pp. 691.e1–691.e8, 2011.

[68] J. G. Arena, R. A. Sherman, G. M. Bruno, and J. D. Smith, "The relationship between situational stress and phantom limb pain: cross-lagged correlational data from six month pain logs," *Journal of Psychosomatic Research*, vol. 34, no. 1, pp. 71–77, 1990.

[69] E. Leskowitz, "Phantom limb pain: an energy/trauma model," *Explore: Journal of Science and Healing*, vol. 10, no. 6, pp. 389–397, 2014.

[70] C. de Roos, A. C. Veenstra, A. de Jongh et al., "Treatment of chronic phantom limb pain using a trauma-focused psychological approach," *Pain Research and Management*, vol. 15, no. 2, pp. 65–71, 2010.

[71] S. P. Cohen, J. M. Gambel, S. N. Raja, and S. Galvagno, "The contribution of sympathetic mechanisms to postamputation phantom and residual limb pain: a pilot study," *Journal of Pain*, vol. 12, no. 8, pp. 859–867, 2011.

[72] J. Schneider, A. Hofmann, C. Rost, and F. Shapiro, "EMDR in the treatment of chronic phantom limb pain," *Pain Medicine*, vol. 9, no. 1, pp. 76–82, 2008.

[73] D. C. Turk, "The role of psychological factors in chronic pain," *Acta Anaesthesiologica Scandinavica*, vol. 43, no. 9, pp. 885–888, 1999.

[74] D. C. Turk, D. Meichenbaum, and M. Genest, *Pain and Behavioral Medicine: A Cognitive-Behavioral Perspective*, Guilford Press, New York, NY, USA, 1983.

[75] A. Vanhaudenhuyse, S. Laureys, and M. E. Faymonville, "Neurophysiology of hypnosis," *Neurophysiologie Clinique/ Clinical Neurophysiology*, vol. 44, no. 4, pp. 343–353, 2014.

[76] M. P. Jensen and D. R. Patterson, "Hypnotic approaches for chronic pain management," *American Psychologist*, vol. 69, no. 2, pp. 167–177, 2014.

[77] P. Mack, A. K. T. Yam, and A. Y. H. Chin, "Hypnotherapy: a forgotten modality in managing chronic post-traumatic upper limb pain," *Annals Academy of Medicine Singapore*, vol. 42, pp. 361-362, 2013.

[78] L. Colloca, R. Klinger, H. Flor, and U. Bingel, "Placebo analgesia: psychological and neurobiological mechanisms," *Pain*, vol. 154, no. 4, pp. 511–514, 2013.

[79] L. Vase, I. Skyt, and K. T. Hall, "Placebo, nocebo, and neuropathic pain," *Pain*, vol. 157, pp. S98–S105, 2016.

[80] L. Vase, L. L. Egsgaard, L. Nikolajsen, P. Svensson, T. S. Jensen, and L. Arendt-Nielsen, "Pain catastrophizing and cortical responses in amputees with varying levels of phantom limb pain: a high-density EEG brain-mapping study," *Experimental Brain Research*, vol. 218, no. 3, pp. 407–417, 2012.

[81] H. Flor, "Maladaptive plasticity, memory for pain and phantom limb pain: review and suggestions for new therapies," *Expert Review of Neurotherapeutics*, vol. 8, no. 5, pp. 809–818, 2008.

[82] R. Melzack, T. J. Coderre, J. Katz, and A. L. Vaccarino, "Central neuroplasticity and pathological pain," *Annals of the New York Academy of Sciences*, vol. 933, no. 1, pp. 157–174, 2001.

[83] J. Sandkühler, "Learning and memory in pain pathways," *Pain*, vol. 88, no. 2, pp. 113–118, 2000.

[84] C. J. Woolf and M. W. Salter, "Neuronal plasticity: increasing the gain in pain," *Science*, vol. 288, no. 5472, pp. 1765–1768, 2000.

[85] H. Flor, "Cortical reorganisation and chronic pain: implications for rehabilitation," *Journal of Rehabilitation Medicine*, vol. 35, pp. 66–72, 2003.

[86] H. Flor, "Extinction of pain memories: importance for the treatment of chronic pain," in *Current Topics in Pain: 12th World Congress on Pain*, pp. 221–244, IASP Press, Seattle, WA, USA, 2009.

[87] J. Katz, "Psychophysical correlates of phantom limb experience," *Journal of Neurology, Neurosurgery and Psychiatry*, vol. 55, no. 9, pp. 811–821, 1992.

[88] V. C. Anderson-Barnes, C. McAuliffe, K. M. Swanberg, and J. W. Tsao, "Phantom limb pain–a phenomenon of proprioceptive memory?," *Medical Hypotheses*, vol. 73, no. 4, pp. 555–558, 2009.

[89] T. S. Jensen, B. Krebs, J. Nielsen, and P. Rasmussen, "Immediate and long-term phantom limb pain in amputees: incidence, clinical characteristics and relationship to preamputation limb pain," *Pain*, vol. 21, no. 3, pp. 267–278, 1985.

[90] L. Nikolajsen, S. Ilkjær, K. Krøner, J. H. Christensen, and T. S. Jensen, "The influence of preamputation pain on postamputation stump and phantom pain," *Pain*, vol. 72, no. 3, pp. 393–405, 1997.

[91] S. Mazza, M. Frot, and A. E. Rey, "A comprehensive literature review of chronic pain and memory," *Progress in Neuro-Psychopharmacology and Biological Psychiatry*, 2017, In press.

[92] C. Berryman, T. R. Stanton, K. Jane Bowering, A. Tabor, A. McFarlane, and G. Lorimer Moseley, "Evidence for working memory deficits in chronic pain: a systematic review and meta-analysis," *Pain*, vol. 154, no. 8, pp. 1181–1196, 2013.

[93] X. Liu, L. Li, F. Tang, S. Wu, and Y. Hu, "Memory impairment in chronic pain patients and the related neuropsychological

mechanisms: a review," *Acta Neuropsychiatrica*, vol. 26, no. 4, pp. 195–201, 2014.

[94] S. J. Linton and W. S. Shaw, "Impact of psychological factors in the experience of pain," *Physical Therapy*, vol. 91, no. 5, pp. 700–711, 2011.

[95] A. K. Rosenstiel and F. J. Keefe, "The use of coping strategies in chronic low back pain patients: relationship to patient characteristics and current adjustment," *Pain*, vol. 17, no. 1, pp. 33–44, 1983.

[96] A. Hill, "The use of pain coping strategies by patients with phantom limb pain," *Pain*, vol. 55, no. 3, pp. 347–353, 1993.

[97] A. Hill, C. A. Niven, and C. Knussen, "The role of coping in adjustment to phantom limb pain," *Pain*, vol. 62, no. 1, pp. 79–86, 1995.

[98] A. T. Hirsh, T. M. Dillworth, D. M. Ehde, and M. P. Jensen, "Sex differences in pain and psychological functioning in persons with limb loss," *Journal of Pain*, vol. 11, no. 1, pp. 79–86, 2010.

[99] A. S. Whyte and C. A. Niven, "Variation in phantom limb pain: results of a diary study," *Journal of Pain and Symptom Management*, vol. 22, no. 5, pp. 947–953, 2001.

[100] H. Flor, D. J. Behle, and N. Birbaumer, "Assessment of pain-related cognitions in chronic pain patients," *Behaviour Research and Therapy*, vol. 31, no. 1, pp. 63–73, 1993.

[101] M. M. Wertli, R. Eugster, U. Held, J. Steurer, R. Kofmehl, and S. Weiser, "Catastrophizing-a prognostic factor for outcome in patients with low back pain–a systematic review," *Spine Journal*, vol. 14, no. 11, pp. 2639–2657, 2014.

[102] M. A. Hanley, M. P. Jensen, D. M. Ehde, A. J. Hoffman, D. R. Patterson, and L. R. Robinson, "Psychosocial predictors of long-term adjustment to lower-limb amputation and phantom limb pain," *Disability and Rehabilitation*, vol. 26, no. 14-15, pp. 882–893, 2004.

[103] M. P. Jensen, D. M. Ehde, A. J. Hoffman, D. R. Patterson, J. M. Czerniecki, and L. R. Robinson, "Cognitions, coping and social environment predict adjustment to phantom limb pain," *Pain*, vol. 95, no. 1, pp. 133–142, 2002.

[104] C. Richardson, S. Glenn, M. Horgan, and T. Nurmikko, "A prospective study of factors associated with the presence of phantom limb pain six months after major lower limb amputation in patients with peripheral vascular disease," *Journal of Pain*, vol. 8, no. 10, pp. 793–801, 2007.

[105] L. Vase, L. Nikolajsen, B. Christensen et al., "Cognitive-emotional sensitization contributes to wind-up-like pain in phantom limb pain patients," *Pain*, vol. 152, no. 1, pp. 157–162, 2011.

[106] D. Kleinböhl, R. Hölzl, A. Möltner, C. Rommel, C. Weber, and P. M. Osswald, "Psychophysical measures of sensitization to tonic heat discriminate chronic pain patients," *Pain*, vol. 81, no. 1, pp. 35–43, 1999.

[107] L. M. Mendell, "Physiological properties of unmyelinated fiber projection to the spinal cord," *Experimental Neurology*, vol. 16, no. 3, pp. 316–332, 1966.

[108] A. S. Whyte and L. Carroll, "The relationship between catastrophizing and disability in amputees experiencing phantom pain," *Disability and Rehabilitation*, vol. 26, no. 11, pp. 649–654, 2004.

[109] G. L. Moseley, A. Gallace, and C. Spence, "Bodily illusions in health and disease: physiological and clinical perspectives and the concept of a cortical 'body matrix'," *Neuroscience and Biobehavioral Reviews*, vol. 36, no. 1, pp. 34–46, 2012.

[110] E. Canzoneri, M. Marzolla, A. Amoresano, G. Verni, and A. Serino, "Amputation and prosthesis implantation shape body and peripersonal space representations," *Scientific Reports*, vol. 3, no. 1, 2013.

[111] P. M. McDonnell, R. N. Scott, J. Dickison, R. A. Theriault, and B. Wood, "Do artificial limbs become part of the user? New evidence," *Journal of Rehabilitation Research and Development*, vol. 26, no. 2, pp. 17–24, 1989.

[112] D. Nico, E. Daprati, F. Rigal, L. Parsons, and A. Sirigu, "Left and right hand recognition in upper limb amputees," *Brain*, vol. 127, no. 1, pp. 120–132, 2004.

[113] S. Preißler, C. Dietrich, K. R. Blume, G. O. Hofmann, W. H. R. Miltner, and T. Weiss, "Plasticity in the visual system is associated with prosthesis use in phantom limb pain," *Frontiers in Human Neuroscience*, vol. 7, p. 311, 2013.

[114] A. Karl, N. Birbaumer, W. Lutzenberger, L. G. Cohen, and H. Flor, "Reorganization of motor and somatosensory cortex in upper extremity amputees with phantom limb pain," *Journal of Neuroscience*, vol. 21, no. 10, pp. 3609–3618, 2001.

[115] S. M. Grüsser, C. Winter, W. Mühlnickel et al., "The relationship of perceptual phenomena and cortical reorganization in upper extremity amputees," *Neuroscience*, vol. 102, no. 2, pp. 263–272, 2001.

[116] E. Bonda, M. Petrides, S. Frey, and A. Evans, "Neural correlates of mental transformations of the body-in-space," *Proceedings of the National Academy of Sciences*, vol. 92, no. 24, pp. 11180–11184, 1995.

[117] A. Reinersmann, G. S. Haarmeyer, M. Blankenburg et al., "Left is where the L is right. Significantly delayed reaction time in limb laterality recognition in both CRPS and phantom limb pain patients," *Neuroscience Letters*, vol. 486, no. 3, pp. 240–245, 2010.

[118] C. K. Wong and C. K. Wong, "Limb laterality recognition score: a reliable clinical measure related to phantom limb pain," *Pain Medicine*, vol. 19, no. 4, pp. 753–756, 2017.

[119] Y. Lyu, X. Guo, R. Bekrater-Bodmann, H. Flor, and S. Tong, "Phantom limb perception interferes with motor imagery after unilateral upper-limb amputation," *Scientific Reports*, vol. 6, no. 1, p. 21100, 2016.

[120] H. Hamada, D. Matsuzawa, C. Sutoh et al., "Comparison of brain activity between motor imagery and mental rotation of the hand tasks: a functional magnetic resonance imaging study," *Brain Imaging and Behavior*, pp. 1–11, 2018.

[121] M. Diers, C. Christmann, C. Koeppe, M. Ruf, and H. Flor, "Mirrored, imagined and executed movements differentially activate sensorimotor cortex in amputees with and without phantom limb pain," *Pain*, vol. 149, no. 2, pp. 296–304, 2010.

[122] M. J. Giummarra and G. L. Moseley, "Phantom limb pain and bodily awareness: current concepts and future directions," *Current Opinion in Anaesthesiology*, vol. 24, no. 5, pp. 524–531, 2011.

[123] G. L. Moseley, "Graded motor imagery for pathologic pain: a randomized controlled trial," *Neurology*, vol. 67, no. 12, pp. 2129–2134, 2006.

[124] K. MacIver, D. M. Lloyd, S. Kelly, N. Roberts, and T. Nurmikko, "Phantom limb pain, cortical reorganization and the therapeutic effect of mental imagery," *Brain*, vol. 131, no. 8, pp. 2181–2191, 2008.

[125] V. S. Ramachandran and D. Rogers-Ramachandran, "Synaesthesia in phantom limbs induced with mirrors," *Proceedings of the Royal Society B: Biological Sciences*, vol. 263, no. 1369, pp. 377–386, 1996.

[126] B. L. Chan, R. Witt, A. P. Charrow et al., "Mirror therapy for phantom limb pain," *New England Journal of Medicine*, vol. 357, no. 21, pp. 2206-2207, 2007.

[127] J. Foell, R. Bekrater-Bodmann, M. Diers, and H. Flor, "Mirror therapy for phantom limb pain: brain changes and the role of body representation," *European Journal of Pain*, vol. 18, no. 5, pp. 729–739, 2014.

[128] M. Lotze, W. Grodd, N. Birbaumer, M. Erb, E. Huse, and H. Flor, "Does use of a myoelectric prosthesis prevent cortical reorganization and phantom limb pain?," *Nature Neuroscience*, vol. 2, no. 6, pp. 501-502, 1999.

[129] T. Weiss, W. H. Miltner, T. Adler, L. Brückner, and E. Taub, "Decrease in phantom limb pain associated with prosthesis-induced increased use of an amputation stump in humans," *Neuroscience Letters*, vol. 272, no. 2, pp. 131–134, 1999.

[130] M. Ortiz-Catalan, R. A. Guðmundsdóttir, M. B. Kristoffersen et al., "Phantom motor execution facilitated by machine learning and augmented reality as treatment for phantom limb pain: a single group, clinical trial in patients with chronic intractable phantom limb pain," *The Lancet*, vol. 388, no. 10062, pp. 2885–2894, 2016.

[131] G. Macauda, R. Bekrater-Bodmann, P. Brugger, and B. Lenggenhager, "When less is more–implicit preference for incomplete bodies in xenomelia," *Journal of Psychiatric Research*, vol. 84, pp. 249–255, 2017.

[132] I. Pucher, W. Kickinger, and O. Frischenschlager, "Coping with amputation and phantom limb pain," *Journal of Psychosomatic Research*, vol. 46, no. 4, pp. 379–383, 1999.

[133] C. Schneider, D. Palomba, and H. Flor, "Pavlovian conditioning of muscular responses in chronic pain patients: central and peripheral correlates," *Pain*, vol. 112, no. 3, pp. 239–247, 2004.

[134] N. Geschwind, M. Meulders, M. L. Peters, J. W. S. Vlaeyen, and A. Meulders, "Can experimentally induced positive affect attenuate generalization of fear of movement-related pain?," *Journal of Pain*, vol. 16, no. 3, pp. 258–269, 2015.

[135] A. Meulders, M. Meulders, and J. W. S. Vlaeyen, "Positive affect protects against deficient safety learning during extinction of fear of movement-related pain in healthy individuals scoring relatively high on trait anxiety," *Journal of Pain*, vol. 15, no. 6, pp. 632–644, 2014.

[136] A. V. Apkarian, M. N. Baliki, and M. A. Farmer, "Predicting transition to chronic pain," *Current Opinion in Neurology*, vol. 26, no. 4, pp. 360–367, 2013.

[137] B. Lenggenhager, C. A. Arnold, and M. J. Giummarra, "Phantom limbs: pain, embodiment, and scientific advances in integrative therapies: phantom limbs," *Wiley Interdisciplinary Reviews: Cognitive Science*, vol. 5, no. 2, pp. 221–231, 2014.

[138] G. L. Moseley and H. Flor, "Targeting cortical representations in the treatment of chronic pain: a review," *Neurorehabilitation and Neural Repair*, vol. 26, no. 6, pp. 646–652, 2012.

[139] D. Senkowski and A. Heinz, "Chronic pain and distorted body image: implications for multisensory feedback interventions," *Neuroscience and Biobehavioral Reviews*, vol. 69, pp. 252–259, 2016.

[140] T. Weiss, "Plasticity and cortical reorganization associated with pain," *Zeitschrift für Psychologie*, vol. 224, no. 2, pp. 71–79, 2016.

6

Preconditioning Contractions Suppress Muscle Pain Markers after Damaging Eccentric Contractions

Hiroshi Nagahisa,[1] Kazumi Ikezaki,[1] Ryotaro Yamada,[2] Takashi Yamada,[2] and Hirofumi Miyata[1]

[1]*Biological Sciences, Graduate School of Sciences and Technology for Innovation, Yamaguchi University, Yoshida 1677-1, Yamaguchi 753-8515, Japan*
[2]*Graduate School of Health Sciences, Sapporo Medical University, Sapporo 060-8556, Japan*

Correspondence should be addressed to Hirofumi Miyata; hiro@yamaguchi-u.ac.jp

Academic Editor: Filippo Brighina

Inexperienced vigorous exercise, including eccentric contraction (ECC), causes muscle pain and damage. Similar prior light exercise suppresses the development of muscle pain (repeated-bout effect), but the molecular mechanisms behind this are not sufficiently understood. In this study, the influence of a nondamaging preconditioning ECC load (Precon) on muscle pain-related molecules and satellite cell-activating factors was investigated at the mRNA expression level. Nine-week-old male Wistar rats ($n = 36$) were divided into 2 groups: a group receiving only a damaging ECC (100 contractions) load (non-Precon) and a group receiving a nondamaging ECC (10 contractions) load 2 days before receiving the damaging ECC load (Precon). ECC was loaded on the left leg, and the right leg was regarded as the intact control (CTL). The medial head of the gastrocnemius muscle from all rats was excised 2 or 4 days after the damaging ECC loading, and the relative mRNA expression levels of muscle pain- and satellite cell-related molecules were quantitated using real-time RT PCR. Precon suppressed increases in MHC-embryonic and MHC-neonatal mRNA expressions. Enhancement of HGF, Pax7, MyoD, and myogenin mRNA expression was also suppressed, suggesting that Precon decreased the degree of muscle damage and no muscle regeneration or satellite cell activation occurred. Similarly, increases in mRNA expression of muscle pain-related molecules (BKB_2 receptor, COX-2, and mPGEC-1) were also suppressed. This study clearly demonstrated that at the mRNA level, prior light ECC suppressed muscle damage induced by later damaging ECC and promoted recovery from muscle pain.

1. Introduction

Inexperienced vigorous exercise, including eccentric contraction (ECC), induces muscle damage, edema, reduction of tension, limitation of the range of motion, and muscle pain. Regarding muscle pain, delayed onset muscle soreness (DOMS) persists for several days after exercise and generally resolves after several days [1–3]. ECC more effectively promotes muscular hypertrophy compared with concentric and isometric contractions [4, 5]. Therefore, ECC is considered to be efficient exercise for rehabilitation and training aiming at improvement of muscle function. On the other hand, ECC-induced symptoms, such as DOMS, may influence activity in daily life, rehabilitation, and motivation of athletes for daily training even though the symptoms are transient. However, it is also known that performing similar exercise several days before training reduces the grade of DOMS and damage and promotes recovery of reduced tension [2, 6, 7]. This effect of pre-exercise is referred to as the repeated-bout effect, and it has been reported to appear within 2 days to one week [6–8] and persist for 6 months [9]. However, the physiological mechanisms concerning the effects of pre-exercise on muscle pain and regeneration remain still unclear.

Experimentally, in a model of muscle pain of inflammation induced by formalin injection into the gastrocnemius muscle, mRNA expression of the B_2 receptor of bradykinin (BK) represents several bioactivities, including induction of increases in muscle pain [10]. As this muscle pain is suppressed by administration of BKB_2 receptor antagonist, the BKB_2 receptor is considered to be involved in muscle pain [8, 10]. Other molecules involved in pain include prostaglandin (PG) E_2. The protein and mRNA expression levels of an enzyme involved in PGE_2 synthesis, cyclooxygenase-2 (COX-2), increase after ECC [11]. Muscle pain and inflammation after ECC and those induced by carrageenan are reduced by administration of a COX-2 inhibitor, and the level of the final product of COX-2, PGE_2, simultaneously decreases [11, 12]. There are several isozymes of PGE synthase, which is the final enzyme of the PGE_2 synthetic pathway, and microsomal PGE synthase-1 (mPGES-1) has been suggested to be closely associated with COX-2 [13]. Accordingly, it is likely that expression of COX-2 and mPGES-1 in the PGE_2 synthetic pathway is involved in muscle pain via PGE_2 production.

Although the BKB_2 receptor or enzymes in the PGE_2 synthetic pathway, such as COX-2 and mPGES-1, may be associated with muscle pain, the influence of pre-exercise on the expression of these muscle pain-related molecules is unclear. In this study, the influence of prior light non-damaging ECC (Precon) on muscle damage, muscle pain-related molecules, and muscle regeneration (satellite cell-activating factors) induced by later damaging ECC was examined at the mRNA expression level.

2. Materials and Methods

2.1. Animals and Experimental Protocol. All rat experiments were performed at Yamaguchi University and Sapporo Medical University and conducted in accordance with approved protocols by the Committee on Animal Experiments of Yamaguchi University (No. 290) and Sapporo Medical University (No. 16-077). Animal care was in accordance with institutional guidelines.

Male Wistar rats (9-week old, $n = 36$) were supplied by Sanyo Labo Service (Sapporo, Japan). Rats were housed in an environmentally controlled room (24 ± 2°C, 12 h : 12 h light-dark cycle) and given food and water ad libitum. Rats were assigned to a Precon group and a non-Precon group ($n = 18$ in each group). In all the groups, ECC was loaded on the left leg, and the right leg was regarded as intact control (CTL) of each experimental group. In the Precon group, the left plantar flexor muscles were exposed to Precon (i.e., 10 repeated ECC) 2 days prior to 100 repeated damaging ECC. Previous studies showed that muscle damage increase progressively with the number of forced ECC [14, 15]. In the preliminary experiments, we confirmed that the maximum isometric torque of the plantar flexor muscles was not reduced 48 hours after 10 repeated ECC (data not shown). The left muscles in the non-Precon group were exposed to damaging ECC without Precon. 0 (Immediately), 2, or 4 days after completion of damaging ECC, the planter flexor muscles were removed from each animal ($n = 6$ in each group). The medial gastrocnemius muscles were used for further analyses.

2.2. Eccentric Contractions. Under isoflurane anesthesia, rats were placed supine on a platform and their left foot was secured in a foot plate connected to a torque sensor (S-14154, Takei Scientific Instruments, Tokyo, Japan) at an angle of 0° dorsiflexion (i.e., 90° relative to the tibia). ECC comprised forced dorsiflexion from 0° to 40° at 150°/s combined with neuromuscular electrical stimulation (ES). Plantar flexor muscles were stimulated supramaximally (45 V) via a pair of surface electrodes every 4 s. Stimulation parameters were set as follows: 1 ms monophasic rectangular pulse and 50 Hz stimulation frequency. The torque production was measured during ES.

2.3. Histochemical Analysis. Cryostat sections (10 μm) were stained with hematoxylin and eosin (H&E). To obtain sections with Evans blue dye (EBD), rats were intraperitoneally injected with 1% (wt/vol) EBD solution (1 mg/10 g body wt) 24 hours before sacrifice. H&E and EBD images were obtained from the serial sections using a fluorescence microscope BIOREVO BZ-9000 (KEYENCE, Osaka, Japan).

2.4. Real-Time RT PCR. The procedure described in the previous study was used for real-time RT PCR analysis [16]. The muscle samples were homogenized with TRIzol reagent (Molecular Probes, Breda, Netherlands) to extract total RNA. Genomic DNA was removed from total RNA by treating for 30 min at 37°C with TURBO DNase (Ambion, Austin, USA). To synthesize first strand cDNA, DNase-treated RNA (0.5 μg) was used with an Exscript RT reagent kit (Takara, Tokyo, Japan). Subsequently, the SYBR Green PCR Master Mix protocol in the StepOne Plus Real-Time PCR system (Applied Biosystems Japan, Tokyo, Japan) was used for real-time PCR analysis of cDNA products.

The amplification program was composed of an initial denaturation step at 95° for 10 min, 40 cycles of denaturation at 95° for 30 sec, and annealing/extension at 58° for 1 min. Glyceraldehyde-3-phosphate dehydrogenase (GAPDH) was used to estimate an internal control. The normalization of each mRNA was calculated from GAPDH by subtracting the cycle threshold (C_t) value of GAPDH from the C_t value of the target gene (ΔC_t (target)). The relative expression of the target gene was calculated as the relative quantification value for the CTL value. No nonspecific amplification in cDNA samples was detected by dissociation curve analysis after the relative expression.

Table 1 shows the sequences of the specific primers used in the present study. Primer Express software (Applied Biosystems Japan) was used for design of each PCR primer. The oligonucleotides were purchased from FASMAC (FASMAC, Kanagawa, Japan).

2.5. Statistical Analyses. All values are expressed as mean ± standard error (SE). Differences in mRNA expressions between groups were compared using one-way ANOVA followed by t-test with Bonferroni adjustment. Statistical significance was set at $P < 0.05$.

Table 1: Real-time RT PCR primer sequences.

Gene	Accession number		Sequence	Primer position
GAPDH	NM_017008.4	Forward	GCTCTCTGCTCCTCCCTGTTC	4–24
		Reverse	GAGGCTGGCACTGCACAA	44–61
MHC-embryonic	NM_012604.1	Forward	CTTCAAACTGAAAAACGCCTATGA	4536–4559
		Reverse	GTTCTAAGTTCTTATTCTCTCGCTTCACA	4584–4612
MHC-neonatal	NM_001100485.1	Forward	ATCAGTGCCAATCCCTTGCT	742–761
		Reverse	CCAAAGCGAGGAGTTGTCA	795–815
HGF	NM_017017.2	Forward	AAAACTACATGGGCAACTTATCCAA	1335–1359
		Reverse	ATGACGGTGTAAATCCTCCATATTC	1396–1420
Pax7	NM_001191984.1	Forward	AAAAGATTGAGGAGTATAAGAGGGAGAA	347–374
		Reverse	GCCGGTCCCGGATTTC	394–409
MyoD	NM_176079.1	Forward	GACGGCTCTCTCTGCTCCTTT	259–279
		Reverse	AGTCGAAACACGGATCATCATAGA	296–319
Myogenin	M24393.1	Forward	GACCCTACAGGTGCCCACAA	604–623
		Reverse	CCGTGATGCTGTCCACGAT	643–661
BKB_2 receptor	M59967.2	Forward	GAGCTTGAAGCATCCTAGGGAAT	1543–1565
		Reverse	CGCTTATGCCGTGAGACAAGA	1583–1603
COX-2	U03389.1	Forward	GGCAAAGGCCTCCATTGAC	1423–1441
		Reverse	GCGTTTGCGGTACTCATTGA	1470–1489
mPGES-1	NM_021583.3	Forward	TGCTCCCCGCCTTTCTG	78–94
		Reverse	CCACCGCGTACATCTTGATG	115–134

GAPDH, glyceraldehydes-3-phosphate dehydrogenase; MHC, myosin heavy chain; HGF, hepatocyte growth factor; Pax7, paired box transcription factor-7; MyoD, myogenic determination factor; BKB_2, bradykinin B_2 receptor; COX-2, cyclooxygenase 2; mPGES-1, microsomal prostaglandin E synthase-1.

3. Results

3.1. Histochemical Properties of Skeletal Muscle after Damaging ECC. There was not obvious histopathological alteration in sections of H&E at 0 day between non-Precon and Precon groups (Figures 1(a) and 1(b)). In sections of H&E at 2 and 4 days after damaging ECC, a number of swollen myofibers with rounded shape and many inflammatory cells surrounding them were observed in the non-Precon group (Figures 1(c) and 1(e)), while these unfavorable changes dramatically were suppressed in the Precon group (Figures 1(d) and 1(f)).

In agreement with these results, EBD-positive fibers which indicate development of membrane damage were not observed in 0 day (Figures 1(g) and 1(h)), increased at 2 and 4 days after damaging ECC in the non-Precon group (Figures 1(i) and 1(k)), and little increased during the same period in the Precon group (Figures 1(j) and 1(l)).

3.2. Expression of Skeletal Muscle Damage- and Regeneration-Related Factors mRNA. The expression level was presented as a value relative to that in CTL muscles of each group at 0 day. MHC-embryonic and MHC-neonatal are expressed during the regeneration process after muscle damage. At 2 days after damaging ECC, the expression level of MHC-embryonic mRNA was significantly increased in the Precon group (Figure 2(a)). At 4 days after damaging ECC, both the non-Precon and Precon groups showed significant increase in MHC-embryonic mRNA expression, whereas the expression of MHC-embryonic in the non-Precon group was significantly greater than in the Precon group.

The expression level of MHC-neonatal, at 0, 2, and 4 days after damaging ECC, was significantly increased in both the non-Precon and Precon groups (Figure 2(b)). However, there was no difference between the non-Precon and Precon groups.

The expression level of HGF mRNA, which is a well-studied activation factor for satellite cells, was significantly increased in the Precon group at 2 and 4 days after damaging ECC (Figure 3(a)). In the non-Precon group, the mRNA expression of HGF was significantly increased at 2 and 4 days after damaging ECC. However, at 2 and 4 days after damaging ECC, the expression level of HGF mRNA was significantly lower in the Precon group compared with the non-Precon group.

The mRNA expression level of Pax7, which is expressed in activation and proliferation state of satellite cells, was significantly increased only in the nonPrecon group at 2 and 4 days after damaging ECC (Figure 3(b)). In addition, at 4 days after damaging ECC, the expression of Pax7 mRNA was significantly lower in the Precon group compared with non-Precon group.

The mRNA expression level of MyoD regulating proliferation and differentiation of satellite cells was significantly increased in the non-Precon group 2 days after damaging ECC (Figure 3(c)). At 4 days after damaging ECC, the expression level of MyoD mRNA in the Precon group was significantly lower than in the non-Precon group.

The mRNA expression level of myogenin, which is expressed in the differentiation state of satellite cells, was significantly increased in the Precon group at 0 and 2 days after damaging ECC (Figure 3(d)). In the non-Precon group, at 2 and 4 days after damaging ECC, the mRNA expression level of myogenin was significantly increased. Furthermore, the expression level of myogenin mRNA was significantly

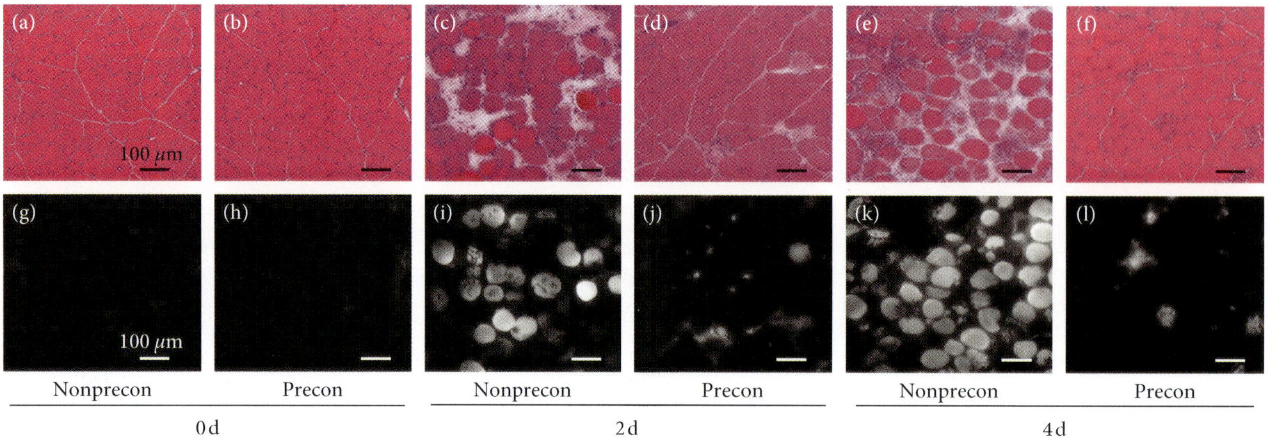

Figure 1: Photomicrograph of hematoxylin and eosin (a–f) and Evans blue dye (g–l) staining on sections of the left medial gastrocnemius muscles after damaging eccentric contractions.

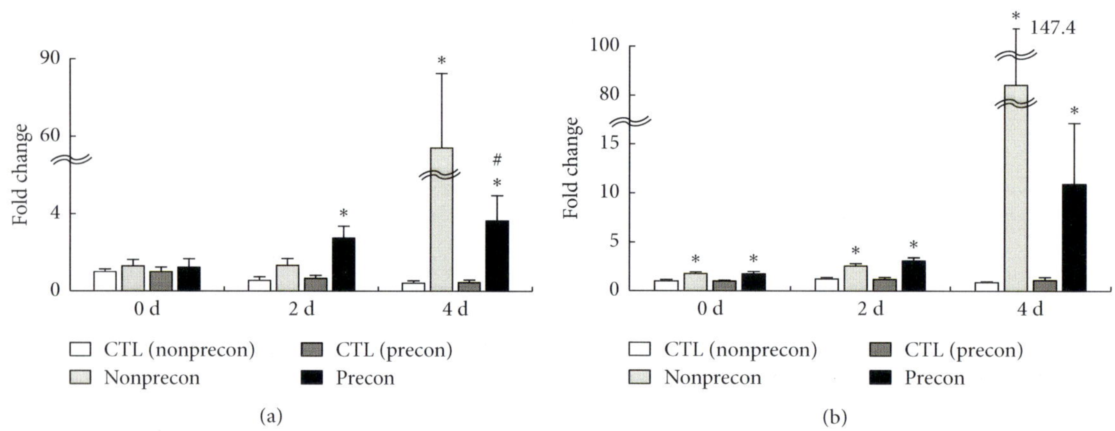

Figure 2: Time course changes in relative expression of MHC-embryonic (a) and MHC-neonatal (b) mRNA. The mRNA expression of each time point was calculated as x-fold change from each CTL value at 0 d. CTL indicates intact right muscle of each experimental group. Values are means ± SE. *significant differences ($P < 0.05$) as compared with each CTL value. #significant differences ($P < 0.05$) as compared with each non-Precon value.

lower in the Precon group compared with non-Precon group at 2 and 4 days after damaging ECC.

3.3. The Expression of Muscle Pain-Related Molecules mRNA. The expression level of BKB_2 receptor mRNA in the Precon group was significantly increased at 0, 2, and 4 days after damaging ECC (Figure 4(a)). In the non-Precon group, the mRNA expression of BKB_2 receptor was significantly increased at 2 and 4 days after damaging ECC. However, at 2 and 4 days after damaging ECC, the expression level of BKB_2 receptor mRNA was significantly lower in the Precon group compared with the non-Precon group.

The mRNA expression level of COX-2 in the Precon and non-Precon group was significantly increased at 2 days after damaging ECC (Figure 4(b)). However, at 4 days after damaging ECC, the expression of COX-2 was significantly increased only in the non-Precon group and its expression in the Precon group was significantly lower than in the non-Precon group.

The expression level of mPGES-1 in the non-Precon group was significantly increased at 2 and 4 days after damaging ECC, whereas there was no marked alteration in the Precon group (Figure 4(c)). In addition, at 4 days after damaging ECC, the expression level of mPGES-1 mRNA was significantly lower in the Precon group compared with the non-Precon group.

4. Discussion

The influence of prior light nondamaging ECC on muscle damage, muscle pain, and muscle regeneration-related molecules induced by later damaging ECC was investigated. In fact, Precon suppressed histopathological alteration induced by damaging ECC, corresponding to our previous results [17]. Furthermore, Precon suppressed increases in MHC-embryonic and MHC-neonatal mRNA expressions, suggesting a decrease in the degree of muscle damage. Similarly, increases in mRNA expression of HGF, Pax7, MyoD, and myogenin were suppressed by Precon,

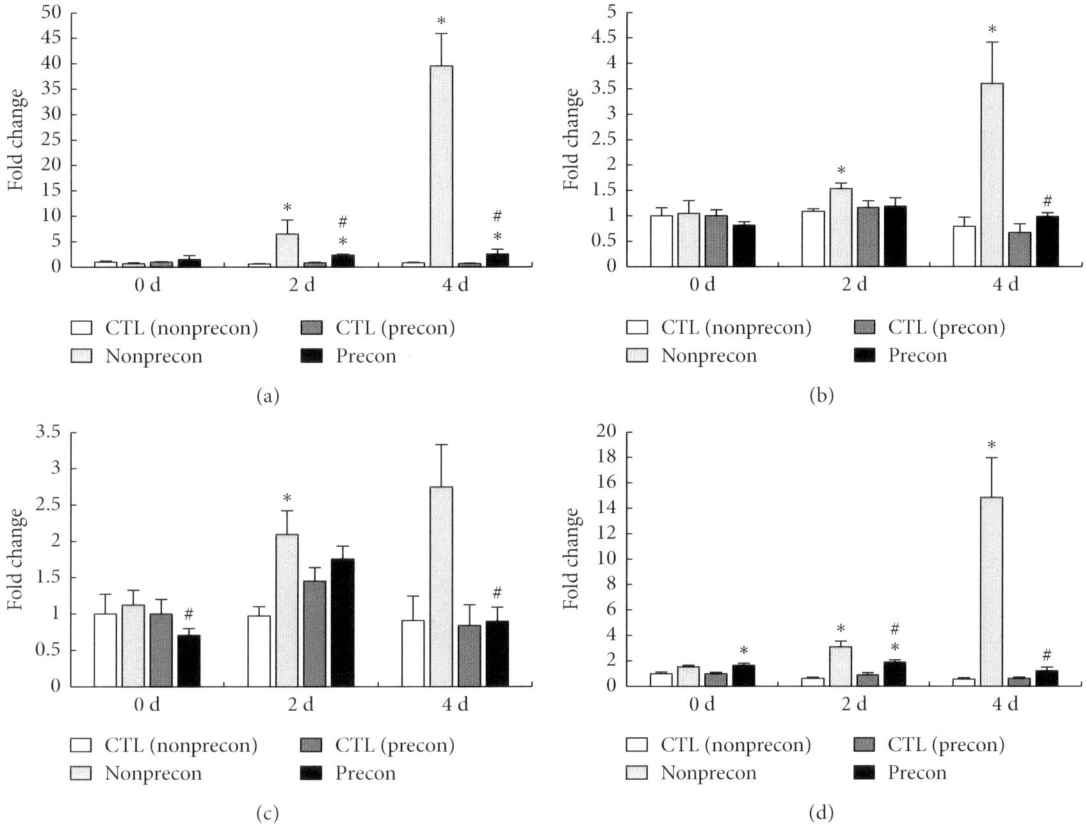

FIGURE 3: Time course changes in relative expression of HGF (a), Pax7 (b), MyoD (c), and myogenin (d) mRNA. The mRNA expression of each time point was calculated as x-fold change from each CTL value at 0 d. CTL indicates intact right muscle of each experimental group. Values are means ± SE. *significant differences ($P < 0.05$) as compared with each CTL value. #significant differences ($P < 0.05$) as compared with each non-Precon value.

suggesting that Precon reduced the degree of muscle damage, negating the need for muscle regeneration. Enhancement of mRNA expression of muscle pain-related molecules was also suppressed. This study demonstrated that prior light ECC reduces muscle damage induced by later damaging ECC and promotes recovery from muscle pain at the mRNA level.

In this study, we did not confirm the effect of Precon itself on mRNA expression. However, most of the mRNA expressions including muscle pain-related molecules in the non-Precon group did not significantly increase compared with its control and Precon groups at 0 day (2 days after Precon). Considering that the Precon itself (10 repeated ECC) has less impact than non-Precon (100 repeated ECC), the effect of Precon itself on mRNA expression was speculated to be little at least 0 and 2 days after the Precon.

4.1. Muscle Damage and Regeneration Induced by Eccentric Contraction. Skeletal muscle expresses developmental MHC, such as MHC-embryonic and MHC-neonatal, in the recovery course after muscle damage, in addition to mature MHC, such as MHC I, IIa, IIx, and IIb [18, 19]. These developmental MHCs are replaced by mature MHC during recovery after muscle damage. MHC-embryonic and MHC-neonatal mRNA expression increased after damaging ECC, but the degree of the increase in MHC-embryonic at 4 days after damaging ECC was reduced by Precon. Muscle satellite cells play an important role in muscle regeneration after muscle damage. Satellite cells are localized between the basement and plasma membranes, but they are normally in the resting state and express Pax7 [20]. When satellite cells are stimulated by muscle damage, they are activated, and they proliferate, differentiate, and supply new muscle fiber and nuclei [20]. Some cells then return to the resting state [20]. Many studies have demonstrated that growth factors such as HGF are associated with activation and proliferation of myoblasts [21]. Furthermore, MyoD and myogenin are expressed when satellite cells are activated, and they proliferate, or differentiate [20]. In the rats that received only damaging ECC, HGF, Pax7, MyoD, and myogenin mRNA expression increased after damaging ECC, suggesting a functional muscle regeneration mechanism, whereas these increases were not observed in the Precon group, suggesting that prior Precon reduced the degree of muscle damage, leading to only a slight need for muscle regeneration. Damage by vigorous ECC has been clarified by indirect analysis (serum creatine kinase) [1, 2] and histological analysis [22–24]. In our study, the muscle was

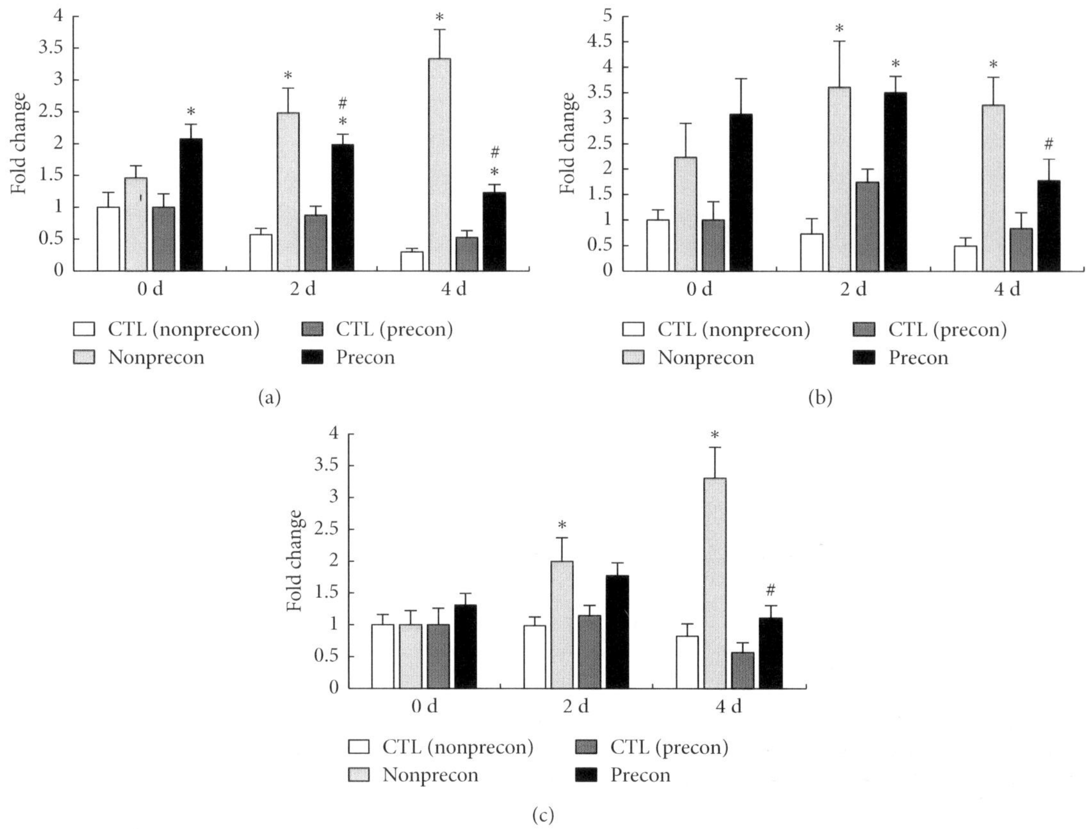

Figure 4: Time course changes in relative expression of BKB_2 receptor (a), COX-2 (b), and mPGES-1 (c) mRNA. The mRNA expression of each time point was calculated as x-fold change from each CTL value at 0 d. CTL indicates intact right muscle of each experimental group. Values are means ± SE. *significant differences ($P < 0.05$) as compared with each CTL value. #significant differences ($P < 0.05$) as compared with each non-Precon value.

damaged in the group only with damaging ECC, confirming that Precon markedly reduced the degree of damage at the mRNA expression level.

4.2. Muscle Pain Markers Induced by Eccentric Contraction. PGE_2 increases in skeletal muscle during dynamic exercise, but it does not increase during static exercise [25]. An enzyme in the PGE_2 synthetic pathway, COX-2, is highly involved in muscle pain. In fact, COX-2 inhibitors can reduce muscle pain when it is applied before lengthening contraction [11, 12]. In addition, the final enzyme of PGE_2 synthesis, mPGES-1, also produces PGE_2 from COX-2-derived metabolites [13] and is also involved in PGE_2-induced pain and inflammation [26]. Therefore, COX-2 and mPGES-1 may induce muscle pain through PGE_2 production. In inflammation, COX-2 is expressed in neutrophils, macrophages, endothelial cells, and muscle nuclei/muscle satellite cells [11, 27, 28]. mPGES-1 has been reported to be localized in macrophages and fibroblasts during inflammation [29, 30]. In the present study, Precon suppressed COX-2 and mPGES-1 mRNA expression, indicating decreased PGE2 production. Accordingly, muscle pain due to PGE_2 may have been reduced in the Precon group compared with in the non-Precon group.

Eccentric exercise elevates the blood [31] and interstitial BK levels in skeletal muscle and tendon tissue [32]. There are 2 types of BK receptors: BKB_1 and BKB_2. The BKB_1 receptor is expressed when tissue is damaged and contributes to chronic inflammation, whereas the BKB_2 receptor is constantly expressed and considered to be involved in acute inflammation [33–35]. BKB_2 receptor mRNA expression was decreased by Precon 2 and 4 days after damaging ECC. In a previous study, muscle pain developed in the intact leg from 1 to 4 days after eccentric contraction, but when a BKB_2 receptor antagonist was administered before eccentric contraction, later muscle pain was suppressed, whereas the BKB_1 receptor antagonist exerted no muscle pain-inhibitory effects [36]. In an inflammation model induced by intramuscular injection of formalin, both BKB_1 and B_2 receptor antagonists demonstrated muscle pain-inhibitory effects from immediately after formalin injection to 7 hours later, but only the B_2 receptor antagonist reduced IL-6 mRNA expression [10]. IL-6 is an inflammatory marker that has been suggested to contribute to muscle pain [37, 38]. Thus, the BKB_2 receptor may be more closely involved in muscle pain from inflammation compared with the B_1 receptor. In addition, administration of a BKB_2 receptor antagonist 30 minutes after ECC did not suppress muscle pain, suggesting that the BKB_2 receptor functions in the development of muscle pain rather than the maintenance of muscle pain [36]. In this study, BKB2 receptor mRNA expression showed significant increase at 0 day (immediately after damaging ECC). However, BKB2 receptor mRNA expression of the non-Precon group gradually increased while those of the Precon group showed gradual decrease, suggesting that the peak of pain marker shifted to the left in the Precon group. Although we could not prove whether the peak shift of BKB2 receptor mRNA expression directly relate to muscle pain, the mRNA expression of the Precon group was suppressed in accordance with other muscle pain-related molecules and histopathological damage at 2 and 4 days after damaging ECC.

In summary, we found that the BKB2 receptor which plays an important role in muscle pain significantly increased after eccentric contraction and the expression of mRNA was suppressed by prior low-load ECC in relatively early stage.

4.3. Influence of Preconditioning on Training Effect. ECC- and pre-exercise-induced muscle damage, muscle regeneration, and muscle pain were investigated. Our results suggest that prior light ECC reduces muscle damage caused by later damaging ECC and accompanying muscle regeneration and suppresses muscle pain at the mRNA expression level. Based on these findings, in order to reduce exercise-induced muscle pain, prior light exercise may be preferable. However, to improve muscle function, prior light exercise may reduce the later training effects because Precon suppressed mRNA expression of a muscle satellite cell marker, Pax7, which plays an important role in muscular hypertrophy, as well as MyoD and myogenin, which are involved in proliferation and differentiation of satellite cells [20]. In addition, the importance of COX-2 for muscular hypertrophy has been reported using a compensatory muscular hypertrophy model with a COX-2 inhibitor [28]. Thus, suppression of COX-2 expression and activity may be a good method to reduce muscle pain, but COX-2 expression and activity may be necessary when the objective is muscular hypertrophy. Further studies on the long-term effects are necessary.

Acknowledgments

This work was supported in part by a grant from the Japanese Ministry of Education, Science and Culture (Nos. 17J08086 and 16H03221).

References

[1] N. Nelson, "Delayed onset muscle soreness: is massage effective?," *Journal of Bodywork and Movement Therapies*, vol. 17, no. 4, pp. 475–482, 2013.

[2] T. C. Chen, H. L. Chen, A. J. Pearce, and K. Nosaka, "Attenuation of eccentric exercise-induced muscle damage by preconditioning exercises," *Medicine & Science in Sports & Exercise*, vol. 44, no. 11, pp. 2090–2098, 2012.

[3] R. D. Hyldahl and M. J. Hubal, "Lengthening our perspective: morphological, cellular, and molecular responses to eccentric exercise," *Muscle & Nerve*, vol. 49, no. 2, pp. 155–170, 2014.

[4] M. Roig, K. O'Brien, G. Kirk et al., "The effects of eccentric versus concentric resistance training on muscle strength and mass in healthy adults: a systematic review with meta-analysis," *British Journal of Sports Medicine*, vol. 43, no. 8, pp. 556–568, 2009.

[5] N. Hedayatpour and D. Falla, "Physiological and neural adaptations to eccentric exercise: mechanisms and considerations for training," *BioMed Research International*, vol. 2015, Article ID 193741, 7 pages, 2015.

[6] A. P. Lavender and K. Nosaka, "A light load eccentric exercise confers protection against a subsequent bout of more demanding eccentric exercise," *Journal of Science and Medicine in Sport*, vol. 11, no. 3, pp. 291–298, 2008.

[7] S. Maeo, M. Yamamoto, H. Kanehisa, and K. Nosaka, "Prevention of downhill walking-induced muscle damage by non-damaging downhill walking," *PLoS One*, vol. 12, no. 3, Article ID e0173909, 2017.

[8] H. Urai, S. Murase, and K. Mizumura, "Decreased nerve growth factor upregulation is a mechanism for reduced mechanical hyperalgesia after the second bout of exercise in rats," *Scandinavian Journal of Medicine & Science in Sports*, vol. 23, no. 2, pp. e96–e101, 2013.

[9] K. Nosaka, K. Sakamoto, M. Newton, and P. Sacco, "How long does the protective effect on eccentric exercise-induced muscle damage last?," *Medicine & Science in Sports & Exercise*, vol. 33, no. 9, pp. 1490–1495, 2001.

[10] F. C. Meotti, R. Campos, K. da Silva, A. F. Paszcuk, R. Costa, and J. B. Calixto, "Inflammatory muscle pain is dependent on the activation of kinin B_1 and B_2 receptors and intracellular kinase pathways," *British Journal of Pharmacology*, vol. 166, no. 3, pp. 1127–1139, 2012.

[11] S. Murase, E. Terazawa, K. Hirate et al., "Upregulated glial cell line-derived neurotrophic factor through cyclooxygenase-2 activation in the muscle is required for mechanical hyperalgesia after exercise in rats," *Journal of Physiology*, vol. 591, no. 12, pp. 3035–3048, 2013.

[12] Y. Zhang, A. Shaffer, J. Portanova, K. Seibert, and P. C. Isakson, "Inhibition of cyclooxygenase-2 rapidly reverses inflammatory hyperalgesia and prostaglandin E2 production," *Journal of Pharmacology and Experimental Therapeutics*, vol. 283, no. 3, pp. 1069–1075, 1997.

[13] B. Samuelsson, R. Morgenstern, and P. J. Jakobsson, "Membrane prostaglandin E synthase-1: a novel therapeutic target," *Pharmacological Reviews*, vol. 59, no. 3, pp. 207–224, 2007.

[14] M. K. Hesselink, H. Kuipers, P. Geurten, and H. Van Straaten, "Structural muscle damage and muscle strength after incremental number of isometric and forced lengthening contractions," *Journal of Muscle Research & Cell Motility*, vol. 17, no. 3, pp. 335–341, 1996.

[15] M. E. Willems and W. T. Stauber, "The effect of number of lengthening contractions on rat isometric force production at

different frequencies of nerve stimulation," *Acta Physiologica*, vol. 196, no. 3, pp. 351–356, 2009.

[16] H. Nagahisa, K. Okabe, Y. Iuchi, J. Fujii, and H. Miyata, "Characteristics of skeletal muscle fibers of SOD1 knockout mice," *Oxidative Medicine and Cellular Longevity*, vol. 2016, Article ID 9345970, 8 pages, 2016.

[17] R. Yamada, K. Himori, D. Tatebayashi et al., "Preconditioning contractions prevent the delayed onset of myofibrillar dysfunction after damaging eccentric contractions," *Journal of Physiology*, vol. 596, no. 18, pp. 4427–4442, 2018.

[18] S. Schiaffino, A. C. Rossi, V. Smerdu, L. A. Leinwand, and C. Reggiani, "Developmental myosins: expression patterns and functional significance," *Skeletal Muscle*, vol. 5, p. 22, 2015.

[19] S. Ciciliot and S. Schiaffino, "Regeneration of mammalian skeletal muscle. Basic mechanisms and clinical implications," *Current Pharmaceutical Design*, vol. 16, no. 8, pp. 906–914, 2010.

[20] N. A. Dumont, Y. X. Wang, and M. A. Rudnicki, "Intrinsic and extrinsic mechanisms regulating satellite cell function," *Development*, vol. 142, no. 9, pp. 1572–1581, 2015.

[21] M. Yamada, R. Tatsumi, K. Yamanouchi et al., "High concentrations of HGF inhibit skeletal muscle satellite cell proliferation in vitro by inducing expression of myostatin: a possible mechanism for reestablishing satellite cell quiescence in vivo," *American Journal of Physiology-Cell Physiology*, vol. 298, no. 3, pp. C465–C476, 2010.

[22] Y. Kano, K. Masuda, H. Furukawa, M. Sudo, K. Mito, and K. Sakamoto, "Histological skeletal muscle damage and surface EMG relationships following eccentric contractions," *Journal of Physiological Sciences*, vol. 58, no. 5, pp. 349–355, 2008.

[23] M. Sudo and Y. Kano, "Myofiber apoptosis occurs in the inflammation and regeneration phase following eccentric contractions in rats," *Journal of Physiological Sciences*, vol. 59, no. 6, pp. 405–412, 2009.

[24] R. D. Hyldahl, T. Olson, T. Welling, L. Groscost, and A. C. Parcell, "Satellite cell activity is differentially affected by contraction mode in human muscle following a work-matched bout of exercise," *Frontiers in Physiology*, vol. 5, p. 485, 2014.

[25] M. Karamouzis, H. Langberg, D. Skovgaard, J. Bulow, M. Kjaer, and B. Saltin, "In situ microdialysis of intramuscular prostaglandin and thromboxane in contracting skeletal muscle in humans," *Acta Physiologica Scandinavica*, vol. 171, no. 1, pp. 71–76, 2001.

[26] M. Dallaporta, E. Pecchi, S. Thirion, A. Jean, and J. D. Troadec, "Toward the management of inflammation: recent developments of mPGES-1 inhibitors," *Recent Patents on CNS Drug Discovery*, vol. 5, no. 1, pp. 70–80, 2010.

[27] T. Bachawaty, S. L. Washington, and S. W. Walsh, "Neutrophil expression of cyclooxygenase 2 in preeclampsia," *Reproductive Sciences*, vol. 17, no. 5, pp. 465–470, 2010.

[28] M. L. Novak, W. Billich, S. M. Smith et al., "COX-2 inhibitor reduces skeletal muscle hypertrophy in mice," *American Journal of Physiology-Regulatory, Integrative and Comparative Physiology*, vol. 296, no. 4, pp. R1132–R1139, 2009.

[29] M. Korotkova, S. B. Helmers, I. Loell et al., "Effects of immunosuppressive treatment on microsomal prostaglandin E synthase 1 and cyclooxygenases expression in muscle tissue of patients with polymyositis or dermatomyositis," *Annals of the Rheumatic Diseases*, vol. 67, no. 11, pp. 1596–1602, 2008.

[30] M. Korotkova and P. J. Jakobsson, "Microsomal prostaglandin e synthase-1 in rheumatic diseases," *Frontiers in Pharmacology*, vol. 1, p. 146, 2011.

[31] C. Blais Jr., A. Adam, D. Massicotte, and F. Péronnet, "Increase in blood bradykinin concentration after eccentric weight-training exercise in men," *Journal of Applied Physiology*, vol. 87, no. 3, pp. 1197–1201, 1999.

[32] H. Langberg, C. Bjørn, R. Boushel, Y. Hellsten, and M. Kjaer, "Exercise-induced increase in interstitial bradykinin and adenosine concentrations in skeletal muscle and peritendinous tissue in humans," *Journal of Physiology*, vol. 542, no. 3, pp. 977–983, 2002.

[33] M. Hamza, X. M. Wang, A. Adam et al., "Kinin B1 receptors contributes to acute pain following minor surgery in humans," *Molecular Pain*, vol. 6, p. 12, 2010.

[34] J. B. Su, "Different cross-talk sites between the renin-angiotensin and the kallikrein-kinin systems," *Journal of the Renin-Angiotensin-Aldosterone System*, vol. 15, no. 4, pp. 319–328, 2014.

[35] R. Couture, M. Harrisson, R. M. Vianna, and F. Cloutier, "Kinin receptors in pain and inflammation," *European Journal of Pharmacology*, vol. 429, no. 1–3, pp. 161–176, 2001.

[36] S. Murase, E. Terazawa, F. Queme et al., "Bradykinin and nerve growth factor play pivotal roles in muscular mechanical hyperalgesia after exercise (delayed-onset muscle soreness)," *Journal of Neuroscience*, vol. 30, no. 10, pp. 3752–3761, 2010.

[37] O. A. Dina, P. G. Green, and J. D. Levine, "Role of interleukin-6 in chronic muscle hyperalgesic priming," *Neuroscience*, vol. 152, no. 2, pp. 521–525, 2008.

[38] M. N. Manjavachi, E. M. Motta, D. M. Marotta, D. F. Leite, and J. B. Calixto, "Mechanisms involved in IL-6-induced muscular mechanical hyperalgesia in mice," *Pain*, vol. 151, no. 2, pp. 345–355, 2010.

7

Physical Activity and Sleep in Chronic Fatigue Syndrome and Fibromyalgia Syndrome: Associations with Symptom Severity in the General Population Cohort LifeLines

Monica L. Joustra,[1] Wilma L. Zijlema,[1] Judith G. M. Rosmalen,[1,2] and Karin A. M. Janssens[1]

[1] *University of Groningen, University Medical Center Groningen, Department of Psychiatry, Groningen, Netherlands*
[2] *University of Groningen, University Medical Center Groningen, Department of Internal Medicine, Groningen, Netherlands*

Correspondence should be addressed to Monica L. Joustra; m.l.joustra@umcg.nl

Academic Editor: Virginia A. Aparicio

Objective. The aim of the current study was to compare physical activity and sleep duration between patients with chronic fatigue syndrome (CFS), patients with fibromyalgia syndrome (FMS), and controls and to examine the association between physical activity level and sleep duration with symptom severity within these patient groups. *Methods.* This study used data of LifeLines, a general population cohort in which 1.0% ($n = 943$, 63.7% female, age 44.9 (SD 11.6) years) reported CFS, 3.0% ($n = 2,714$; 91.6% female; age 48.4 (SD 10.7) years) reported FMS, and 95.7% ($n = 87,532$; 57.9% female; age 44.3 (SD 12.4) years) reported neither CFS nor FMS. Physical activity, sleep duration, and symptom severity were assessed by questionnaires and analysed using ANCOVA and regression analyses, adjusted for age, sex, body mass index, smoking, and educational level. *Results.* Patients with CFS and FMS had significantly lower physical activity scores (8834 ± 5967 and 8813 ± 5549 MET $*$ minutes) than controls (9541 ± 5533; $p < 0.001$). Patients with CFS had the longest sleep duration (466 ± 86 minutes) compared to patients with FMS and controls (450 ± 67 and 446 ± 56; $p < 0.001$). A linear association between physical activity, sleep duration, and symptom severity was only found in controls, in whom higher physical total activity scores and longer sleep duration were associated with a lower symptom severity. In contrast, quadratic associations were found in all groups: both relatively low and high physical activity scores and relatively short and long sleep duration were associated with higher symptom severity in CFS, FMS, and controls. *Conclusion.* This study indicates that patients with CFS or FMS sleep longer and are less physically active than controls on average. Both low and high levels of physical activity and short and long sleep duration are associated with higher symptom severity, suggesting the importance of patient-tailored treatment.

1. Introduction

Functional somatic syndromes (FSS), including chronic fatigue syndrome (CFS) and fibromyalgia syndrome (FMS), are common, disabling, and costly health conditions without known underlying organic pathology [1–4]. CFS is an illness characterised by profound disabling unexplained fatigue [5], while the primary complaint of patients with FMS is unexplained musculoskeletal pain [6]. Both core symptoms are typically accompanied by various additional symptoms. The etiology of CFS and FMS is assumed to be multifactorial including biological, psychological, and social contributing factors [7].

The role of physical activity and sleep in the pathophysiology of CFS and FMS is not well understood. Regarding physical effort, various studies have evaluated the ability of patients with CFS or FMS to perform physical activity, but the results are conflicting [8–10]. There are also different approaches in the way individuals with CFS and FMS cope with physical activity. Recent research suggests that both avoidance of activity and overactivity are associated with an increase in symptom severity, including pain and fatigue [9, 11, 12]. This indicates that, in patients with CFS and FMS, both high and low levels of physical activity may result in higher symptom severity, comparable to what is observed in the general population [13]. Regarding recovery, sleep difficulties have been associated with negative effects on pain and fatigue [14, 15]. A study found that nights with an unusually long or short sleep duration resulted in greater fatigue and that moderate sleep duration was associated with the least fatigue [15]. As with physical activity, an association between sleep duration and symptom severity may thus exist in these patient groups [16].

CFS and FMS are known for substantial clinical and diagnostic overlap. The two conditions are comorbid: 35% to 75% of patients with CFS met the criteria for FMS [17]. This phenomenon resulted in the lumper-splitter discussion [18]. "Lumpers" believe that all FSS result from the same etiology, and "splitters" take the approach that every separate FSS has its own specific background. It is not known to which extent patients with CFS and FMS differ with regard to physical activity and sleep. Studies that compare these associations between patients of one population-based cohort are, to the best of our knowledge, lacking.

The aim of this study was to examine whether patients with CFS, patients with FMS, and controls have different levels of physical activity and sleep duration. Furthermore, we will examine the degree to which physical activity or sleep duration is associated with the severity of physical symptoms, in CFS, FMS, or controls. We hypothesize that both too much and too little physical activity and sleep are related to symptom severity and expect this association to be stronger in patients with CFS and FMS than controls. Furthermore, we hypothesize that CFS is more strongly related to sleep difficulties and FMS is more strongly related to physical activity. These hypotheses were tested within LifeLines, a large population-based cohort study.

2. Materials and Methods

2.1. The Sample. This study is conducted within the sampling frame of the LifeLines cohort study [19–21], a general population cohort in which 1.0% ($n = 943$; 63.7% female; age 44.9 (SD 11.6) years) reported CFS, 3.0% ($n = 2,714$; 91.6% female; age 48.4 (SD 10.7) years) reported FMS, and 95.7% ($n = 87,532$; 57.9% female; age 44.3 (SD 12.4) years) reported neither CFS nor FMS. The LifeLines cohort study is a multidisciplinary prospective population-based cohort study with a unique three-generation design. LifeLines aims to examine the health and health-related behaviours of more than 167,000 persons living in the North East region of the Netherlands, with a special focus on multimorbidity and complex genetics. It uses a broad range of research procedures to assess biomedical, sociodemographics behavioural, physical, and psychological factors that contribute to health and/or disease of the general population.

2.1.1. Participants. Participants were recruited in two different ways. First, participants aged 25–50 years were invited through a number of general practitioners from the three northern provinces of the Netherlands. Second, persons who were interested to participate in the study could register themselves via the LifeLines website. Patients who agreed to participate were asked to invite their partner, parents, parents-in-law, and children to as well participate in the LifeLines cohort study. Therefore, participants of all age were included in the study. General practitioners evaluated eligibility for participation, whereby persons with severe psychiatric or physical illness, and those not being able to visit the general practitioner and to fill in the LifeLines questionnaires, and/or persons those who did not understand the Dutch language were excluded from the study. However, children and parents were not excluded in the case of the mentioned exclusion criteria, when a representative was willing to assist these persons in the performance of the study. In case of pregnancy, participation was rescheduled until 6 months after pregnancy or 3 months after breastfeeding.

The LifeLines cohort study obtained approval by the Medical Ethical Committee of the University Medical Center Groningen. All participants received written information on the purpose and methods of the LifeLines cohort study. Written informed consent of participants was obtained after the procedure of the LifeLines cohort study was fully explained. Data of the LifeLines cohort study are kept confidential and are only used for medical research.

2.2. Measures

2.2.1. Chronic Fatigue Syndrome and Fibromyalgia Syndrome. CFS and FMS were assessed by means of a self-report questionnaire, including a list of chronic disorders including CFS and FMS. The participants were asked to indicate which of these disorders they had or have had. More than one answer to this question was allowed. Participants who reported both CFS and FMS were excluded ($n = 264$), since we were interested in differences between both conditions. Controls were defined by the absence of CFS and FMS.

2.2.2. Physical Activity and Sleep Duration. Physical activity was assessed by means of the validated Short Questionnaire to Assess Health-enhancing physical activity (SQUASH) [22]. This self-report questionnaire assesses physical activity undertaken in an average week in the past months across a set of domains. These domains include commuting activities (walking or bicycling to/from work or school), leisure-time activities (walking, bicycling, gardening, and odd jobs), sports activities, household activities, and activities at work and school. It is a reliable and valid questionnaire [22]. The SQUASH discusses three questions per activity: days per week of the activity (frequency), average time per day (duration in minutes), and intensity of the activity. The intensity of the physical activity was scored on a 3-point scale ranging between (1) "*Slow*," (2) "*Moderate*," and (3) "*Fast*."

The answers collected with the SQUASH can be examined as a continuous measure by weighting each type of activity by its energy requirements defined in intensity scores, also referred to as metabolic equivalent of tasks (METs). METs are defined as multiples of the resting metabolic rate, thus the energy expenditure at rest. Selected MET values are derived using the Ainsworth's Compendium of Physical Activities [23]. Based on age and assigned MET values, physical activities were subdivided into three intensity categories: light, moderate, and vigorous. For adults aged 18–54 years, the following cutoff values were used: <4.0 MET (light intensity), 4.0 to 6.5 MET (moderate intensity), and ≥6.5 MET (vigorous intensity), and for adults aged ≥55 years, these cutoff values were <3.0 MET (light), 3.0 to 5.0 MET (moderate), and ≥5.0 MET (vigorous). The three MET categories were combined with self-reported intensity for each activity, resulting in a combined intensity score ranging from 1 to 9, with 1 being light MET and light self-reported intensity and 9 being vigorous MET and vigorous self-reported intensity. The classification of physical activities according to the combined intensity score was <3 (light intensity), 3 to 6 (moderate intensity), and ≥6 (vigorous intensity). The physical activity scores of the different domains were calculated by multiplying duration (minutes per week) with the MET value, taking into account the combined intensity score. Subjects with unlikely values were excluded if separate activity categories exceeded plausible values, more than two activity categories of the questionnaire were missing, and/or ≥18 hours/day were spent on all activities together.

Sleep duration was assessed using the question: "How many minutes do you sleep on average per day?"

2.2.3. Symptom Severity. Symptom severity was assessed with the 12-item somatization scale of the Symptom CheckList-90 (SCL-90 SOM) [24]. The SOM scale measures self-reported intensity of somatic symptoms. This scale consists of 12 somatic symptoms, including a lump in your throat, faintness or dizziness, feeling weak in parts of your body, headaches, heavy feelings in arms or legs, hot or cold spells, nausea or upset stomach, numbness or tingling in your body, pains in heart or chest, pains in lower back, soreness of your muscles, and trouble getting your breath. Participants were asked to what extent they have been limited by these somatic symptoms in the past seven days. The somatic symptoms were scored on a 5-point scale ranging from (1) "*Not at all*" to (5) "*Extremely.*" An additional item assessing fatigue was used from the RAND-36 [25]: "How much of the time during the past four weeks did you feel tired?" This item was scored on a six-point scale ranging from (1) "*All of the time*" to (6) "*None of the time.*" The fatigue score was transformed to a 5-point scale with (1) "*None of the time*" to (5) "*All of the time,*" with a combined score of (3) "*A good bit of the time*" and (4) "*Some of the time*" into (3) "*quite a bit*" to obtain consistency with the SOM scale. Symptom severity was calculated by taking the mean score of the 13 somatic symptoms. Therefore, the total symptom severity ranged from (1) all symptoms endorsed as "*Not at all or none of the time*" to (5) all symptoms endorsed as "*Extremely or all of the time.*"

2.2.4. Covariates. Length in centimetres and weight in kilograms were assessed during a basic medical examination at a local LifeLines research facility. Subsequently, body mass index (BMI) was calculated as kg/m^2. The smoking status was assessed using the following question: "Do you smoke now, or have you smoked in the past month?" Participants could fill in "*yes*" or "*no.*" Educational level was assessed using the following question: "What is your highest completed education?," resulting in information about low, middle, and high educational level. Low educational level was defined as lower secondary education or less, middle educational level was defined as higher secondary education, and high educational level was defined as tertiary education.

2.3. Statistical Analyses. For all continuous variables, means ± standard deviations (SDs) were calculated. One-way analyses of variance (ANOVA) were performed for continuous data, to test the differences in sample characteristics. Differences in symptom severity were also investigated between males and females within the different study groups. In addition, χ^2 tests were performed for categorical data. For continuous variables, analyses of covariance (ANCOVA) with post hoc Bonferroni correction were performed to examine differences in physical activity level and sleep duration between patients with CFS, patients with FMS, and controls. In addition, sex differences in physical activity and sleep duration were explored. Linear and quadratic regression analyses were conducted using standardized variables to examine how physical activity and sleep duration were associated with symptom severity in the different groups. Four regression models were performed: both linear and regression analyses for physical activity and for sleep duration. All analyses were adjusted for age, sex, BMI, smoking status, and educational level, since they are known to be related to CFS [26, 27], FMS [28–30], physical activity [31, 32], and sleep [33, 34]. All analyses were performed using SPSS version 20. Statistical significance was defined as $p < 0.05$.

3. Results

3.1. Sample Characteristics. Data were available for 91,453 participants; descriptives, including age, BMI, education, SOM score, sex, and smoking, are shown in Table 1. Of these participants, 1.0% ($n = 943$) reported CFS, 3.0% ($n = 2,714$) reported FMS, and 95.7% ($n = 87,532$) reported neither CFS nor FMS. Women were most prevalent in all groups. The mean age varied between 44.3 ± 12.4 for controls, 44.9 ± 11.9 for patients with CFS, and 48.4 ± 10.7 years for patients with FMS. Female CFS patients and controls reported significantly higher symptom severity (2.1 ± 0.6 and 1.5 ± 0.4, respectively) compared to males (1.9 ± 0.6 and 1.4 ± 0.3), while no difference in symptom severity was found in female FMS patients (2.0 ± 0.5) compared to male FMS patients (1.9 ± 0.5).

3.2. Physical Activity and Sleep Duration. Physical activity levels in patients with CFS, patients with FMS, and controls

TABLE 1: Sample characteristics.

	CFS	FMS	Controls	Pairwise comparisons[c]; p value: CFS vs FMS	CFS vs controls	FMS vs controls
Mean (SD)						
Number (%)	943 (1.0)	2714 (3.0)	87532 (95.7)			
Age[a]	44.9 (11.6)	48.4 (10.7)	44.3 (12.4)	<0.001	0.137	<0.001
BMI (kg/m^2)[a]	26.4 (4.8)	27.8 (5.3)	26.0 (4.3)	<0.001	0.407	<0.001
Symptom severity (1–5)[a]	2.0 (0.6)	2.0 (0.5)	1.5 (0.4)	0.038	<0.001	<0.001
n (%)						
Education[b]						
Low	319 (33.8)	1193 (44.0)	25,418 (29.0)	<0.001	<0.001	<0.001
Middle	377 (40.0)	1055 (38.9)	34,211 (39.1)			
High	213 (22.6)	377 (13.9)	25,697 (29.7)			
Female[b]	601 (63.7)	2485 (91.6)	50,705 (57.9)	<0.001	<0.001	<0.001
Smoking[b]	257 (27.3)	609 (22.4)	18,520 (21.2)	0.002	<0.001	0.145

CFS = chronic fatigue syndrome; FMS = fibromyalgia syndrome. [a]ANOVA; [b]χ^2 test; [c]Bonferroni correction for continuous and χ^2 test for categorical variables.

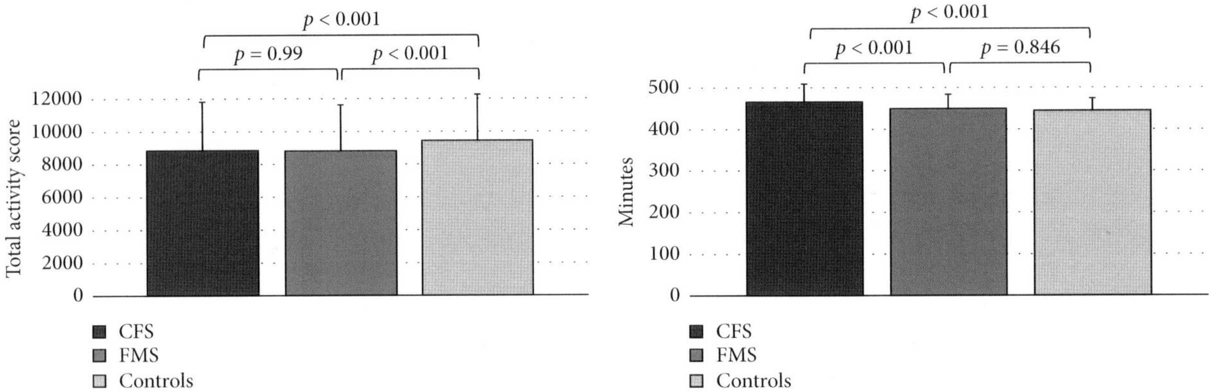

(a) (b)

FIGURE 1: (a) Physical activity. (b) Sleep duration. CFS = chronic fatigue syndrome; FMS = fibromyalgia syndrome. Analyses of covariance and Bonferroni correction were done, adjusted for age, sex, BMI, smoking, and education.

are shown in Figure 1(a). ANCOVA analysis revealed significant groups' differences ($F(7, 76182) = 303$, $p < 0.001$). Post hoc comparisons with Bonferroni correction indicated that patients with CFS and FMS had a significantly lower physical total activity score than controls (8834 ± 5967 and 8813 ± 5549 MET ∗ minutes, respectively, versus 9541 ± 5533; both $p < 0.001$). There was no significant difference in physical total activity score between patients with CFS and FMS ($p = 0.99$). Lastly, males were significantly more physically active than females among all three study groups.

Sleep duration in patients with CFS, patients with FMS, and controls is shown in Figure 1(b). ANCOVA analysis revealed significant groups' differences ($F(7, 39438) = 222$, $p \leq 0.001$). Post hoc comparisons with Bonferroni correction indicated that patients with CFS had the longest sleep duration (466 ± 86 minutes) compared to patients with FMS and controls (450 ± 67 and 446 ± 56, respectively, both $p < 0.001$), while no difference was found between patients with FMS and controls ($p = 0.846$). Furthermore, female CFS patients and controls reported significantly longer sleep duration (474 ± 84 and 453 ± 59 minutes, respectively) than males in the corresponding groups (453 ± 87 and 437 ± 50 minutes), while no difference in sleep duration was found between female FMS patients (451 ± 66 minutes) and male FMS patients (442 ± 80 minutes).

3.3. Physical Activity or Sleep Duration Associated with Symptom Severity. Physical activity and sleep duration showed both linear and quadratic associations with symptom severity. Results of both linear and quadratic regression analyses are shown in Table 2. Linear regression analyses showed that, only in controls, physical total activity score (model 1) and sleep duration (model 2) were related to symptom severity; controls with a higher physical total activity score or longer sleep duration reported a slightly lower symptom severity. No significant linear associations were found in patients with CFS or FMS between physical total activity score or sleep duration and symptom severity.

Quadratic regression analyses indicated a significant association between total physical activity score in CFS, FMS, and controls (model 3). Both linear and quadratic terms were significant in FMS and controls, and only the quadratic term, but not the linear, was significant in CFS. Thus, patients with CFS, patients with FMS, and controls

Table 2: Associations between physical activity, sleep duration, and symptom severity.

	CFS		FMS		Controls	
	B	95% CI	*B*	95% CI	*B*	95% CI
Linear						
(1) Physical total activity score	−0.007	−0.047, 0.032	−0.009	−0.031, 0.012	−0.007**	−0.009, −0.004
(2) Sleep duration	−0.005	−0.045, 0.036	−0.009	−0.036, 0.017	−0.004*	−0.008, −0.001
Quadratic						
(3) Physical total activity score (linear term)	−0.042	−0.091, 0.008	−0.046**	−0.073, −0.020	−0.009**	−0.012, −0.006
Physical total activity score (quadratic term)	0.020*	0.003, 0.038	0.019**	0.011, 0.027	0.001**	0.001, 0.002
(4) Sleep duration (linear term)	−0.045*	−0.089, 0.00	−0.021	−0.047, 0.005	−0.007**	−0.011, −0.003
Sleep duration (quadratic term)	0.017**	0.008, 0.025	0.040**	0.031, 0.049	0.00**	0.00, 0.00

CFS = chronic fatigue syndrome; FMS = fibromyalgia syndrome. $^{*}p \leq 0.05$; $^{**}p \leq 0.001$. Multivariable regression analyses were done, adjusted for age, sex, BMI, smoking, and education.

with relatively low and high physical activity scores reported higher symptom severity than those with moderate physical activity scores. Furthermore, all three groups showed significant quadratic associations between sleep duration and symptom severity (model 4). Both linear and quadratic sleep terms were significant in patients with CFS and controls, while only the quadratic but not the linear sleep term was significant in patients with FMS. Thus, patients with CFS, patients with FMS, and controls with short or long sleep duration reported a higher symptom severity than those with moderate sleep duration.

4. Discussion

This study revealed that patients with CFS and FMS were significantly less physically active than controls. Furthermore, patients with CFS reported longer sleep duration than patients with FMS and controls. Only in controls, physical total activity score and sleep duration were linearly related to symptom severity, with both higher physical total activity score and higher sleep duration being associated with slightly lower symptom severity. Quadratic associations were present in all groups; both relatively high and low physical activity levels were associated with higher symptom severity in patients with CFS, patients with FMS, and controls; and both relatively long and short sleep duration were associated with higher symptom severity in patients with CFS, patients with FMS, and controls.

The main strength of this study is the large population cohort. To the best of our knowledge, this is the first study that evaluates physical activity and sleep duration in patients with CFS and FMS in one large population cohort. A sufficient number of patients with CFS and FMS were identified, allowing for meaningful statistical comparisons. Moreover, the large number of patients enabled examining the association between sleep duration, physical activity, and symptom severity in CFS, FMS, and controls. Both patients and controls with different physical activity or sleep duration outcomes were therefore present in the cohort. Finally, since LifeLines is a large cohort study with extensive measurements, adjusting for important covariates such as age, sex, BMI, smoking status, and educational level was possible.

Our study also contained limitations, including the use of a self-report questionnaire for the assessment of CFS and FMS. Instead of current diagnoses, our questionnaire asked for a history of CFS and FMS. A previous study in a general population cohort from the same geographical area indicated that about 75% and 100% of the participants that reported a history of CFS and FMS, respectively, still had this syndrome at the time of reporting [35]. In addition, self-reports may underestimate the amount of persons with FSS. This seems not likely in our study because the prevalence rates for CFS and FMS were comparable to previous studies [27, 29]. Moreover, the majority of the patients with CFS and FMS in the current study recently experienced fatigue and musculoskeletal pain. Furthermore, subjective measurements were used to assess sleep duration and physical activity, instead of objective measures. For example, sleep duration was assessed using a single question, so participants may have interpreted this differently (e.g., time in bed, actual time sleep, and inclusion of naps). A final limitation is that the cross-sectional design did not allow conclusions on cause-and-effect relationships.

In line with previous findings, this study revealed that both patients with CFS and FMS were significantly less physically active than controls [36, 37]. However, it should be mentioned that self-reported questionnaires to assess physical activity levels in these patient groups have shown a low reliability [38, 39]. In contrast to our hypothesis, no difference in physical activity was found between patients with CFS and FMS. Lower activity levels in patients with CFS or FMS might be explained by the substantial limitations in physical functioning that may be caused by their symptoms [9]. In addition, a lack of physical activity might also contribute to physical deconditioning, further increasing symptom severity [12, 40]. We found that both low and high physical activity levels in patients with CFS, patients with FMS, and controls were associated with the reporting of more symptoms. This finding stresses the close relationship between physical activity and the experience of symptoms. Thus, on the one hand, low activity levels may be associated with the experience of more and more severe symptoms, while on the other hand, high physical activity level may exacerbate symptoms in CFS and FMS [9, 11, 12].

Differences between patients with CFS and FMS were found for sleep duration, since patients with CFS were found to report longer sleep duration than patients with FMS and controls. However, misestimation of sleep duration appears common in patients with CFS and FMS, particularly in patients having a poor sleep quality [41, 42]. Nevertheless, our results are in accordance with our hypothesis and might be due to the primary complaint of disabling fatigue in patients with CFS [5, 43, 44]. Furthermore, our results are in line with a recent study that reported that nights with an unusually long or short sleep duration resulted in greater fatigue, and that moderate sleep duration was associated with the least fatigue [15].

Our study also revealed differences between patients, as illustrated by the finding of quadratic associations of symptom severity with physical activity and sleep. These quadratic associations indicate that the pathophysiological role of physical activity and sleep varies not only between but also within patient groups with CFS or FMS. Treatment aimed at reducing symptoms might therefore better be tailored to individual patients. This is mainly important since both CFS and FMS are characterised both by non-restorative sleep and intolerance to physical exercise. Since the LifeLines cohort is a large population cohort study that aims to study a wide spectrum of mental and somatic disorders, it was not feasible to more extensively assess lifestyle factors such as physical activity and sleep in CFS and FMS during the baseline assessment because of practical limitations. We aim to include objectively measured lifestyle factors in CFS and FMS in future assessment waves. Further studies will be necessary to determine the effect of objectively measured physical activity or sleep duration, by using, for instance, polysomnography or accelerometers. Furthermore, the association between sleep duration and symptom severity was found to vary between different patients. Therefore, studies that evaluate how sleep duration and physical activity are related to symptom severity within individual patients, so called idiographic research [45], is recommended to further study the role of sleep and physical activity in patients with CFS and FMS.

5. Conclusion

This study revealed that, on average, patients with CFS and FMS sleep longer and are less physically active than controls and that both high and low levels of physical activity and sleep duration are associated with higher symptom severity. Differences were found within patient groups, suggesting etiological heterogeneity in these patients and thus the importance of patient-tailored treatment.

Abbreviations

FSS: Functional somatic syndromes
CFS: Chronic fatigue syndrome
FMS: Fibromyalgia syndrome.

Disclosure

An earlier version of this manuscript has been presented as a master thesis at the University Medical Center Groningen. Wilma L. Zijlema is currently working at ISGlobal, Doctor Aiguader 88, 08003 Barcelona, Spain; Universitat Pompeu Fabra (UPF), Doctor Aiguader 88, 08003 Barcelona, Spain; CIBER Epidemiología y Salud Pública (CIBERESP), Melchor Fernández Almagro, 3-5, 28029 Madrid, Spain.

Acknowledgments

LifeLines has been funded by a number of public sources, notably the Dutch Government, the Netherlands Organization of Scientific Research NWO, the Northern Netherlands Collaboration of Provinces (SNN), European Fund for Regional Development, the Dutch Ministry of Economic Affairs, Pieken in de Delta, Provinces of Groningen and Drenthe, the Target project, BBMRI-NL, the University of Groningen, and the University Medical Center Groningen, the Netherlands.

References

[1] M. W. De Waal, I. A. Arnold, J. A. Eekhof, and A. M. Van Hemert, "Somatoform disorders in general practice: prevalence, functional impairment and comorbidity with anxiety and depressive disorders," *British Journal of Psychiatry*, vol. 184, no. 6, pp. 470–476, 2004.

[2] J. L. Jackson and K. Kroenke, "Prevalence, impact, and prognosis of multisomatoform disorder in primary care: a 5-year follow-up study," *Psychosomatic Medicine*, vol. 70, no. 4, pp. 430–434, 2008.

[3] R. Hoedeman, A. H. Blankenstein, B. Krol, P. C. Koopmans, and J. W. Groothoff, "The contribution of high levels of somatic symptom severity to sickness absence duration, disability and discharge," *Journal of Occupational Rehabilitation*, vol. 20, no. 2, pp. 264–273, 2010.

[4] A. Konnopka, C. Kaufmann, H. König et al., "Association of costs with somatic symptom severity in patients with medically unexplained symptoms," *Journal of Psychosomatic Research*, vol. 75, no. 4, pp. 370–375, 2013.

[5] K. Fukuda, S. E. Straus, I. Hickie, M. C. Sharpe, J. G. Dobbins, and A. Komaroff, "The chronic fatigue syndrome: a comprehensive approach to its definition and study," *Annals of Internal Medicine*, vol. 121, no. 12, pp. 953–959, 1994.

[6] F. Wolfe, D. J. Clauw, M. Fitzcharles et al., "The American College of Rheumatology preliminary diagnostic criteria for fibromyalgia and measurement of symptom severity," *Arthritis Care and Research*, vol. 62, no. 5, pp. 600–610, 2010.

[7] C. T. Buffington, "Developmental influences on medically unexplained symptoms," *Psychotherapy and Psychosomatics*, vol. 78, no. 3, pp. 139–144, 2009.

[8] C. D. Black, P. J. O'Connor, and K. K. McCully, "Increased daily physical activity and fatigue symptoms in chronic fatigue syndrome," *Dynamic Medicine*, vol. 4, no. 1, p. 3, 2005.

[9] W. J. Kop, A. Lyden, A. A. Berlin et al., "Ambulatory monitoring of physical activity and symptoms in fibromyalgia and chronic fatigue syndrome," *Arthritis and Rheumatism*, vol. 52, no. 1, pp. 296–303, 2005.

[10] S. P. Bailey, "TIRED OF BEING TIRED: exercise as a treatment for chronic fatigue syndrome," *ACSM's Health and Fitness Journal*, vol. 15, no. 1, pp. 20–25, 2011.

[11] N. E. Andrews, J. Strong, and P. J. Meredith, "Activity pacing, avoidance, endurance, and associations with patient functioning in chronic pain: a systematic review and meta-analysis," *Archives of Physical Medicine and Rehabilitation*, vol. 93, no. 11, pp. 2109.e7–2121.e7, 2012.

[12] J. Nijs, N. Roussel, J. Van Oosterwijck et al., "Fear of movement and avoidance behaviour toward physical activity in chronic-fatigue syndrome and fibromyalgia: state of the art and implications for clinical practice," *Clinical Rheumatology*, vol. 32, no. 8, pp. 1121–1129, 2013.

[13] J. H. O'Keefe, H. R. Patil, C. J. Lavie, A. Magalski, R. A. Vogel, and P. A. McCullough, "Potential adverse cardiovascular effects from excessive endurance exercise," *Mayo Clinic Proceedings*, vol. 87, no. 6, pp. 587–595, 2012.

[14] S. M. Bigatti, A. M. Hernandez, T. A. Cronan, and K. L. Rand, "Sleep disturbances in fibromyalgia syndrome: relationship to pain and depression," *Arthritis Care and Research*, vol. 59, no. 7, pp. 961–967, 2008.

[15] N. A. Hamilton, G. Affleck, H. Tennen et al., "Fibromyalgia: the role of sleep in affect and in negative event reactivity and recovery," *Health Psychology*, vol. 27, no. 4, pp. 490–497, 2008.

[16] K. L. Knutson and F. W. Turek, "The U-shaped association between sleep and health: the 2 peaks do not mean the same thing," *Sleep*, vol. 29, no. 7, pp. 878-879, 2006.

[17] L. A. Aaron, M. M. Burke, and D. Buchwald, "Overlapping conditions among patients with chronic fatigue syndrome, fibromyalgia, and temporomandibular disorder," *Archives of Internal Medicine*, vol. 160, no. 2, pp. 221–227, 2000.

[18] S. Wessely, C. Nimnuan, and M. Sharpe, "Functional somatic syndromes: one or many?," *The Lancet*, vol. 354, no. 9182, pp. 936–939, 1999.

[19] R. P. Stolk, J. G. Rosmalen, D. S. Postma et al., "Universal risk factors for multifactorial diseases," *European Journal of Epidemiology*, vol. 23, no. 1, pp. 67–74, 2008.

[20] M. L. Joustra, K. A. Janssens, U. Bültmann, and J. G. Rosmalen, "Functional limitations in functional somatic syndromes and well-defined medical diseases. Results from the general population cohort LifeLines," *Journal of Psychosomatic Research*, vol. 79, no. 2, pp. 94–99, 2015.

[21] M. L. Joustra, "*Physical activity and sleep duration in chronic fatigue syndrome and fibromyalgia. Results from the general population cohort LifeLines*," M.S. thesis, University of Groningen, Groningen, Netherlands, 2014.

[22] G. Wendel-Vos, A. J. Schuit, W. H. Saris, and D. Kromhout, "Reproducibility and relative validity of the short questionnaire to assess health-enhancing physical activity," *Journal of Clinical Epidemiology*, vol. 56, no. 12, pp. 1163–1169, 2003.

[23] B. E. Ainsworth, W. L. Haskell, M. C. Whitt et al., "Compendium of physical activities: an update of activity codes and MET intensities," *Medicine & Science in Sports & Exercise*, vol. 32, no. 9, pp. S498–S504, 2000.

[24] L. Derogatis, *SCL-90. Administration, Scoring and Procedures Manual-I for the R (Revised) Version and Other Instruments of the Psychopathology Rating Scales Series*, Johns Hopkins University School of Medicine, Chicago, IL, USA, 1977.

[25] R. D. Hays and L. S. Morales, "The RAND-36 measure of health-related quality of life," *Annals of Medicine*, vol. 33, no. 5, pp. 350–357, 2001.

[26] K. Kroenke, R. L. Spitzer, and R. Swindle, "A symptom checklist to screen for somatoform disorders in primary care," *Psychosomatics*, vol. 39, no. 3, pp. 263–272, 1998.

[27] M. van't Leven, G. A. Zielhuis, J. W. van der Meer, A. L. Verbeek, and G. Bleijenberg, "Fatigue and chronic fatigue syndrome-like complaints in the general population," *European Journal of Public Health*, vol. 20, no. 3, pp. 251–257, 2010.

[28] A. Assumpção, A. B. Cavalcante, C. E. Capela et al., "Prevalence of fibromyalgia in a low socioeconomic status population," *BMC Musculoskeletal Disorders*, vol. 10, no. 1, p. 64, 2009.

[29] J. C. Branco, B. Bannwarth, I. Failde et al., "Prevalence of fibromyalgia: a survey in five European countries," *Seminars in Arthritis and Rheumatism*, vol. 39, no. 6, pp. 448–453, 2010.

[30] K. Kroenke and R. L. Spitzer, "Gender differences in the reporting of physical and somatoform symptoms," *Psychosomatic Medicine*, vol. 60, no. 2, pp. 150–155, 1998.

[31] B. R. Belcher, D. Berrigan, K. W. Dodd, B. A. Emken, C. Chou, and D. Spuijt-Metz, "Physical activity in US youth: impact of race/ethnicity, age, gender, and weight status," *Medicine & Science in Sports & Exercise*, vol. 42, no. 12, pp. 2211–2221, 2010.

[32] H. Valkeinen, K. Harald, K. Borodulin et al., "Educational differences in estimated and measured physical fitness," *European Journal of Public Health*, vol. 23, no. 6, pp. 998–1002, 2013.

[33] S. J. Thomas, K. L. Lichstein, D. J. Taylor, B. W. Riedel, and A. J. Bush, "Epidemiology of bedtime, arising time, and time in bed: analysis of age, gender, and ethnicity," *Behavioral Sleep Medicine*, vol. 12, no. 3, pp. 169–182, 2014.

[34] F. P. Cappuccio, F. M. Taggart, N. Kandala, and A. Currie, "Meta-analysis of short sleep duration and obesity in children and adults," *Sleep*, vol. 31, no. 5, pp. 619–626, 2008.

[35] E. M. Kingma, P. de Jonge, J. Ormel, and J. G. Rosmalen, "Predictors of a functional somatic syndrome diagnosis in patients with persistent functional somatic symptoms," *International Journal of Behavioral Medicine*, vol. 20, no. 2, pp. 206–212, 2012.

[36] M. J. McLoughlin, L. H. Colbert, A. J. Stegner, and D. B. Cook, "Are women with fibromyalgia less physically active than healthy women," *Medicine & Science in Sports & Exercise*, vol. 43, no. 5, pp. 905–912, 2011.

[37] R. M. Evering, M. G. van Weering, K. C. Groothuis-Oudshoorn, and M. M. Vollenbroek-Hutten, "Daily physical activity of patients with the chronic fatigue syndrome: a systematic review," *Clinical Rehabilitation*, vol. 25, no. 2, pp. 112–133, 2011.

[38] V. Segura-Jiménez, I. C. Álvarez-Gallardo, A. Romero-Zurita et al., "Comparison of physical activity using questionnaires (leisure time physical activity instrument and physical activity at home and work instrument) and accelerometry in fibromyalgia patients: the Al-Ándalus project," *Archives of Physical Medicine and Rehabilitation*, vol. 95, no. 10, pp. 1903.e2–1911.e2, 2014.

[39] J. Benítez-Porres, M. Delgado, and J. R. Ruiz, "Comparison of physical activity estimates using International Physical Activity Questionnaire (IPAQ) and accelerometry in fibromyalgia patients: the Al-Andalus study," *Journal of Sports Sciences*, vol. 31, no. 16, pp. 1741–1752, 2013.

[40] E. Bazelmans, G. Bleijenberg, J. Van Der Meer, and H. Folgering, "Is physical deconditioning a perpetuating factor in chronic fatigue syndrome? A controlled study on maximal exercise performance and relations with fatigue, impairment and physical activity," *Psychological Medicine*, vol. 31, no. 1, pp. 107–114, 2001.

[41] V. Segura-Jimenez, D. Camiletti-Moiron, D. Munguia-Izquierdo et al., "Agreement between self-reported sleep patterns and actigraphy in fibromyalgia and healthy women," *Clinical and Experimental Rheumatology*, vol. 33, no. 88, pp. S58–S67, 2015.

[42] N. F. Watson, V. Kapur, L. M. Arguelles et al., "Comparison of subjective and objective measures of insomnia in monozygotic twins discordant for chronic fatigue syndrome," *Sleep*, vol. 26, no. 3, pp. 324–328, 2003.

[43] D. Neu, O. Mairesse, G. Hoffmann et al., "Sleep quality perception in the chronic fatigue syndrome: correlations with sleep efficiency, affective symptoms and intensity of fatigue," *Neuropsychobiology*, vol. 56, no. 1, pp. 40–46, 2007.

[44] M. Majer, J. F. Jones, E. R. Unger et al., "Perception versus polysomnographic assessment of sleep in CFS and non-fatigued control subjects: results from a population-based study," *BMC Neurology*, vol. 7, p. 40, 2007.

[45] J. G. Rosmalen, A. M. Wenting, A. M. Roest, P. de Jonge, and E. H. Bos, "Revealing causal heterogeneity using time series analysis of ambulatory assessments: application to the association between depression and physical activity after myocardial infarction," *Psychosomatic Medicine*, vol. 74, no. 4, pp. 377–386, 2012.

8

Jaw Exercise Therapy and Psychoeducation to Reduce Oral Parafunctional Activities for the Management of Persistent Dentoalveolar Pain

Izumi Makino,[1] Young-Chang Arai,[1,2] Shuichi Aono,[1] Masayuki Inoue,[1,2] Hiroki Sakurai,[3] Yusuke Ohmichi,[1] Kazuhiro Shimo,[1,2] Makoto Nishihara,[1] Jun Sato,[1] Noboru Hatakeyama,[1] Takako Matsubara,[1,3] Tatsunori Ikemoto,[1,2] and Takahiro Ushida[1,2]

[1]*Multidisciplinary Pain Center, Aichi Medical University School of Medicine, Aichi, Japan*
[2]*Institute of Physical Fitness, Sports Medicine and Rehabilitation, Aichi Medical University School of Medicine, Aichi, Japan*
[3]*Faculty of Health and Medical Sciences, Tokoha University, Shizuoka, Japan*
[4]*Rehabilitation, Nihon Fukushi University, Aichi, Japan*

Correspondence should be addressed to Izumi Makino; cosmosdc3666@gmail.com

Academic Editor: Simona Tecco

Objective. To retrospectively analyze the effects of our original combination therapy treatment on patients with nonodontogenic persistent dentoalveolar pain. *Methods.* Twenty-one patients suffering from persistent dentoalveolar pain (nineteen females and two males; mean age ± standard deviation: 55.7 ± 19.6 years) participated in this study. They were treated with a therapy combination of jaw exercise and psychoeducation to reduce oral parafunctional activities every month. The intensity of pain in these subjects was evaluated using a numerical rating scale (NRS) before and after treatment. *Results.* The NRSs at the baseline ranged from 5 to 10 (median, 8), from 0 to 10 (median, 2) at one month after treatment, from 0 to 10 (median, 1) at three months after treatment, and from 0 to 10 (median, 0) at the end of treatment. Pain intensity after treatment improved significantly. *Conclusion.* There was a significant reduction in pain after our combination of therapies as nonpharmacological treatments, and therefore this treatment could be useful in the management of NPDP patients.

1. Introduction

Patients suffering from nonodontogenic persistent dentoalveolar pain (NPDP) continue to seek pain treatment from several doctors, not only dentists but also several kinds of medical practitioners. NPDP is known as idiopathic periodontalgia [1], phantom tooth pain [2], atypical odontalgia (AO) [3], persistent idiopathic facial pain [4], and persistent dentoalveolar pain disorder (PDAP) as recently reported by Nixdorf and Moana-Filho [5]. NPDP is described as a pain that persists in the dentoalveolar region without any evidence of clinical disease. Malacarne et al. reported PDAP is likely to be neuropathic in origin, but pathophysiological mechanisms to explain the onset and persistence of the pain are still far from understood in their review [6]. Dentists and medical practitioners treating NPDP frequently fail to provide adequate pain relief and improve patient's quality of life [7].

Several studies have shown that, in many cases of NPDP, the pain occurred after dental treatment, including endodontic treatment or surgical procedure [8, 9]. However, NPDP can also occur spontaneously in sound teeth [10]. Some reports suggested that NPDP was caused by central sensitization mechanisms [10–13]. Moreover, NPDP has been regarded as a psychological problem because the psychiatric prevalence of the PDAP patient was high since chronic pain disorder could be associated with psychological problems [1, 2, 5, 14]. Otherwise, NPDP might occur from cracked teeth or from myofascial pain syndrome [15], because it is difficult to differentiate the diagnoses.

Effective treatments for NPDP have yet to be established. General treatments for NPDP are the pharmacological treatments used to treat neuropathic pain. However, these treatments are not actually always effective in alleviating NPDP, and some patients experience severe side effects [7, 16]. Furthermore, several reports highly recommend avoiding irreversible treatments for NPDP [5, 8]. The current treatment target might be to improve quality of life (QOL) but not to provide adequate pain relief [6].

Recently, there are many reports that therapies including exercise therapy, cognitive-behavioral therapy or progressive relaxation, and intensive interdisciplinary rehabilitation are moderately effective for chronic pain. Therefore, we tried to treat NPDP patients using our original combination therapy (exercise of jaw movement and psychoeducation to reduce oral parafunction activities (OPAs)) that was effective on craniocervical chronic pain in a previous study [17].

The aim of this study was to retrospectively analyze the effects of treatment of our original combination therapy for patients with NPDP.

2. Materials and Methods

Data were collected in a test battery using an iPad and through interviews conducted by a dentist. The same dentist treated the patients using our original combination therapy. The intensity of pain was rated by the patient using a Numerical Rating Scale (NRS), where 0 indicated no pain and 10 indicated the greatest pain possible. Patients were asked about the pain intensity at every visit, and inquiries about their pain condition were made by telephone call for the follow-up.

All patients were referred from other hospitals to the Pain Center for treatment of NPDP. Treatment protocols used in the present report were based on institutional policy and clinical guidelines approved by the IRB of Aichi Medical University, and written consent was obtained from all patients (Reference number 13-083).

2.1. Participants. Participants were the patients who visited the Multidisciplinary Pain Center (Pain Center) of Aichi Medical University from December 2010 to June 2012. Twenty-one patients were chosen as participants at first, but six patients dropped out during treatment. Nineteen patients were female and two were male, and their mean age was 55.7 ± 19.6 years. They were selected according to the following inclusion and exclusion criteria:

Inclusion criteria:

(i) Nonodontogenic persistent dentoalveolar pain (NPDP)
(ii) Pain duration more than 3 months
(iii) Age >18 years

Exclusion criteria:

(i) Clear case of odontogenic pain
(ii) Rheumatic disease or general inflammatory condition
(iii) Fibromyalgia
(iv) Language difficulties and communication difficulties
(v) Closed locking jaw

2.2. Procedure of Treatment. The patients were administered our combination therapy under the supervision of a dentist (Makino) at our pain center at every visit. They were instructed to continue the exercises at home.

2.2.1. Listening and Explanation. After checking the medical history of each patient, we listened to the patient's complaints regarding NPDP and reconfirmed their pain. We confirmed that there was no clinical or radiographic evidence of relevant pathology in their pain and explained this to the patients.

2.2.2. Exercise for Jaw Movement. Patients were instructed to perform the jaw movement exercise at home. The exercise consists of ten sets of protrusion-retrusion (anterior-posterior) jaw movements, a lateral jaw movement with the right side, and then a lateral jaw movement on the left side. Protrusion-retrusion (anterior-posterior) jaw movements were performed while biting on a cotton roll with the front teeth. A lateral jaw movement with the right side was performed while biting on a cotton roll with the right canine, and then a lateral jaw movement on the left side was performed while biting on a cotton roll with the left canine. One set exercise: a cotton roll goes up from below to the occlusal plane at first, secondly, a cotton roll maintains position at the occlusal plane, and finally, a cotton roll goes down in each exercise. These exercises were performed once a day. It was important for the patients to concentrate on the jaw exercise while watching their jaws move in a small mirror and to move the jaw slowly. They were also advised to perform the exercise carefully so as not to induce pain (Figure 1).

2.2.3. Psychoeducation

(1) Recognition of OPAs. We informed patients to understand that it was important to recognize both OPAs and the frequency of OPAs during the daytime. We advised them not to be obsessed with OPAs or attempt to avoid them, but just to recognize that it had occurred. In addition, our other instruction was that when they felt pain, they had to recognize what kind of OPAs they were doing and how frequently they were doing them.

(2) Relaxation of Masticatory System Method. Patients were trained to relax their tongue, their masticatory muscles, and their jaw. This form of relaxation involved taking a breath with their mouth wide open and then closing the mouth and trying to relax the tongue and jaw, without allowing the teeth to clench together. They were instructed to perform this

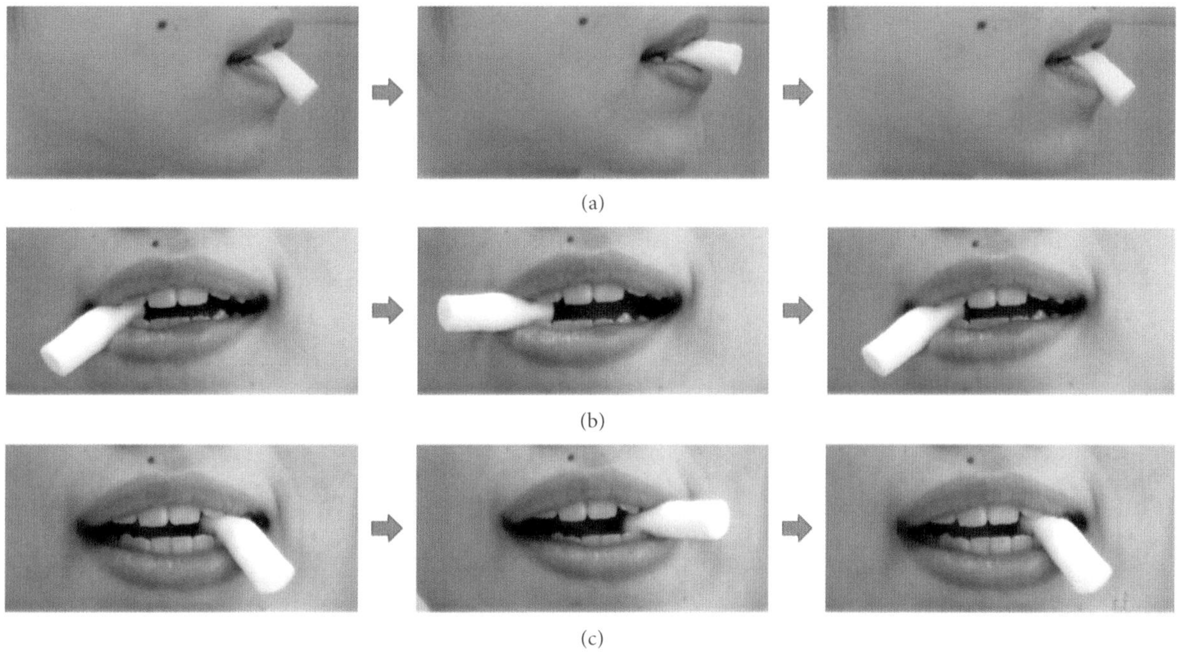

FIGURE 1: Jaw exercise. (a) Protusion-retrusion jaw movements while biting on a cotton roll with the front teeth. (b) Right jaw movement while biting on a cotton roll with the right canine. (c) Left jaw movement while biting on a cotton roll with the left canine.

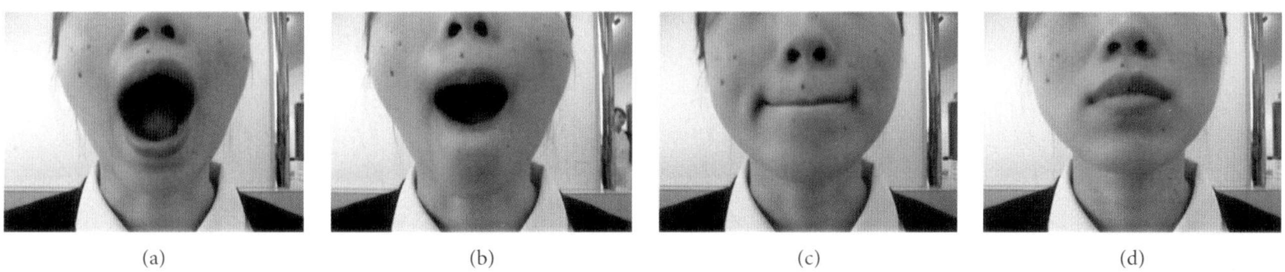

FIGURE 2: Mouth exercise and relaxation. (a) Take a breath with the mouth wide open. (b) Roll the lips back inside the mouth. (c) Close the mouth until the lips touch. (d) Relax the masticatory muscles, tongue, and jaw without letting the teeth touch.

system of relaxation when they noticed their pain and OPAs (Figure 2).

2.3. One-Year Follow-Up. In the follow-up 1 year after the patient's last visit, we followed up on their pain condition over a telephone call.

2.4. Statistical Analysis. The pain intensities in the patients gained at every visit to the pain center. The data of the initial pain and the pain intensity one month later, three months later, and at the end of treatment were first analyzed by Friedman test followed by Wilcoxon signed-rank test between the initial pain and the pain intensity one month later, three months later, and at the end of treatment. The level of significance for each test was set at $P = 0.01$.

3. Results

The characteristics and the dental treatment histories of the patients are described in Table 1. The mean duration of pain was 37.7 ± 48.6 months. At first, 21 participants were recruited for this study, but six participants (patient number: 16-21) dropped out during treatment. Finally the number for statistical analysis was 15 out of 21 participants. Only 12 participants could be contacted by telephone call for the follow-up.

3.1. Intensity of Pain. The individual changes in NRS are listed in Table 2. The NRSs of the baseline ranged from 5 to 10 (Median, 8). The NRS ranged from 0 to 10 (Median, 0) at one month after treatment, from 0 to 10 (Median, 0) at three months after treatment, and from 0 to 10 (Median, 0) at the end of treatment. The data of the 4 groups were significantly different by the Friedman test ($P < 0.01$). Pain intensity after treatment improved significantly ($P < 0.01$) (Wilcoxon test) (Table 2; Figure 3).

3.2. Follow-Up. One year later, we evaluated 11 patients by telephone call after the patient's last visit. Three patients out

Table 1: Characteristics and treatment used in 21 patients.

Patientnumber	Sex	Age (years)	Duration (months)	Pain location	History of present illness	Phamacological treatment	OPA	HADS (anxiety)	HADS (depression)	PCS
1	F	70	30	34	rct	NSAIDs	c, t	14	15	—
2	F	37	4	14.15	none	Tizanidine hydrochloride NSAIDs	c	6	5	36
3	F	58	7	(21) area	ext and cur	NSAIDs	t	7	5	23
4	F	27	7	16.26.36.46	rct	Mirtazapine-lorazepam	c, t	16	16	40
5	F	59	48	36.37	none	Flunitrazepam-etizolam	c, t	18	18	51
6	F	71	6	36.37	cr	Etizolam	c, t	9	3	40
7	F	39	48	26.27	none	Lorazepam	c	10	6	32
8	F	37	36	(26) area	ext and cur	Clonazepam-gabapentin carbamazepine-pregabalin	c, t	9	8	19
9	F	74	36	(46) area	rct and ext	NSAIDs	—	12	10	47
10	F	75	240	(24.25.26) area	ext	NSAIDs	c, t	8	4	42
11	F	82	24	11.14.21	none	NSAIDs	c	3	13	31
12	M	58	24	6.17.26.27.36.37.46.47	none	Pregabalin-brotizolam	j	13	14	37
13	M	78	24	37	br	NSAIDs	t	8	8	38
14	F	89	3	16 (44.45.46.47) area	ext and cur	Mirtazapine	t	15	18	50
15	F	72	3	11.12.13 (16) area	none	Pregabalin-carbamazepine NSAIDs	c, t	12	16	45
16	F	44	36	25 (26) area	ext	Drugs for bipolar disorder	c	18	18	—
17	F	39	30	26	rct and ext	Drugs for schizophrenia	c, t	7	11	22
18	F	46	36	13.38	none	Drugs for schizophrenia	c	11	18	44
19	F	69	36	(37.38) area	ext	Amitriptyline-NSAIDs-pregabalin	—	3	2	15
20	F	24	18	All teeth	none	Drugs for obsessive-compulsive disorder	—	13	9	46
21	F	21	96	26	None → pulpectomy	Amitriptyline	c	14	9	40
Mean		55.7	37.7					10.8	10.8	36.7

Tooth number is shown by two-digit notation (FDI). (Number) area is in situ after extraction of tooth. History of present illness: none = nontreatment; ext = extraction of tooth; rct = root canal treatment; cur = curettage of alveolar bone. cr = crown, br = bridge, OPA: c = diurnal tooth clenching; t = touching tooth by tongue; j = jaw moving; HADS = Hospital Anxiety and Depression Scale to determine the levels of anxiety and depression. PCS = Pain Catastrophizing Scale to determine the levels of physical and emotional distress associated with their pain.

Table 2: The pain intensity in each visiting time at pain center.

Patient number	Before	1 month	3 months	End
1	8	5	5	0
2	8	2	2	0
3	5	3	0	0
4	8	10	0	0
5	8	8	4	1
6	5	2	1	1
7	7	0	0	0
8	10	10	10	10
9	9	9	5	5
10	8	0	6	5
11	8	0	0	0
12	8	1	0	0
13	8	8	2	0
14	10	0	0	0
15	10	0	0	0
Mean	8	4	2	1
Median	8	2	1	0
P value		0.0051	0.007	0.007

The NRSs of the baseline ranged from 5 to 10 (median, 8). The NRS ranged from 0 to 10 (median, 0) at one month after treatment. The NRS ranged from 0 to 10 (median, 0) at three month after treatment. The NRS ranged from 0 to 10 (median, 0) at the end of treatment. *P* value: the data were analyzed by Wilcoxon signed-rank test between the initial pain and the pain intensity at one month later, three month later, and end of treatment.

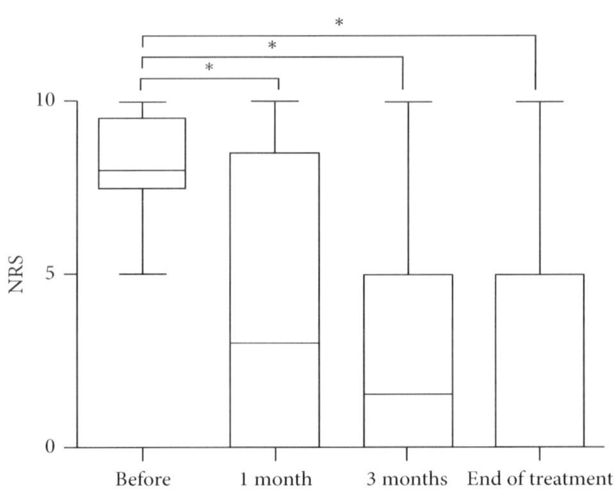

Figure 3: The pain intensity in each visiting time at pain center. Horizontal bar represents medians, boxes represent the 25th and 75th percentile ranges, and T bars represent the 5th and 95th percentile ranges. *Difference between before and after treatment ($P < 0.01$) (Wilcoxon test).

of 11 had no pain, seven patients had a recurrence of less pain, and one patient displayed no improvement. Ten patients took no medication, while one patient occasionally took medication. However, one patient took medication everyday with no improvement of pain (Table 3).

4. Discussion

Generally, patients with NPDP are suffering from their pain for a long time because available treatments fail to provide adequate pain relief. However, this study found that our treatment significantly improved the pain intensity of NPDP and their QOL at follow-up. To date, therapeutic algorithm for NPDP [8] includes mainly pharmacological treatments, which are tricyclic antidepressants [14], serotonin and norepinephrine reuptake inhibitors [18], anticonvulsants [19], or pregabaline [20] as used for neuropathic pain. Although these treatments could have serious side effects, the effectiveness is not so high for NPDP [16]. In our study, three patients said that they felt a little decrease in pain intensity after taking anxiolytics, but almost no patients experienced any pain relief through pharmacological treatments. These NPDP patients might include patients with persistent periodontitis without bacterial inflammation, myofascial pain syndrome, neuropathic pain, and PDAP because diagnostic criteria have not yet been established. But, the present results apparently showed the benefits of our original therapy for NPDP patients.

Table 3: The condition in the follow-up.

Patient number	NRS	Medicine
1	3~6	None
2	1~2	None
3	0	None
4	2~3	None
5	0	None
6	3~5	Sometime
7	0	None
8	10	Usual
9	—	—
10	0~1	None
11	3~8	None
12	3~5	None
13	0~5	None
14	—	—
15	—	—

The NRS ranges from 0 to 10, and ten patients took no medication, one patient occasionally took medication in the follow-up.

Our original therapy consists of exercise and psychoeducation that have become common therapies for chronic pain. Recently, there are many reports of moderately effective nonpharmacologic therapies for TMD [21, 22], and nonspecific chronic low back pain includes exercise therapy, cognitive-behavioral therapy or progressive relaxation, and intensive interdisciplinary rehabilitation [23]. Moreover, we have been focusing on the fact that many NPDP patients performed OPAs such as tongue touching of teeth and area of pain, and teeth clenching while experiencing pain or not. Many studies reported that chronic pain disorders including NPDP have been linked to psychological factors [5, 24]. And, a study reported that OPAs are associated with emotional stress induced by social factors [25]. Vickers et al. hypotheses that activation of low-threshold mechanoreceptors by bruxism, which is another form of OPA, may modulate nociception through gate-control mechanisms; bruxism may thus be a potential pain-coping mechanism for AO [24]. In this study, almost all patients claimed that they were always doing OPAs to pay attention to their pain area during the day. We announce that NPDP patients have been doing

OPAs more frequently than dentists recognize, and OPAs keep stimulating teeth or pain area by hard pressure. That is, OPAs (teeth clenching or touching teeth by tongue) may be major triggers in NPDP, and highly frequent OPAs might have a bad influence on masticatory muscles. We think that psychoeducation to reduce the frequency of OPAs could decrease OPAs and change the facilitating muscles with exercise. An additionally important point is that we, as medical professionals, must sufficiently recognize the patients' pain and explain it to them, because of the importance of the relation between the patient and the clinician [21].

The Hospital Anxiety (median, 11) and Depression Scale (median, 10) and Pain Catastrophizing Scale (Median, 40) of the participants in this study showed high score tendencies. Four out of the 6 subjects who dropped out in this study had mental diseases (bipolar disorder, schizophrenia, and obsessive-compulsive disorder). Medical practitioners may need to be careful of mental conditions or mental diseases of NPDP patients.

Based on the present results, we could generate a hypothesis about the onset mechanisms of NPDP. NPDP patients are iterating OPAs (clenching and tongue habit) pressure teeth or area where a tooth once resists. If these pressures continue, c-fibers on periodontal ligament space will keep receiving the stimulation at first, and wind-up phenomena will occur subsequently at the central nervous system. This could be why local anesthesia for NPDP patients leads to complete or incomplete pain relief, as seen on a previous study [11]. And, most NPDP patients in this study said that they have more OPAs than they had thought, and their pain intensity became lower the second time they visited the pain center after they had controlled the OPAs. It seemed that the NPDP improved as the frequency of OPAs decreased. As NPDP is chronic pain that means a plastic change in the central nervous system, the pain could not be relieved immediately and psychoeducation is needed for the treatment. That is, in NPDP, inflammation on periodontium is processed under disrupted psychosocial conditions, thereby leading to plastic changes of the central nervous system.

There are several limitations to this study. First of all, the participants in this study were an undefined group having NPDP because correct diagnosis and pathophysiological mechanisms of NPDP have yet to be established. The number of participants in this study is small. The further studies of NPDP are needed but these studies are difficult because the population of NPDP patients is small.

5. Conclusion

This study reported a significant reduction in pain after our own combination of therapies to improve jaw movement and psychoeducation to reduce OPAs as forms of non-pharmacological treatment. Therefore, this treatment could be useful in the management of NPDP patients.

Acknowledgments

The authors thank Matthew James McLaughlin for reviewing and editing our final manuscript.

References

[1] M. Harris, "Psychogenic aspects of facial pain," *British Dental Journal*, vol. 136, no. 5, pp. 199–202, 1974.

[2] J. J. Marbach, "Phantom tooth pain," *Journal of Endodontics*, vol. 4, no. 12, pp. 362–372, 1978.

[3] R. T. Rees and M. Harris, "Atypical odontalgia," *British Journal of Oral Surgery*, vol. 16, no. 3, pp. 212–218, 1979.

[4] Headache Classification Committee of the International Headache Society, "The international classification of headache disorders, 3rd edition (beta version)," *Cephalalgia*, vol. 33, no. 9, pp. 629–808, 2013.

[5] D. Nixdorf and E. Moana-Filho, "Persistent dento-alveolar pain disorder (PDAP): working towards a better understanding," *British Journal of Pain*, vol. 5, no. 4, pp. 18–27, 2011.

[6] A. Malacarne, E. L. H. Spierings, C. Lu, and G. E. Maloney, "Persistent dentoalveolar pain disorder: a comprehensive review," *Journal of Endodontics*, vol. 44, no. 2, pp. 206–211, 2018.

[7] J. Durham and D. R. Nixdorf, "Healthcare pathway and biopsychosocial impact of persistent dentoalveolar pain disorder: a qualitative study," *International Endodontic Journal*, vol. 47, no. 12, pp. 1151–1159, 2014.

[8] L. Baad-Hansen, "Atypical odontalgia–pathophysiology and clinical management," *Journal of Oral Rehabilitation*, vol. 35, no. 1, pp. 1–11, 2008.

[9] N. Polycarpou, D. Canavan, R. Moles, and K. Gulabivala, "Prevalence of persistent pain after endodontic treatment and factors affecting its occurrence in cases with complete radiographic healing," *International Endodontic Journal*, vol. 38, no. 8, pp. 169–178, 2005.

[10] T. List, G. Leijon, M. Helkimo, S. F. Dworkin, and P. Svensson, "Clinical findings and psychosocial factors in patients with atypical odontalgia: a case-control study," *Journal of Orofacial Pain*, vol. 21, no. 2, pp. 89–98, 2007.

[11] T. List, G. Leijon, M. Helkimo, A. Öster, and P. Svensson, "Effect of local anesthesia on atypical odontalgia: a randomized controlled trial," *Pain*, vol. 122, no. 3, pp. 306–314, 2006.

[12] T. List, G. Leijon, and P. Svensson, "Somatosensory abnormalities in atypical odontalgia: a case-control study," *Pain*, vol. 139, no. 2, pp. 333–341, 2008.

[13] L. Baad-Hansen, M. Pigg, S. E. Ivanovic et al., "Intraoral somatosensory abnormalities in patients with atypical odontalgia: a controlled multicenter quantitative sensory testing study," *Pain*, vol. 154, no. 8, pp. 1287–1294, 2013.

[14] L. Baad-Hansen, G. Leijon, P. Svensson, and T. List, "Comparison of clinical findings and psychosocial factors in patients with atypical odontalgia and temporomandibular disorders," *Journal of Orofacial Pain*, vol. 22, pp. 7–14, 2008.

[15] D. G. Simons, J. G. Travell, and L. S. Simons, *Travell & Simons' Myofascial Pain and Dysfunction: Upper Half of Body*, Lippincott Williams & Wilkins, Philadelphia, PA, USA, 1999.

[16] M. Pigg, P. Svensson, M. Drangsholt, and T. List, "Seven-year follow-up of patients diagnosed with atypical odontalgia:

a prospective study," *Journal of Orofacial Pain*, vol. 27, no. 2, pp. 151–164, 2013.

[17] I. Makino, Y.-C. P. Arai, S. Aono, K. Hayashi, A. Morimoto, and M. Nishihara, "The effects of exercise therapy for the improvement of jaw movement and psychological intervention to reduce parafunctional activities on chronic pain in the craniocervical region," *Pain Practice*, vol. 14, pp. 413–418, 2014.

[18] M. Ito, H. Kimura, K. Yoshida, Y. Kimura, N. Ozaki, and K. Kurita, "Effectiveness of milnacipran for the treatment of chronic pain in the orofacial region," *Clinical Neuropharmacology*, vol. 33, no. 2, pp. 79–83, 2010.

[19] W. J. J. M. Martin and T. Forouzanfar, "The efficacy of anticonvulsants on orofacial pain: a systematic review," *Oral Surgery, Oral Medicine, Oral Pathology, Oral Radiology, and Endodontology*, vol. 111, no. 5, pp. 627–633, 2011.

[20] J. M. Zakrzewska, "Medical management of trigeminal neuropathic pains," *Expert Opinion on Pharmacotherapy*, vol. 11, no. 8, pp. 1239–1254, 2010.

[21] B. Craane, P. U. Dijkstra, K. Stappaerts, and A. De Laat, "One-year evaluation of the effect of physical therapy for masticatory muscle pain: a randomized controlled trial," *European Journal of Pain*, vol. 16, no. 5, pp. 737–747, 2012.

[22] C. R. Carlson, P. M. Bertrand, A. D. Ehrlich, A. W. Maxwell, and R. G. Burton, "Physical self-regulation training for the management of temporomandibular disorders," *Journal of Orofacial Pain*, vol. 15, no. 1, pp. 47–55, 2001.

[23] R. Chou, A. Qaseem, V. Snow et al., "Diagnosis and treatment of low back pain: a joint clinical practice guideline from the American College of Physicians and the American Pain Society," *Annals of Internal Medicine*, vol. 147, no. 7, pp. 478–491, 2007.

[24] E. R. Vickers, M. J. Cousins, S. Walker, and K. Chisholm, "Analysis of 50 patients with atypical odontalgia: a preliminary report on pharmacological procedures for diagnosis and treatment," *Oral Surgery, Oral Medicine, Oral Pathology, Oral Radiology, and Endodontology*, vol. 85, no. 1, pp. 24–32, 1998.

[25] S. K. Rao, M. Bhat, and J. David, "Work, stress, and diurnal bruxism: a pilot study among information technology professionals in Bangalore City, India," *International Journal of Dentistry*, vol. 2011, Article ID 650489, 5 pages, 2011.

The Impact of Pain Invisibility on Patient-Centered Care and Empathetic Attitude in Chronic Pain Management

Emilie Paul-Savoie,[1] **Patricia Bourgault**,[1] **Stéphane Potvin**,[2] **Emilie Gosselin**,[1] **and Sylvie Lafrenaye**[3]

[1]*School of Nursing, Faculty of Medicine and Health Sciences, Université de Sherbrooke, Sherbrooke, QC, Canada*
[2]*Centre de Recherche de L'Institut Universitaire en Santé Mentale de Montréal, Department of Psychiatry, Faculty of Medicine, Université de Montréal, Montreal, QC, Canada*
[3]*Department of Pediatrics, Faculty of Medicine and Health Sciences, Université de Sherbrooke, Sherbrooke, QC, Canada*

Correspondence should be addressed to Sylvie Lafrenaye; sylvie.lafrenaye@usherbrooke.ca

Academic Editor: Carlo Lai

Objectives. The use of interdisciplinary patient-centered care (PCC) and empathetic behaviour seems to be a promising avenue to address chronic pain management, but their use in this context seems to be suboptimal. Several patient factors can influence the use of PCC and empathy, but little is known about the impact of pain visibility on these behaviours. The objective of this study was to investigate the influence of visible physical signs on caregiver's patient-centered and empathetic behaviours in chronic pain context. *Methods.* A convenience sample of 21 nurses and 21 physicians participated in a descriptive study. PCC and empathy were evaluated from self-assessment and observer's assessment using a video of real patients with chronic pain. *Results.* The results show that caregivers have demonstrated an intraindividual variability: PCC and empathetic behaviours of the participants were significantly higher for patients who have visible signs of pain (rheumatoid arthritis and complex regional pain syndrome) than for those who have no visible signs (Ehler–Danlos syndrome and fibromyalgia) ($p < 0.001$). Participants who show a greater difference in their patient-centered behaviour according to pain visibility have less clinical experience. *Discussion.* The pain visibility in chronic pain patients is an important factor contributing to an increased use of PCC and empathy by nurses and physicians, and clinical experience can influence their behaviours. Thus, pain invisibility can be a barrier to quality of care, and these findings reinforce the relevance to educating caregivers to these unconscious biases on their behaviour toward chronic pain patients.

1. Introduction

Chronic pain is a common public global health problem, associated with significant disability and many social consequences [1]. Chronic pain affects people of all ages, with a particularly high prevalence in adults, ranging from 10 to 55% [2]. People with chronic pain are known to consult health professional frequently, leading in a heavy economic burden [3, 4]. To be effective, the treatment of chronic pain must consider biological, psychological, and social factors simultaneously [5]. Thus, the use of interdisciplinary patient-centered care (PCC) seems to be a promising avenue to address chronic pain management [6, 7].

There are many definitions of PCC in the context of nursing and medicine, but four dimensions are common to most cited definitions: patient-as-person, biopsychosocial perspective, sharing power and responsibility, and therapeutic alliance [8–10]. The use of this approach is related with many clinical benefits for patients with chronic pain [7, 11–13]. More specifically, researchers have shown that PCC resulted in a decrease in the number of tender points and psychological distress in fibromyalgia patients [11]. Qualitative findings support that PCC allows nurses to improve their assessment and to provide better anticipatory guidance and coaching [12].

In addition, many researchers suggest that empathy is necessary for the use of PCC [8, 14, 15]. In the model of Bilodeau et al., "having an empathetic presence" is an important dimension of PCC [8]. In healthcare, empathy is defined as a cognitive attribute involving an understanding of the patient's experience and perspective, as a separate individual, combined with an ability to communicate that understanding to the patient [16]. Interestingly, it has been suggested that high levels of empathy were related to positive outcomes for patients [17–19] and especially with chronic pain patients [20].

Although many studies support the benefits of PCC, [21] its use in chronic pain management seems to be challenging and suboptimal [20, 22]. Patient-centered behaviour or communication does not necessarily translate into a "unique recipe," and caregivers seem to use a flexible style according to patient characteristics [23]. Over the last years, it has been suggested that several patient factors can influence the use of PCC, such as age, gender, and level of education [24–26]. For example, caregivers would tend to use more PCC behaviour with women, older, and nonsmoker patients [24, 26]. Moreover, some authors have shown that physicians tend to use more PCC when patients reported more physical symptoms, such as nausea, dry mouth, or constipation, and when they rated patients' health condition as more severe [26]. However, in chronic pain context, little is known about the impact of the "visibility" of physical signs on patient-centered behaviour.

Patient factors may also influence caregivers' empathy. Indeed, both behavioral and functional neuroimaging measures have demonstrated that some stigma or prejudice could modulate empathy [27]. Since many patients with chronic pain do not display any visible physical symptoms and remain stoic when they feel pain [28], it is important to assess the impact of this specific factor on patient-centered care and empathetic behaviour.

Various methods have been used for measuring the use of PCC and empathy, such as self-rating and observer rating [9, 23, 29]. Self-assessment instruments are the most common strategy used for measuring PCC and empathy, but they do not consider the influence of different patient factors such as the presence or absence of visible physical signs. The observation of PCC and empathy in real clinical encounters may raise some ethical and methodological issues, including the inability to have standardized visits, which introduces confounding variables. The use of standardized patient simulations is a very expensive strategy [30]. Videos of real patients with chronic pain could overcome these limitations by allowing a standardized and repetitive assessment of attitudes and behaviours of caregivers [31].

Thus, the main objective of this study was to investigate the influence of the presence of visible physical signs on patient-centered and empathetic behaviours of nurses and physicians using videos of real patients suffering from chronic pain. In view of the limited knowledge on the topic, we also sought to identify, in an exploratory fashion, the characteristics of the caregivers who respond differently to the presence or absence of visible signs of pain.

2. Materials and Methods

2.1. Study Design and Settings. This study is part of a larger study which investigated PCC and empathy in chronic pain management [32]. A descriptive design was used, conducted from May to November 2013, in the province of Quebec, Canada. The Scientific and Human Ethics Committee of the institution where the study took place approved the research protocol. A population composed of nurses and physicians has been targeted since interdisciplinary pain management is recommended [8]. A convenience sampling approach was chosen, and participants were recruited through advertisements and referrals. Participants were recruited from 16 different healthcare centres, including urban, semiurban, and rural centres, in the province of Quebec, Canada.

2.2. Participants. All participants gave their written, informed consent, and a coding system was used to keep the data confidential. To take part in the study, the participants need to (i) be active members of the Quebec Board of Nurses or the Quebec College of Physicians, (ii) have chronic pain patients in their routine practice, and (iii) speak French. After signing the informed consent, a sample of 21 nurses and 21 physicians took part in the study. A minimum of 38 participants was needed to detect a moderate difference ($d = 0.5$) between visible and invisible pain conditions with a power of 85% and a type-1 error of 5%. Participants did not know the detailed purpose of the study to avoid social desirability bias, but they were informed that pain management was investigated.

2.3. Self-Assessment Measures. The practice orientation of each participant was measured with the French version of the Patient Practitioner Orientation Scale (F-PPOS) [33]. This self-administrated questionnaire is designed for the assessment of practitioners' or future-practitioners' attitudes and orientations in their care approach. This scale contains 18 items divided into two subscales: "sharing" and "caring," and the four dimensions of PCC are represented. For each item, the caregiver is asked to indicate his or her level of agreement on a 6-point Likert scale (strongly agree to strongly disagree). A total score, ranging from patient-centered (a score of 6.00) to disease-centered (a score of 1.00), can be calculated with the addition of the two subscales. The original version of the PPOS has good face validity and acceptable internal consistency for the total scale (an alpha of 0.89) [34]. The French version of the PPOS has good content validity and acceptable internal consistency for the total scale an (alpha of 0.60) [34], since the minimum threshold is 0.50 [35].

The self-rated empathy was measured with the French version of the Jefferson Scale of Physician Empathy (F-JSPE) (P. Bourgault, S. Lavoie, and M. Grégoire et al., unpublished data, June 2009). This self-administrated questionnaire comprises 20 items divided into 4 dimensions: (i) adopting the patient's perspective, (ii) understanding the patient's experiences, feelings, and signals, (iii) ignoring the patient's perspective, and (iv) adopting the patient's way of thinking. The F-JSPE also includes a single item measuring the value placed on empathy. Participants respond to items on a 7-Likert scale. The total score, ranging from not empathic (a score of 20) to empathic (score of 140), can be calculated with the addition of all the items. The original version of the

JSPE has good criterion-related validity with the Empathic Concern Scale of the Interpersonal Reactivity Index ($r = 0.40$), internal consistency (an alpha of 0.87 to 0.89), test-retest reliability (test-retest reliability coefficient = 0.65), and construct validity [16, 36]. The F-JSPE has good content validity and acceptable internal consistency (an alpha of 0.77) (P. Bourgault, S. Lavoie, and M. Grégoire et al., unpublished data, June 2009).

2.4. Observers' Assessment Measures. The PCC behaviour of each participant was measured with the Sherbrooke Observation Scale of patient-centered care (SOS-PCC) [31]. This instrument has been developed for the assessment of PCC behaviour of a professional caregiver by a trained observer, in the experimental clinical setting. Nine items divided into 4 dimensions (patient-as-person, biopsychosocial perspective, sharing power and responsibility, and therapeutic alliance) are measured on a 4-points Likert scale. The instrument was originally developed in French for a population of nurses and physicians. A total score, ranging from disease-centered (a score of 9) to patient-centered (a score of 36), can be calculated by the addition of all items. This instrument has good content validity, internal consistency (an alpha of 0.88), and inter-rater reliability (an intraclass coefficient (ICC) of 0.93) [31].

An adapted French version of Reynolds Empathy Scale (F-RES) has been used for the assessment of empathetic behaviour by a trained observer [37]. The F-RES consists of 9 items with a categorical rating scale ("yes," "no," or "incomplete"). This instrument has good internal consistency (an alpha of 0.70) and inter-rater reliability (an ICC of 0.85) [38]. In this study, we used a 7-item version with a 4-point Likert scale to make it more responsive to the context of videos. A total score, ranging from not empathetic (a score of 7) to empathetic (a score of 28), can be calculated by adding all items.

2.5. Procedure. All study participants watched four videos of real patients with chronic pain and were subsequently interviewed individually. These 4-minute videos showed female patients aged between 16 and 45 years-old, with different pathologies in which chronic pain was experienced (rheumatoid arthritis, complex regional pain syndrome (CRPS), Ehlers–Danlos syndrome, and fibromyalgia). A more detailed description of the development and content of these videos is available elsewhere [31]. In these videos, some patients had no visible physical signs (Ehlers–Danlos syndrome and fibromyalgia) and others had obvious visible deformities in the upper limb (rheumatoid arthritis and CRPS). After viewing the videos, participants had to describe the management plan that they would provide for each patient, and these answers were video recorded. At the end of the session, each participant responded to the self-administrated questionnaires. After the data collection ($n = 42$ participants), three external observers watched the recorded interviews of each participant (4 interviews/participant). The group of observers consisted of a resident in psychiatry, a nurse, and a PhD student in the healthcare field. The observers were selected based on their experience in the healthcare field (more than five years) and their complementary expertise (medicine, nursing, and research). To ensure the standardization in their assessment, they had previously been trained by the research team to complete the observation scale. They evaluated the PCC and empathetic behaviour demonstrated by participants for each video using the SOS-PCC and the F-RES. Figure 1 showed the conduct of the study.

2.6. Data Analysis. Statistical analyzes were performed using the software SPSS version 18.0. To describe continuous variables, mean (standard deviation) was used, whereas frequency (percentage) was used for nominal and categorical variables. To compare patient-centered and empathetic behaviour of the participants ($n = 42$) according to the presence or absence of visible physical signs in the patients presented in the videos, paired T-tests were used on the mean score of the three observers.

To investigate if the clinical experience can influence the modification of the behaviours according to the pain visibility, for each study participant, we calculated the difference of SOS-PCC and F-RES between the his/her behaviour for the patients with visible signs and the patients without visible signs. We divided the participants into two groups according to these differences: the participants who rated the two groups of patients similarly and those who rated the two groups of patients differently. To determine whether a participant showed similar or different behaviours, we have used the mean scores of SOS-PCC and F-RES for the thresholds. We used paired T-tests to compare the differences in clinical experience between the two groups study participants. The statistical level of significance was set at $p < 0.05$. We do not have any missing data.

3. Results and Discussion

3.1. Participants' Characteristics. The sample included 42 native French-speaking caregivers ranging from 27 to 67 years ($M = 46.12$ years; $SD = 10.84$) and the majority was women (69%). Twenty-one (50%) of the participants were nurses, and 21 (50%) were physicians. Our sample was composed of nurses working in different settings, general practitioners, and medical specialists (physiatrist, rheumatologist, orthopaedist, radiologist, nephrologist, neurologist, and psychiatrist). The nurses and physicians had an average of 19.74 years of clinical experience. In this group, participants self-reported a mean overall orientation for PPC of 4.82. More specifically, the mean was 4.49 for the sharing subscale and 5.16 for the caring subscale. The participants self-reported a mean of 116.53 for empathy. These results suggest moderate levels of PCC and empathy when participants assess themselves. For the observer's assessment with observation scales, the results are presented for each video. For observed PCC, the mean for the 4 videos was 25.94, and for observed empathy, the mean was 20.70. Table 1 shows the characteristics of these participants.

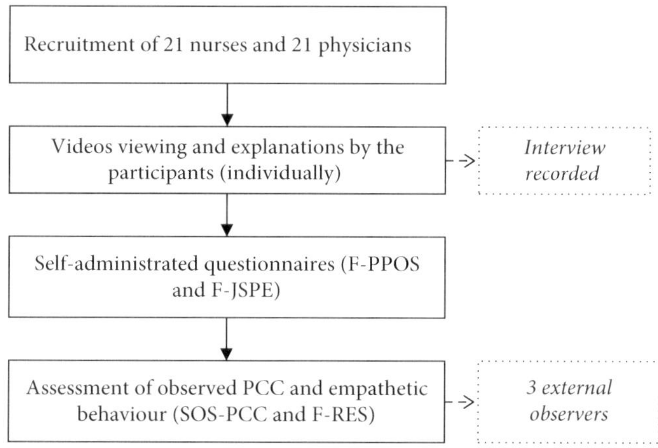

Figure 1: Conduct of the study. F-PPOS indicates the French version of the Patient-Practitioner Orientation Scale, F-JSPE indicates the French version of the Jefferson Scale of Physician Empathy, PCC indicates patient-centered care, SOS-PCC indicates Sherbrooke Observation Scale of patient-centered care, and F-RES indicates the French version of the Reynolds Empathy Scale.

3.2. Patient-Centered and Empathetic Behaviour according to the Presence or Absence of Visible Physical Signs. In total, 168 interviews in response to the videos were videotaped successfully. We divided these interviews in two groups: (i) interviews in response to the videos presenting patients with visible physical signs (rheumatoid arthritis and CRPS) and (ii) interviews in response to the videos presenting patients without visible physical signs (Ehlers–Danlos syndrome and fibromyalgia). Regarding the observed patient-centered and empathetic behaviours, the mean for SOS-PCC and F-RES was calculated for both groups. The results support that patient-centered and empathetic behaviour was significantly higher for the group of patients with visible physical signs ($p < 0.001$) (Figure 2). The group of participants who show a greater difference in their patient-centered behaviour according to pain visibility have less clinical experience than the group that had similar behaviour for both patients with and without physical visible signs ($p = 0.03$). For empathetic behaviour, the difference is not statistically significant ($p = 0.23$) (Table 2).

4. Discussion

The results suggest that our sample of caregivers have moderate levels of self-reported PCC and empathy. In comparison with other studies, nurses and physicians who have participated in our study used more PCC than other groups of nurses and physicians with similar sociodemographic characteristics [38, 39]. For self-reported empathy, our sample was comparable to other nurses and physicians [40].

The main purpose of this descriptive study was to investigate the influence of the presence or absence of visible physical signs on caregiver behaviours and attitudes in chronic pain management. PCC and empathy were assessed from two perspectives, using a combination of self-administrated questionnaires and observation scales using innovative videos of real patients with chronic pain. Our results show that nurses and physicians show intraindividual variability. Indeed, we found that PCC and empathetic behaviour of nurses and physicians vary according to the presence or absence of visible physical signs in patients with chronic pain.

Interestingly, another research team have demonstrated that residents in internal medicine have displayed more patient-centered behaviour when they consider that the patient has a more severe health condition and more visible physical symptoms [26]. In the same vein, another research group has demonstrated that patient-centered practice style of physicians was positively related with higher patient self-reported physical health status [24]. Although the severity of the disease is not automatically associated with the presence of visible physical symptoms, the results of clinical observations have shown that patients with more severe diseases were given longer consultations and the opportunity to talk more about their medical condition [41]. These observations have a great importance in the context of chronic pain, since these patients often have no visible physical signs, and can remain stoic when they feel pain [28] because their condition is often present for several years. For example, patients with neuropathic pain suffer from allodynia and hyperalgesia, but they often have no obvious physical signs. Moreover, some authors have suggested that professional caregivers were baffled by the lack of correlation between pain intensity verbally and nonverbally expressed by chronic pain patients and their medical condition [42].

It has been shown that physicians tend to rely on their initial assessment of the pain of their patients with chronic pain even when this initial assessment underestimates the pain subsequently reported verbally by the patients [43]. Thus, if chronic pain patients are not asked about their preoccupations and their medical condition's severity, stoic patients and those with less visible physical signs are more likely to receive suboptimal personalized care, with a more disease-centered orientation and less empathetic behaviour. These findings suggest that nurses and physicians adjust their practice orientation and empathy according to the clinical condition. It could explain why many patients with chronic pain are frustrated after their clinical encounters. This has a particular impact since these interactions are prominent in their experience [43].

Table 1: Results of self-administrated questionnaires.

	Participants ($n = 42$)
Age, mean (SD)	46.12 (10.84)
Gender, n (%)	
Male	13 (31)
Female	29 (69)
Profession, n (%)	
Nurse	21 (50)
Physician	21 (50)
Clinical experience, mean (SD)	19.74 (10.34)
F-PPOS total, mean (SD)	4.82 (0.39)
Sharing, mean (SD)	4.49 (0.59)
Caring, mean (SD)	5.16 (0.37)
F-JSPE, mean (SD)	116.53 (9.80)
SOS-PCC, mean (SD)	25.94 (3.86)
Patient with rheumatoid arthritis, mean (SD)	27.12 (3.88)
Patient with CRPS, mean (SD)	27.38 (4.30)
Patient with Ehlers–Danlos syndrome, mean (SD)	26.02 (4.38)
Patient with fibromyalgia, mean (SD)	24.87 (5.11)
F-RES, mean (SD)	20.70 (3.41)
Patient with rheumatoid arthritis, mean (SD)	21.89 (3.59)
Patient with CRPS, mean (SD)	22.30 (3.25)
Patient with Ehlers–Danlos syndrome, mean (SD)	20.34 (3.81)
Patient with fibromyalgia, mean (SD)	18.94 (4.05)

SD = standard deviation; F-PPOS = French version of Patient-Practitioner Orientation Scale; F-JSPE = French version of Jefferson Scale of Physician Empathy; SOS-PCC = Sherbrooke Orientation Scale of patient-centered care; CRPS = complex regional pain syndrome; F-RES = French version of Reynolds Empathy Scale.

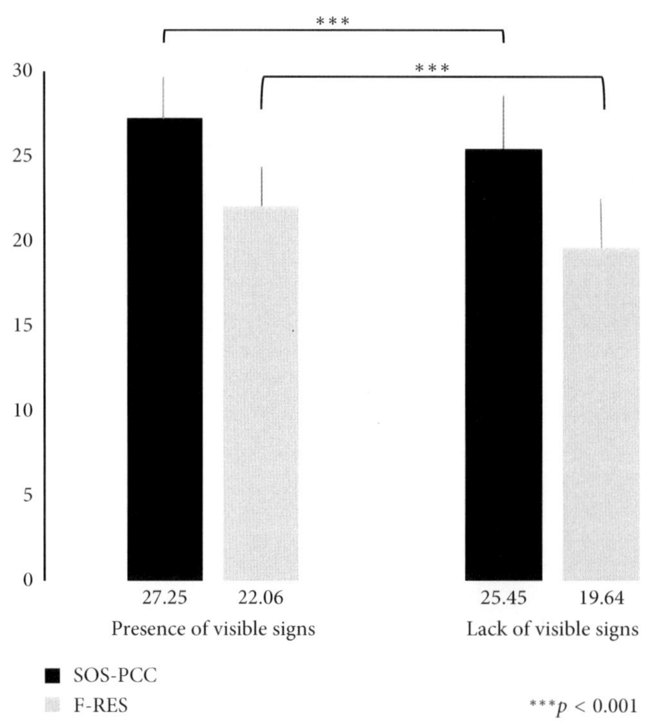

Figure 2: Influence of pain visibility on patient-centered care and empathy. Patient-centered care and empathy behaviours were observed by external raters. SOS-PCC indicates Sherbrooke Orientation Scale of patient-centered care, and F-RES indicates French version of the Reynolds Empathy Scale.

Interestingly, we found that the clinical experience can influence the behaviours of nurses and physicians. Indeed, caregivers with more years of experience are less likely to change their behaviour were according to the presence or absence of physical visible signs. Many studies have investigated the influence of clinical experience on PCC and

TABLE 2: Influence of clinical experience on caregivers' behaviours in the presence or absence of physical visible signs.

	Similar ratings	Different ratings	p value
Patient-centered behaviour			
n	14	28	
Clinical experience, years (SD)	24.64 (8.68)	17.29 (10.36)	0.03
Empathetic behaviour			
n	20	22	
Clinical experience, years (SD)	20.35 (9.73)	19.18 (11.05)	0.23

SD = standard deviation.

empathy [44, 45], but little is known about how clinical experience could modulate these variables. A brain imaging study showed that clinical exposure could reduce empathy for pain [46]. More specifically, the authors investigated cortical activity among physicians and control subjects exposed to a series of visual stimuli with body parts in painful and painless situations. Their results indicated that the cortical structures associated with empathy for pain were significantly activated in the control subjects, but not in physicians. It is suggested that these observations are the consequence of a protective regulatory mechanism in people who work daily with pain in order to prevent their distress [46]. Thus, it is possible to believe that the behaviours of the most experienced caregivers are less influenced by the presence of visible signs of pain. However, our results show no difference in PCC and empathy levels according to the clinical experience ($p > 0.05$). It is also possible that the most experienced caregivers are more aware of the impact of pain visibility, and they consider this potential bias in their interventions.

One potential limitation of our study is the lack of a real interaction between participants and patients in the videos. As a result of its methodological advantages and low cost, we used standardized videos of real chronic pain patients. However, the observation scales used for the assessment of PCC and empathetic behaviours were adapted for this kind of situation. Another potential limitation is the reactivity bias. It is possible that participants have positively modified their answers regarding the treatment plan that they would provide in reality. However, many efforts have been made to mitigate this potential bias. First, the participants did not know the variables under study at the time of data collection. Secondly, the questionnaires were distributed at the end of the experimental session in order to avoid a modification in behaviour, conscious or not, from participants.

5. Conclusions

In the last years, several studies have shown that practice orientation and empathy of professional caregivers could be influenced by many patients' factors [43, 45, 46], and our results are consistent with these previous findings. To our knowledge, this is the first study showing a direct influence of visible physical signs on PCC and empathy in the context of chronic pain management. Those observations are to be considered, since chronic pain patients often do not show any apparent physical signs. Thus, these patients are more likely to receive suboptimal pain management, more disease centered and devoid of empathic behaviour. This raises the importance of educating caregivers and future caregivers to these unconscious biases and the potential impact on chronic pain patients. The impact of the presence or absence of apparent physical signs must also be considered for research in chronic pain since it is a potential confounding factor. Future studies could utilize real clinical encounters and other populations to replicate these results.

Disclosure

This work is part of a doctoral study. This article is based on the thesis "Paul-Savoie E, Identification des caractéristiques des soignants liées à l'utilisation d'une approche centrée sur le patient dans un contexte de douleur chronique" (published doctoral thesis; https://doi.org/10.13039/100009874) (Université de Sherbrooke, Sherbrooke, Canada, https://savoirs.usherbrooke.ca/handle/11143/6974).

Acknowledgments

E. Paul-Savoie had at the time of the study a doctoral scholarship from the Canadian Institute of Health Research (CIHR) and was supported by the medicine and health science faculty of the Université de Sherbrooke. P. Bourgault was at the time of the study a Junior 1 Clinician Investigator with the Quebec Fund for Health Research (FRQS) and a researcher at the Centre de recherche du Centre hospitalier universitaire de Sherbrooke (CR-CHUS). S. Potvin was at the time of the study a Junior 1 Young Investigator from the FRQS and was supported by the Centre de recherche de l'Institut universitaire en santé mentale de Montréal and the Louis-H Lafontaine Hospital Foundation. E. Gosselin had doctoral scholarships from the FRQS, the Ministère de l'éducation supérieure, de la recherche et des sciences (MESRS)-Universités, and the Réseau de recherche en interventions en sciences infirmières du Québec. S. Lafrenaye was supported by the medicine and health science faculty of the Université de Sherbrooke and a researcher at the CR-CHUS.

References

[1] D. S. Goldberg and S. J. McGee, "Pain as a global public health priority," *BMC Public Health*, vol. 11, no. 1, p. 770, 2011.

[2] R. A. Elzahaf, O. A Tashani, B. A Unsworth et al., "The prevalence of chronic an analysis of countries with a human development index less than 0.9: a systematic review without meta-analysis," *Current Medical Research and Opinion*, vol. 28, no. 7, pp. 1221–1229, 2012.

[3] D. J. Gaskin and P. Richard, "The economic costs of pain in the United States," *Journal of Pain*, vol. 13, no. 8, pp. 715–724, 2012.

[4] P. A. Pizzo and N. M. Clark, "Alleviating suffering 101–pain relief in the United States," *New England Journal of Medicine*, vol. 366, no. 3, pp. 197–199, 2012.

[5] L. Jacobson and A. J. Mariano, "General considerations of chronic pain," in *Bonica's Management of Pain*, J. D. Loeser, S. H. Butler, R. Chapman, and D. C. Turk, Eds., pp. 241–254, Lippincott Williams & Wilkins, Philadelphia, PA, USA, 2001.

[6] J. Carter, A. C. Watson, and P. V. Sminkey, "Pain management: screening and assessment of pain as part of a comprehensive case management process," *Professional Case Management*, vol. 19, no. 3, pp. 126–134, 2014.

[7] C. M. Goertz, S. A. Salsbury, C. R. Long et al., "Patient-centered professional practice models for managing low back pain in older adults: a pilot randomized controlled trial," *BMC Geriatrics*, vol. 17, pp. 235–248, 2017.

[8] K. Bilodeau, S. Dubois, and J. Pepin, "Contribution des sciences infirmières au développement des savoirs interprofessionnels," *Recherches en soins infirmiers*, vol. 113, no. 2, pp. 43–50, 2013.

[9] C. Hudon, M. Fortin, J. L. Haggerty et al., "Measuring patients' perceptions of patient-centered care: a systematic review of tools for family medicine," *Annals of Family Medicine*, vol. 9, no. 2, pp. 155–164, 2011.

[10] B. McCormack and T. McCance, "Developing a conceptual framework for person-centred nursing," *Journal of Advanced Nursing*, vol. 56, no. 5, pp. 472–479, 2006.

[11] M. M. Alamo, R. R. Moral, and L. A. P. de Torres, "Evaluation of a patient-centred approach in generalized musculoskeletal chronic pain/fibromyalgia patients in primary care," *Patient Education and Counseling*, vol. 48, no. 1, pp. 23–31, 2002.

[12] D. B. Monsivais and J. C. Engebretson, "Cultural cues: review of qualitative evidence of patient-centered care in patients with nonmalignant chronic pain," *Rehabilitation Nursing*, vol. 36, no. 4, pp. 166–171, 2011.

[13] T. Taverner, S. J. Closs, and M. Briggs, "The journey to chronic pain : a grounded theory of older adults' experience of pain associated with leg ulceration," *Pain Management Nursing*, vol. 15, pp. 186–198, 2014.

[14] M. S. Krasner, R. M. Epstein, H. Beckman et al., "Association of an educational program in mindful communication with burnout, empathy, and attitudes among primary care physicians," *JAMA*, vol. 302, no. 12, pp. 1284–1293, 2009.

[15] S. A. Passalacqua and C. Segrin, "The effect of resident physician stress, burnout, and empathy on patient-centered communication during the long-call shift," *Health Communication*, vol. 27, no. 5, pp. 449–456, 2011.

[16] M. Hojat, J. S. Gonnella, T. J. Nasca et al., "Physician empathy: definition, components, measurement, and relationship to gender and specialty," *American Journal of Psychiatry*, vol. 159, no. 9, pp. 1563–1569, 2002.

[17] E. B. Larson and X. Yao, "Clinical empathy as emotional labor in the patient-physician relationship," *JAMA*, vol. 293, no. 9, pp. 1100–1106, 2005.

[18] M. Neumann, M. Wirtz, E. Bollschweiler et al., "Determinants and patient-reported long-term outcomes of physician empathy in oncology: a structural equation modelling approach," *Patient Education and Counseling*, vol. 69, no. 1–3, pp. 63–75, 2007.

[19] D. P. Rakel, T. J. Hoeft, B. P. Barrett et al., "Practitioner empathy and the duration of the common cold," *Family Medicine*, vol. 41, no. 7, pp. 494–501, 2009.

[20] L. Canovas, A. J. Carrascosa, M. Garcia et al., "Impact of empathy in the patient-doctor relationship on chronic pain relief and quality of life: a prospective study in Spanish pain clinics," *Pain Medicine*, vol. 19, no. 7, pp. 1304–1314, 2017.

[21] P. Haidet, J. E. Dains, D. A. Paterniti et al., "Medical student attitudes toward the doctor-patient relationship," *Medical Education*, vol. 36, no. 6, pp. 568–574, 2002.

[22] S. Parsons, G. Harding, A. Breen et al., "Will shared decision making between patient with chronic musculoskeletal pain and physiotherapists, osteopaths and chiropractors improve patient care?," *Family Practice*, vol. 29, no. 2, pp. 203–212, 2012.

[23] R. M. Epstein, P. Franks, K. Fiscella et al., "Measuring patient-centered communication in patient-physician consultations: theoretical and practical issues," *Social Science and Medicine*, vol. 61, no. 7, pp. 1516–1528, 2005.

[24] K. D. Bertakis and R. Azari, "Determinants and outcomes of patient-centered care," *Patient Education and Counseling*, vol. 85, no. 1, pp. 46–52, 2011.

[25] S. Willems, S. De Maesschalck, M. Deveugele et al., "Socio-economic status of the patient and doctor-patient communication: does it make a difference?," *Patient Education and Counseling*, vol. 56, no. 2, pp. 139–146, 2005.

[26] L. C. Zandbelt, E. M. Smets, F. J. Oorf et al., "Determinants of physicians' patient-centred behaviour in the medical specialist encounter," *Social Science and Medicine*, vol. 63, no. 4, pp. 899–910, 2006.

[27] J. Decety, S. Echols, and J. Correll, "The blame game: the effect of responsibility and social stigma on empathy for pain," *Journal of Cognitive Neuroscience*, vol. 22, no. 5, pp. 985–997, 2009.

[28] D. B. Monsivais, "Decreasing the stigma burden of chronic pain," *Journal of the American Association of Nurse Practitioners*, vol. 25, no. 10, pp. 551–556, 2013.

[29] J. M. Hemmerdinger, S. Stoddart, and A. Lilford, "A systematic review of tests of empathy in medicine," *BMC Medical Education*, vol. 7, no. 1, p. 24, 2007.

[30] J. Childs, "Clinical resource centers in nursing programs," *Nurse Educator*, vol. 27, no. 5, pp. 232–235, 2002.

[31] E. Paul-Savoie, P. Bourgault, E. Gosselin et al., "Assessing patient-centered care for chronic pain: validation of a new research paradigm," *Pain Research and Management*, vol. 20, no. 4, pp. 183–188, 2015.

[32] E. Paul-Savoie, "Identification des caractéristiques des soignants liées à l'utilisation d'une approche centrée sur le patient dans un contexte de douleur chronique,"Sherbrooke, Canada, (Published doctoral thesis).

[33] E. Paul-Savoie, P. Bourgault, E. Gosselin et al., "Assessing patient-centered care: validation of the French Version of the Patient-Practitioner Orientation Scale (PPOS)," *European Journal for Person Centered Healthcare*, vol. 3, no. 3, pp. 295–302, 2015.

[34] E. Krupat, S. L. Rosenkranz, C. M. Yeager et al., "The practice orientations of physicians and patients: the effect of doctor-patient congruence on satisfaction," *Patient Education and Counseling*, vol. 39, no. 1, pp. 49–59, 2000.

[35] C. A. McHorney, J. E. Ware, J. F. R. Lu et al., "The MOS 36-item short-form health survey (SF-36): III. Tests of data

quality, scaling assumptions, and reliability across diverse patient groups," *Medical Care*, vol. 32, no. 1, pp. 40–66, 1994.

[36] M. Hojat, J. S. Gonnella, S. Mangione et al., "Physician empathy in medical education and practice: experience with the Jefferson scale of physician empathy," *Seminars in Integrative Medicine*, vol. 1, no. 1, pp. 25–41, 2003.

[37] E. Gosselin, E. Paul-Savoie, S. Lavoie et al., "Reliability and validity of the French version of the Reynolds Empathy Scale in nursing," *Journal of Nursing Measurement*, vol. 23, pp. E16–E26, 2015.

[38] C. M. H. Chan and W. A. W. Ahmad, "Differences in physician attitudes towards patient-centredness: across four medical specialties," *International Journal of Clinical Practice*, vol. 66, no. 1, pp. 16–20, 2011.

[39] A. M. Grilo, M. C. Santos, J. S. Rita et al., "Assessment of nursing students and nurses' orientation toward patient-centeredness," *Nurse Education Today*, vol. 34, no. 1, pp. 35–39, 2014.

[40] S. K. Fields, M. Hojat, J. S. Gonnella et al., "Comparisons of nurses and physicians on an operational measure of empathy," *Evaluation and the Health Professions*, vol. 27, no. 1, pp. 80–94, 2004.

[41] P. K. Graugaard, K. Holgersen, H. Eide et al., "Changes in physician-patient communication from initial to return visits: a prospective study in a haematology outpatient clinic," *Patient Education and Counseling*, vol. 57, no. 1, pp. 22–29, 2005.

[42] A. Allaz, *Le Messager Boiteux: Approche Pratique des Douleurs Chroniques Rebelles, Genève: Médecine et Hygiène*, in French, Lavoisier S.A.S, Chêne-Bourg, Switzerland, 2003.

[43] P. Riva, P. Rusconi, L. Montali et al., "The influence of anchoring on pain judgement," *Journal of Pain and Symptom Management*, vol. 42, no. 2, pp. 265–277, 2011.

[44] M. Neumann, F. Edelhauser, D. Tauschel et al., "Empathy decline and its reasons: a systematic review of studies with medical students and residents," *Academic Medicine*, vol. 86, no. 8, pp. 996–1009, 2011.

[45] Z. Tsimtsiou, A. Benos, A. A. Garyfallos et al., "Predictors of physicians' attitudes toward sharing information with patients and addressing psychosocial needs: a cross-sectional study in Greece," *Health Communication*, vol. 27, no. 3, pp. 257–263, 2012.

[46] Y. Cheng, C. P. Lin, H. L. Li et al., "Expertise modulates the perception of pain in others," *Current Biology*, vol. 17, no. 19, pp. 1708–1713, 2007.

Relationship between Cervical Spine and Skeletal Class II in Subjects with and without Temporomandibular Disorders

Paola Di Giacomo, Valeria Ferrara, Ettore Accivile, Giacomo Ferrato, Antonella Polimeni, and Carlo Di Paolo

Department of Oral and Maxillofacial Sciences, Sapienza University of Rome, Rome, Italy

Correspondence should be addressed to Paola Di Giacomo; p.digiacomo@uniroma1.it

Academic Editor: Fabio Antonaci

Aim. To assess changes in the craniocervical structure and in hyoid bone position in skeletal Class II subjects with and without temporomandibular disorders (TMD). *Materials and Methods.* The cephalometric analysis of 59 subjects with skeletal Class II was evaluated and compared. The measurements considered were ANB as a parameter of Class II and C0-C1 distance, C1-C2 distance, craniocervical angle, and hyoid bone position for the cervical spine analysis. Patients were divided into patients with TMD (group A) and patients without TMD (group B). TMD were evaluated with Diagnostic Criteria for TMD (DC/TMD). Descriptive statistics and Pearson's and Spearman's correlation analysis, with p value <0,005, were performed. *Results.* C0-C1 and C1-C2 distance values and hyoid bone position resulted within the normal range in the majority of patients examined. Craniocervical angle was altered in 33 patients. The reduction of this angle with the increase of the ANB value resulted to be statistically significant in group A, according to Pearson's correlation index. No other data were statistically significant. *Conclusions.* The significant relationship between skeletal Class II and cervical spine cannot be highlighted. The alteration of craniocervical angle seems to be mildly present, with backward counterclockwise rotation of the head upon the neck in the sample (groups A and B). The presence of TMD as a key factor of changes in neck posture could explain the different result between the two groups about the relationship between ANB and craniocervical angle. This result should be further analyzed in order to better understand if cervical spine changes could be related to mandibular postural ones in the craniocervical space or to temporomandibular joint retropositioning, more recognizable in Class II with TMD, which could determine functional changes in other structures of this unit; neck posture could be the result of a compensatory/antalgic mechanism in response to TMD.

1. Introduction

The stomatognathic system is composed of several structures which, acting in synergy, provide the complex functions of swallowing, sucking, chewing, speech, and breathing. Functionality of these components has a cybernetic and integrated control, and it depends on the specific individual adaptability and response to perturbing factors. This system correlates with the cervical spine and hyoid bone, forming a functional craniocervical mandibular unit. For this reason, the principles of head and neck biomechanics are of great interest both in the dental field (particularly in the orthodontic and gnathologic field) and in the physical rehabilitation one.

Because of the impossibility to record functions in the same moment in which they are performed, anatomical relationships among the examined structures are analyzed in order to evaluate functional and dysfunctional aspects of the craniocervical mandibular system.

Many studies found support for anatomical [1, 2] and functional [3, 4] relationship between the cranial region, the temporomandibular joint, the cervical spine, and the hyoid bone. Although there is presence of suggestive results in these studies, the mechanism of this relationship is still unclear.

In the literature, cervical posture is related to different factors of the body such as craniofacial morphology [5, 6] and functional factors such as nasorespiratory function [7]

and temporomandibular dysfunction [2]. Previous studies were focused on the relationship between the cervical spine and skeletal class of the subjects [2, 5, 6], but results were contrasting. Skeletal Class II malocclusions were chosen for this study, needing to analyze a specific skeletal category to compare with data obtained in the literature [6, 8, 9] and needing to have a homogeneous sample under the point of view of skeletal class, within which a large subgroup of dysfunctional patients could be collected. In fact, skeletal Class II subjects are more easily linked to temporomandibular disorders [10, 11].

The choice to deal also with TMD is because the relationship between temporomandibular joint "status" and head-neck posture should be investigated, within the craniocervical mandibular unit. Temporomandibular disorders are often associated with headache and neck pain. The relation between TMD and the head and neck posture changes is still controversial and unclear [12]. Some studies [13, 14] found correlation between the presence of symptoms of craniocervical dysfunction and temporomandibular disorders. On the contrary, others [11, 15] found no relationship between TMD and head-neck posture.

In this study, means that are scientifically appropriate, easy to use, and produce measurable results were used. For this reason, data were gathered from cephalometric analysis, carried out on lateral X-ray of the skull (lateral skull radiographs) which, together with orthopantomography, represents basic X-ray imaging in orthodontic and gnathologic fields. In fact, this allows to evaluate possible changes in the physiological curve of the cervical spine, head position, and hyoid bone position, in addition to standard orthodontic skeletal assessment.

2. Materials and Methods

2.1. Study Design. To address the research purpose, patients were recruited among those who came under our observation at the Gnathology Section of the Department of Oral and Maxillo-facial Sciences, Sapienza University of Rome, and at the Clinical Operative Unit of Orthodontics of the George Eastman Hospital, Sapienza University of Rome, between October 2017 and March 2018, according to the inclusion and exclusion criteria.

The study was approved by the Institutional Human Ethics Committee, Sapienza University of Rome.

2.1.1. Inclusion Criteria

(i) Patients with presence of skeletal Class II

(ii) Patients at least 18 years old

(iii) Patients who provided signed informed consent, according to the World Medical Association's Declaration of Helsinki

2.1.2. Exclusion Criteria

(i) Loss of posterior teeth

(ii) History of trauma

(iii) Previous orthodontic and/or gnathologic and/or physical therapies

(iv) Presence of further structural malformations in the areas of interest

(v) Presence of uncontrolled systemic disease

On the basis of these criteria, the sample comprised 59 individuals, 38 females and 21 males, with an average age of 33.65 years.

The sample was divided into two subgroups: group A—patients with dysfunctions, and group B—patients without dysfunctions. The integrated DC/TMD method was used for the screening of temporomandibular disorders [16] and to assess which patients belonged to group A and which to group B. Group A comprised 26 patients, 24 females and 2 males, with an average age of 44.69 years. Only patients with the following disorders were considered: disc displacement with reduction; myalgia and myofascial pain; subluxation; headache associated with TMD; arthralgia; and osteoarthrosis. Disc displacements without reduction were not taken into account because the complexity of pathology has many confounding factors.

Group B comprised 33 individuals, 14 females and 19 males, with an average age of 24.33 years.

2.2. Cephalometric Assessment. All cephalograms were made upon a standardized lateral radiograph (18 Å~24 cm film; Kodak, Germany) on the basis of natural head position (patients' midplane-X-ray source distance 146 cm; patients' midplane-film distance 13.5 cm; enlargement factor 1%; and exposure 4–21 mAs, 60–80 kV) by a single technician in the Radiology Unit of George Eastman Hospital, Policlinico Umberto I, Rome.

Specific linear and angular measures from the cephalometric analysis performed on the lateral skull radiographs were assessed. The cephalometric analysis used was chosen among those proposed in the literature and scientifically validated for the study of the relationships between skull bones, in particular jaw and mandible, and between these and the cervical spine and the hyoid bone. McNamara's modified cephalometric analysis was used, and linear and angular measures were performed. Among the various affected measures, the cephalometric parameter considered for the evaluation of presence of skeletal Class II was ANB angle, according to Steiner (normal value $2^\circ \pm 2^\circ$) [17].

The standard cephalometric analysis was associated with the method proposed by Rocabado [18] for the study of the other cervical parameters. The parameters considered in the study were as follows:

(i) The craniocervical angle which is the inner angle formed by the intersection of McGregor's plane (line passing through the occiput and nasal spine) and odontoid plane (line passing through the inferior-anterior point of the odontoid process and its superior apex) with a normal value of 101 ± 5.

(ii) The C0-C1 vertebrae distance with a normal range of 6.5 ± 2.5 mm.

(iii) The C1-C2 vertebrae distance with a normal range of 6.5 ± 2.5 mm.

(iv) Hyoid bone position defined by the relationship between the H point (superoanterior point of the hyoid bone) and H′ line (conjunction line between retrognathion and C3 vertebra). The distance H-H′ should be 5 ± 2 mm.

2.3. Statistics. Data taken from the cephalometric analysis were interpreted using basic descriptive statistical analysis and Pearson's correlation index for random variables and the nonparametric Spearman's ordinary measures to evaluate the correlation between parameters.

2.3.1. Correlation Scores

(i) $0 < \rho_{XY} < 0.3$–weak correlation

(ii) $0.3 < \rho_{XY} < 0.7$–moderate correlation

(iii) $\rho_{XY} > 0.7$–strong correlation

The level of significance (p value) is 0.005, verified according to Student's t tables (for Pearson's correlation results and Spearman's correlation analysis with $N > 30$) and according to Spearman's rho value for Spearman's correlation analysis with $N < 30$.

3. Results

Data obtained were primarily organized in tables and analyzed with descriptive statistics. Only significant results were presented, considering the great amount of data.

The absolute frequency distribution of each ANB value (5 to 9°/10°) was reported. For each ANB value, the absolute and percent frequency distribution of the values of the measured cervical variables, divided on the basis of the severity as abnormally low, normal, and abnormally high, was considered.

Furthermore, these results were divided into two subgroups, on the basis of the presence or not of temporomandibular disorders. Percent frequencies of DC/TMD diseases are reported in Table 1.

For what concerning skeletal Class II and cervical alterations, independently from the presence of temporomandibular disorders, the following results were found: 65% of all subjects examined (38 subjects) showed normal values of C0-C1 space on the vertical plane. The C1-C2 space was normal in 73% of the patients (43 subjects), as shown in Tables 2 and 3. The hyoid bone was found to be in a normal limit position in 51% (30 subjects) of the subjects examined and in an outside positive position in 49% of the cases (29 subjects) (Table 4).

Craniocervical angle measurement was out of standard in 56% of the patients (33 subjects); 13 of them (40%) were found to be positive to TMD. It was reduced in 51% of the patients (30 subjects), normal in 44% (26 subjects), and increased in 5% of them (3 subjects) (Table 5).

In our work, the descriptive analysis found that 35.60% of the patients presented an ANB angle of 5° (21), and these subjects showed the highest number of abnormal values of all cervical measurements considered.

Table 1: Absolute frequency and percentage (n (%) values) of DC/TMD diseases.

DC/TMD disease	Prevalence (%) ($N = 26$)
Muscle/myofascial pain	50 (13)
Arthralgia	82 (21)
Disc dislocation with reduction	8 (2)
Subluxation	13 (3)
Headache associated with TMD	31 (8)
Osteoarthrosis	8 (2)

For what concerning skeletal Class II, temporomandibular disorders, and cervical anomalies, the C0-C1 space was altered in 30% of not-dysfunctional patients and in 42% of dysfunctional patients and the C1-C2 space was altered in 27% of both not-dysfunctional and dysfunctional patients. Craniocervical angle in not-dysfunctional patients showed some anomalies in 20 of 33 subjects (61%), while in the dysfunctional group, it was altered in 13 of 26 subjects (50%). Hyoid bone position was altered in 54% of the dysfunctional patients (14 subjects); this result was similar in 45% of nondysfunctional subjects (15 of 18). There are not significant percent differences between the two groups.

There are no statistically significant data (Tables 6–8) except for the moderate inverse correlation between the increase of ANB and the reduction of craniocervical angle in the dysfunctional group, in Pearson's correlation test (Table 9).

4. Discussion

From the analysis of the entire sample, there were not particular significant results in percentage terms for what concerning the relationship between skeletal Class II in adult patients and neck structure and posture, within the limits of the sample examined. The statistical correlations did not show significance between the variables, either in positive or in negative sense. Correlation indexes were always very close to zero, and these proved that distributions were independent of the previous associations. This is not in line with the results obtained in some publications of the scientific literature, which support a correlation between skeletal class II and morphologic and postural cervical spine alterations [6, 9, 19]. Festa [6] found the relationship between cervical lordosis and cranial base and mandibular length. Hosseinzadeh Nik and Aciyabar [9] found significant correlation between cervical column posture angles and the parameters ANB and Wits in Class II patients. Sonnessen [18] found associations between fusions of the cervical column and mandibular retrognathia, large cranial base angle, and large horizontal overjet, and Miyuki et al. [20] found that Class II subjects have significantly lower atlas dorsal arch heights. On the contrary, Bebnowski et al. [21] found that cervical anomalies (CVAs) did not correlate to any cephalometric values nor they could be confirmed by CBCT, the gold standard for assessing CVA.

TABLE 2: Absolute and percent frequencies of the C0-C1 distance value for each ANB score. ANB scores are 5 to 9°/10°. C0-C1 values are divided into abnormally low, normal, and abnormally high. Class II is divided on the basis of the presence or not of TMD.

TMD	ANB Value	C0-C1 space: Abnormally low (<4.5 mm)	Normal	Abnormally high (>4.5 mm)	Total.
Absent	5	2	14	1	17
	6	1	2	5	8
	7	0	3	1	4
	9	0	4	0	4
	Total	3	23	7	33
		0.09	0.70	0.21	1.0
Present	5	6	8	0	14
	6	3	4	2	9
	7	0	1	0	1
	9	0	1	0	1
	10	0	1	0	1
	Total	9	15	2	26
		0.35	0.58	0.08	1.0

TABLE 3: Absolute and percent frequencies of the C1-C2 distance value for each ANB score. ANB scores are 5 to 9°/10°. C1-C2 values are divided into abnormally low, normal, and abnormally high. Class II is divided on the basis of the presence or not of TMD.

TMD	ANB Value	C1-C2 space: Abnormally low (<4.5 mm)	Normal	Abnormally high (>4.5 mm)	Total
Absent	5	2	11	4	17
	6	2	5	1	8
	7	0	4	0	4
	9	0	4	0	4
	Total	4	24	5	33
		0.12	0.73	0.15	1.0
Present	5	3	11	0	14
	6	3	5	1	9
	7	0	1	0	1
	9	0	1	0	1
	10	0	1	0	1
	Total	6	19	1	26
		0.23	0.73	0.04	1.0

TABLE 4: Absolute and percent frequencies of hyoid bone position for each ANB score. ANB scores are 5 to 9°/10°. Values are divided into abnormally low and normal. Class II is divided on the basis of the presence or not of TMD.

TMD	ANB Value	Hyoid bone position: Abnormally low (<3 mm)	Normal	Total
Absent	5	8	9	17
	6	5	3	8
	7	1	3	4
	9	1	3	4
	Total	15	18	33
		0.45	0.55	1.0
Present	5	7	7	14
	6	6	3	9
	7	1	0	1
	9	0	1	1
	10	0	1	1
	Total	14	12	26
		0.54	0.46	1.0

These studies represented the starting point of this research which should be verified in our sample. The data obtained do not confirm what has been said in these previous research studies. The only alteration which can be reported is about craniocervical angle, but it is present only in 56% of the patients, so it cannot be considered to be representative.

TABLE 5: Absolute and percent frequencies of the craniocervical angle value for each ANB score. ANB scores are 5 to 9°/10°. Values are divided into abnormally low, normal, and abnormally high. Class II is divided on the basis of the presence or not of TMD.

TMD	ANB Value	Craniocervical angle: Abnormally low (<96°)	Normal	Abnormally high (>106°)	Total
Absent	5	8	7	2	17
	6	4	4	0	8
	7	3	1	0	4
	9	3	1	0	4
	Total	18	13	2	33
		0.55	0.39	0.06	1.0
Present	5	6	7	1	14
	6	4	5	0	9
	7	0	1	0	1
	9	1	0	0	1
	10	1	0	0	1
	Total	12	13	1	26
		0.46	0.50	0.04	1.0
		1.0	1.0	1.0	1,0

TABLE 6: Pearson's and Spearman's correlation analysis between C0-C1 distance and ANB scores.

TMD	Pearson's correlation index	Student's t test ($p < 0.005$)	Spearman's correlation index	Student's t test ($p < 0.005$)
Absent ($N = 33$)	0.147 (L)	0.830 (NS)	0.158 (L)	0.890 (NS)
Present ($N = 26$)	0.113 (L)	0.5 (NS)	0.152 (L)	NS according to critical values table for the nonparametric test

L: low correlation; NS: nonsignificant. Student's t test is used for the evaluation of significance, with a p value <0.005.

TABLE 7: Pearson's and Spearman's correlation analysis between C1-C2 distance and ANB scores.

TMD	Pearson's correlation index	Student's t test ($p < 0.005$)	Spearman's correlation index	Student's t test ($p < 0.005$)
Absent	0.043 (L)	0.241 (NS)	0.100 (L)	0.560 (NS)
Present	−0.039 (L)	−0.190 (NS)	0.134 (L)	NS according to critical values table for the nonparametric test

L: low correlation; NS: nonsignificant. Student's t test is used for the evaluation of significance, with a p value <0.005.

TABLE 8: Pearson's and Spearman's correlation analysis between hyoid bone position and ANB scores.

TMD	Pearson's correlation index	Student's t test ($p < 0.005$)	Spearman's correlation index	Student's t test ($p < 0.005$)
Absent	0.024 (L)	0.135 (NS)	0.072 (L)	0.403 (NS)
Present	−0.109 (L)	−0.535 (NS)	−0.145 (L)	NS according to critical values table for the nonparametric test

L: low correlation; NS: nonsignificant. Student's t test is used for the evaluation of significance, with a p value <0.005.

TABLE 9: Pearson's and Spearman's correlation analysis between craniocervical angle and ANB scores.

TMD	Pearson's correlation index	Student's t test ($p < 0.005$)	Spearman's correlation index	Student's t test ($p < 0.005$)
Absent	−0.085 (L)	−0.475 (NS)	−0.169 (L)	−0.954 (NS)
Present	−0.547 (M)	−3.198 (S)	−0.212 (L)	NS according to critical values table for the nonparametric test

L: low correlation; M: moderate correlation; NS: nonsignificant. Student's t test is used for the evaluation of significance, with a p value <0.005.

Significance is the inverse correlation, according to Pearson's analysis, between the increase of ANB and the reduction of craniocervical angle. These data are not recognizable in the entire sample, but only in the dysfunctional subgroup. The different result between the two groups could be explained by the fact that the factor related to postural neck changes is not so much represented by the sagittal skeletal pattern of the jaws but the presence of temporomandibular disorders. The relationship between TMD and cervical spine is debated, but cervical painful symptomatology is often referred by dysfunctional patients. The mechanism underlying these data is probably linked to close spatial relationships among these structures [22, 23] and due to the fact that they are parts of the same functional unit [23].

There are cephalometric parameters that should be investigated to better understand the results obtained in this study and to verify that there are not other differences between the two groups, except for temporomandibular disorders. A comparison between SNA and SNB values in order to evaluate the prevalent component of Class II in each group should be done; a comparison between SNB and mandibular length in both groups is needed in order to analyze the presence of a retropositioned mandible or of reduction of the lengthy one. Lippold et al. [24] argue that the mandible seems to have a greater effect on body posture than other craniofacial parameters. Some studies [2, 6] report the relationship between mandibular length and cervical posture. However, from what emerged from Pearson's correlation analysis, the mandibular component of Class II more often associated with TMD should be analyzed. And this component is the retropositioning of the mandible, as said in the literature [25]. Retropositioned mandible, which could be the cause or effect of TMD itself, is associated with Class II and linked to the increase of ANB value and of severity of TMD, as said previously [25]. The increased severity of temporomandibular disorders also could lead to a compensatory or antalgic posture of the neck, as confirmed by the literature [2].

The anatomical change in a specific district could not justify the anatomical change in other districts. Instead functional/dysfunctional changes, determined by "anatomical links" such as muscles, ligaments, and joints, could influence other structures. The analysis of Class II components could be important in order to verify that it is not the mandibular length or the maxillary protrusion in skeletal Class II but the spacial postural changes in the mandible, such as retropositioning or divergence, which could lead to other changes. These do not necessarily have the pathologic mean as seen in this study; in fact, also in the dysfunctional group, only 40% had an alteration of craniocervical angle.

5. Conclusions

The findings of this study, within the limits of the sample, may be useful to understand that significant data are not emerged in relation to Class II and cervical spine alterations in both groups. Structures should be better investigated under a functional point of view, although there is an intrinsic limit for the record of the functional aspects.

Cervical spine assessment could be influenced by functional changes in the mandible, rather than the anatomical one, but further studies in larger samples and according to previous indications are requested. Anyway, these changes do not seem to have a great pathologic mean from what have been emerging from the study.

References

[1] A. Bedoya, Z. Landa Nieto, L. L. Zuluaga, and M. Rocabado, "Morphometry of the cranial base and the cranial-cervical-mandibular system in young patients with type II, division 1 malocclusion, using tomographic cone beam," *Cranio*, vol. 32, no. 3, pp. 199–207, 2014.

[2] M. D'Attilio, E. Epifania, F. Ciuffolo et al., "Cervical lordosis angle measured on lateral cephalograms; findings in skeletal class II female subjects with and without TMD: a cross sectional study," *Cranio*, vol. 22, no. 1, pp. 27–44, 2004.

[3] R. La Touche, A. París-Alemany, H. von Piekartz, J. S. Mannheimer, J. Fernández-Carnero, and M. Rocabado, "The influence of cranio-cervical posture on maximal mouth opening and pressure pain threshold in patients with myofascial temporomandibular pain disorders," *Clinical Journal of Pain*, vol. 27, no. 1, pp. 48–55, 2011.

[4] R. A. Matheus, F. M. Ramos-Perez, A. V. Menezes et al., "The relationship between temporomandibular dysfunction and head and cervical posture," *Journal of Applied Oral Science*, vol. 17, no. 3, pp. 204–208, 2009.

[5] J. V. Huggare and M. Tellervo Laine-Alava, "Nasorespiratory function and head posture," *American Journal of Orthodontics and Dentofacial Orthopedics*, vol. 112, no. 5, pp. 507–511, 1997.

[6] F. Festa, S. Tecco, M. Dolci et al., "Relationship between cervical lordosis and facial morphology in Caucasian women with a skeletalclass II malocclusion: a cross-sectional study," *Cranio*, vol. 21, no. 2, pp. 121–129, 2003.

[7] B. Solow, S. Siersb.k-Nielsen, and E. Greve, "Airway adequacy, head posture and craniofacial morphology," *American Journal of Orthodontics*, vol. 86, no. 3, pp. 214–222, 1984.

[8] Z. Hedayati, M. Paknahad, and F. Zorriasatine, "Comparison of natural head position in different anteroposterior malocclusions," *Journal of Dentistry*, vol. 10, no. 3, pp. 210–220, 2013.

[9] T. Hosseinzadeh Nik and P. Janbaz Aciyabar, "The relationship between cervical column curvature and sagittal position of the jaws: using a new method for evaluating curvature," *Iranian Journal of Radiology*, vol. 8, no. 3, pp. 161–166, 2011.

[10] D. Manfredini, M. Segù, N. Arveda, L. Lombardo, G. Siciliani, and A. Rossi, "Temporomandibular joint disorders in patients with different facial morphology: a systematic review of the literature," *Journal of Oral and Maxillofacial Surgery*, vol. 74, no. 1, pp. 29–46, 2016.

[11] G. Farronato, G. Rosso, L. Giannini, G. Galbiati, and C. Maspero, "Correlation between skeletal Class II and

temporomandibular disorders: a literature review," *Minerva Stomatologica*, vol. 65, no. 4, pp. 239–247, 2016.
[12] C. P. Rocha and C. S. Croci, "Caria PH is there relationship between temporomandibular disorders and head and cervical posture? A systematic review," *Journal of Oral Rehabilitation*, vol. 40, pp. 875–881, 2013.
[13] C. M. Visscher, F. Lobbezoo, W. de Boer, and J. van der Zaag, "Naeije M Prevalence of cervical spinal pain in craniomandibular pain patients," *European Journal of Oral Sciences*, vol. 109, no. 2, pp. 76–80, 2001.
[14] S. Armijo-Olivo, K. Rappoport, J. Fuentes et al., "Head and cervical posture in patients with temporomandibular disorders," *Journal of Orofacial Pain*, vol. 25, no. 3, pp. 199–209, 2011.
[15] E. F. Faulin, C. G. Guedes, P. P. Feltrin, and C. M. Joffiley, "Association between temporomandibular disorders and abnormal head postures," *Brazilian Oral Research*, vol. 29, no. 1, pp. 1–6, 2015.
[16] E. Schiffman, R. Ohrbach, E. Truelove et al., "Diagnostic criteria for temporomandibular disorders (DC/TMD) for clinical and research applications: recommendations of the international RDC/TMD consortium Network* and orofacial pain special interest group," *Journal of Oral and Facial Pain and Headache*, vol. 28, no. 1, pp. 6–27, 2014.
[17] C. C. Steiner, "Cephalometrics for you and me," *American Journal of Orthodontics*, vol. 39, no. 10, pp. 729–775, 1953.
[18] M. Rocabado, "Analisis biomecânico craneo cervical atraves de una teleradiografia lateral," *Revista Chilena de Ortodoncia*, vol. 1, no. 1, pp. 42–52, 1984.
[19] L. Sonnesen and I. Kjaer, "Anomalies of the cervical vertebrae in patients with skeletal Class II malocclusion and horizontal maxillary overjet," *American Journal of Orthodontics and Dentofacial Orthopedics*, vol. 133, no. 2, pp. 188.e15–188.e20, 2008.
[20] M. Watanabea, T. Yamaguchib, and K. Makic, "Cervical vertebra morphology in different skeletal classes A three-dimensional computed tomography evaluation," *Angle Orthodontist*, vol. 80, no. 4, pp. 719–724, 2010.
[21] D. Bebnowski, M. P. Hänggi, G. Markic, M. Roos, and T. Peltomäki, "Cervical vertebrae anomalies in subjects with Class II malocclusion assessed by lateral cephalogram and cone beam computed tomography," *European Journal of Orthodontics*, vol. 34, no. 2, pp. 226–231, 2012.
[22] H. Korbmacher, G. Eggers-Stroeder, L. Koch, and B. Kahl-Nieke, "Correlations between anomalies of the dentition and pathologies of the locomotor system—a literature review," *Journal of Orofacial Orthopedics*, vol. 65, no. 3, pp. 190–203, 2004.
[23] M. Rocabado, "Biomechanical relationship of the cranial, cervical, and hyoid regions," *Journal of Craniomandibular Practice*, vol. 1, no. 3, pp. 61–66, 1983.
[24] C. Lippold, G. Danesh, G. Hoppe, B. Drerup, and L. Hackenberg, "Sagittal spinal posture in relation to craniofacial morphology," *Angle Orthodontist*, vol. 76, no. 4, pp. 625–631, 2006.
[25] J. A. Bósio, J. G. Burch, R. H. Tallents, D. B. Wade, and F. M. Beck, "Lateral cephalometric analysis of asymptomatic volunteers and symptomatic patients with and without bilateral temporomandibular joint disk displacement," *American Journal of Orthodontics and Dentofacial Orthopedics*, vol. 114, no. 3, pp. 248–255, 1998.

11

Effects of Physical-Agent Pain Relief Modalities for Fibromyalgia Patients: A Systematic Review and Meta-Analysis of Randomized Controlled Trials

Yuichiro Honda,[1,2] Junya Sakamoto,[1] Yohei Hamaue,[3,4] Hideki Kataoka,[1,5] Yasutaka Kondo,[6] Ryo Sasabe,[1,2] Kyo Goto,[1,5] Takuya Fukushima,[1,2] Satoshi Oga,[1,7] Ryo Sasaki,[1,8] Natsumi Tanaka,[1,3] Jiro Nakano,[1] and Minoru Okita[1]

[1]*Department of Physical Therapy Science, Nagasaki University Graduate School of Biomedical Sciences, Sakamoto 1-7-1, Nagasaki 852-8520, Japan*
[2]*Department of Rehabilitation, Nagasaki University Hospital, Sakamoto 1-7-1, Nagasaki 852-8520, Japan*
[3]*Department of Physical Therapy, Niigata University of Health and Welfare, Shimami-cho 1398, Kitaku, Niigata 950-3198, Japan*
[4]*Institute for Human Movement and Medical Sciences, Niigata University of Health and Welfare, Shimami-cho 1398, Kitaku, Niigata 950-3198, Japan*
[5]*Department of Rehabilitation, Nagasaki Memorial Hospital, Fukahori 1-11-5, Nagasaki 851-0301, Japan*
[6]*Department of Rehabilitation, Japanese Red Cross Nagasaki Atomic Bomb Hospital, Mori 3-15, Nagasaki 852-8104, Japan*
[7]*Department of Rehabilitation, Saiseikai Nagasaki Hospital, Kitafuchi 2-5-1, Nagasaki 850-0003, Japan*
[8]*Department of Rehabilitation, Juzenkai Hospital, Kago 7-18, Nagasaki 850-0905, Japan*

Correspondence should be addressed to Junya Sakamoto; jun-saka@nagasaki-u.ac.jp

Academic Editor: Shinya Kasai

Purpose. We conducted a systematic review and meta-analysis to investigate the effects of the following physical-agent modalities for pain relief in fibromyalgia (FM) patients. *Methods*. We identified randomized controlled studies of adults with FM in the MEDLINE, CINAHL, and PEDro databases. The primary outcome measure was pain relief measured by a visual analogue scale (VAS), and the secondary outcome measures of interest were subjective improvements in the number of tender points, Fibromyalgia Impact Questionnaire (FIQ), and quality of life (QOL) scores. *Results*. Eleven studies were included in our review. The studies' physical-agent modalities were low-level laser therapy (LLLT), thermal therapy, electromagnetic field therapy, and transcutaneous electrical nerve stimulation (TENS). LLLT did not reduce VAS scores, but it significantly reduced both the number of tender points and FIQ score. Thermal therapy was associated with significantly reduced VAS scores, tender points, and FIQ scores. Electromagnetic field therapy was associated with significantly reduced VAS score and FIQ score. TENS significantly reduced VAS scores. *Conclusion*. Our analyses revealed that thermal therapy and LLLT had a partial effect on pain relief in FM patients, and this beneficial effect may have a positive influence on FM patients' health status.

1. Introduction

Fibromyalgia (FM) is an idiopathic, common, and complex syndrome, defined as long-lasting, widespread, and symmetrical nonarticular musculoskeletal pain with generalized tender points at specific anatomical sites [1, 2]. The pain that individuals with FM experience interferes with their performance of activities of daily life (ADLs) and results in a decreased quality of life (QOL) [2–5].

There are many possible treatments for FM that can be classified as pharmacological and nonpharmacological therapies [6–8]. The authors of a 2014 meta-analysis reported that very few drugs in well-designed clinical trials have demonstrated significant relief for multiple FM symptom domains, whereas nonpharmacologic treatments with weaker study designs have demonstrated multidimensional effects [8]. Nonpharmacological therapies such as physical exercise including strength training, aerobic training, and yoga [9, 10] and multicomponent therapy interventions [11, 12] have been used for FM. Physical-agent modalities are defined as passive treatments such as thermotherapy, cryotherapy, massage, electrotherapy, laser treatment, and others are nonpharmacological interventions used for FM patients [10]. Even though several placebo-controlled trials assessing the effects of physical-agent modalities on pain, ADLs, and QOL in patients with FM have been published in recent years, some studies had small sample sizes and have presented controversial results. A further elucidation of the effects of each physical-agent modality for FM is needed. We conducted the present study to systematically review the effects of physical-agent modalities for the treatment of FM, especially for the improvement of pain, ADLs, and QOL.

2. Methods

2.1. Search Strategy. We performed electronic searches of three databases—MEDLINE (the US National Library of Medicine bibliographic database), CINAHL (the Cumulative Index to Nursing and Allied Health Literature), and PEDro (the Physiotherapy Evidence Database)—up to February 28, 2017. A primary search with the term "fibromyalgia" was combined with the following terms: "cryotherapy," "icing," "low-level laser," "laser therapy," "electronical stimulation," "TENS," "electrotherapy," "magnetic therapy," "ultrasound," "ultrasonic," "thermotherapy," "heat therapy," "thermal therapy," "shortwave," "microwave," "hot pack," "wrapping," and "traction," and secondly, with "randomized controlled trial." Reference lists of included articles were scanned for additional citations. The full search strategy is available upon request.

2.2. Study Criteria and Selection. Studies were included if (1) the participants were fibromyalgia patients; (2) the design was a randomized controlled trial (RCT) including crossover designs, published in peer-reviewed journals; (3) treatment using physical-agent modalities was compared with a pure control or placebo; and (4) the full text was available. Five independent reviewers screened the titles and abstracts of all retrieved citations for eligibility. Full-text articles were retrieved for review when they showed potential inclusion criteria or when there was insufficient information in the abstract and title to make a decision. Disagreements regarding selected articles were discussed between reviewers until a consensus was achieved, or a fifth reviewer was included to reach a majority decision. This systematic review is in accordance with the Preferred Reporting Items for Systematic Reviews and Meta-Analyses (PRISMA) statement.

2.3. Outcome Measures. The primary outcome measure was pain relief. The criterion that we used for the study's measurement of pain intensity was that the pain intensity had to be measured by a visual analogue scale (VAS) at the baseline and again after treatment. The secondary outcome measures of interest were subjective improvements in the number of tender points, the score on a Fibromyalgia Impact Questionnaire (FIQ), and the score for quality of life (QOL). The FIQ measures physical functioning, work status, depression, anxiety, sleep, pain, stiffness, fatigue, and well being. The studies' patients' QOL had to be measured by the Short Form 36 Health Survey (SF-36), Health Assessment Questionnaire (HAQ), or Arthritis Impact Measurement Scale (AIMS).

2.4. Data Extraction. The goal of our data extraction was to determine the differences between the studies' treatment groups regarding the mean outcome differences before and after treatment, and the standard error of these differences. The data were extracted independently by five investigators. The following data were extracted from each included study: participant demographics, the study design, the interventions, and the evaluation methods used for each group.

In studies in which multiple periods of treatment for pain were set, we analyzed the data for the longest period. In studies in which pain (as measured by a VAS) was treated in multiple body parts, the data for the part that had the strongest pain were analyzed. For the study's analysis, we required the mean difference between the baseline and the final data and the standard deviation of that difference for each group of subjects. When the required data were not described in studies, we calculated the mean difference and standard deviation using the study's data as described [13, 14]. Studies in which the required data could not be calculated were excluded.

2.5. Evaluation of the Studies' Methodological Quality. Two independent reviewers performed a quality assessment of each study by using the PEDro scale (Physiotherapy Evidence Database, 1999). This scale has shown good reliability for scoring RCTs [15]. The PEDro scale consists of 11 items related to scientific rigor. The scale's items 2 to 11 contribute to internal validity, and the study is given 1 point for each of these items that is met. The first item relates to external validity and is not included in the final score. The quality assessment was performed independently by the two reviewers, and any disagreement was discussed until consensus was reached.

2.6. Data Synthesis and Analyses. We performed the meta-analysis using Review Manager software, ver. 5.0 (Copenhagen, The Nordic Cochrane Centre, the Cochrane Collaboration, 2008) to determine whether the treatments using physical-agent modalities decreased the FM patients' pain. Outcomes were analyzed as continuous outcomes using a fixed-effect model to calculate the weighted mean difference and 95% confidence interval (95% CI). A p value ≤ 0.05 indicated significance for an overall effect. Heterogeneity was investigated using the chi-square test, and a $p$value $\leq$ 0.05 was accepted as significant. Subgroup analyses were also performed according to the physical-agent modalities.

3. Results

3.1. Database Search and Study Selection. Figure 1 illustrates the different stages of the search and the selection of studies included in our review. The initial search of the three electronic databases identified 227 titles and abstracts, of which 30 were retrieved for full-text review. When the exclusion criteria were applied, 11 studies satisfied the criteria to be included in this review [16–26]. The main reasons for exclusion were as follows: (1) outcomes of the pain scale were not reported or (2) the interventions and the comparison groups did not include a control group.

3.2. Quality Assessment of the Included Studies. A detailed description of the 11 studies' PEDro scores is shown in Table 1. Seven studies [17, 18, 21–23, 25, 26] showed a PEDro score >5, two studies [16, 17] scored 5, and the remaining two studies [19, 24] scored 4. The most frequent omissions in the studies were the lack of blinding of therapists (10 studies). The allocation of patients was not described in sufficient detail to ascertain whether the allocation was concealed in the randomization method (eight studies), and an "intention to treat" analysis was applied for least one key outcome (eight studies).

3.3. Characteristics of the Studies' Participants. The characteristics of the participants of the 11 studies are summarized in Table 2. The total number of participants was 498. Because two studies [23, 26] had a double treatment design, 28 subjects were excluded in this meta-analysis. The total number of participants included in the meta-analysis was thus 470. The treatment groups comprised a total of 236 FM patients and the control groups were a total of 234 participants. Detailed demographic data were not reported in all studies, but the majority of the participants were adults; one study [22] did not report the ages of the participants. The male: female ratio varied among the five studies [19–23], and the other six studies included only female participants [16–18, 24–26]. All participants (including the control group subjects) were patients with FM.

3.4. Characteristics of the Studies' Interventions and Physical-Agent Modalities. The interventions (i.e., the physical-agent modalities) applied in the 11 studies are summarized in Table 2. The most common intervention was low-level laser therapy, used in five studies [16, 21, 22, 24, 26]. Thermal therapy (which included balneotherapy, mudpack, and thermal bath) was used in four studies [16, 18–20]. TENS [23] and pulsed electromagnetic field therapy [25] were used in one study each.

The intervention protocols varied among the studies. The amplitude and irradiation density of the LLLT [16, 21, 22, 24, 26] were, respectively, applied to the tender point and the trigger point from 28 sec to 3 min. In thermal therapy [16, 18–20], the temperature ranged from 30°C to 45°C, and the adaptation time was from 10 to 30 min; several studies used 20 min. The TENS [23] was applied for 20 min, 2×/day for 7 days, and the intervention conditions were 200 μsec, 2 and 100 Hz, and 60 mA. Pulsed electromagnetic field therapy [25] was applied for 30 min, 2×/day for 7 days, and the intervention condition was 40 μT, 0.1–64 Hz.

3.5. Effects of Interventions

3.5.1. Pain (as Measured by VAS). Six of the 11 studies evaluated the participants' pain by means of a VAS and were included in the meta-analysis. Figure 2 illustrates the mean difference and 95% CI values for pain relief as measured by VAS in these six studies for the physical-agent modalities LLLT, thermal therapies, TENS, and electromagnetic field therapy. The five studies' LLLT was not associated with the reduction of pain compared with the control group (mean difference: −4.00; 95% CI, −23.4 to 15.4, $p = 0.69$). In contrast, the TENS (−23.00; 95% CI, −43.28 to −2.72, $p = 0.03$), the electromagnetic field therapy (−30.30; 95% CI, −35.19 to −25.41, $p < 0.00001$), and thermal therapy (−29.74; 95% CI, −37.29 to −22.19, $I^2 = 75\%$, $p = 0.02$) were associated with a significant reduction of VAS score compared with the respective control group.

3.5.2. The Number of Tender Points. Six studies evaluated pain by evaluating the number of tender points and were included in the meta-analysis. As illustrated in Figure 3, the LLLT (−2.21; 95% CI, −3.51 to −0.92, $I^2 = 42\%$, $p = 0.0008$) and thermal therapy (−5.71; 95% CI, −7.26 to −4.51, $I^2 = 0\%$, $p < 0.00001$) were both associated with a significant reduction of the number of tender points compared with the control group.

3.5.3. The Fibromyalgia Impact Questionnaire (FIQ) Score. Ten studies evaluated the FIQ score and were included in the meta-analysis. As shown in Figure 4, electromagnetic field therapy (−24.80; 95% CI, −31.23 to −18.37, $p < 0.00001$), LLLT (−4.35; 95% CI, −6.69 to −2.01, $I^2 = 62\%$, $p = 0.03$), and thermal therapy (−24.67; 95% CI, −28.94 to −20.39, $I^2 = 84\%$, $p = 0.0004$) were all associated with a significant reduction of FIQ score compared with the control group.

3.5.4. Quality of Life (QOL). Two studies evaluated the participants' QOL and were included in the meta-analysis. The LLLT as evaluated by SF-36 demonstrated no significant difference compared with the control group (5.80; 95% CI, −4.72 to 16.32, $p = 0.28$). Thermal therapy, evaluated by HAQ and AIMS, demonstrated no significant difference compared with the control group (HAQ: −0.30; 95% CI, −0.93 to 0.33, $p = 0.35$, AIMS: −0.40; 95% CI, −1.67 to 0.87, $p = 0.54$).

4. Discussion

Fibromyalgia is defined as chronic pain, tenderness, and pain amplification [1, 27]. Increased levels of inflammatory cytokines and changes in neurotropic growth factors in the central nervous system and peripherally may influence the development and maintenance of central pain hypersensitivity by affecting adaptation and neuroplasticity [28–30]. The chronic painful lesions of fibromyalgia lead to limitations of activities of daily life and have been very difficult to treat effectively.

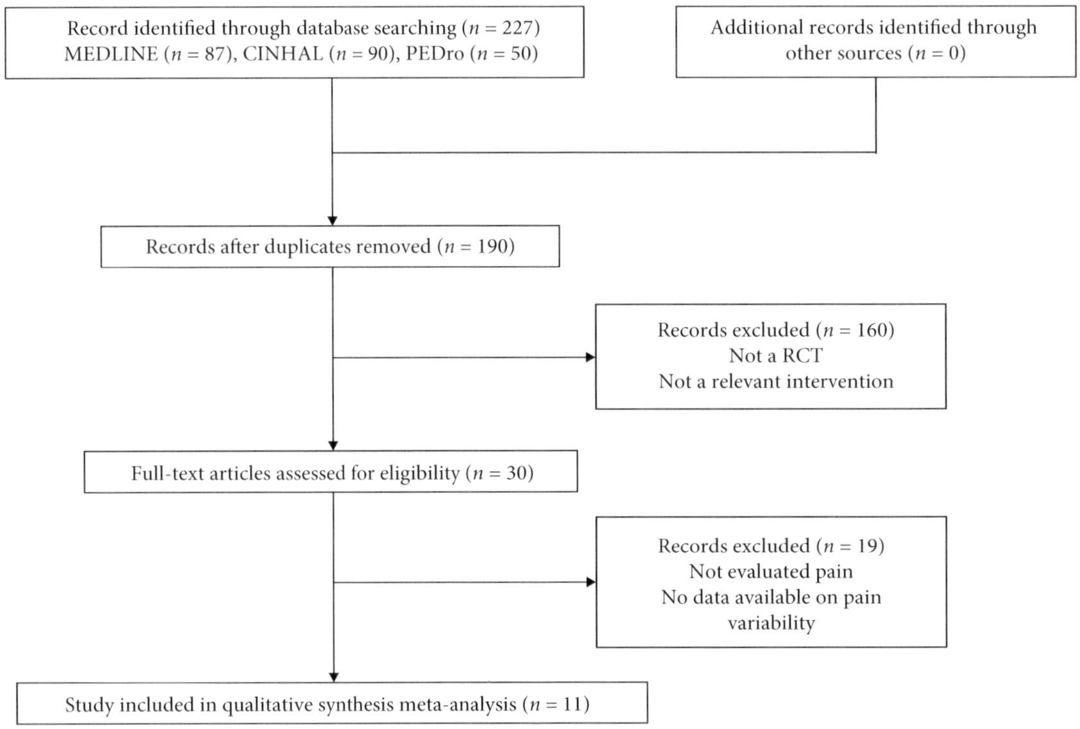

Figure 1: The different phases of the search of the three databases and the selection of the studies included in the present analyses.

Table 1: Detailed description of PEDro scores.

Study (year published)	PEDro scores											
	1	2	3	4	5	6	7	8	9	10	11	Total of 2–11
Ardic et al. (2007) [16]	Yes	1	0	0	0	0	1	1	0	1	1	5
Armagan et al. (2006) [17]	Yes	1	0	1	1	0	1	1	0	1	1	7
Bagdatli et al. (2015) [18]	Yes	1	0	1	0	0	1	1	1	1	1	7
Evcik et al. (2002) [19]	No	1	0	1	0	0	0	0	0	1	1	4
Fioravanti et al. (2007) [20]	Yes	1	0	1	0	0	0	1	0	1	1	5
Gür et al. (2002) [21]	Yes	1	1	1	1	0	0	1	0	1	1	7
Gür et al. (2002) [22]	Yes	1	0	1	1	0	1	1	0	1	1	7
Lauretti et al. (2013) [23]	Yes	1	1	1	1	1	1	1	0	1	1	9
Ruaro et al. (2014) [24]	No	1	0	0	1	0	0	0	0	1	1	4
Sutbeyaz et al. (2009) [25]	Yes	1	1	1	1	0	1	0	1	1	1	8
Vayvay et al. (2016) [26]	Yes	1	0	1	0	0	0	1	1	1	1	6
Total for each item		11	3	9	6	1	6	8	3	11	11	69

Fibromyalgia is characterized by a clinical syndrome whose primary symptoms include chronic widespread pain [1], and nonpharmacological options for fibromyalgia-induced pain may be as important as pharmacological treatment. Our meta-analysis revealed that TENS, electromagnetic therapy, and thermal therapy had positive effects on fibromyalgia-induced pain. These positive effects of nonpharmacological treatment may be due to physiological and biochemical changes in fibromyalgia patients. In two studies [23, 31], one of which was part of the present meta-analysis, the application of a TENS device improved pain relief in FM patients, and the effectiveness was suggested to be derived from a reduction in leukocyte migration, local action at peripheral opioids, and a decrease in local inflammatory reaction in the painful muscles. Low-frequency pulsed electromagnetic field therapy may improve pain in fibromyalgia patients, and several factors might mediate the therapeutic effects, such as alteration in pain perception, increases in the pain threshold and hormone levels, the inhibition of inflammatory edema, and vascular changes [25, 32]. Notably, only one RCT for TENS and one RCT for electromagnetic field therapy were identified. A further accumulation of RCT data regarding the effects of TENS and electromagnetic field therapy on fibromyalgia is needed. Ardic et al. [16] indicated that balneotherapy can effectively treat patients with fibromyalgia by relieving their clinical chronic pain, and they proposed that the suppression of inflammatory mediators with balneotherapy is related to its beneficial effect. Studies that examined hyperthermia showed that balneotherapy with mudpack and hot-pool

TABLE 2: Characteristics of the studies' participants and interventions.

Study (year published) [ref.]	Participants	Age (intervention, control, or placebo group)	Modality	Treatments	Evaluation
Ardic et al. (2007) [16]	24 women with FM	43.5 ± 10.2, 48.8 ± 8.9	*Balneotherapy* 30°C, 20 min	Once daily, 5 days/wk for 3 wks, whole body; control	Pain (VAS), NTP, algometric score, FIQ, BDI, serum PGE2, LTB4, and IL-1 levels
Armagan et al. (2006) [17]	32 women with FM	38.9 ± 4.9, 37.6 ± 5.9	*Low-level laser therapy* 50 mW, 830 nm, 1 min each tender point	Once daily, 5 days/wk for 10 days; control	NTP, morning stiffness, VSGI, FIQ, and total myalgia score
Bagdatli et al. (2015) [18]	70 women with FM	45.2 ± 9.1, 42.8 ± 9.6	*Balneotherapy and mudpack* 38°C, 20 min and 45°C, 20 min	10 times within 2 wks, whole body; control	PGASc, IGASc, FIQ, pain, fatigue, sleep, stiffness, anxiety, depression, and BDI
Evcik et al. (2002) [19]	42 patients with FM	42.0 ± 6.8, 41.5 ± 7.1	*Balneotherapy* 36°C, 20 min	Once daily, 5 days/wk for 3 wks, whole body; control	Pain (VAS), FIQ, NTP, and BDI
Fioravanti et al. (2007) [20]	80 patients with FM	46.2 ± 10.5, 48.6 ± 9.4	*Mudpack and thermal bath* 40°C–45°C, 10 min and 37°C–38°C, 15 min	Once daily, for 2 wks, whole body; control	FIQ, VAS (headache, fatigue, sleep disturbances), NTP, HAQ, and AIMS
Gür et al. (2002) [21]	50 patients with FM	30.4 ± 6.9, 28.5 ± 6.3	*Low-level laser therapy* 2 J/cm^2, 3 min each tender point	Once daily, 5 days/wk for 2 wks; placebo	Pain, NTP, skinfold tenderness, stiffness, sleep disturbance, muscle spasm, fatigue, and FIQ
Gür et al. (2002) [22]	40 patients with FM	—	*Low-level laser therapy* 11.2 mW, 3 min each tender point	Once daily, 5 days/wk for 2 wks; placebo	Pain, NTP, skinfold tenderness, stiffness, sleep disturbance, muscular spasm, and fatigue
Lauretti et al. (2013) [23]	39 patients with FM	32 ± 8, 35 ± 8	*TENS* 200 μsec, 2 and 100 Hz, 60 mA, 20 min	Twice a day, for 7 days; placebo	Pain (VAS), daily analgesic consumption, quality of sleep, and fatigue
Ruaro et al. (2014) [24]	20 women with FM	43.4, 39.4	*Low-level laser therapy* 20 mW, 670 nm,7 s ×4 for 18 trigger points	3 times/wk for 4 wks; placebo	NTP, FIQ, McGill pain questionnaire, and VAS
Sutbeyaz et al. (2009) [25]	56 women with FM	43.0 ± 9.6, 40.9 ± 6.9	*Pulsed electromagnetic field therapy* 40 μT, 0.1–64 Hz, 30 min	Twice a day, for 3 wks, whole body; control	FIQ, pain (VAS), BDI, SF-36, and PGART
Vayvay et al. (2016) [26]	45 women with FM	36.4 ± 8.3, 38.0 ± 8.4	*Laser therapy* 2 J/cm^2, 3 min each trigger points	Once daily, 5 days/wk for 3 wks; placebo	Pain (VAS), body flexibility, FIQ, SF-36, and BDI

VAS: visual analogue scale; NTP: no. of tender points; BDI: Beck's depression index; FIQ: Fibromyalgia Impact Questionnaire; PGE2: prostaglandin E2; LTB4: leukotriene B4; IL: interleukin; VSGI: global improvement as reported on a verbal scale; PGASc: patient's global assessment score; IGASc: investigator's global assessment score; HAQ: health assessment questionnaire; AIMS: arthritis impact measurement scale; HDRS: Hamilton depression rate scale; DSM: diagnostic and statistical manual of mental disorders; SF-36: 36-item short form health survey; PGART: patient's global assessment of response to therapy.

treatments described a pain-relieving effect, which may be explained by a mitigation of muscle tone, increase in the pain threshold in the nerve endings, and/or peripheral vasodilatation [19, 20, 33].

Tender points were defined by the American College of Rheumatology criteria, which is the standard method for evaluating tenderness in fibromyalgia patients [34]. Our meta-analysis showed that the LLLT and thermal therapy were effective treatments for tenderness in fibromyalgia patients. That is, although Armagan et al. indicated that the numbers of tender points in their LLLT and placebo groups were not significantly different [17], the other two studies showed that the patients' tender point numbers decreased after LLLT [21, 24]. Our meta-analysis showed favors plot in LLLT group and that LLLT was thus an effective therapeutic method to reduce the number of tender points in FM patients. However, our meta-analysis indicated that LLLT did not effectively reduce the patients' VAS pain scores. On the other hand, three of the 11 studies in our meta-analysis that evaluated balneotherapy showed tender points' count was significantly different between the treatment group and nontreatment group, in addition to decrease in pain

Study of subgroup	Experimental Mean	SD	Total	Control Mean	SD	Total	Mean difference IV, fixed, 95% CI
TENS							
Lauretti (2013)	−25.0	14.1	13	−2.0	30.3	10	−23.00 (−43.28, −2.72)
Subtotal (95% CI)			13			10	−23.00 (−43.28, −2.72)
Heterogeneity: not applicable							
Test for overall effect: $Z = 2.22$ ($P = 0.03$)							
Electromagnetic field therapy							
Sutbayaz (2009)	−35.3	10.7	25	−5.0	6.3	24	−30.30 (−35.19, −25.41)
Subtotal (95% CI)			25			24	−30.30 (−35.19, −25.41)
Heterogeneity: not applicable							
Test for overall effect: $Z = 12.14$ ($P < 0.00001$)							
Low-level laser therapy							
Vayvay (2016)	−21.0	32.4	15	−17.0	20.5	15	−4.00 (−23.40, 15.40)
Subtotal (95% CI)			15			15	−4.00 (−23.40, 15.40)
Heterogeneity: not applicable							
Test for overall effect: $Z = 0.40$ ($P = 0.69$)							
Thermal therapy							
Ardic et al. (2007)	−41.7	23.3	12	2.5	12.8	9	−44.20 (−59.81, −28.59)
Bagdatli et al. (2015)	−23.5	28.4	35	−7.7	26.7	35	−15.80 (−28.71, −2.89)
Evcik (2002)	−45.0	20.6	22	−12.0	17.7	20	−33.00 (−44.59, −21.41)
Subtotal (95% CI)			69			64	−29.74 (−37.29, −22.19)
Heterogeneity: $\chi^2 = 8.08$, $df = 2$ ($P = 0.02$); $I^2 = 75\%$							
Test for overall effect: $Z = 7.72$ ($P < 0.00001$)							

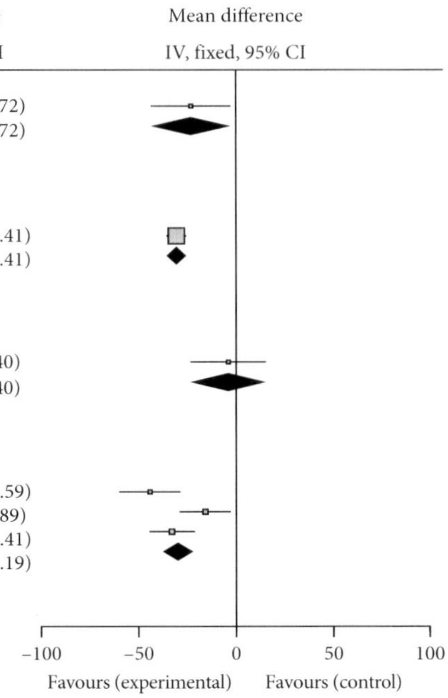

Figure 2: The mean difference and 95% CI of pain relief as measured using a VAS in 6 of the 11 studies for the physical-agent modalities: LLLT, thermal therapies, TENS, and electromagnetic field therapy.

Study of subgroup	Experimental Mean	SD	Total	Control Mean	SD	Total	Mean difference IV, fixed, 95% CI
Low level laser therapy							
Armagan (2006)	−1.9	2.8	16	−1.1	3.0	16	−0.80 (−2.81, 1.21)
[a]Gür (2002)	−7.5	4.5	25	−3.9	4.5	25	−3.60 (−6.09, −1.11)
Ruaro (2014)	−4.3	3.1	10	−1.4	2.1	10	−2.90 (−5.22, −0.58)
Subtotal (95% CI)			51			51	−2.21 (−3.51, −0.92)
Heterogeneity: $\chi^2 = 3.42$, $df = 2$ ($P = 0.18$); $I^2 = 42\%$							
Test for overall effect: $Z = 3.34$ ($P = 0.0008$)							
Thermal therapy							
Ardic et al. (2007)	−3.8	3.6	12	1.1	3.1	9	−4.90 (−7.77, −2.03)
Evcik (2002)	−7.6	3.4	22	−1.1	3.5	20	−6.50 (−8.59, −4.41)
Fioravanti (2007)	−4.2	6.0	13	0.2	3.6	10	−4.40 (−8.35, −0.45)
Subtotal (95% CI)			47			39	−5.71 (−7.26, −4.15)
Heterogeneity: $\chi^2 = 1.28$, $df = 2$ ($P = 0.53$); $I^2 = 0\%$							
Test for overall effect: $Z = 7.20$ ($P < 0.00001$)							

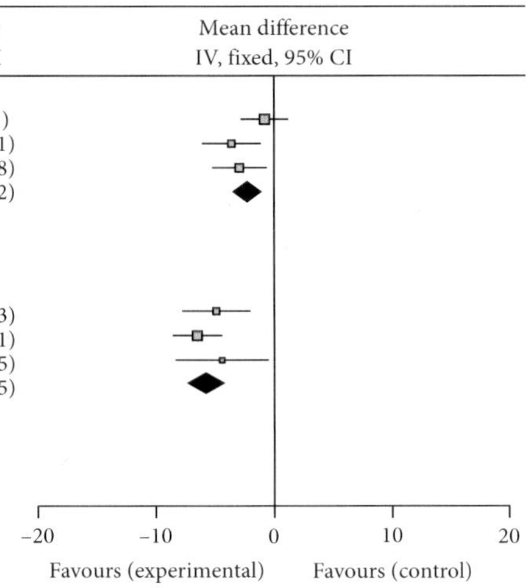

Figure 3: The mean difference and 95% confidence interval (CI) of tender points for physical-agent modalities.

intensity [16, 19, 20]. This difference between physical-agent modalities may be derived from effective area of each modality. Many thermal therapies influence the body surface widely compared with the LLLT in the same therapeutic time; thermal therapy can treat multiple pain locations at a session. This has an advantage for treatment widespread pain of fibromyalgia patients. Therefore, thermal therapy reduces both pain intensity and the number of tender points. By contrast, LLLT may be ruled unfit to widespread pain of fibromyalgia patients because of narrow range of effective irradiated area. In the case of short-term treatment, LLLT may fail to decrease pain intensity in some painful areas, and then VAS in the patients remain persistently high. For this reason, LLLT may be more effective for decreasing the number of tender points than reducing the pain intensity. The therapeutic mechanism underlying LLLT remains to be elucidated in further studies.

The Fibromyalgia Impact Questionnaire (FIQ) comprised ten items in a self-administered instrument that measure physical functioning, work status, anxiety, pain, fatigue, sleep, depression, stiffness, well being, and evaluates activities of daily living (ADLs) in fibromyalgia patients [35]. EULAR guidelines emphasized that the goals of treatment are to improve the quality of life, maintain function (functional ability in everyday situations), and reduce symptoms [36]. In our meta-analysis, electromagnetic field therapy, LLLT, and thermal therapy were all associated with a significant reduction of the FIQ score. Three RCTs

Study of subgroup	Experimental Mean	Experimental SD	Experimental Total	Control Mean	Control SD	Control Total	Mean difference IV, fixed, 95% CI
Electromagnetic field therapy							
Sutbayaz (2009)	−33.5	13.3	25	−8.7	9.4	24	−24.80 (−31.23, −18.37)
Subtotal (95% CI)			25			24	−24.80 (−31.23, −18.37)
Heterogeneity: not applicable							
Test for overall effect: $Z = 7.56$ ($P < 0.00001$)							
Low level laser therapy							
Armagan (2016)	−7.0	13.7	16	−1.8	13.5	16	−5.20 (−14.62, 4.22)
[a]Gür (2002)	−23.3	14.2	25	−9.6	12.1	25	−13.70 (−21.01, −6.39)
[b]Gür (2002)	−6.6	4.5	20	−4.2	4.2	20	−2.40 (−5.10, 0.30)
Ruaro (2014)	−18.6	15.0	10	−5.2	15.5	10	−13.40 (−26.77, −0.03)
Vayvay (2016)	−23.8	14.4	15	−16.2	13.4	15	−7.60 (−17.55, 2.35)
Subtotal (95% CI)			86			86	−4.35 (−6.69, −2.01)
Heterogeneity: $\chi^2 = 10.49$, $df = 4$ ($P = 0.03$); $I^2 = 62\%$							
Test for overall effect: $Z = 3.65$ ($P = 0.0003$)							
Thermal therapy							
Ardic et al. (2007)	−9.8	15.4	12	2.3	14.7	9	−12.10 (−25.07, 0.87)
Bagdatli et al. (2015)	−19.6	17.6	35	−2.8	18.8	35	−16.80 (−25.33, −8.27)
Evcik (2002)	−35.7	10.4	22	−1.8	9.6	20	−33.90 (−39.95, −27.85)
Fioravanti (2007)	−14.2	26.7	40	1.4	25.4	40	−15.60 (−27.02, −4.18)
Subtotal (95% CI)			109			104	−24.67 (−28.94, −20.39)
Heterogeneity: $\chi^2 = 18.25$, $df = 3$ ($P = 0.0004$); $I^2 = 84\%$							
Test for overall effect: $Z = 11.31$ ($P < 0.00001$)							

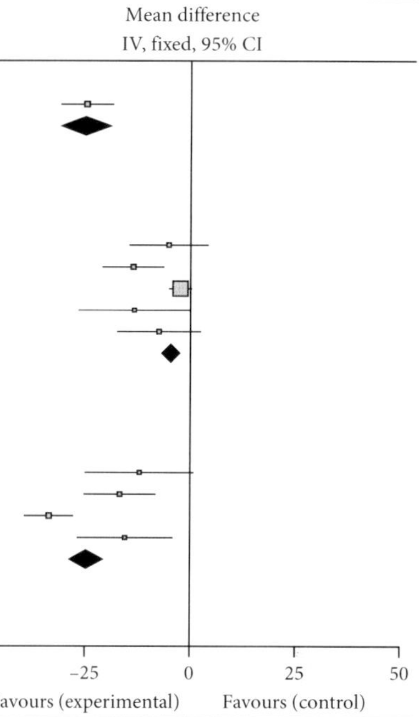

FIGURE 4: The mean difference and 95% CI values on the FIQ for the physical-agent modalities.

indicated that thermal therapy, including balneotherapy, mud baths, and mudpacks, had a positive effect on the FM patients' FIQ score, suggesting that thermal therapy ameliorated fibromyalgia-induced pain, and the improvement of fibromyalgia symptoms thus had a positive effect on the FIQ total score [10, 11, 13]. On the other hand, three of the five RCTs of LLLT reported that LLLT did not effectively reduce the FIQ score. Fibromyalgia-induced pain was not significantly changed in our meta-analysis, and this noneffectiveness may have led to the unchanged FIQ score. In addition, Bennett et al. suggested that a 14% change in the FIQ total score is clinically relevant [37]. In the results of LLLT, change in the FIQ total score is small compared with the clinically relevant value. Therefore, the positive effect of LLLT for fibromyalgia patients is smaller compared with thermal therapy and may be definite for the treatment of fibromyalgia.

Regarding the quality of the studies' evidence, although the PEDro score in nine studies was >5 (max. score = 9, min. score = 4), all nine studies were small-scale (the largest treatment group consisted of 40 participants). The intervention period in all nine studies was short (max. treatment period of 4 weeks). The quality of evidence according to Grades of Recommendation, Assessment, Development, and Evaluation (GRADE) for all outcomes of efficacy, tolerability, and safety was low, downgraded for the reasons given in the following description of study limitations.

The limitations are as follows. First, our review used only the MEDLINE, CINAHL, and PEDro databases for the search for studies, and we selected only English-language publications for the meta-analysis. We also selected only studies that included a pure control group or placebo groups (i.e., no other intervention). There are few reports on each physical-agent modality for fibromyalgia, and the heterogeneity analysis revealed a high score in the meta-analysis. Our meta-analysis did not evaluate the total effect of all of the physical-agent modalities since we searched for each modality's effect. Finally, the RCTs did not provide much data regarding the patients' QOL, and our search was thus unable to reveal adequate findings about posttreatment QOL in fibromyalgia patients. These restrictions are tasks to address in future studies.

5. Conclusions

In summary, our findings suggest that thermal therapy has a positive effect on fibromyalgia-induced pain, tender point, and FIQ. Thermal therapy is a more effective physical-agent modality for fibromyalgia patient treatment. Effect of electromagnetic therapy and TENS for the treatment of FM on pain intensity was observed. However, there are few reports on these physical-agent modalities. We speculate that this effectiveness has underlying mechanisms involving both the central nervous system and the peripheral nervous system. Clinically, nonpharmacological treatment for peripheral organization in fibromyalgia patients is important, and physicians need to consider both central and peripheral tissue as therapeutic targets.

References

[1] F. Wolfe, D. J. Clauw, M. A. Fitzcharles et al., "The American College of Rheumatology preliminary diagnostic criteria for fibromyalgia and measurement of symptom severity," *Arthritis Care & Research*, vol. 62, no. 5, pp. 600–610, 2010.

[2] D. J. Clauw, "Fibromyalgia and related conditions," *Mayo Clinic Proceedings*, vol. 90, no. 5, pp. 680–692, 2015.

[3] J. Jones, D. N. Rutledge, K. D. Jones, L. Matallana, and D. S. Rooks, "Self-assessed physical function levels of women with fibromyalgia: a national survey," *Women's Health Issues*, vol. 18, no. 5, pp. 406–412, 2008.

[4] C. Henriksson and C. Burckhardt, "Impact of fibromyalgia on everyday life. A study of women in the USA and Sweden," *Disability and Rehabilitation*, vol. 18, no. 5, pp. 241–248, 1996.

[5] J. A. Verbunt, D. H. Pernot, and R. J. Smeets, "Disability and quality of life in patients with fibromyalgia," *Health and Quality of Life Outcomes*, vol. 6, no. 1, p. 8, 2008.

[6] K. Kroenke, E. E. Krebs, and M. J. Bair, "Pharmacotherapy of chronic pain: a synthesis of recommendations from systematic reviews," *General Hospital Psychiatry*, vol. 31, no. 3, pp. 206–219, 2009.

[7] C. Sommer, W. Häuser, R. Alten et al., "Drug therapy of fibromyalgia syndrome. Systematic review, meta-analysis and guideline," *Der Schmerz*, vol. 26, no. 3, pp. 297–310, 2012.

[8] S. Perrot and I. J. Russell, "More ubiquitous effects from non-pharmacologic than from pharmacologic treatments for fibromyalgia syndrome: a meta-analysis examining six core symptoms," *European Journal of Pain*, vol. 18, no. 8, pp. 1067–1080, 2014.

[9] J. Langhorst, P. Klose, G. J. Dobos, K. Bernardy, and W. Häuser, "Efficacy and safety of meditative movement therapies in fibromyalgia syndrome: a systematic review and meta-analysis of randomized controlled trials," *Rheumatology International*, vol. 33, no. 1, pp. 193–207, 2013.

[10] A. Winkelmann, W. Häuser, E. Friedel et al., "Physiotherapy and physical agent therapies for fibromyalgia syndrome, systematic review, meta-analysis and guidelines," *Der Schmerz*, vol. 26, no. 3, pp. 276–286, 2012.

[11] B. Arnold, W. Häuser, M. Arnold et al., "Multicomponent therapy of fibromyalgia syndrome. Systematic review, meta-analysis and guideline," *Der Schmerz*, vol. 26, no. 3, pp. 287–290, 2012.

[12] V. Köllner, W. Häuser, K. Klimczyk et al., "Psychotherapy for patients with fibromyalgia syndrome. Systematic review, meta-analysis and guideline," *Der Schmerz*, vol. 26, no. 3, pp. 291–296, 2012.

[13] D. Follmann, P. Elliott, I. Suh, and J. Cutler, "Variance imputation for overviews of clinical trials with continuous response," *Journal of Clinical Epidemiology*, vol. 45, no. 7, pp. 769–773, 1992.

[14] K. R. Abrams, C. L. Gillies, and P. C. Lambert, "Meta-analysis of heterogeneously reported trials assessing change from baseline," *Statistics in Medicine*, vol. 24, no. 24, pp. 3823–3844, 2005.

[15] C. G. Maher, C. Sherrington, R. D. Herbert, A. M. Moseley, and M. Elkins, "Reliability of the PEDro scale for rating quality of randomized controlled trials," *Physical Therapy*, vol. 83, no. 8, pp. 713–721, 2003.

[16] F. Ardic, M. Ozgen, H. Aybek, S. Rota, D. Cubukcu, and A. Gokgoz, "Effects of balneotherapy on serum IL-1, PGE2 and LTB4 levels in fibromyalgia patients," *Rheumatology International*, vol. 27, no. 5, pp. 441–446, 2007.

[17] O. T. F. Armagan, A. Ekim, and C. Oner, "Long-term efficacy of low level laser therapy in women with fibromyalgia: a placebo-controlled study," *Journal of Back and Musculoskeletal Rehabilitation*, vol. 19, no. 4, pp. 135–140, 2006.

[18] A. O. Bagdatli, A. Donmez, R. Eroksuz, G. Bahadir, M. Turan, and N. Erdogan, "Does addition of 'mud-pack and hot pool treatment' to patient education make a difference in fibromyalgia patients? A randomized controlled single blind study," *International Journal of Biometeorology*, vol. 59, no. 12, pp. 1905–1911, 2015.

[19] D. Evcik, B. Kizilay, and E. Gokcen, "The effects of balneotherapy on fibromyalgia patients," *Rheumatology International*, vol. 22, no. 2, pp. 56–59, 2002.

[20] A. Fioravanti, G. Perpignano, G. Tirri et al., "Effects of mud-bath treatment on fibromyalgia patients: a randomized clinical trial," *Rheumatology International*, vol. 27, no. 12, pp. 1157–1161, 2007.

[21] A. Gür, M. Karakoc, K. Nas, R. Cevik, J. Sarac, and S. Ataoglu, "Effects of low power laser and low dose amitriptyline therapy on clinical symptoms and quality of life in fibromyalgia: a single-blind, placebo-controlled trial," *Rheumatology International*, vol. 22, no. 5, pp. 188–193, 2002.

[22] A. Gür, M. Karakoc, K. Nas, R. Cevik, J. Saraç, and E. Demir, "Efficacy of low power laser therapy in fibromyalgia: a single-blind, placebo-controlled trial," *Lasers in Medical Science*, vol. 17, no. 1, pp. 57–61, 2002.

[23] G. R. Lauretti, E. F. Chubaci, and A. L. Mattos, "Efficacy of the use of two simultaneously TENS devices for fibromyalgia pain," *Rheumatology International*, vol. 33, no. 8, pp. 2117–2122, 2013.

[24] J. A. Ruaro, A. R. Frez, M. B. Ruaro, and R. A. Nicolau, "Low-level laser therapy to treat fibromyalgia," *Lasers in Medical Science*, vol. 29, no. 6, pp. 1815–1819, 2014.

[25] S. T. S. N. Sutbeyaz, F. Koseoglu, and S. Kibar, "Low-frequency pulsed electromagnetic field therapy in fibromyalgia: a randomized, double-blind, sham-controlled clinical study," *Clinical Journal of Pain*, vol. 25, no. 8, pp. 722–728, 2009.

[26] E. S. Vayvay, D. Tok, E. Turgut, and V. B. Tunay, "The effect of Laser and taping on pain, functional status and quality of life in patients with fibromyalgia syndrome: a placebo-randomized controlled clinical trial," *Journal of Back and Musculoskeletal Rehabilitation*, vol. 29, no. 1, pp. 77–83, 2016.

[27] E. Kosek, J. Ekholm, and P. Hansson, "Sensory dysfunction in fibromyalgia patients with implications for pathogenic mechanisms," *Pain*, vol. 68, no. 2, pp. 375–383, 1996.

[28] D. Kadetoff, J. Lampa, M. Westman, M. Andersson, and E. Kosek, "Evidence of central inflammation in fibromyalgia-increased cerebrospinal fluid interleukin-8 levels," *Journal of Neuroimmunology*, vol. 242, no. 1-2, pp. 33–38, 2012.

[29] C. Morgado, L. Silva, P. Pereira-Terra, and I. Tavares, "Changes in serotoninergic and noradrenergic descending pain pathways during painful diabetic neuropathy: the preventive action of IGF1," *Neurobiology of Disease*, vol. 43, no. 1, pp. 275–284, 2011.

[30] J. L. Bjersing, M. Erlandsson, M. I. Bokarewa, and K. Mannerkorpi, "Exercise and obesity in fibromyalgia. Beneficial roles of insulin-like growth factor 1 and resistin?," *Arthritis Research & Therapy*, vol. 15, no. 1, p. R34, 2013.

[31] H. W. Kim, D. H. Roh, S. Y. Yoon et al., "The anti-inflammatory effects of low- and high-frequency electroacupuncture are mediated by peripheral opioids in a mouse air pouch inflammation model," *Journal of Alternative and Complementary Medicine*, vol. 12, no. 1, pp. 39–44, 2006.

[32] N. M. Shupak, F. S. Prato, and A. W. Thomas, "Therapeutic uses of pulsed magnetic field exposure: a review," *Radio Science Bulletin*, vol. 307, pp. 9–32, 2003.

[33] K. L. Schmidt, "Scientific basis of spa treatment in rheumatic diseases," *Rheumatology in Europe*, vol. 24, pp. 136–140, 1995.

[34] F. Wolfe, H. A. Smythe, M. B. Yunus et al., "The american college of rheumatology 1990 criteria for the classification of

fibromyalgia. Report of the multicenter criteria committee," *Arthritis & Rheumatism*, vol. 33, no. 2, pp. 160–172, 1990.
[35] C. S. Burckhardt, S. R. Clark, and R. M. Bennett, "The fibromyalgia impact questionnaire: development and validation," *Journal of Rheumatology*, vol. 18, no. 5, pp. 728–733, 1991.
[36] G. J. Macfarlane, C. Kronisch, L. E. Dean et al., "EULAR revised recommendations for the management of fibromyalgia," *Annals of the Rheumatic Diseases*, vol. 76, no. 2, pp. 318–328, 2017.
[37] R. M. Bennett, A. G. Bushmakin, J. C. Cappelleri, G. Zlateva, and A. B. Sadosky, "Minimal clinically important difference in the fibromyalgia impact questionnaire," *Journal of Rheumatology*, vol. 36, no. 6, pp. 1304–1311, 2009.

12

Difference in Response to a Motor Imagery Task: A Comparison between Individuals with and without Painful Temporomandibular Disorders

Daisuke Uritani,[1] Tomoko Nishida,[2] Nanami Sakaguchi,[3] Tetsuji Kawakami,[4] Lester E. Jones,[5] and Tadaaki Kirita[4]

[1]*Department of Physical Therapy, Faculty of Health Science, Kio Univeristy, 4-2-2 Umaminaka, Koryocho, Kitakatsuragigun, Nara 6350832, Japan*
[2]*Department of Rehabilitation, Japanese Red Cross Kyoto Daiichi Hospital, 15-749 Honmachi, Higashiyamaku, Kyoto 6050981, Japan*
[3]*Department of Rehabilitation, Higashiosaka Yamaji Hospital, 1-7-5 Inaba, Higashiosaka, Osaka 5780925, Japan*
[4]*Department of Oral and Maxillofacial Surgery, Nara Medical University, 840 Shijo-Cho, Kashihara, Nara 6348521, Japan*
[5]*Judith Lumley Centre, La Trobe University, Plenty Road, Bundoora, Melbourne, VIC 3086, Australia*

Correspondence should be addressed to Daisuke Uritani; d.uritani@kio.ac.jp

Academic Editor: Minoru Okita

The aim of the study was to investigate the difference in response to a motor imagery task between individuals with and without painful temporomandibular disorders (TMDs). The participants were 24 adults with and without TMD (TMD and control group, resp.). A set of photographic images of the profile view of a person's head and neck and a hand and a foot were presented in a random order. The set consisted of six different orientations with rotations of each image at 0, 60, 120, 180, 240, and 300 degrees and included left and right representations. The participants were required to view the image and make a decision as to whether it was a left or a right side presented, that is, mental rotation (MR) task. Data were collected on 48 tasks (including left and right) at each orientation for each body part. Reaction times (RTs) for correct answers and accuracy in making the left or right judgements were recorded. The RT was slower in the TMD group than in the control group. The RT for the profile image was slower than those for the hand and foot images. For images that were 180 degrees, the RT was slower and the accuracy was lower than those for five of the other image orientations. The judgements made about the 180-degree rotated image were more inaccurate compared to images of all other orientations among all types of stimuli.

1. Introduction

Temporomandibular disorder (TMD) is a collective term used for explaining a group of conditions in the temporomandibular joint (TMJ) and its related structures [1]. Orofacial pain is the most common symptom of TMD and is usually concentrated in masticatory muscles and/or TMJ [2]. TMDs are also frequently accompanied by limitation of mouth opening and pain-related disability [2]. Among those with acute presentation of TMD, approximately 15% will develop chronic TMD [3].

A recent review of evidence supports the role of physiotherapy in the treatment of TMD including the use therapeutic exercise [4, 5]. However, in clinical practice, some patients with TMD cannot move their TMJ actively because of pain, restricted range of mouth opening, or fear of movement. The resultant immobility can enhance pain and lead to further restriction to range of movement. As a result, a vicious cycle involving pain and immobility can develop and lead to a persistent pain condition [6].

Mental rotation (MR) describes a motor imagery task [7], where rotated images of a body part are presented and the participant is required to make a judgement about whether the image is of a left side or a right side. The assumption is that participants will make their decision by mentally orientating their own body part to match the picture. Although no actual movement takes place, it appears that MR may be a valuable model for exploring the central processes involved in the control of movement.

In support of this, when MR was used with images of hands [8–11] and feet [12], the relevant area of motor cortex was shown to be activated. When images of the side that corresponds to the person's dominant hand are presented, the judgements tend to be made faster [10]. Interestingly it has also been found that when someone has persistent pain, responses to the MR task are impaired [13–16].

As a result of these findings, MR is considered to have potential for early stage musculoskeletal physiotherapy for patients with motion pain or pain-related fear of movement because it can be performed without movement. In fact, MR has already been successfully applied in physiotherapy for patients with musculoskeletal disorders, especially for extremities [17]. In one example, Moseley [15] described the beneficial effect of motor imagery including MR on functional improvement of hands for CRPS patients.

There are few reports about physiotherapy using motor imagery of the orofacial region. von Piekartz et al. [18] performed a left/right facial posture judgement task using MR. They asked people with chronic facial pain to respond to the images by identifying the positioning of facial features, including jaw or tongue position. In the images, these were positioned either towards the left or right side of the face. The order of presentation of the left and right images was randomly presented and images were also rotated. They concluded that people with chronic facial pain were less accurate than controls at a left/right facial posture judgement task [18].

Regarding TMJ, the region in the human precentral gyrus responsible for the execution of voluntary jaw opening movements has been found to be activated during observation of simple jaw opening movements [19]. In addition, functional magnetic resonance imaging studies in humans have revealed somatotopic activation of the premotor cortex during observation of the actions of the mouth, arm/hand, and foot [20]. In people with TMD, alterations in brain activity have been noted in a range of tasks [21–25]. Hence, it has been considered that MR of a particular part, including TMJ, would activate the motor cortex somatotopically, and there might be value in determining the impact of TMD on performance of a MR task.

Applying MR to TMD patients with orofacial pain presents a challenge. Usually MR of the body parts involves the left-right judgement of disoriented body parts in extremities [26]. However, TMJ has different anatomical and kinesiological characteristics compared to joints in extremities. Also, for axial parts of the body, such as trunk and face, it is less clear how to recognize preferred sides compared to the dominant side in extremities such as hand and foot. Where the task involves the referred or dominant side, there may be an influence on the reaction speed and accuracy of left and right judgements. Identifying how these variations may influence the application of MR to TMD pain needs further clarification.

This study aimed at comparing the responses of participants with and without TMD with orofacial pain when undertaking MR tasks for affected (head and neck profile including TMJ) and nonaffected (hand and foot) body parts. We included MR tasks for hands and feet to discriminate the difference of reaction in MR tasks between affected and nonaffected body parts. Research has demonstrated observation of mouth and hand action activated the mouth- and hand-area of the primary motor cortex, respectively [25, 27, 28]. It was hypothesized that reaction in the MR task for the head and neck profile images would be delayed and inaccurate selectively in the TMD patients compared with the healthy controls.

2. Materials and Methods

The participants were 24 adults (23 women) with TMD including orofacial pain, diagnosed based on the criteria for TMD by the Japanese Society for Temporomandibular Joint (TMD group), and 24 adults (21 women) without TMD (control group). No participants in the TMD group had surgery in the orofacial region. Clinical information on the TMD group is provided in Table 1. The Research Ethics Committee of Kio University (H28-59) and Nara Medical University (497-3) approved this study, and all participants provided written informed consent.

Anthropometric data, pain intensity, and passive range of mouth opening (mouth ROM) were collected from medical records. Pain intensity was assessed using a visual analogue scale (VAS), and participants were verbally instructed that the left hand end of the scale represented "no pain" and the right end of the scale represented "worst imaginable pain." Mouth opening was measured using a standardized measure (Keisei Kaikoudo scale, Keisei Medical Industrial Co., Ltd. Tokyo, Japan) by a dentist.

All participants were tested in the left and right judgements of body parts (head and neck side profiles, hands, and feet) using MR. The order of presentation of these three body parts was determined by a simple process, where the participant blindly selected from a collection of sticks, and each stick was named with a body part.

The testing was performed in a consultation room in a university hospital. Participants sat in front of a laptop computer (LAVIE HZ750, NEC, Japan, with screen size 16.5 cm by 29.0 cm) and were asked to put their right and left index finger on the "M" and "Z" key, respectively. They were asked to maintain their position, gaze at the screen, and maintain their posture during testing (Figure 1). Participants' viewing distance from the laptop screen and the horizontal screen angle were not set in advance and adjusted so each participant could operate the laptop keyboard comfortably.

SuperLab (Cedrus Corporation, USA), psychological experiment software for presenting experimental imagery, was used for the MR task. The images consisted of realistic photos (11 cm square) of a head and neck profile of a young woman, a hand, and a foot presented on the laptop screen

Table 1: Characteristics of the participants.

	TMD group	Control group	Overall
Age (years)	49.2 (11.7)	42.5 (19.2)	45.9 (16.1)
Woman (%)	95.8	83.3	89.6
Right-handed (%)	88.0	96.0	91.7
Right-footed (%)	84.0	96.0	89.6
Height (cm)	156.7 (9.6)	161.0 (7.9)	158.8 (8.9)
Weight (kg)	52.2 (9.9)*	58.8 (10.6)	55.5 (10.7)
Range of mouth opening (mm)	39.6 (5.8)*	47.3 (6.4)	43.4 (7.2)
Pain described by VAS (mm)	39.4 (30.2)	NA	
Subtype of TMD	Myalgia of the masticatory muscle: 11 TMJ disc derangement with reduction: 5 TMJ disc derangement without reduction: 2 Myalgia + disc derangement with reduction: 2 Unknown: 4		

*$p < 0.05$ (TMD group versus control group); TMD, temporomandibular disorders; VAS, visual analog scale; TMJ, temporomandibular joint; NA, not available.

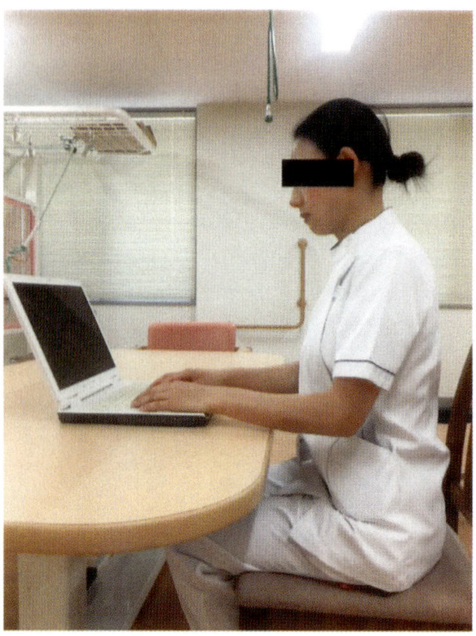

Figure 1: Experimental setting. Participants sat in front of a laptop computer and were asked to put their right and left index fingers on the "M" and "Z" keys, respectively. They were asked to maintain their position, gaze at the screen, and maintain their posture during testing.

(Figure 2). Left and right photographic images were mirror images of each other. Photographic images of hands and feet were taken from the dorsal surface. All stimuli were presented at six different degrees of orientations (0°, 60°, 120°, 180°, 240°, and 300°) for both sides. Photographic images were rotated in a clockwise direction from 0°.

A total of 36 different images, including different orientations, were delivered: 12 for the profile, 12 for the hand, and 12 for the foot image. Testing was completed in three sets so that each body part was tested separately. The sequence of orientation and side of photographic images for each part was randomized between subjects. After each image was presented on the laptop screen, participants had to make a judgement to determine if the image represented a left or right side (i.e., for profile) or a left or right body part (i.e., for hand and for foot). Participants were asked to answer as quickly and accurately as possible using the laptop keyboard. If the answer was right, the participants pressed the "M" key, if left, the participants pressed the "Z" key. Reaction time (RT) was defined as the time between the appearance of the image on the laptop screen and pushing the key. Whether the participant's response was correct or incorrect was also recorded. Stimuli remained on the screen until participants pushed the key. The trigger for computer to present the next picture was when the M or Z key was pressed. As with previous research, if a RT was more than three standard deviations above the mean for a particular stimulus type and image orientation (e.g., profile and 60 degrees), the trial was eliminated and considered as an "incorrect" answer (13 out of 852 trials (1.5%) in the TMD group and 15 out of 864 trials (1.7%) in the control group) [10]. This is because the person has more time to think about the process and so their response to MR is not capturing the desired automatic response. This meant these slow reactions times were not included in the RT analysis, as only correct answers were considered in the RT analysis.

Forty-eight responses, provided by 24 participants for left and right sides, were attained for each cell (defined by stimulus type and side) for the profile and foot stimulus types in both groups and the hand stimulus type in the control group. Only 46 responses, provided by 23 participants, were attained for each cell in the hand stimulus type in the TMD group because the data from one participant in TMD group could not be recorded correctly and were excluded before statistical analysis. Subsequently, accuracy was calculated as the percentage of the number of the correct answers to 48 responses in the profile and foot stimulus type in both groups and the hand stimuli type in the control group and to 46 responses in the hand stimuli in the TMD group. We analyzed RTs and accuracy using analysis of variance (ANOVA) with a post hoc test. When analyzing RTs, ANOVA included a between-subjects factor, "group" (TMD and control), and two within-subjects factors, "stimulus type" (profiles, hands, and feet), and "stimulus orientation" (0°, 60°, 120°, 180°, 240°, and 300°). Post hoc comparisons were carried out using Tukey's test, the Games-Howell test, or unpaired t test, when necessary. In addition, we explored correlations between mean RT and accuracy of response for the profile stimulus type, and pain intensity and mouth ROM were calculated in the TMD group. Statistical analysis was performed using IBM SPSS statistics 22 (IBM Japan, Tokyo, Japan). Significance level was set at 5%.

3. Results

Participants' characteristics for each group are presented in Table 1. The participants were mostly women with a right sided dominance. The TMD group mean pain for the VAS was 39.4 (standard deviation 30.2). Predictably, mouth ROM in the TMD group was smaller than that in the control group ($p < 0.05$).

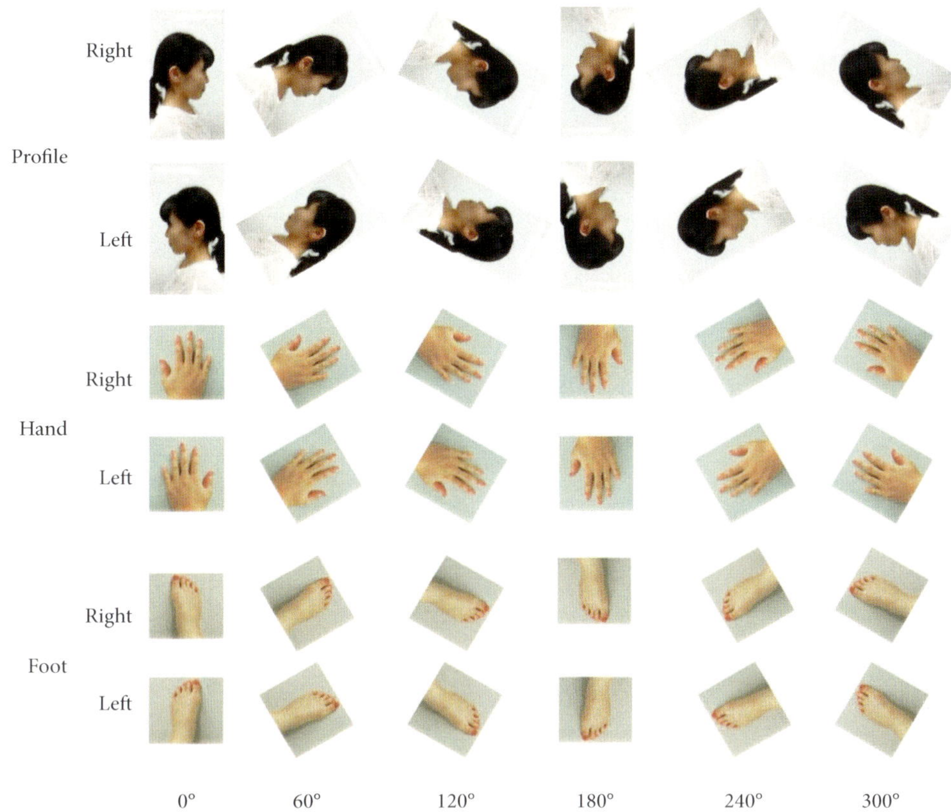

FIGURE 2: Photographic images of three types of experimental stimuli (profile, hand, and foot) in the six orientations (0°, 60°, 120°, 180°, 240°, and 300°) used in mental rotation. Left stimuli were mirror images of right stimuli.

TABLE 2: Mean RTs (msec) in the two groups for each stimulus type and orientation.

	0	60	120	180	240	300	Overall
Profile							
Control	1076.4	1125.8	1383.8	1632.1	1484.9	1113.2	1274.6
TMD	1322.6	1329.0	1698.7	1971.0	1567.3	1222.3	1471.8
Hand							
Control	1037.6	1091.4	1189.5	1602.6	1193.7	1102.6	1175.4
TMD	1076.9	1130.1	1347.2	2304.8	1336.8	1189.4	1336.1
Foot							
Control	858.7	936.1	1169.7	1346.8	1049.3	969.3	1047.2
TMD	965.9	1030.0	1347.5	1701.9	1285.0	1026.2	1212.1
Overall	1054.3	1104.1	1344.9	1722.3	1308.6	1101.8	

3.1. Reaction Time to Mental Rotation (MR) Task. Left and right judgement RTs of the two groups are presented in Table 2. The following highlights the significant results drawing on information from both of these tables.

In ANOVA for the group factor, RT of the TMD group (1333.8 ± 702.8 ms) was significantly slower than that of the control group (1161.3 ± 517.6 ms) (F (1. 1478) = 43.1, $p < 0.01$). Regarding the stimulus type factor, RT for profile (1371.0 ± 743.6 ms) was significantly slower than that for hand (1252.8 ± 601.2 ms) and foot (1128.9 ± 483.9 ms), and RT for hand was significantly slower than that for foot (F (2. 1478) = 29.0, $p < 0.01$). Regarding the stimulus orientation factor, the overall RT for images rotated by 180 degrees (1722.3 ± 818.3 ms) was significantly slower than RTs for five of the other image orientations (0 degree = 1054.3 ± 457.9 ms; 60 degrees = 1104.1 ± 444.3 ms; 120 degrees = 1344.9 ± 713.4 ms; 240 degrees = 1308.6 ± 612.0 ms; 300 degrees = 1101.8 ± 459.9 ms). RTs for 120 and 240 degrees were significantly slower than those for 0, 60, and 300 degrees (F (5. 1478) = 45.2, $p < 0.01$).

The interaction between group and stimulus orientation factors was significant (F (5. 1478) = 3.1, $p = 0.01$). The TMD group was slower than the control group at all stimulus orientations except 300 degrees (Figure 3). Within both groups, RT for 180 degrees was slower than those for all other image orientations. Within the TMD group, RTs for 120 and 240 degrees were slower than those for 0, 60, and 300 degrees. Within the control group, RTs for 120 and

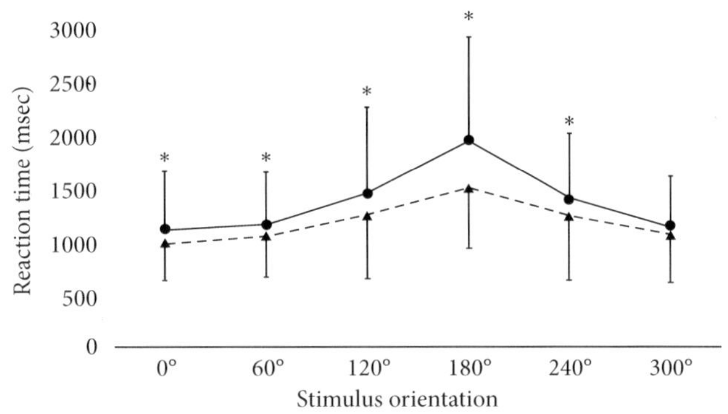

Figure 3: Mean reaction times of three stimulus types of TMD group (circles) and control group (triangle). Error bars indicate standard deviations. Asterisks indicate significant differences between two groups ($p < 0.05$).

240 degrees were slower than those for 0 and 60 degrees (Figure 3). Group and stimulus type factors, stimulus type and stimulus orientation factors, and group, stimulus type, and stimulus orientation factors were not significant (F (2. 1478) = 0.2, $p = 0.82$; F (10. 1478) = 1.8, $p = 0.06$; F (10. 1478) = 0.7, $p = 0.68$, resp.).

Mean RT for profile in the TMD group was significantly correlated with mouth ROM ($r = 0.42$, $p = 0.04$), but not with pain intensity ($r = -0.24$, $p = 0.25$).

3.2. Accuracy in Response to Mental Rotation (MR) Task. Accuracies are presented in Table 3. For the stimulus type factor, the accuracy for profile (83.2%) and hand (86.9%) was significantly lower than that for foot (94.6%) (F (2. 27) = 14.5, $p < 0.01$). In the stimulus orientation factor, the accuracy for 180 degrees (65.0%) was significantly lower than those for all other image orientations (0 degree = 94.4%; 60 degrees = 96.2%; 120 degrees = 90.6%; 240 degrees = 87.0%; 300 degrees = 96.2%) (F (5. 27) = 30.2, $p < 0.01$). No significant difference was presented in the group factor (TMD group = 86.9%; control group = 89.6%) (F (1. 27) = 2.4, $p = 0.14$).

No significant differences were found between the TMD group (86.9%) and the control group (89.6%) for accuracy. Mean accuracy for profile stimulus type in the TMD group was not correlated with mouth ROM ($r = -0.06$, $p = 0.79$) or pain intensity ($r = -0.20$, $p = 0.35$).

4. Discussion

The result in this study showed that the RT in the MR was slower in the TMD group than in the control group. In addition, the RT for profiles was slower than those for hands and feet. Furthermore, for the inverted image (i.e., 180 degree rotation), the RT was slower, and the accuracy was lower than those for more familiar orientations (i.e., more upright). The response for the inverted image was more inaccurate compared to images of all other orientations, among all stimulus types. The significant interaction between group and stimulus orientation factors means between-group differences occur only at specific degrees of image orientation. In this study, RT between the TMD and the control group presented significant difference at 0 to 240 degrees orientation, but not at 300 degrees orientation. This result could be expected given what is known of brain activation in people with TMD [21–25].

Table 3: Accuracy (%) in the two groups for each stimulus type and orientation.

	0	60	120	180	240	300	Overall
Profile							
Control	91.7	95.8	83.3	58.3	85.4	95.8	85.1
TMD	93.8	91.7	79.2	50.0	79.2	93.8	81.3
Hand							
Control	93.8	95.8	93.8	58.3	91.7	95.8	88.2
TMD	93.5	95.7	93.5	58.7	76.1	95.7	85.5
Foot							
Control	97.9	97.9	97.9	83.3	95.8	100.0	95.5
TMD	95.8	100.0	95.8	81.3	93.8	95.8	93.8
Overall	94.4	96.2	90.6	65.0	87.0	96.2	

Mouth ROM in the TMD group was smaller than that in the control group. Average heights in both group did not have a significant difference, though average weights did. It is inferred that normal mouth ROM is associated with height rather than weight. Therefore, it is considered that the TMD group had functional limitation in the TMJ compared with the control group because average heights had no significant difference.

Previous studies described the delayed RT and/or decreased accuracy in MR of body parts in people with chronic leg pain [12], chronic shoulder/arm pain [13], and other musculoskeletal pain and dysfunction, such as complex regional pain syndrome [14], carpal tunnel syndrome [16], and cervical dystonia [10]. The results in this study correspond to the results in these studies. Therefore, as has been shown with painful conditions in the extremities, painful TMD appears to disturb reaction in MR compared with healthy controls.

It might be expected that response to MR tasks is affected for the stimulus type associated with the area of pain (e.g., profile and painful TMD). Previous research has shown delayed reaction in MR was found in the affected quadrant selectively among people with pain in extremities [14, 16]. However, in this study, RT in the TMD group was slower, not only for the profile stimulus type but also for hand and foot stimulus types, compared to the control group. Similarly, Fiorio et al. [10] revealed that the response to MR by people with cervical dystonia was affected not only for face but also for hand and foot. Therefore, processing of left and right judgement in MR may be different between extremities, where the effects might be limited to the affected body part and axial parts of the body, such as TMJ.

The results in this study might result from different processing of motor imagery or body perception between TMJ and extremities. Gandevia and Phegan [29] demonstrated that anesthesia of the lips caused distorted perception of the size of thumbs. People with back or neck pain presented altered pain sensitivity and/or tactile spatial acuity in their extremities [30–32]. Distorted sensory processing in the axial part of the body may have influence on the perception of the orientation of the extremities. This might provide an explanation for the results in this study but needs to be clarified with further research, in particular, an investigation into the explicit link between the left and right judgement process and body perception, in people with TMD.

Shibukawa et al. [25] reported that deficit or marked attenuation of the neuromagnetic responses was found during observing jaw opening movement in TMD group compared to healthy subjects, but no significant difference was found during observing palm-opening movements between two groups. That is, they demonstrated that cortical dysfunction associated with jaw-movement observation was specific phenomena in the patients of TMD. Their result does not correspond with our results. This difference may be due to the difference of the way to present image. Our study applied MR using static photographic images while Shibukawa et al. [25] used dynamic video image. Therefore, there may be different visuomotor integration processes between static and dynamic images among TMD patients though we cannot clarify it in the current study.

The difference of accuracy between groups was not significant, while the RT presented between-group difference. A previous study in people with chronic shoulder/arm pain and complex regional pain syndrome also presented results that showed an increased RT but comparable accuracy compared to the control subjects [13]. The process of left and right judgement in MR of the body parts can be described by 3 stages [16, 26]. At first, people make an initial decision on the side of the body pictured [26]. Second, the decision is followed by a mental rotation of the involved body part into the pictured position [26]. At last, people confirm the accuracy of the initial decision via comparing the mentally rotated body part with the actual image [26]. Weissman-Fogel et al. [24] suggested that the slow behavioral responses in people with TMD may be due to functional deficit in recruitment of attention and/or cognition processing areas. Delayed RT may correspond to a disturbance of the initial decision as a correction during the confirmation stage result in a delayed RT while maintaining accuracy [16].

Mean RT of profile stimulus type in the TMD group showed significant positive correlation with passive range of mouth opening. That is, people with larger range of mouth opening had slower RT when presented with the profile stimulus type. The reason why larger range of mouth opening was related to slower RT was not able to be revealed by the results in this study. Indeed, it might be expected the opposite to be the case in patients where mouth opening is painful. The passive range of mouth measurements used might have excluded any guarding due to pain, and the association between active range of mouth opening and RT of profile stimulus type may have presented different result.

The association between mean RT of profile and pain intensity and that between mean accuracy and passive range of mouth opening and pain intensity were not significant. This is not the first study to report RT and pain intensity are not correlated. Two studies using MR found no correlation between RT and accuracy with pain intensity and disability [16, 33]. These results may imply that pain intensity is not associated with disturbance of motor imagery.

This study has several limitations. First, in the TMD group, we did not analyze the association between the painful side and the side presented in the image. There is some evidence in the motor imagery literature that this may be important when evaluating responses [10]. Second, as we mentioned, we have to clarify the possibility of difference of left and right judgement process and/or body perception between people with TMD and with pain in extremities. For example, sensory testing at peripheral sites should be considered in conjunction with MR in future studies. Third, we did not take into account symptom duration because previous research has described no association between RT and accuracy and symptom duration [16, 33]. However, these studies were not investigating painful TMD, and as there seems to be some differences between responses to MR where the location of pain is axial, compared to in the extremities, we would consider that future research might explore duration of symptoms as an influencing factor on RT and accuracy. Fourth, we did not have the resources to capture brain activity as has been done on some studies involving MR, and this would enhance the data supporting findings using RT and accuracy alone. Fifth, most of participants in this study were women. Sex differences were reported in MR [34]. Therefore, the results in this study may be influenced by the rate of participants of women, and we will have to consider the sex difference in future studies. Finally, the number of participants recruited for this study was relatively small. To have greater confidence in the findings, we will need to calculate and recruit the appropriate sample size. More research on motor imagery tasks and specifically involving participants with TMD will help to guide this.

Despite these limitations, we consider the findings of this study to suggest that the use of motor imagery in physiotherapy, for clinical examination and treatment, in TMD patients with chronic pain may be worth investigating. MR has been used for clinical examination for those with chronic pain in extremities, where patients were slower to identify extremities depicted in postures that they find difficult to attain with their own body part [12, 13]. MR also presented a beneficial effect on pain in the extremities when used in physiotherapy treatment [15]. Therefore, our findings which showed that responses to MR by those with pain in the TMJ may be similar to responses by those with pain in the extremities give support for further clinical research into the use of motor imagery for patients with chronic painful TMD.

5. Conclusions

The RTs in the MR for profile were more delayed in the individuals with TMD than in those without TMD. When the MR task involved an inverted image, the reaction time was slower and the accuracy was lower than those for other image orientations. Therefore, TMD may influence the motor imagery in the orofacial region. In addition, MR may be useful for assessment and treatment for the TMD patients as well as people with pain in extremities, but further research is needed.

Acknowledgments

This study was funded by Kio University.

References

[1] L. LeResche, "Epidemiology of temporomandibular disorders: implications for the investigation of etiologic factors," *Critical Reviews in Oral Biology and Medicine*, vol. 8, no. 3, pp. 291–305, 1997.

[2] F. Luther, S. Layton, and F. McDonald, "Orthodontics for treating temporomandibular joint (TMJ) disorders," *Cochrane Database of Systematic Reviews*, no. 7, p. CD006541, 2010.

[3] National Institute of Dental and Craniofacial Research, *Facial Pain*, National Institute of Dental and Craniofacial Research, Bethesda, MD, USA, 2014, https://www.nidcr.nih.gov/DataStatistics/FindDataByTopic/FacialPain/.

[4] S. M. Shaffer, J.-M. Brismée, P. S. Sizer, and C. A. Courtney, "Temporomandibular disorders. Part 2: conservative management," *Journal of Manual and Manipulative Therapy*, vol. 22, no. 1, pp. 13–23, 2014.

[5] S. Armijo-Olivo, L. Pitance, V. Singh, F. Neto, N. Thie, and A. Michelotti, "Effectiveness of manual therapy and therapeutic exercise for temporomandibular disorders: systematic review and meta-analysis," *Physical Therapy*, vol. 96, no. 1, pp. 9–25, 2016.

[6] M. Leeuw, M. E. J. B. Goossens, S. J. Linton, G. Crombez, K. Boersma, and J. W. S. Vlaeyen, "The fear-avoidance model of musculoskeletal pain: current state of scientific evidence," *Journal of Behavioral Medicine*, vol. 30, no. 1, pp. 77–94, 2007.

[7] R. N. Shepard and J. Metzler, "Mental rotation of three-dimensional objects," *Science*, vol. 171, no. 3972, pp. 701–703, 1971.

[8] F. P. de Lange, R. C. Helmich, and I. Toni, "Posture influences motor imagery: an fMRI study," *Neuroimage*, vol. 33, no. 2, pp. 609–617, 2006.

[9] M. Fiorio, M. Tinazzi, and S. M. Aglioti, "Selective impairment of hand mental rotation in patients with focal hand dystonia," *Brain: a Journal of Neurology*, vol. 129, no. 1, pp. 47–54, 2006.

[10] M. Fiorio, M. Tinazzi, S. Ionta et al., "Mental rotation of body parts and non-corporeal objects in patients with idiopathic cervical dystonia," *Neuropsychologia*, vol. 45, no. 10, pp. 2346–2354, 2007.

[11] T. Wolbers, C. Weiller, and C. Buchel, "Contralateral coding of imagined body parts in the superior parietal lobe," *Cerebral Cortex*, vol. 13, no. 4, pp. 392–399, 2003.

[12] H. B. Coslett, J. Medina, D. Kliot, and A. Burkey, "Mental motor imagery and chronic pain: the foot laterality task," *Journal of the International Neuropsychological Society*, vol. 16, no. 4, pp. 603–612, 2010.

[13] H. B. Coslett, J. Medina, D. Kliot, and A. R. Burkey, "Mental motor imagery indexes pain: the hand laterality task," *European Journal of Pain*, vol. 14, no. 10, pp. 1007–1013, 2010.

[14] G. L. Moseley, "Why do people with complex regional pain syndrome take longer to recognize their affected hand?," *Neurology*, vol. 62, no. 12, pp. 2182–2186, 2004.

[15] G. L. Moseley, "Graded motor imagery for pathologic pain: a randomized controlled trial," *Neurology*, vol. 67, no. 12, pp. 2129–2134, 2006.

[16] A. B. Schmid and M. W. Coppieters, "Left/right judgment of body parts is selectively impaired in patients with unilateral carpal tunnel syndrome," *Clinical Journal of Pain*, vol. 28, no. 7, pp. 615–622, 2012.

[17] R. Dickstein and J. E. Deutsch, "Motor imagery in physical therapist practice," *Physical Therapy*, vol. 87, no. 7, pp. 942–953, 2007.

[18] H. von Piekartz, S. B. Wallwork, G. Mohr, D. S. Butler, and G. L. Moseley, "People with chronic facial pain perform worse than controls at a facial emotion recognition task, but it is not all about the emotion," *Journal of Oral Rehabilitation*, vol. 42, no. 4, pp. 243–250, 2015.

[19] Y. Shibukawa, T. Ishikawa, Y. Kato et al., "Cortical dysfunction in patients with temporomandibular disorders," *Journal of Oral Biosciences*, vol. 51, no. 2, pp. 65–71, 2009.

[20] G. Buccino, F. Binkofski, G. R. Fink et al., "Action observation activates premotor and parietal areas in a somatotopic manner: an fMRI study," *European Journal of Neuroscience*, vol. 13, no. 2, pp. 400–404, 2001.

[21] S. S. He, F. Li, F. Song et al., "Spontaneous neural activity alterations in temporomandibular disorders: a cross-sectional and longitudinal resting-state functional magnetic resonance imaging study," *Neuroscience*, vol. 278, pp. 1–10, 2014.

[22] E. Ichesco, A. Quintero, D. J. Clauw et al., "Altered functional connectivity between the insula and the cingulate cortex in patients with temporomandibular disorder: a pilot study," *Headache*, vol. 52, no. 3, pp. 441–454, 2012.

[23] M. Moayedi, I. Weissman-Fogel, T. V. Salomons et al., "White matter brain and trigeminal nerve abnormalities in temporomandibular disorder," *Pain*, vol. 153, no. 7, pp. 1467–1477, 2012.

[24] I. Weissman-Fogel, M. Moayedi, H. C. Tenenbaum, M. B. Goldberg, B. V. Freeman, and K. D. Davis, "Abnormal cortical activity in patients with temporomandibular disorder evoked by cognitive and emotional tasks," *Pain*, vol. 152, no. 2, pp. 384–396, 2011.

[25] Y. Shibukawa, T. Ishikawa, Y. Kato et al., "Cerebral cortical dysfunction in patients with temporomandibular disorders in association with jaw movement observation," *Pain*, vol. 128, no. 1-2, pp. 180–188, 2007.

[26] L. M. Parsons, "Integrating cognitive psychology, neurology and neuroimaging," *Acta Psychologica*, vol. 107, no. 1-3, pp. 155–181, 2001.

[27] R. Hari, N. Forss, S. Avikainen, E. Kirveskari, S. Salenius, and G. Rizzolatti, "Activation of human primary motor cortex during action observation: a neuromagnetic study," *Proceedings of the National Academy of Sciences*, vol. 95, no. 25, pp. 15061–15065, 1998.

[28] J. Jarvelainen, M. Schürmann, S. Avikainen, and R. Hari, "Stronger reactivity of the human primary motor cortex during observation of live rather than video motor acts," *Neuroreport*, vol. 12, no. 16, pp. 3493–3495, 2001.

[29] S. C. Gandevia and C. M. Phegan, "Perceptual distortions of the human body image produced by local anaesthesia, pain and cutaneous stimulation," *Journal of Physiology*, vol. 514, no. 2, pp. 609–616, 1999.

[30] M. Linari-Melfi, I. Cantarero-Villanueva, C. Fernández-Lao, C. Fernández-de-las-Peñas, R. Guisado-Barrilao, and M. Arroyo-Morales, "Analysis of deep tissue hypersensitivity to pressure pain in professional pianists with insidious mechanical neck pain," *BMC Musculoskeletal Disorders*, vol. 12, p. 268, 2011.

[31] A. Steinmetz and G. A. Jull, "Sensory and sensorimotor features in violinists and violists with neck pain," *Archives of Physical Medicine and Rehabilitation*, vol. 94, no. 12, pp. 2523–2528, 2013.

[32] A. M. Zamorano, I. Riquelme, B. Kleber, E. AltenmÃller, S. M. Hatem, and P. Montoya, "Pain sensitivity and tactile spatial acuity are altered in healthy musicians as in chronic pain patients," *Frontiers in Human Neuroscience*, vol. 8, p. 1016, 2014.

[33] R. Pelletier, J. Higgins, and D. Bourbonnais, "Laterality recognition of images, motor performance, and aspects related to pain in participants with and without wrist/hand disorders: An observational cross-sectional study," *Musculoskeletal Science and Practice*, vol. 35, pp. 18–24, 2018.

[34] T. D. Parsons, P. Larson, K. Kratz et al., "Sex differences in mental rotation and spatial rotation in a virtual environment," *Neuropsychologia*, vol. 42, no. 4, pp. 555–562, 2004.

13

The Impact of Chronic Discogenic Low Back Pain: Costs and Patients' Burden

José W. Geurts, [1,2] **Paul C. Willems**, [3] **Jan-Willem Kallewaard**, [2] **Maarten van Kleef**, [1] **and Carmen Dirksen** [4]

[1] *Department of Anesthesiology and Pain Medicine, Maastricht University Medical Centre, Maastricht, Netherlands*
[2] *Department of Anesthesiology and Pain Management, Rijnstate Hospital, Arnhem, Netherlands*
[3] *Department of Orthopedic Surgery, Maastricht University Medical Centre, Maastricht, Netherlands*
[4] *Department of Clinical Epidemiology and Medical Technology, Maastricht University Medical Centre, CAPHRI—Care and Public Health Research Institute, Maastricht, Netherlands*

Correspondence should be addressed to José W. Geurts; jwjmgeurts@rijnstate.nl

Academic Editor: Parisa Gazerani

Introduction. Chronic discogenic low back pain (CDP) is frequently diagnosed in patients referred to specialized pain clinics for their back pain. The aim of this study is to assess the impact of CDP both on the individual patient and on society. *Materials and Methods.* Using the baseline records of 80 patients in a randomized trial assessing the effectiveness of a new intervention for CDP, healthcare and societal costs related to back pain are calculated. Furthermore, the impact of the condition on perceived pain, disability, health-related quality of life, Quality of life Adjusted Life Years (QALY), and QALY loss is assessed. *Results.* Using the friction costs approach, we found that the annual costs for society are €7,911.95 per CDP patient, 51% healthcare and 49% societal costs. When using the human capital approach, total costs were €18,940.58, 22% healthcare and 78% societal costs. Healthcare costs were mainly related to pain treatment. Mean pain severity was 6.5 (0–10), and 46% suffered from severe pain (≥7/10). Mean physical limitations rate was 43.7; 13.5% of the patients were very limited to disabled. QALY loss compared to a healthy population was 64%. *Discussion.* This study shows that in patients with CDP referred to a pain clinic, costs for society are high and the most used healthcare resources are pain therapies. Patients suffer severe pain, are physically limited, and experience a serious loss in quality of life.

1. Introduction

Low back pain is one of the most common disabling conditions worldwide [1]. Approximately 70 to 85% of the western population will develop low back pain at least once during their lifetime [2]. Of the people that consult their general practitioner for low back pain, one year later about 60% still report pain [3]. The prevalence of chronic low back pain (CLBP) is globally calculated to be 9442.5 per 100,000 (9%) [4]. CLBP is a common, long-lasting, and disabling condition with high costs for society [5–7]. In 2007, the costs for CLBP represented 0.6% of the gross national product in the Netherlands [7]. Direct healthcare costs are, for instance, caused by patients searching for pain treatment [2, 5, 8, 9]. Indirect (societal) costs represent secondary consequences of CLBP, the losses resulting from morbidity or disability, mainly caused by work absenteeism and informal caregiving [10, 11]. Although indirect costs are known to be the highest cost factor for CLBP, direct healthcare costs, like medical specialist care and hospital costs, for low back pain are high as well [5, 8, 11].

CLBP may emerge from several different etiologies but about 40 to 50% of CLBP, treated in specialized pain or orthopedic clinics, is alleged to be of discogenic origin [12–14]. Disk degeneration involves structural disruption and cell-mediated changes in composition of the disk, particularly annular fissures reaching the outer annulus [15]. Provocation discography is, up to now, the only test that with some reliability can distinguish pain of discogenic origin from other sources of CLBP [15, 16]. Patients with chronic discogenic low back pain (CDP) in clinical practice differ from other CLBP patients in that the chronic pain is located more axial and the pain is severe [17]. There is evidence that CDP more often starts at a younger age than other types of chronic pain. A study reports that if the CLBP starts at a young age, the more likely the pain is discogenic in origin [14, 18]. Although most CDP patients are amenable for pain intervention therapies, up till now there is no evidence for a longer term beneficial treatment [19].

Little is known about the specific impact of CDP on patients and its burden for society. About the impact of CLBP in general, there is more information [12, 13, 20] and some is known about the impact of radicular syndromes [21].

Therefore, the first aim of this study is to provide healthcare and societal cost information about CDP patients who have been referred to pain specialized care. The second aim is to assess the impact of CDP on patients' pain, disability, health-related quality of life, and QALY loss.

2. Methods

2.1. Design. This study is a CDP evaluation with both a cost of illness analysis and assessment of outcome [22].

There are two methods available to estimate costs of disease. Top-down healthcare cost data can be obtained from central data collecting sources like medical insurance agencies [8, 23]. The other method is bottom-up data collection that uses individual patient-level information collected by surveys and diaries from a single study or multiple smaller studies. Our approach is the bottom-up method using data obtained in a multicenter study. This study was performed from 2013 to 2016 in 4 pain centres throughout the Netherlands. Patients with CLBP were predominantly referred from primary care, and sometimes from neurologic or orthopedic settings. Baseline data were collected during the IMBI RCT [24] that was conducted to assess the efficacy and cost effectiveness of a minimal interventional procedure for CDP. The diagnosis of CDP cannot be made with a reasonable amount of certainty with conventional clinical tests [13]. Therefore, data from this study were used to obtain information from CDP patients for whom a provocation discography had been performed to confirm the suspected diagnosis of CDP [17].

2.2. Participants. Eighty consecutive patients with CDP, as diagnosed by clinical history, physical examination, magnetic resonance imaging, and provocation discography, were eligible for the IMBI study and were included in this evaluation. Inclusion and exclusion criteria were described in detail in the study protocol of the RCT [24]. Patients had to be above 18, have a BMI of ≤ 35, and had to rate at least a 5 for their low back pain on an 11 box (0–10) numeric rating scale after at least 6 months of pain treatment. Facet pain was excluded by negative facet blocks. The diagnosis of discogenic pain was confirmed by a positive provocative discography along with morphologic signs of disc degeneration, that is, annular tear grade II to IV according to the modified Dallas Classification [24, 25].

2.3. Assessment of Impact. The baseline data used for this study included sociodemographic characteristics, pain severity and pain medication use, disability, and health-related quality of life [26]. Furthermore, cost information over the last 3 months, e.g., healthcare utilisation, medication, and lost working hours, was collected from each patient entering the study. Health-related quality of life at baseline and 3-month cost information were projected over a full year for calculation of QALY (loss) and annual societal costs.

2.4. Pain. Patients rated their low back pain in a pain diary, 3 times a day during 4 days, using 11 box (0–10) numeric rating scales (PNRS); zero represents no pain and 10 excruciating pain [26].

2.5. Disability. Physical functioning was measured with the Oswestry Disability Index (ODI) [27]. The value of the ODI scale represents the physical limitations rate (0–100%):

(i) 0–20% minimally limited: patient can get along with most daily activities. There is normally no treatment indicated except advice about sitting, lifting, and exercises.

(ii) 21–40% moderately limited: patient experiences pain when lifting, sitting, and standing. Travel and social life is sometimes difficult, and absenteeism can occur. Normally, there are no limitations in daily activities, sexual activity, or sleeping.

(iii) 41–60% clearly limited: pain is problem in activities. Treatment is indicated.

(iv) 61–80% very limited to disabled: back pain affects all aspects of life of the patient. Treatment is very desirable.

(v) 81–100% disabled. These patients are often bedridden.

2.6. Health-Related Quality of Life. Health-related quality of life was assessed with the Rand-36 and the EuroQol (EQ-5D-3L) [28–30]. The Rand-36 measures eight domains of quality of life: physical functioning, social functioning, role limitations (physical problem), role limitations (emotional problems), mental health, pain, general health perception, and health change. Furthermore, two summary scores were calculated from the Rand-36: the physical component summary (PCS) and the mental health component summary (MCS). A higher score relates to a better health status. The EQ-5D-3L was used to measure health state, it contains 5 domains: mobility, self-care, usual activities, pain/discomfort, and anxiety/depression, and a general health score measured with a visual analogue scale 0–100 (VAS) [31, 32]. Each domain has three levels: no limitations, some limitations, and severe limitations. This results in 243 possible sets of health states. A selection of these health states has been valued by the general public in the U.K. using the time-trade-off method. This resulted in an algorithm which allows calculation of a utility value (i.e., quality of life score) for each possible health state [31]. The utility values range from −0.549 to 1, where 1 is perfect health and ≤ 0 is a health state equal to death or a health state considered worse than death.

2.7. Quality of Life Adjusted Life Years (QALY). The QALY is a composite measure which multiplies life years with the quality of these life years. One QALY represents one life year in perfect health. QALYs lived in one year were calculated based on the EQ-5D-3L at baseline, using the UK algorithm [31]. It was assumed that the utility score at baseline represented the utility score for a full year. Furthermore, because CDP is not a fatal disease, it was assumed that the QALY loss was fully attributed to the loss in health-related quality of life.

2.8. Costs. Health care and societal costs were measured with cost questionnaires with a recall period of 3 months, which were filled out by patients online [33].

The patients were asked to record the resource use specifically related to their treatment of back pain, such as visits to primary care, medical specialists, physical therapists, and complementary and alternative medicine. Furthermore, the questionnaire queried specifically about back pain-related medication costs, extra requirements such as adaptations to home or equipment for their mobility, and professional caregiving costs. Moreover, patients were asked to report societal costs that included lost productivity and informal caregiving costs. Work absenteeism was measured with the productivity and disease questionnaire (PRODISQ) [34].

2.9. Statistical Methods. With the exception of the pain diary and the EQ-5D-3L, which were presented to the patient in a booklet, all data were collected by web-based questionnaires software, SelectSurvey (NETv4.075.011© Copyright 2008 ClassApps.com) and MACRO (version 4.1.2.3750© 1999–2012 InferMed Limited, London, UK) [24]. Before the intervention, the booklets were inspected for missing data, and completion of the online questionnaires was checked. After these preparations, we assumed that patients filled in the relevant questions correctly, and no correction was made for missing baseline data of the 80 patients used for this study. Costs were calculated by multiplying resource use by the cost price using Dutch guideline prices for the resources, reference year 2014 [35]. If a guideline price was not readily available, an assumption was made on the basis of an existing guideline price. We used mean hourly labor costs for employees across all sectors of €37.50 [35]. Informal care and unpaid productivity loss was valued at €14/hour [35].

All costs-related information from the baseline questionnaires in which patients were asked about information covering a period of 3 months before entering the study were

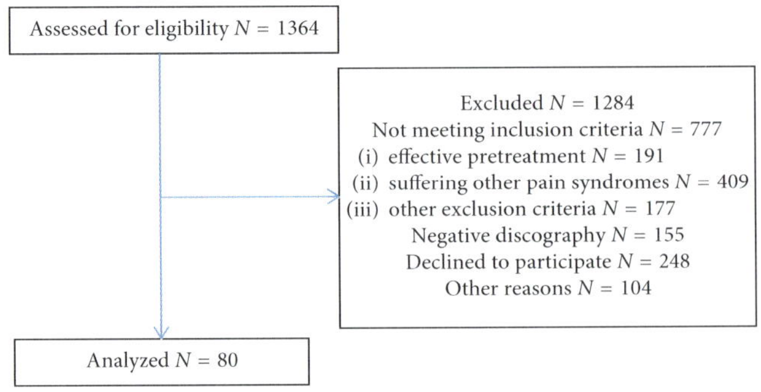

FIGURE 1: Flow diagram.

TABLE 1: Patient characteristics.

	N = 80	Male	Female
Gender, N (%)		23 (29%)	57 (71%)
	Mean (SD)	Mean (SD)	Mean (SD)
Age (years)	41.8 (9.9)	41.5 (8.7)	41.9 (10.5)
Low back pain (0–10)	6.5 (1.5)	6.7 (1.7)	6.4 (1.4)
Pain duration (years)	10.6 (8.0)	9.7 (5.6)	10.9 (8.8)
Treatment duration (years)	5.7 (5.7)	3.5 (2.5)	6.6 (6.3)
Education, N (%)			
Low	8 (10%)	2 (9%)	6 (11%)
Middle	45 (55%)	14 (61%)	31 (54%)
High	27 (35%)	7 (30%)	20 (35%)
Employment/work, N (%)			
Full time	31	12 (52%)	19 (33)
<30 hours a week	26	2 (9%)	24 (42%)
Unemployed	13	4 (17%)	9 (16%)
Disability payment (DIA)	10	5 (22%)	5 (9%)

Data presented as total group and divided by gender. DIA = Disablement Insurance Act; SD = standard deviation.

multiplied by 4 to calculate annual costs per patient. Study-related costs, like costs made for informed consent consults, were not included in the cost analysis. The cost of work absence (productivity losses) was calculated using the friction cost method, which assumes that each worker is replaceable within 85 workdays or 12 weeks [6, 11, 35, 36]. Additionally, the human capital approach was used, as this method is applied in many cost studies as well [6, 37]. Both approaches assume that the individual's level of earnings reflects their productivity. However, in the human capital approach, lost productivity due to long-term absenteeism is valued, even until the age of retirement [10].

In this study, we estimated the costs of absenteeism due to CDP for each patient by multiplying the total number of sick days by the mean number of daily working hours and the costs per hour [35]. Using the human capital approach, disability wages were calculated to be 75% of the average working costs per hour with a maximum of €52.766 a year according to the Employee Insurance Agency (UWV) in the Netherlands [38].

Results are presented as means, range, and standard deviation. Costs results are presented as bootstrapped means and 95% confidence intervals of means (CI). Statistical analyses were performed using SPSS version 24 (SPSS Inc., Chicago IL, USA).

Table 2: Health-related quality of life of patients with discogenic low back pain.

	Mean	Std. deviation
Rand (36)		
Physical functioning	48.25	18.25
Social functioning	52.37	23.60
Role limitations physical	15.31	26.23
Role limitations emotional	59.16	43.40
Mental health	65.10	20.08
Bodily pain	32.88	17.22
Vitality	44.62	17.92
General health	35.62	20.96
Physical sum score	32.52	6.05
Mental sum score	44.67	10.96
EQ-5D-3L		
EQ-5D overall health (VAS)	52.51	17.74
UK utility value (EQ-5D)	0.36	0.34

VAS = visual analogue scale.

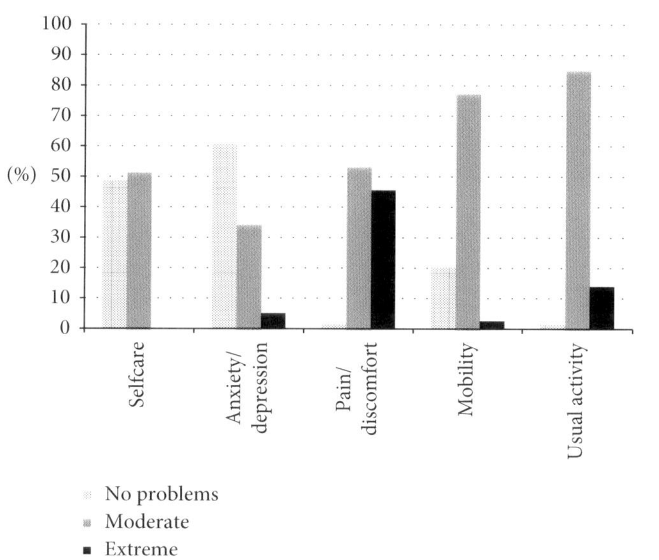

Figure 2: Baseline EQ-5D health profile (percent patients' response categories per domain).

3. Results

Eighty patients included in the IMBI study [24] were assessed for baseline information. Figure 1 shows the flow diagram of the IMBI study. More than 1300 patients were assessed for eligibility in the participating centres. Fifty-seven percent did not meet the inclusion criteria. More than 50% of discographies were negative. Table 1 shows the patient characteristics. The study group comprised 57 (71%) female and 23 (29%) male patients. Mean age was 42 (21 to 65). Mean BMI was 25.3 (18 to 35), length 174 (154 to 196) cm, and weight 77.3 (42 to 118) kg.

3.1. Pain. Table 1 shows that the patients scored the severity of their low back pain on mean at 6.5 (PNRS: 0 to 10). Maximum mean pain was 8.8 (SD: 1.0). Low back pain duration was mean 10.6 (1 to 40) years.

3.2. Disability. The mean physical limitations rate was 43.7 (SD: 14.9) as measured by the ODI [27]. All patients showed some physical limitations of their CDP. Thirty-seven patients (46%) had clear physical limitations, 30 (38%) showed moderate limitations, 9 (11%) patients were very limited to disabled, and 2 (2.5%) patients were disabled by the CDP. Two patients (2.5%) had minimal physical limitations.

3.3. Health-Related Quality of Life. Health-related quality of life as measured with the Rand-36 and EQ-5D-3L is shown in Table 2 and Figure 2. Using the EQ_5D_3L, when perfect health is scored at 100 and death is scored at zero, this CDP population scored on mean 52.5 (SD: 17.7). Figure 2 compares the outcome of the 5 health subscores of the EQ-5D-3L. This figure shows that most CDP patients score on average low on the domains pain, mobility, and usual activity. The Rand-36 shows the same results. The lowest scores were shown on the item "role limitations due to physical functioning" mean 15.3 (SD: 26.3) and bodily pain 32.9 (SD: 17.2).

3.4. Quality-Adjusted Life Years (QALY) and QALY Loss. Table 1 shows that the mean utility for the health state of CDP patients was 0.36 (SD: 0.34), resulting in a mean QALY of 0.36. Compared to a year in full health, this can be translated as a QALY loss of 64% [39].

3.5. Costs. Table 3 shows the mean CDP-related healthcare costs. Mean annual costs were calculated to be €4,015.38. Patients' visits for their back pain to the daycare clinic generated the most costs, mean €1,955.00 (CI: 1,565–2,353) per patient followed by back pain-related consults physical therapy, i.e., €461.10 (CI: 245–676).

Sixty-seven patients (84%) regularly used analgesics for their low back pain: 33% of patients regularly used paracetamol, 31% used nonsteroidal anti-inflammatory drugs, 14% used weak opioids analgesics, and 11% of patients used strong opioids. The mean yearly cost for medication was calculated at €144.56 (CI: 89–200). Approximately 80% of healthcare cost are targeted at pain therapies and related therapies like physical therapy (12%), psychosocial therapy (6%), and 4% for complementary and alternative medicine (CAM). Daycare clinic and pain clinic both made up for 53.5% of the healthcare costs.

The total mean societal costs were composed out of informal caregiving and costs related to work absence (see Table 4). Thirty-seven (46%) patients reported costs for informal caregiving, and 20 patients (25%) noted work absence. The mean absence from work (friction) costs per patient was €3,778.32 versus €14,806.95 using the human capital approach.

Using the friction cost approach, the mean annual total costs per patient with CDP were €7,911.95: €4,015.38 (51%) healthcare cost and €3,896.57 (49%) societal costs.

When the human capital cost approach is used, the total mean annual cost per CDP patient was calculated to be

TABLE 3: Healthcare costs per CDP patient in euros divided by cost type.

Cost type	*N* visits[e]	*N* patients	Mean^ costs per resource user (CI)	Mean^ cost per patient* (CI)	Cum. %
Daycare clinic	340	53	2,950.94 (2574–3328)	1,955.00 (1565–2353)	48
Physical therapy	1112	27	1,475.52 (965–1986)	461.10 (245–676)	60
Travel costs	964	79	303.03 (232–374)	299.24 (229–370)	67
Psychosocial therapy	208	17	1,703.63 (615–2792)	234.25 (51–417)	73
Pain clinic	888	60	292.37 (227–358)	219.27 (163–275)	78.5
CAM therapies	224	10	1,330.80 (427–2234)	166.35 (30–303)	82.5
Medication	126	67	172.62 (108–237)	144.56 (89–200)	86
Extra requirements	36	9	1,128.89 (−36 to 2294)	127.00 (−6 to 260)	89
Rehabilitation	264	4	2,524.50 (−2273 to 7322)	126.23 (−53 to 305)	92
Home care	1056[h]	37	3.210 (1490–5010)	118.25 (−3 to 325)	95
Occupational physician	228	29	259.45 (173–345)	94.05 (53–135)	97
Primary care	164	18	300.67 (220–381)	67.65 (35–100)	98
Hospital nights	40	10	528.89 (407–651)	59.50 (20–99)	99
Policlinic other	92	4	523.25 (−852 to 1899)	26.16 (−19 to 72)	99.5
Intensive care	4	1	2,015	25.18 (−24 to 75)	100
Total healthcare costs		80	4,015.38 (3251–4779)	4,015.38 (3251–4779)	

[e]Visits/events/services/volumes; [h]volume in hours; ^bootstrapped mean; *mean costs per patient = costs for all patients including cost per patients without visit/event/service (0€); CI = 95% confidence interval for mean: lower bound-upper bound.

TABLE 4: Societal costs per patient in euros divided by cost type (results of the friction cost and human capital cost approach).

Cost type friction costs approach	*N*[e]	Mean^ costs per resource user (CI)	Mean^ cost per patient* (CI)	Cum. %
Informal caregiving	37	255.68 (143–368)	118.25 (60–177)	3
Absence work; friction costs	20	15,113 (11090–19135)	3,778.32 (2038–5518)	100
Societal cost per patient: Friction			3,896.57 (2157–5636)	
Cost type human capital approach				
Informal caregiving	37	255.68 (143–368)	118.25 (60–177)	0.8
Absence work; human capital	31	38,212 (28520–47903)	14,806,95 (9283–20330)	100
Disability wages	11	46,720 (39447–53994)	6,424.03 (2720–10128)	
Societal cost per patient: human capital			14,925.20 (9389–20460)	

[e]Number of patients per event/service; ^bootstrapped mean; *mean costs per patient = costs for all patients including cost per patients without event/service (0€); CI = 95% confidence interval for mean: lower bound-upper bound.

€18,940.58: €4,015.38 (22%) healthcare cost and €14,925.20 (78%) societal costs.

4. Discussion

The main objective of this study was to assess the costs of CDP for patients and society. Furthermore, we assessed the impact of CDP on patients' pain, disability, health-related quality of life, QALYs, and QALY loss.

Almost half (46%) of CDP patients reported severe pain (>7 of PNRS 0 to 10), 54% suffered moderate pain. A European prevalence study in chronic pain suffering patients showed that 34% had severe pain and 66% had moderate pain [40]. In agreement with clinical practice, this study shows that CDP patients suffer more severe pain in relation to the general chronic pain suffering patients [40].

In this study, we found that the annual cost per patient for the society is €7,911.95: €4,015.38 (51%) healthcare cost and €3,896.57 (49%) societal costs, using the friction costs approach. Using the human capital approach, the mean cost is €18,940.58: €4,015.38 (22%) for the healthcare cost and €14,925.20 (78%) societal costs per patient.

Costs are on average 56% lower in studies using the friction cost approach than in studies using the human capital approach, because it takes into account that employees can be replaced after a certain time period, i.e., for this study, 85 workdays or 12 weeks [11, 36]. In contrast with the human capital method, long-term absenteeism and disability do not induce additional costs when applying the friction cost method.

The cost for disability wages (€6,424.03) was only considered in the human capital approach [41]. Including work disability in the estimation of productivity costs was done with the assumption that the disability was caused by CDP. Although one of the basic principles of the human capital method is the assumption that there is full use of labor (i.e., no unemployment), the policy in the Netherlands is to provide for 75% of the last earned wages, and therefore, for the disability cost calculations, 75% of the mean hourly labor costs was used instead of 100%.

The inclusion and exclusion criteria for the RCT, from which this study retrieved information, could have an effect on the outcome considering that the patients with more than 35 BMI, or degeneration of multiple discs (>2) were excluded. Furthermore, patients with very severe disc degeneration (Grade V Modified Dallas Scale) were excluded in the RCT, and this study used data from [24, 25]. It is therefore likely that the burden and costs are even higher for the total CDP suffering population. This study shows that almost all CDP patients were physically disabled. This was not only shown with the ODI, but also the domain measuring role limitations physical functioning of the Rand-36 showed a very low score, 15.3 (SD: 26.3).

In comparison, a study in rheumatoid arthritis [42] patients showed a score of 48 for this domain, and in migraine suffering patients showed 60 in role physical functioning [29]. Furthermore, the domain physical functioning in our study was 48.3 (SD: 18.3), and a Dutch patient group suffering rheumatoid arthritis scored 62.3 (SE: 2.0) for physical functioning [42].

The HRQoL was not only low in the scores for physical functioning but also general health and bodily pain scores were low. The mean utility value (i.e., quality of life score) based on the EQ-5D was extremely low (0.36) in the CDP patients. General population score of people in Europe around 45 years of age is approximately 0.85; for instance, a chronic low back pain population in Finland scored mean 0.74 [43]. Similar low quality of life utility scores were reported in a population with major depressive disorders, 0.33 versus 0.36 in our population [44].

The lowest scores of the Rand-36 were shown on the item "role limitations due to physical functioning" mean 15.3 (SD: 26.3) and bodily pain 32.9 (SD: 17.2). In comparison, the Dutch general population scored, respectively, 79.5 (SD: 35.4) and 80.5 (SD: 24.4) [29]. Overall, the burden of disease resulted in a QALY loss of 64% compared to a person in full health.

Our study showed that the patients with CDP in our study suffered moderate to severe pain for on average 10 years (Table 1), are physically disabled, and have a low quality of life due to the bodily pain and functional limitations. This study also shows that unemployment is high in the CDP population: 16% in women and 17% in men (Table 1). On average, in the Netherlands 5% of the working population is unemployed according to the CBS Statistics, the Netherlands (CBS). Eleven (14%) patients in our study population received disability wages (DIA), 22% of the males and 9% of the females. In the Netherlands, on average 10% of the population receives DIA (CBS).

This study was performed in 4 pain centres across the Netherlands: 3 general hospitals and 1 university pain clinic. Only patients with a confirmed diagnosis of chronic discogenic low back pain were included in this study. Our study comprised 57/80 (71%) female patients. Although this seems a disproportional amount of the female gender, research shows that a larger part of the female CLBP suffering population has back pain with impairment: 70% in women versus 57% in men [2]. Our study records showed that apart from women having a longer treatment history (Table 1), mean 6.6 years in women and 3.5 in men, patient characteristics showed no obvious differences between the sexes.

The prevalence of CLBP is estimated to be 9% [4] in the general population, and approximately 50% of CLBP patients in a pain clinic are alleged to suffer discogenic pain [12–14]. However, this does not mean that the population prevalence of CDP is 4.5% (half of the CLBP population prevalence of 9%) because not all CLBP patients are referred to a pain clinic. It is likely that the average CLBP patient referred to a pain clinic is suffering more, and less episodic, severe pain. Therefore, we assume that the incidence of CDP within the CLBP of a pain clinic population is higher than in the general population. A recent study confirms this assumption by showing that only 13% of the CLBP in a nonpain clinic (an outpatient orthopedic clinic) could be diagnosed with discogenic pain [45]. Because the prevalence of CDP in the general population is uncertain, no efforts were made to extrapolate the costs to population level.

As far as we know, this is the first study that shows the economic burden for society and the impact of CDP on patients. A comparable study with bottom-up information conducted with patients from a pain clinic showed that the total costs of chronic pain suffering patients was US$24,043 using the human capital cost approach [46]. In this study, the hospital stay (nights) took the largest share of healthcare costs (44%). For CDP patients in our study, hospital nights due to CDP are rare, i.e., mean €59.50 (1%) per patient (Table 3). In contrast with the aforementioned study, more costs are made by our study population for therapies like physical therapy, psychotherapy, pain medication, and CAM therapies. Another study assessing cost effectiveness of steroid injections in radicular pain syndrome showed that the mean societal (friction) costs were €4,414 to €6,943 [21].

On average, CDP patients are in the middle of their productive life at the age of 40, have growing up children, have to pay off mortgage and plan ahead for the studies of their children. Patients suffering low back pain tend to return to work within 6 weeks to 3 months after the acute phase of the condition [38]. However, this does not always mean that the back pain suffering has stopped [3], and most CDP patients remain searching for an effective pain treatment. Our study shows that patients reported CLBP duration for a mean of 10.6 (1 to 40) years and pain treatment of on average six years. Despite all treatment received, before inclusion into the study assessing efficacy of a new treatment, the mean pain was still high (mean PNRS 6.5 (11box)) [24].

Although many healthcare resources are used (and much money is spent each year), the patients included in this trial at baseline still suffer pain and experience loss in quality of life. Innovations and further development of effective treatments are essential to better manage CDP and diminish associated patient burden and societal costs in the future.

5. Conclusion

Society spends €7,911.95 (friction costs approach) or €18,940.58 (human capital approach) each year per CDP patient. Societal costs are for a large part caused by work absence. In patients with CDP, healthcare resources are mostly used for pain therapies. Despite these efforts, baseline patients for this study suffer severe pain, are physically limited, and experience serious loss of quality of life.

Acknowledgments

The original RCT used for the present study was funded by "The Netherlands Organization for Health Research and Development" (ZonMw) (Project number 836011026_JG_CD_JG). This study sponsor has no role in, and no authority over, data collection, management, analyses, interpretation of data, writing the report, and the decision to submit the report for publication.

References

[1] T. Vos, A. D. Flaxman, M. Naghavi et al., "Years lived with disability (YLDs) for 1160 sequelae of 289 diseases and injuries 1990-2010: a systematic analysis for the Global Burden of Disease Study 2010," *The Lancet*, vol. 380, no. 9859, pp. 2163–2196, 2012.

[2] G. B. J. Andersson, "Epidemiological features of chronic low-back pain," *The Lancet*, vol. 354, no. 9178, pp. 581–585, 1999.

[3] C. J. Itz, J. W. Geurts, M. van Kleef et al., "Clinical course of non-specific low back pain: a systematic review of prospective cohort studies set in primary care," *European Journal of Pain*, vol. 17, no. 1, pp. 5–15, 2013.

[4] T. Vos, R. M. Barber, B. Bell et al., "Global, regional, and national incidence, prevalence, and years lived with disability for 301 acute and chronic diseases and injuries in 188 countries, 1990–2013: a systematic analysis for the Global Burden of Disease Study 2013," *The Lancet*, vol. 386, no. 9995, pp. 743–800, 2015.

[5] N. Maniadakis and A. Gray, "The economic burden of back pain in the UK," *Pain*, vol. 84, no. 1, pp. 95–103, 2000.

[6] S. Dagenais, J. Caro, and S. Haldeman, "A systematic review of low back pain cost of illness studies in the United States and internationally," *The Spine Journal*, vol. 8, no. 1, pp. 8–20, 2008.

[7] L. C. Lambeek, M. W. Van Tulder, I. C. Swinkels et al., "The trend in total cost of back pain in The Netherlands in the period 2002 to 2007," *Spine*, vol. 36, no. 13, pp. 1050–1058, 2011.

[8] C. J. Itz, B. L. Ramaekers, M. van Kleef et al., "Medical specialists care and hospital costs for low back pain in the Netherlands," *European Journal of Pain*, vol. 21, no. 4, pp. 705–715, 2017.

[9] H. Liedgens, M. Obradovic, J. De Courcy et al., "A burden of illness study for neuropathic pain in Europe," *ClinicoEconomics and Outcomes Research*, vol. 8, pp. 113–126, 2016.

[10] S. S. Tan, C. A. Bouwmans, F. F. Rutten et al., "Update of the Dutch manual for costing in economic evaluations," *International Journal of Technology Assessment in Health Care*, vol. 28, no. 2, pp. 152–158, 2012.

[11] R. C. Hutubessy, M. W. van Tulder, H. Vondeling et al., "Indirect costs of back pain in the Netherlands: a comparison of the human capital method with the friction cost method," *Pain*, vol. 80, no. 1, pp. 201–207, 1999.

[12] S. D. Kuslich, C. L. Ulstrom, and C. J. Michael, "The tissue origin of low back pain and sciatica: a report of pain response to tissue stimulation during operations on the lumbar spine using local anesthesia," *Orthopedic Clinics of North America*, vol. 22, no. 2, pp. 181–187, 1991.

[13] A. C. Schwarzer, C. N. Aprill, R. Derby et al., "The prevalence and clinical features of internal disc disruption in patients with chronic low back pain," *Spine*, vol. 20, no. 17, pp. 1878–1883, 1995.

[14] M. J. DePalma, J. M. Ketchum, and T. Saullo, "What is the source of chronic low back pain and does age play a role?," *Pain Medicine*, vol. 12, no. 2, pp. 224–233, 2011.

[15] R. D. Guyer, D. D. Ohnmeiss, and A. Vaccaro, "Lumbar discography," *The Spine Journal*, vol. 3, no. 3, pp. 11–27, 2003.

[16] C. D. Collins, J. P. Stack, D. J. O'Connell et al., "The role of discography in lumbar disc disease: a comparative study of magnetic resonance imaging and discography," *Clinical Radiology*, vol. 42, no. 4, pp. 252–257, 1990.

[17] N. Bogduk, C. Aprill, and R. Derby, "Lumbar discogenic pain: state-of-the-art review," *Pain Medicine*, vol. 14, no. 6, pp. 813–836, 2013.

[18] J. Cid, J. L. De La Calle, E. Lopez et al., "A modified delphi survey on the signs and symptoms of low back pain: indicators for an interventional management approach," *Pain Practice*, vol. 15, no. 1, pp. 12–21, 2013.

[19] Y. Zhou and S. Abdi, "Diagnosis and minimally invasive treatment of lumbar discogenic pain—a review of the literature," *Clinical Journal of Pain*, vol. 22, no. 5, pp. 468–481, 2006.

[20] E. Jonsson, G. Olafsson, P. Fritzell et al., "Profile of low back pain: treatment and costs associated with patients referred to orthopaedic specialists in Sweden," *Spine*, vol. 42, no. 17, pp. 1302–1310, 2017.

[21] A. Spijker-Huiges, K. Vermeulen, J. C. Winters et al., "Costs and cost-effectiveness of epidural steroids for acute lumbosacral radicular syndrome in general practice: an economic evaluation alongside a pragmatic randomized control trial," *Spine*, vol. 39, no. 24, pp. 2007–2012, 2014.

[22] S. Byford, D. J. Torgerson, and J. Raftery, "Economic note: cost of illness studies," *BMJ*, vol. 320, no. 7245, p. 1335, 2000.

[23] M. W. van Tulder, B. W. Koes, and L. M. Bouter, "A cost-of-illness study of back pain in the Netherlands," *Pain*, vol. 62, no. 2, pp. 233–240, 1995.

[24] J. W. Geurts, J. W. Kallewaard, A. Kessels et al., "Efficacy and cost-effectiveness of intradiscal methylene blue injection for chronic discogenic low back pain: study protocol for a randomized controlled trial," *Trials*, vol. 16, no. 1, p. 532, 2015.

[25] B. L. Sachs, H. Vanharanta, M. A. Spivey et al., "Dallas discogram description. A new classification of CT/discography in low-back disorders," *Spine*, vol. 12, no. 3, pp. 287–294, 1987.

[26] R. H. Dworkin, D. C. Turk, J. T. Farrar et al., "Core outcome measures for chronic pain clinical trials: IMMPACT recommendations," *Pain*, vol. 113, no. 1, pp. 9–19, 2005.

[27] J. C. Fairbank and P. B. Pynsent, "The oswestry disability index," *Spine*, vol. 25, no. 22, pp. 2940–2952, 2000.

[28] P. Kind, *The EuroQoL Instrument: An Index of Health-Related Quality of Life*, Lippincott-Raven Publishers, Philadelphia, PA, USA, 1996.

[29] N. K. Aaronson, M. Muller, P. D. Cohen et al., "Translation, validation, and norming of the Dutch language version of the SF-36 Health Survey in community and chronic disease populations," *Journal of Clinical Epidemiology*, vol. 51, no. 11, pp. 1055–1068, 1998.

[30] K. I. Vander Zee, R. Sanderman, J. W. Heyink et al., "Psychometric qualities of the rand 36-item health survey 1.0: a multidimensional measure of general health status,"

International Journal of Behavioral Medicine, vol. 3, no. 2, pp. 104–122, 1996.

[31] P. Dolan, "Modeling valuations for EuroQol health states," *Medical Care*, vol. 35, no. 11, pp. 1095–1108, 1997.

[32] L. M. Lamers, J. McDonnell, P. F. Stalmeier et al., "The Dutch tariff: results and arguments for an effective design for national EQ-5D valuation studies," *Health Economics*, vol. 15, no. 10, pp. 1121–1132, 2006.

[33] M. E. Goossens, M. P. Rutten-van Molken, J. W. Vlaeyen et al., "The cost diary: a method to measure direct and indirect costs in cost-effectiveness research," *Journal of Clinical Epidemiology*, vol. 53, no. 7, pp. 688–695, 2000.

[34] M. A. Koopmanschap, "PRODISQ: a modular questionnaire on productivity and disease for economic evaluation studies," *Expert Review of Pharmacoeconomics & Outcomes Research*, vol. 5, no. 1, pp. 23–28, 2005.

[35] N. Zorginstituut, *Manual for Cost Research. Methods and Standard Cost Prices for Economic Evaluations in Health Care*, in Dutch, Zorginstituut Nederland, Diemen, 2015.

[36] M. A. Koopmanschap, F. F. Rutten, B. M. van Ineveld et al., "The friction cost method for measuring indirect costs of disease," *Journal of Health Economics*, vol. 14, no. 2, pp. 171–189, 1995.

[37] S. Dagenais, D. M. Roffey, E. K. Wai et al., "Can cost utility evaluations inform decision making about interventions for low back pain?," *The Spine Journal*, vol. 9, no. 11, pp. 944–957, 2009.

[38] J. Bowey-Morris, S. Davis, G. Purcell-Jones et al., "Beliefs about back pain: results of a population survey of working age adults," *Clinical Journal of Pain*, vol. 27, no. 3, pp. 214–224, 2011.

[39] P. Dolan, D. Torgerson, and T. K. Kakarlapudi, "Health-related quality of life of Colles' fracture patients," *Osteoporosis International*, vol. 9, no. 3, pp. 196–199, 1999.

[40] H. Breivik, B. Collett, V. Ventafridda et al., "Survey of chronic pain in Europe: prevalence, impact on daily life, and treatment," *European Journal of Pain*, vol. 10, no. 4, pp. 287–333, 2006.

[41] A. D. van Asselt, C. D. Dirksen, A. Arntz et al., "Difficulties in calculating productivity costs: work disability associated with borderline personality disorder," *Value in Health*, vol. 11, no. 4, pp. 637–644, 2008.

[42] H. S. Picavet and N. Hoeymans, "Health related quality of life in multiple musculoskeletal diseases: SF-36 and EQ-5D in the DMC3 study," *Annals of the Rheumatic Diseases*, vol. 63, no. 6, pp. 723–729, 2004.

[43] R. Rabin and F. de Charro, "EQ-5D: a measure of health status from the EuroQol Group," *Annals of Medicine*, vol. 33, no. 5, pp. 337–343, 2001.

[44] C. Sapin, B. Fantino, M. L. Nowicki et al., "Usefulness of EQ-5D in assessing health status in primary care patients with major depressive disorder," *Health and Quality of Life Outcomes*, vol. 2, no. 1, p. 20, 2004.

[45] H. Suzuki, T. Kanchiku, Y. Imajo et al., "Diagnosis and characters of non-specific low back pain in Japan: the Yamaguchi low back pain study," *PLoS One*, vol. 11, no. 8, Article ID e0160454, 2016.

[46] B. Gannon, D. P. Finn, D. O'Gorman et al., "The cost of chronic pain: an analysis of a regional pain management service in Ireland," *Pain Medicine*, vol. 14, no. 10, pp. 1518–1528, 2013.

Association of Depression/Anxiety Symptoms with Neck Pain: A Systematic Review and Meta-Analysis of Literature in China

Fushui Liu[1] **Ting Fang**[1] **Fanyuan Zhou,**[1] **Meimei Zhao**[1] **Mei Chen**[1] **Jianyu You,**[1] **Yuli Jin,**[1] **Jinmei Xie,**[1] **and Zhongyong Liu**[2]

[1]*School of Moxibustion, Jiangxi University of Traditional Chinese Medicine, Nanchang, China*
[2]*College of Clinical Medicine, Jiangxi University of Traditional Chinese Medicine, Nanchang, China*

Correspondence should be addressed to Zhongyong Liu; lzyongmail@163.com

Academic Editor: Panagiotis Zis

Background. Due to its high morbidity and prevalence, the potential relationships of depression/anxiety symptoms in neck pain (NP) are not well demonstrated. *Objectives.* This study aimed to conduct a comprehensive estimation of controlled trials of psychological problems and to test hypotheses concerning whether NP was statistically relative to anxiety/depression symptoms. *Methods.* Chinese literature databases such as the China National Knowledge Infrastructure (CNKI), VIP Information (VIP), Chinese Biomedicine (CBM), and Wanfang Data (WANFANG) were scientifically searched for reports published until February 5, 2018. Controlled trials incorporating NP patients with anxiety/depression versus healthy people were contained. Two researchers screened each article and extracted data, respectively, and blinded to the findings of each other. Meta-analysis was conducted by the Cochrane Collaboration's RevMan 5.3 and Stata 14.0 (Stata Corp LP, USA) software. *Results.* We identified 13 eligible studies involving 2339 patients and 3290 healthy people. Compared with healthy control participants, the findings indicated that depression/anxiety symptoms were more common or severe in NP patients (respectively, SMD = 0.89; 95% CI = (0.58, 1.20); $P < 0.01$ and SMD = 0.92; 95% CI = (0.65, 1.20); and $P < 0.01$), results from the pooled data demonstrated no statistical significance between depression/anxiety symptoms and gender in NP patients (resp., SMD = 0.16; 95% CI = (−0.18, 0.51); $P = 0.35$ and SMD = −0.08; 95% CI = (−0.42, 0.27); and $P = 0.67$), and the combined data of the incidence of depression or anxiety symptoms revealed significant difference between NP patients and healthy persons (resp., RR = 4.81; 95% CI = (3.30, 7.01); $P < 0.01$ and RR = 3.29; 95% CI = (2.16, 5.00); and $P < 0.01$). In addition, we did not find articles that met the inclusion criteria, which compared NP patients with other physical illnesses in terms of anxiety/depression symptoms. *Conclusions.* This meta-analysis suggests that anxiety/depression symptoms are associated with high morbidity in NP patients. We consider these reports support the viewpoint that nonspecific mechanisms mediate mental disturbances in NP. This study may have clinical value for NP, offering an underlying target for the prevention and treatment of anxiety/depression.

1. Introduction

Neck pain (NP) has become a common public health problem all over the world, with a high rate of disability, presents a negative impact on the health and quality of life in people, and exerts great pressure on individuals, families, health systems, and social economy [1–3]. Reportedly, NP was ranked the fourth leading cause of disability next to ischemic heart disease, cerebrovascular disease, and lower respiratory infection, with an annual prevalence rate exceeding 30% [4, 5]. In 2005, over a third of a billion had experienced neck pain more than 3 months of duration [4, 5]. Preliminary statistics showed that the incidence of NP in China ranged between 3.8% and 17.6%, and it affected nearly 15% of the global population [6, 7]. NP has obvious financial problems and the annual economic losses caused by NP are as high as $5 billion in America, while it can reach $800 million just for the treatment cost per year in China [6]. The prevention and treatment of NP has attracted the wide attention of people from all walks of life and has important practical significance for the study of NP.

The clinical symptoms of NP are complicated, which mainly include neck, shoulder and back pain, stiffness and weakness of upper limbs, numbness of fingers, dizziness, nausea, vomiting, and even blurred vision [8]. According to its clinical symptoms, it is divided into three syndromes, namely, cervical radiculopathy, cervical myelopathy, and axial neck pain [9]. By contrast, it contains seven types in China, including neck type, nerve root type, vertebral artery type, sympathetic type, spinal cord type, mixed type, and other type (mainly include esophageal compression type) [10]. The clinical diagnosis of NP is established on the basis of the identification of positive symptoms via diagnostic criteria and the exclusion of organic illness, for instance, unexplained dizziness and numbness [10]. Treatment for NP mainly depends on lifestyle intervention, medications, and physical therapies [11].

Research has found that mental health disorders are always connected with physical illness [12, 13] and is also more common in developing than developed countries [14]. What is particularly exciting here is the abundant description of depression/anxiety symptoms in NP. However, scholars differ in opinions on the nature of their relationships [15, 16]. In short, at present, it exists two opposing schools of thought: one considers that NP may be tied closely to depression/anxiety through some pathogenesis and the other considers the associations between NP and mental disorders as nonspecific or chance events.

Despite plentiful descriptions have been reported about mental disturbs in NP patients, no systematic evaluation of the relationship between NP and depression/anxiety symptoms has been found. This article is to systematically review prospective cohort or case-control studies and investigate the association between NP and anxiety/depression symptoms. We completed the quality assessment of included studies to analyze any inconsistencies in data. The research questions are (1) whether depression/anxiety symptoms are more common or serious in NP patients than in healthy people or patients with other medical diseases? and (2) does depression/anxiety symptoms differ from gender in NP patients?

2. Methods

2.1. Search Strategy. According to Cochrane Reviews' Handbook, we developed a study protocol for this systematic review and meta-analysis [17]. Electronic searches were systematically performed in CNKI, VIP, CBM, and WANFANG databases up to February 5, 2018, by two authors (Ting Fang and Mei Chen). Medical subject headings (MeSH) terms relevant to neck pain, anxiety, and depression was utilized in the search, and the same terms in Chinese databases. Then, we browsed the abstracts and full-text articles, respectively, and picked the eligible studies in line with the inclusion criteria. Additionally, we also manually searched the relevant lists of all eligible studies to identify further potential studies and contacted reference authors for additional data if necessary.

2.2. Criteria for Selecting Articles. Inclusion criteria include (1) prospective cohort or case-control studies that concerned anxiety/depression symptoms measured at baseline and their relationship with neck pain; (2) population-based studies that have compared a group of persons with neck pain with another group of either healthy persons or persons with other medical illness; (3) studies that evaluated depression and anxiety symptoms via validated psychometric testings or a structured clinical interview; (4) people diagnosed with neck pain utilizing a certain diagnostic criterion and patients' gender, age, the source of the case, and duration of illness were not limited; and (5) studies must have provided reasonable data for estimating effect size and confidence intervals.

Exclusion criteria include duplicate studies, animal experiments, no clear diagnostic criteria for NP, the measures of anxiety/depression symptoms were not standardized, studies that included treatment measures; and studies that only included NP patients as a subgroup of a large sample and not compared, respectively, from the other participants.

2.3. Data Extraction. Data were independently extracted from the eligible studies by two authors (Ting Fang and Mei Chen) and cross checked. Any discrepancies were discussed among Fushui Liu, Meimei Zhao, and Fanyuan Zhou. The key information was collected systematically using a predefined Excel template. It mainly included first author, year of publication, case source, baseline characteristics for participants (age, sex, and number of participants), diagnostic criteria of NP, assessment standards of depression and anxiety symptoms, and outcome assessments. Where possible, we contacted the first author for clarifying the ambiguous information that provided in some studies.

2.4. Quality Assessment. For detecting bias of included studies, the methodological quality was assessed according to a validated rating scale [18], which was used in psychiatric case-control studies. For this meta-analysis, we regulated this scale and researched selection bias of cases (seven items), selection of bias of controls (six items), and information bias (one item). The quality assessments were completed independently by two reviewers (Ting Fang and Mei Chen). Disagreements would be settled by discussing and analyzing between reviewers.

2.5. Data Analysis. We used RevMan 5.3 statistical software (the Nordic Cochrane Centre, Copenhagen; the Cochrane Collaboration, 2014) for meta-analysis. We defined $P \leq 0.05$ as statistically significant between studies. We calculated combined risk ratio (RR) with 95% confidence intervals (CI) for the categorical data; as continuous variables, we estimated combined standard mean difference (SMD) with 95% CI. The studies' heterogeneity was evaluated by the chi-square test and Higgins I^2 test, and when $I^2 \leq 50\%$ and $P \geq 0.10$, the fixed effect model was used or else the random effect model was applied.

2.6. Ethical Statement. All analyses were based on previously published studies, and so ethical approval was superfluous.

3. Results

3.1. Search Results. Totally, 378 potential literature citations were initially obtained through database examinations. We removed 164 duplicates with EndNote software. 78 articles were ruled out through scanning the title and abstracts. And 118 articles were eliminated according to the exclusion and inclusion criteria. In the rest 18 articles, 3 of them did not compare with healthy people or patients with other medical disease, 2 studies failed to have assessment standards of depression and anxiety symptoms, and 13 eligible articles [7, 19–30] were included finally. The whole selection process is shown in Figure 1.

3.2. Basic Characteristics of Eligible Studies. The eligible studies were published between 2002 and 2017 in China, and 2339 patients and 3290 healthy controls were included. In these studies, regarding the source of cases, three studies [7, 22, 24] were multiple-center controlled trials, two studies [19, 26] were ambiguous, and the remaining studies were single-center controlled trials. Also, they were all completed in outpatients and inpatients, except one [29] which was completed in college students. As for the source of cases in control groups, seven groups [7, 19, 20, 25–28] were from domestic normal population, and the others were healthy people.

NP was diagnosed in 4 studies [22, 25, 29, 30] using the diagnostic criteria acknowledged in China, and the others used self-rating criteria which were validated and reliable. As for the diagnostic criteria of depression and anxiety symptoms, all the studies reported validated scale. Seven studies [7, 19–21, 23, 25, 26] utilized the symptom check list-90 (SCL-90), and 1 study [24] used the symptom check list-290 (SCL-290) to assess depression and anxiety symptoms levels; among them, one study [19] also used the state-trait anxiety inventory (STAI). One study [30] utilized generalized anxiety disorder-7 (GAD-7) and patient health questionnaire-9 (PHQ-9) as the evaluation standard, 4 studies [22, 24, 27, 28] utilized self-rating depression scale (SDS), 2 studies [24, 27] used self-rating depression scale (SAS), and the criteria in the last one [29] were unclear. Table 1 shows the key characteristics of the included studies: study design, sample sizes, design, mean ages, diagnosis criteria for NP, and scales utilized for assessments of the levels of anxiety and depression.

3.3. Quality Assessment. Table 2 reports the methodological quality of the included studies. The clinical setting used for recruitment was frequently reported eligible information, so were the inclusion/exclusion criteria for cases. As for controls, one item concerning the using of students or employees of the research institution was always rated as "no," indicating good methodological practice. Few studies provided sufficient information about the using of advertising for recruitment. The rest questionnaire items for cases and controls were poorly described. Approximately half studies could not offer enough information on whether the investigators were "masked" or not.

3.4. Depression/Anxiety Symptoms Levels in NP Patients: Continuous. Depression and anxiety scores were, respectively, achieved in 13 and 10 studies that included SCL score and other depression rating scores. Data extracted from both reported significantly heterogeneity in the consistency of study results (respectively, $I^2 = 97\%$, $P < 0.01$, and $I^2 = 94\%$, $P < 0.01$), and the random effects model was applied. Overall, the depression and anxiety symptoms' scores were distinctly higher in NP patients compared to healthy control groups (resp., SMD = 0.89; 95% CI = (0.58, 1.20); $P < 0.01$ and SMD = 0.92; 95% CI = (0.65, 1.20); $P < 0.01$) (Figures 2 and 3).

3.5. Relationship between Anxiety/Depression Symptoms and Gender in NP Patients: Continuous. Only 2 studies [25, 30] reported the relationship between depression/anxiety scores and gender in NP patients. No heterogeneity exist in this analysis, and the fixed effects model was used. The overall results demonstrated no significant difference (resp., SMD = 0.16; 95% CI = (−0.18, 0.51); $P = 0.35$ and SMD = −0.08; 95% CI = (−0.42, 0.27); $P = 0.67$) (Figure 4).

3.6. The Incidence of Depression/Anxiety Symptoms in NP Patients: Categorical. 5 studies [22, 24, 27, 28, 30] provided categorical data for depression and anxiety, but only 2 of them [22, 24] presented categorical data in detail. The combined data revealed significant difference between NP patients and healthy persons, indicated that depression and anxiety were closely linked to NP patients (resp., RR = 4.81; 95% CI = (3.30, 7.01); $P < 0.01$ and RR = 3.29; 95% CI = (2.16, 5.00); $P < 0.01$) (Figure 5).

3.7. Sensitivity Analysis for Continuous Data. We completed the same meta-analysis for depression symptoms level in NP patients excluding 6 studies [22, 24, 27–30] whose psychiatric diagnostics were distinctly different from the remaining studies. The level of depression symptoms of NP patients was still higher than healthy control groups (SMD = 0.52; 95% CI = (0.45, 0.58); $P < 0.01$). More importantly, the I^2 showed no heterogeneity between studies (I2 = 0%, $P = 0.59$). We also conducted the same meta-analysis for anxiety level in NP patients excluding 3 studies [24, 27, 30], as the psychiatric diagnostics were different from the remaining studies. The I^2 drops from 95 to 44%, $P = 0.10$, and the level of anxiety remained practically stable (SMD = 0.73; 95% CI = (0.62, 0.84); $P < 0.01$). Totally, our different sensitivity analyses presented similar findings and indicated that the different psychiatric diagnostic criteria resulted high risk for the results.

4. Discussion

In this study, we identified 13 eligible studies involving 2339 patients and 3290 healthy people that intended to evaluate possible links between NP and mental disorders. According to our findings, compared to healthy control groups, the depression and anxiety symptoms scores were distinctly

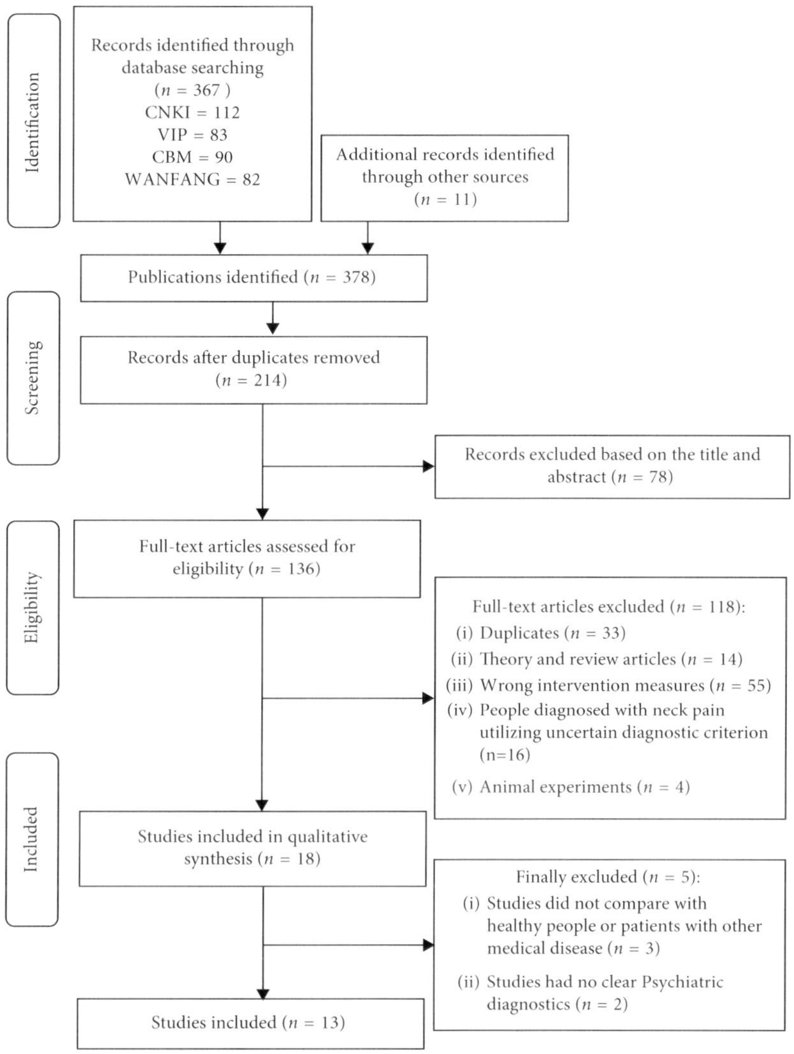

Figure 1: Flow diagram outlining the selection of studies for the review.

higher in NP patients. However, there was no significant difference between depression/anxiety symptoms and gender in NP patients. And we failed to obtain case reports to confirm whether NP patients differ from other chronic diseases in terms of anxiety and depression symptoms. But we found articles from PubMed which testified significant difference between NP patients and other chronic physical illnesses in terms of anxiety and depression symptoms [31, 32], and this conclusion deserved further exploration in future. Also, this study suggested that the morbidity of depression and anxiety symptoms was higher in NP patients. Wen and Liu [28] reported that the morbidity of depression symptoms in 336 cases of NP patients was 36.31%, Huang et al. [27] found that incidence of anxiety and depression symptoms in 38 NP patients was 60.53% and 92.11%, respectively, while it was 77% and 84%, respectively, in Sun's survey of 100 NP patients [30].

Neck pain is a common and frequently occurring disease with complicated clinical etiology, which is mainly related to people's bad living habits, such as long-term head bending posture. It is easy to relapse and lasts for a long time [33]. Long-term chronic pain has a profound impact on patients' mental health, and they are prone to negative emotions such as anxiety and depression, which seriously affect patients' quality of life. Reportedly, the longer the chronic pain lasts, the more severe it becomes and the more anxious or depressive it becomes [34]. Meanwhile, anxiety and depression can also promote psychological responses to chronic pain [34].

Some authors investigated the effects of depression and anxiety symptoms in NP patients and found NP and poor quality of life were two factors leading to depression and anxiety [35]. Instead, Galbusera and Gorter reported depression and anxiety symptoms were two major factors affecting the quality of life in patients with musculoskeletal pain [36, 37]. Relatively, few were currently known about causal mechanisms for depression and anxiety symptoms in NP patients. Different mechanisms perhaps could explain the relationship between pain and anxiety from different aspects of biology, psychology, and sociology [38]. Functional imaging studies showed the affective processing area of brain in patients with anxiety and depression symptoms

Table 1: Summary of studies included in the meta-analyses on anxiety and depression in NP.

Study	Sample sizes	Design	Group comparison	Mean age	NP diagnostics	Psychiatric diagnostics
He et al. [19]	58 vs. 1 388	Case-control	NP vs. Np	49.5	Self-rating	SCL-90/STAI
Wang et al. [20]	52 vs. 1 338	Case-control	NP vs. Np	48.25 ± 13.36	Self-rating	SCL-90
Lou et al. [21]	60 vs. 56	Case-control	NP vs. HC	54.31 ± 8.18	Self-rating	SCL-90
Chen et al. [22]	106 vs. 76	Case-control	NP vs. HC	51 ± 8 vs. 48 ± 7	Chinese acknowledged diagnostic criteria	SDS
Fang et al. [23]	89 vs. 60	Case-control	NP vs. HC	49.3 vs. 47.6	Self-rating	SCL-90
Yao et al. [24]	122 vs. 122	Case-control	NP vs. HC	58.86 ± 8.28 vs. 59.36 ± 7.04	Self-rating	SCL-290/SDS/SAS
Zhang et al. [25]	30 vs. 1 338	Case-control	NP vs. Np	52	Chinese acknowledged diagnostic criteria	SCL-90
Wei et al. [26]	217 vs. 1 338	Case-control	NP vs. Np	38.00 ± 5.67	Self-rating	SCL-90
Huang et al. [27]	38 vs. 1 340	Case-control	NP vs. Np	/	Self-rating	SDS/SAS
Wen and Liu [28]	336 vs. 1 340	Case-control	NP vs. Np	/	Self-rating	SDS
Wang et al. [29]	105 vs. 198	Prospective cohort	NP vs. HC	/	Chinese acknowledged diagnostic criteria	Self-rating
Chen et al. [7]	1 026 vs. 1 338	Case-control	NP vs. Np	/	Self-rating	SCL-90
Sun et al. [30]	100 vs. 100	Case-control	NP vs. HC	45.98 ± 8.54 vs. 45.86 ± 8.43	Chinese acknowledged diagnostic criteria	GAD-7/PHQ-9

NP, neck pain; HC, healthy controls; Np, normal population; SCL, symptom check list; STAI, state-trait anxiety inventory; SDS, self-rating depression scale; SAS, self-rating anxiety scale; GAD-7, generalized anxiety disorder-7; and PHQ-9, patient health questionnaire-9.

Table 2: Methodological quality of the case-control studies ($N = 12$).

Question	Answer		
	Yes *N*	No *N*	Unclear *N*
Cases			
Was the clinical setting used for recruitment made clear?	10	1	1
Was the denominator from which cases were recruited described?	8	1	3
Was duration of illness adequately described?	4	8	0
Was adequate information given on the total number of patients approached?	3	9	0
Was information given on participants and nonparticipants?	2	10	0
Was information given on the differences between participants and refusers?	0	12	0
Were the inclusion and exclusion criteria described well enough to be replicable?	10	2	0
Controls			
Did the study use controls who were students/employees of the research institution?*	0	11	1
Were controls selected from an explicit sampling frame?	9	2	1
Did the study recruit through advertisements?*	0	11	1
Were similar exclusion criteria applied for controls as for cases?	4	0	8
Was information given on number of controls approached?	6	6	0
Was adequate information given on differences between controls refusing and agreeing?	0	12	0
Information bias			
Were the investigators who rated the exposure masked to participants' status?	9	3	0

*"no" is the answer indicative of good methodological practice.

Study or subgroup	Experimental Mean	Experimental SD	Experimental Total	Control Mean	Control SD	Control Total	Weight (%)	Std.mean difference IV, random, 95% CI
Chen et al. [22]	48.69	13.2	106	32.76	8.6	76	7.5	1.38 (1.05, 1.71)
Chen et al. [7]	1.81	0.67	1026	1.5	0.59	1338	8.1	0.50 (0.41, 0.58)
Fang et al. [23]	0.54	0.11	89	0.48	0.05	60	7.5	0.66 (0.32, 0.99)
He et al. [19]	1.86	0.64	58	1.5	0.59	1338	7.7	0.61 (0.34, 0.87)
Huang et al. [27]	52.76	8.33	38	33.46	8.55	1340	7.5	2.26 (1.92, 2.59)
Lou et al. [21]	1.85	0.67	60	1.48	0.62	56	7.3	0.57 (0.20, 0.94)
Sun et al. [30]	10.62	5.9	100	9.23	2.1	100	7.7	0.31 (0.03, 0.59)
Wang et al. [20]	1.8	0.92	52	1.5	0.59	1338	7.7	0.50 (0.22, 0.77)
Wang et al. [29	0.64	0.21	105	0.36	0.18	198	7.7	1.46 (1.20, 1.73)
Wei et al. [26]	1.83	0.49	217	1.5	0.59	1338	8.0	0.57 (0.43, 0.72)
Wen and Liu [28]	48.73	12.3	336	33.46	8.55	1340	8.1	1.62 (1.49, 1.75)
Wang et al. [24]	43.46	12.74	122	33.78	8.33	122	7.7	0.90 (0.63, 1.16)
Zhang et al. [25]	1.63	0.53	30	1.5	0.59	1338	7.4	0.22 (−0.14, 0.58)
Total (95% CI)			2339			9982	100.0	0.89 (0.58, 1.20)

Heterogeneity: $\tau^2 = 0.31$, $\chi^2 = 351.81$, $df = 12$ ($P < 0.00001$); $I^2 = 97\%$

Test for overall effect: $Z = 5.57$ ($P < 0.00001$)

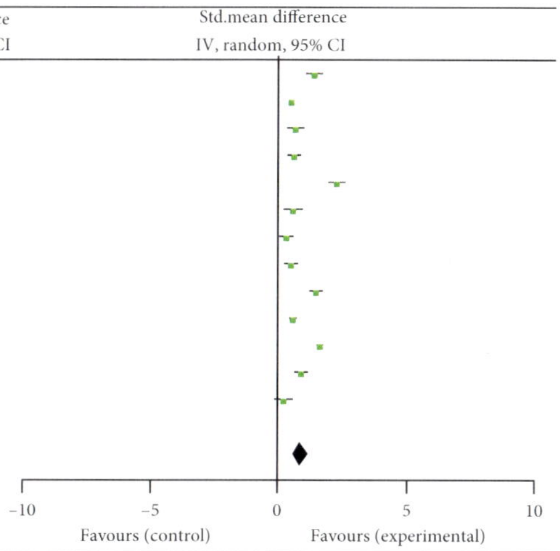

FIGURE 2: Meta-analysis of 13 studies about depression in NP.

Study or subgroup	Experimental Mean	Experimental SD	Experimental Total	Control Mean	Control SD	Control Total	Weight (%)	Std.mean difference IV, random, 95% CI
Chen et al. [7]	1.76	0.58	1026	1.39	0.43	1338	11.1	0.74 (0.65, 0.82)
Fang et al. [23]	0.48	0.12	89	0.42	0.09	60	9.6	0.55 (0.21, 0.88)
He et al. [19]	1.8	0.68	58	1.39	0.43	1338	10.1	2.60 (2.26, 2.94)
Huang et al. [27]	51.76	8.15	38	29.78	8.46	1340	9.6	0.93 (0.66, 1.19)
Lou et al. [21]	1.98	0.45	60	1.46	0.48	56	9.1	1.11 (0.72, 1.50)
Sun et al. [30]	9.71	5.93	100	7.89	4.01	100	10.0	0.36 (0.08, 0.64)
Wang et al. [20]	1.73	0.83	52	1.39	0.43	1338	10.0	0.75 (0.47, 1.03)
Wei et al. [26]	1.65	0.51	217	1.39	0.43	1338	10.9	0.59 (0.44, 0.73)
Wang et al. [24]	42.24	10.38	122	32.26	8.36	122	10.1	1.06 (0.79, 1.32)
Zhang et al. [25]	1.67	0.59	30	1.39	0.43	1338	9.4	0.64 (0.28, 1.01)
Total (95% CI)			1792			8368	100.0	0.92 (0.65,1.20)

Heterogeneity: $\tau^2 = 0.18$, $\chi^2 = 138.92$, $df = 9$ ($P < 0.00001$); $I^2 = 94\%$

Test for overall effect: $Z = 6.54$ ($P < 0.00001$)

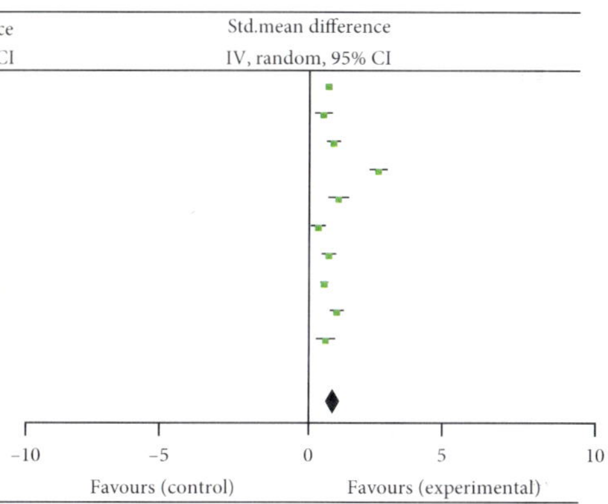

FIGURE 3: Meta-analysis of 10 studies about anxiety in NP patients.

Study or subgroup	Male Mean	Male SD	Male Total	Female Mean	Female SD	Female Total	Weight (%)	Std.mean difference IV, fixed, 95% CI
Relationship between depression and gender in NP patients.								
Sun et al. [30]	10.29	5.75	16	10.89	6.06	14	23.3	−0.10 (−0.82, 0.62)
Zhang et al. [25]	1.53	0.44	45	1.42	0.45	55	76.7	0.24 (−0.15, 0.64)
Subtotal (95% CI)			61			69	100.0	0.16 (−0.18, 0.51)
Heterogeneity: $\chi^2 = 0.68$, $df = 1$ ($P = 0.41$); $I^2 = 0\%$								
Test for overall effect: $Z = 0.93$ ($P = 0.35$)								
Relationship between anxiety and gender in NP patients.								
Sun 2017	9.07	5.91	16	10.24	5.96	14	23.1	−0.19 (−0.91, 0.53)
Zhang 2010	1.54	0.49	45	1.56	0.48	55	76.9	−0.04 (−0.43, 0.35)
Subtotal (95% CI)			61			69	100.0	−0.08 (−0.42, 0.27)
Heterogeneity: $\chi^2 = 0.13$, $df = 1$ ($P = 0.72$); $I^2 = 0\%$								
Test for overall effect: $Z = 0.43$ ($P = 0.67$)								

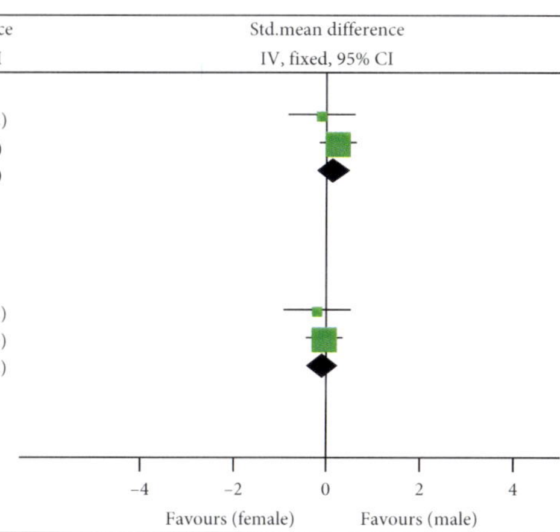

FIGURE 4: Relationship between depression/anxiety and gender in NP patients.

that changed from the insula topology to the prefrontal area of weight-bearing pain management [35]. Besides, it was also found patients with depression and anxiety symptoms had dysfunction of autonomic nervous function and inflammation and activity hyperactivity of the hypothalamic-pituitary-adrenal (HPA) axis [38–41]. Interestingly, when neurotransmitters such as norepinephrine (NE) and 5-hydroxytryptamine (5-HT) decrease, the inhibitory mechanism of pain can be impeded and the development of affective disorders can be promoted [42]. Additionally, studies found an increase in systemic inflammatory markers in the blood of patients with pain disorders and affective

Study or subgroup	Experimental		Control		Weight (%)	Risk Ratio
	Events	Total	Events	Total		M-H, random, 95% CI
The incidence of depression in NP patients.						
Chen et al. [22]	35	106	6	76	21.3	4.18 (1.85, 9.44)
Wang et al. [24]	95	122	19	122	78.7	5.00 (3.27, 7.64)
Subtotal (95% CI)		228		198	100.0	4.81 (3.30, 7.01)
Total events	130		25			
Heterogeneity: $\tau^2 = 0.00$; $\chi^2 = 0.15$, $df = 1$ ($P = 0.70$); $I^2 = 0\%$						
Test for overall effect: $Z = 8.19$ ($P < 0.00001$)						
The incidence of anxiety in NP patients.						
Wang et al. [24]	69	122	21	122	100.0	3.29 (2.16, 5.00)
Subtotal (95% CI)		122		122	100.0	3.29 (2.16, 5.00)
Total events	69		21			
Heterogeneity: Not applicable						
Test for overall effect: $Z = 5.56$ ($P < 0.00001$)						

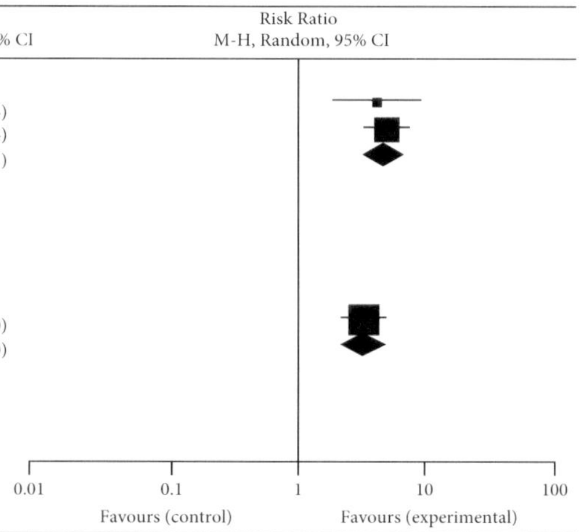

FIGURE 5: The incidence of depression/anxiety in NP patients.

disturbances, which suggests that there is the same basic pathogenetic pathway between the two diseases [43–45]. Similarly, consideration from the view of psychological sociology, pain, and mental disorders are also closely related. Many studies point out that psychological stress and potential obstacles caused by pain can possibly cause immunological changes that eventually results in depression and anxiety [40, 45–47]. In addition, a study had shown that both depression and pain might be risk factors for each other [48].

Anyhow, we should notice potential restrictions of this article. It included first that although we assessed the methodological quality of the included studies via a rating scale [18] for case-control studies, we cannot declare that the rating scale is valid even if the score presented high credibility. Second, few studies provided categorical data, despite 5 studies [22, 24, 27, 28, 30] had involved it, and none of them provided complete data except 2 [22, 24]. The incomplete data may not draw definite conclusion. Furthermore, there were no uniform inclusion and exclusion criteria, which may be a source of heterogeneity.

Despite these limitations, there are still many advantages in our study. In order to improve the accountability of the systematic procedure of this systematic review, we had taken several steps. Two reviewers (Ting Fang and Mei Chen) conducted the electronic searches and picked the suitable studies after browsing the abstracts and full-text articles, respectively, according to the inclusion criteria. Data extraction was also completed, respectively, by two authors. And the methodological quality of the included studies was still evaluated by two authors, and the results were counted.

5. Conclusions

Overall, NP is characterized as a kind of chronic degenerative disease, which has a series of serious influences on body and psychology and severely reduces the quality of life of patients. Therefore, attention should be cautiously attached to the psychological problems in the treatment of NP patients. And clinicians should give the necessary psychological counseling and psychological treatment, which may help alleviate the mental pain of patients and relieve their physical pain at the same time. Moreover, clinicians who treat pain syndromes should not only improve the patients' correct understanding of disease and treatment but also strengthen patients' confidence to overcome the disease.

Authors' Contributions

All authors made substantial contributions to the conception and design of the work, acquisition, analysis, or interpretation of the data, drafting of the manuscript, and/or critical revision for important intellectual content. All authors approved the final version of the manuscript accepted for publication and agree to be accountable for the integrity of all aspects of the work.

Acknowledgments

This study was supported by grants from the National Natural Science Foundation of China (81560792).

References

[1] M. Vassilaki and E. L. Hurwitz, "Insights in public health: perspectives on pain in the low back and neck: global burden, epidemiology, and management," *Hawaii Journal of Medicine & Public Health*, vol. 73, no. 4, pp. 122–126, 2014.

[2] D. Hoy, L. March, A. Woolf et al., "The global burden of neck pain: estimates from the global burden of disease 2010 study," *Annals of the Rheumatic Diseases*, vol. 73, no. 7, pp. 1309–1315, 2014.

[3] E. L. Hurwitz, L. Dongmei, G. Jenni et al., "Variations in patterns of utilization and charges for the care of neck pain in North Carolina, 2000 to 2009: a statewide claims' data analysis," *Journal of Manipulative and Physiological Therapeutics*, vol. 39, no. 4, pp. 240–251, 2016.

[4] E. L. Hurwitz, K. Randhawa, H. Yu, P. Côté, and S. Haldeman, "The Global Spine Care Initiative: a summary of the global

burden of low back and neck pain studies," *European Spine Journal*, 2018.

[5] Disease and Injury Incidence and Prevalence Collaborators, "Global, regional, and national incidence, prevalence, and years lived with disability for 310 diseases and injuries, 1990–2015: a systematic analysis for the Global Burden of Disease Study 2015," *The Lancet*, vol. 388, no. 10053, pp. 1545–1602, 2016.

[6] S. Kang, *A Full Strategy for the Rescue of Cervical Spondylosis*, Jilin Science and Technology Press, Changchun, China, 2008.

[7] X. Chen, C. L. Ma, and Y. R. Xue, "Study on preoperative mental health level of patients with cervical spondylosis," *Journal of Qilu Nursing*, vol. 23, no. 6, pp. 48–50, 2017.

[8] M. Su, "Basic research and progress in acupuncture and moxibustion treatment of neck type cervical spondylosis," *Guide of China Medicine*, vol. 14, no. 23, pp. 34–36, 2016.

[9] M. D. Connell and S. W. Wiesel, "Natural history and pathogenesis of cervical disk disease," *Orthopedic Clinics of North America*, vol. 23, no. 3, pp. 369–380, 1992.

[10] L. Lu, "Clinical study on dose-effect of elaborate-moxibustion on neck pain in cervical spondylosis," M. S. thesis, Guangzhou university of Chinese medicine, Guangzhou, China, 2017.

[11] V. S. H. Madhavee, "Western and Chinese medicine approach on treatment of cervical spondylosis," M. S. thesis, Beijing university of Chinese medicine, Beijing, China, 2017.

[12] J. S. Olver and M. J. Hopwood, "Depression and physical illness," *Medical Journal of Australia*, vol. 199, no. 6, pp. S9–12, 2013.

[13] W. Katon, E. H. Lin, and K. Kroenke, "The association of depression and anxiety with medical symptom burden in patients with chronic medical illness," *General Hospital Psychiatry*, vol. 29, no. 2, pp. 147–155, 2007.

[14] A. Tsang, M. Von Korff, S. Lee S et al., "Common chronic pain conditions in developed and developing countries: gender and age differences and comorbidity with depression-anxiety disorders," *Journal of Pain*, vol. 9, no. 10, pp. 883–891, 2008.

[15] Z. Dimitriadis, E. Kapreli, N. Strimpakos et al., "Do psychological states associate with pain and disability in chronic neck pain patients?," *Journal of Back and Musculoskeletal Rehabilitation*, vol. 28, no. 4, pp. 797–802, 2015.

[16] F. Kayhan, İ. A. Gezer, A. Kayhan, S. Kitiş, and M. Gölen, "Mood and anxiety disorders in patients with chronic low back and neck pain caused by disc herniation," *International Journal of Psychiatry in Clinical Practice*, vol. 20, no. 1, pp. 19–23, 2016.

[17] A. Liberati, D. G. Kltman, J. Tetzlaff et al., "The PRISMA statement for reporting systematic reviews and meta-analyses of studies that evaluate health care interventions: explanation and elaboration," *Annals of Internal Medicine*, vol. 151, no. 4, pp. W65–W94, 2009.

[18] L. William, B. Jonathan, F. Tamsin et al., "Bias in psychiatric case-control studies: literature survey," *British Journal of Psychiatry*, vol. 190, pp. 204–209, 2007.

[19] X. He, J. H. Lin, and J. Hong, "Analysis of sleep quality and mental health status of patients with cervical spondylosis," *Chinese Journal of Clinical Rehabilitation*, vol. 6, no. 16, pp. 2428-2429, 2002.

[20] H. L. Wang, Y. M. Lou, and R. Xue, "Psychological analysis of 52 patients with cervical spondylosis," *Journal of Henan University of Science & Technology: Medical Science*, vol. 21, no. 3, pp. 187-188, 2003.

[21] Y. M. Lou, S. H. Han, and J. H. Guo, "Analysis of mental health status and quality of life of patients with cervical spondylosis," *Journal of Traditional Chinese Orthopedics and Traumatology*, vol. 18, no. 11, pp. 15-16, 2006.

[22] C. L. Chen, Y. Wang, and G. P. He, "Study on depressive disorders of cervical spondylosis," *Shanghai Archives of Psychiatry*, vol. 19, no. 2, pp. 106-107, 2007.

[23] Z. Fang, F. Li, Q. Yang et al., "Study of the psychological and social factors in patients with cervical spondylotic myelopathy," *China Journal of Modern Medicine*, vol. 17, no. 5, pp. 583–585, 2007.

[24] X. Yao, K. Yao, J. J. Fan et al., "Research on the incidence of depression & anxiety of patients with cervical spondylopathy and psychological & ethical intervention," *Chinese Medical Ethics*, vol. 23, no. 5, pp. 61-62, 2010.

[25] D. J. Zhang, T. X. Cheng, J. G. Wang et al., "Investigation and analysis on the mental health status of 30 patients with cervical spondylosis," *China Journal of Health Psychology*, vol. 18, no. 2, pp. 149-150, 2010.

[26] J. Wei, P. Zhao, L. J. Chen et al., "Influence of social support and personality traits on psychological characteristic of patients with chronic cervicodynia and lumbodynia," *Chinese Journal of Traumatology*, vol. 25, no. 3, pp. 216–219, 2012.

[27] C. L. Huang, Q. M. Lu, L. X. Huang et al., "Investigation and analysis of relationship among medical uncertainty, anxiety and depression of cervical spondylosis patients," *China Medical Herald*, vol. 10, no. 9, pp. 109–113, 2013.

[28] J. Wen and M. J. Liu, "Investigation research and nursing measures on depression and social supports for cervical spondylosis patients," *Nursing Practice and Research*, vol. 10, no. 3, pp. 6–9, 2013.

[29] C. L. Wang, C. M. Yang, J. Y. Yun et al., "Investigation and analysis of related factors of 330 college students' sub—health cervical spine," *Journal of Liaoning Medical University*, vol. 35, no. 5, pp. 71–73, 2014.

[30] Z. X. Sun, Y. X. Sun, and X. F. Yu, "Correlative analysis of the quality of sleep and anxiety and depression in patients with cervical spondylosis," *Journal of Shandong Medical College*, vol. 39, no. 3, pp. 161–165, 2017.

[31] F. Altug, E. Kavlak, M. P. Kurtca et al., "Comparison of pain intensity, emotional status and disability level in patients with chronic neck and low back pain," *Journal of Back and Musculoskeletal Rehabilitation*, vol. 28, no. 3, pp. 505–508, 2015.

[32] M. Soysal, B. Kara, and M. N. Arda, "Assessment of physical activity in patients with chronic low back or neck pain," *Turk Neurosurgery*, vol. 23, no. 1, pp. 75–80, 2013.

[33] A. Y. Q. Xiao and Z. P. Hu, "Joint anti-anxiety treatment clinical observation in patients with cervical spondylosis anxiety," *Journal of Medical Practice Management*, vol. 28, no. 8, pp. 993-994, 2015.

[34] G. L. Chen, M. Wang, G. J. Lu et al., "Investigation of anxiety and depression in chronic pain patients and analysis of related factors," *China Journal of Pain Medicine*, vol. 20, no. 4, pp. 226–230, 2014.

[35] X. Y. Chen, "Clinical observation on 30 cases of cervical spondylosis with anxiety treated by Zhen-fu Tuina," M. S. thesis, Beijing University of Chinese Medicine, Beijing, China, 2017.

[36] F. Galbusera, M. van Rijsbergen, K. Ito et al., "Ageing and degenerative changes of the intervertebral disc and their impact on spinal flexibility," *European Spine Journal*, vol. 23, no. 3, pp. S324–S332, 2014.

[37] K. Gorter, "Influence of laminectomy on the course of cervical myelopathy," *Acta Neurochirurgica*, vol. 33, no. 3-4, pp. 265–281, 1976.

[38] S. A. Vreeburg, W. J. Hoogendijk, J. van Pelt et al., "Major depressive disorder and hypothalamic-pituitary-adrenal axis activity: results from a large cohort study," *Archives of General Psychiatry*, vol. 66, no. 6, pp. 617–626, 2009.
[39] M. J. Bair, R. L. Robinson, W. Katon et al., "Depression and pain comorbidity: a literature review," *Archives of Internal Medicine*, vol. 163, no. 20, pp. 2433–2445, 2003.
[40] D. A. Fishbain, R. Cutler, H. L. Rosomoff et al., "Chronic pain-associated depression pressure: antecedent or consequence of chronic pain? A review," *Clinical Journal of Pain*, vol. 13, no. 2, pp. 116–137, 1997.
[41] M. R. Andrew, "What works for whom? Determining the efficacy and harm of treatments for pain," *Pain*, vol. 154, no. 1, pp. S77–S86, 2013.
[42] J. Dersh, P. B. Polatin, and R. J. Gatchel, "Chronic pain and psychopathology: research findings and theoretical considerations," *Psychosomatic Medicine*, vol. 64, no. 5, pp. 773–786, 2002.
[43] Y. Sun and G. C. Li, "Summary of the second symposium on cervical spondylosis," *Chinese Journal of Surgery*, vol. 31, no. 8, pp. 472–476, 1993.
[44] Y. F. Liu and B. Y. Wang, "The significance of X-ray examination in the diagnosis of cervical spondylosis—appending clinical analysis of 158 cases," *Journal of Traditional Chinese Orthopedics and Traumatology*, vol. 19, no. 3, pp. 17–19, 2007.
[45] N. Vogelzangs, A. T. F. Beekman, P. de Jonge, and B. W. J. H. Penninx, "Anxiety disorders and inflammation in a large adult cohort," *Translational Psychiatry*, vol. 3, no. 4, p. e249, 2013.
[46] P. C. Ren, "Comparative study on the application of X-ray, CT and MRI in the diagnosis of cervical spondylosis," *China Medicine and Pharmacy*, vol. 3, no. 24, pp. 113-114, 2013.
[47] D. E. Battle, "Diagnostic and statistical manual of mental disorders (DSM)," *Codas*, vol. 25, no. 2, pp. 191-192, 2013.
[48] P. Zis, A. Daskalaki, I. Bountouni et al., "Depression and chronic pain in the elderly: links and management challenges," *Clinical Interventions in Aging*, vol. 12, pp. 709–720, 2017.

15

Targeting the Endocannabinoid System for Prevention or Treatment of Chemotherapy-Induced Neuropathic Pain: Studies in Animal Models

Willias Masocha

Department of Pharmacology and Therapeutics, Faculty of Pharmacy, Kuwait University, Safat 13110, Kuwait

Correspondence should be addressed to Willias Masocha; masocha@hsc.edu.kw

Academic Editor: Anna Maria Aloisi

There is a scarcity of drugs to either prevent or properly manage chemotherapy-induced neuropathic pain (CINP). Cannabis or cannabinoids have been reported to improve pain measures in patients with neuropathic pain. For this review, a search was done in PubMed for papers that examined the expression of and/or evaluated the use of cannabinoids or drugs that prevent or treat established CINP in a CB receptor-dependent manner in animal models. Twenty-eight articles that fulfilled the inclusion and exclusion criteria established were analysed. Studies suggest there is a specific deficiency of endocannabinoids in the periphery during CINP. Inhibitors of FAAH and MGL, enzymes that degrade the endocannabinoids, CB receptor agonists, desipramine, and coadministered indomethacin plus minocycline were found to either prevent the development and/or attenuate established CINP in a CB receptor-dependent manner. The studies analysed suggest that targeting the endocannabinoid system for prevention and treatment of CINP is a plausible therapeutic option. Almost 90% of the studies on animal models of CINP analysed utilised male rodents. Taking into consideration clinical and experimental findings that show gender differences in the mechanisms involved in pain including CINP and in response to analgesics, it is imperative that future studies on CINP utilise more female models.

1. Introduction

Chemotherapy-induced peripheral neuropathy (CIPN) is a dose-limiting side effect of some anticancer drugs, such as bortezomib, cisplatin, oxaliplatin, paclitaxel, thalidomide, and vincristine. The incidence of CIPN in patients varies from as low as 12.1% to as high as 96.2% depending on the chemotherapeutic agent and possibly the type of cancer in which the drug is used. Some chemotherapeutic drugs are associated with high incidence of CIPN; for example, in patients treated with oxaliplatin, it is around 72.3% (95% CI 59.7–86.8) and with paclitaxel it is around 70.8% (95% CI 43.5–98.1) [1]. Some patients who experience CIPN also experience neuropathic pain; for example, amongst patients who experienced CIPN during paclitaxel treatment, 27% of these patients had neuropathic pain [2], and neuropathic pain occurred in the majority of those treated with bortezomib [3]. Some of the symptoms of the painful CIPN, also referred to as chemotherapy-induced neuropathic pain (CINP), include hyperalgesia, allodynia, and spontaneous sensations such as burning, shooting, numbness, spasm, and prickling, and these can significantly reduce the patient's quality of life [4–6]. Regrettably, there is a scarcity of drugs to either prevent or manage CINP. Currently, only duloxetine has a recommendation for the management of CINP, whilst other drugs used for other neuropathic pain conditions may be given because of the limited CINP treatment options [7]. Thus, studies to understand the pathophysiology and to develop novel treatment options for CINP treatment are essential.

Cannabis or cannabinoids have been reported to improve pain measures in patients with neuropathic or cancer pain [8–11]. A recent study recommends studying the effects of a cannabinoid agent, nabiximols, against CINP in a full randomised, placebo-controlled trial [12].

Phytocannabinoids, synthetic cannabinoids, and endogenous cannabinoids (endocannabinoids), such as *N*-arachidonoylethanolamine (AEA, anandamide) and 2-arachidonoylglycerol (2-AG), produce their effects via activation of cannabinoid receptors, CB1 and CB2 receptors [13]. Endocannabinoids are lipid-based neurotransmitters produced on demand [14–17] from cell membrane phospholipid precursors [18, 19] through various pathways [20]. Endocannabinoid homeostasis is maintained by transporters that transport AEA and 2-AG from the synaptic space back into the cells or by enzymes that degrade the endocannabinoids. Fatty acid amide hydrolase (FAAH) hydrolyses AEA to arachidonic acid and ethanolamine [21]. Monoacylglycerol lipase (MGL) hydrolyses 2-AG to arachidonic acid and glycerol [22, 23].

In this minireview, changes that occur in the endocannabinoid system during CINP and the possibility of targeting the endocannabinoid enzymes and cannabinoid receptors to manage CINP will be discussed. This minireview deals only with results obtained from animal studies.

2. Methods and Selection of Articles to Include in the Analysis of Endocannabinoid Expression and Compounds Utilising the Endocannabinoid System to Prevent or Treat CINP in Animal Models

The U.S. National Library of Medicine, Washington, DC (MEDLINE-PubMed), was used to search for appropriate papers for this study, without limitations of date of publication, using different combinations of the words or phrases: chemotherapy-induced neuropathy, chemotherapy-induced neuropathic pain, cannabinoid, endocannabinoid, pain, expression, cisplatin, paclitaxel, and vincristine. The search strategy was designed to include any published paper that examined the expression of endocannabinoids in animal models of CINP and/or evaluated the use of cannabinoids or drugs that prevent or treat established hyperalgesia, hypersensitivity, or allodynia in animal models of CINP in a cannabinoid receptor-dependent manner. Articles that were found in more than 1 search combination were counted only once. Studies that did not use animals, did not evaluate CINP, or evaluated noncannabinoid compounds without using cannabinoid receptor antagonists, reviews, commentaries, and *in vitro* studies were excluded.

From the electronic search, a total of 48 articles were identified, and of these, 20 articles were excluded because they were reviews, human studies, *in vitro* studies, did not evaluate CINP, and evaluated noncannabinoid compounds without using cannabinoid receptor antagonists. Twenty-eight articles fulfilled the inclusion and exclusion criteria described above and are discussed in the sections below.

3. Expression of Endocannabinoids during Chemotherapy-Induced Neuropathic Pain

Four studies were found that measured the expression of the endocannabinoids 2-AG and AEA in rodent models of CINP [24–27]. All these studies were done in male rodents of cisplatin CINP (Table 1). Treatment of mice with cisplatin reduced the expression of AEA but not 2-AG in the paw skin [25, 27]. Guindon et al. measured the expression of endocannabinoids in the spinal cord and paw skin in rats with cisplatin-induced mechanical and cold allodynia [24]. Rats treated with cisplatin had increased levels of 2-AG and AEA in the lumbar spinal cord, whilst 2-AG, but not AEA, was decreased in the dorsal hind paw skin [24]. In another study, Khasabova et al. showed that treatment of mice with cisplatin resulted in decreased levels of AEA and 2-AG in the paw skin and dorsal root ganglia (DRGs), increased levels of AEA and 2-AG in the spinal cord, but no change in the brain [26]. These studies suggest there is a specific deficiency of endocannabinoids in the periphery during CINP. Thus, increasing the levels of these endocannabinoids in the periphery by inhibiting either their degradation or transport from the synaptic space back into the cells is a potential therapeutic target for managing CINP.

4. Effect of Inhibitors of Endocannabinoid Metabolism on Chemotherapy-Induced Neuropathic Pain

Taking into consideration that FAAH and MGL degrade the endocannabinoids, their inhibitors have been evaluated in animal models of CINP. All of the five studies carried out utilised male rodents of CINP (Table 2). An FAAH inhibitor ST4070 suppressed established mechanical allodynia in rats with vincristine-induced mechanical allodynia [28]. Another FAAH inhibitor URB597 delayed the onset and decreased the magnitude of mechanical and heat hyperalgesia and also suppressed established mechanical and thermal hyperalgesia in mice with cisplatin-induced hyperalgesia in a CB1, but not CB2, receptor-dependent manner [25]. Two FAAH inhibitors URB597 and URB937 and an MGL inhibitor JZL184 suppressed established cisplatin-induced mechanical and cold allodynia in rats. The antiallodynic effects of the FAAH inhibitors and MGL inhibitor were blocked by CB1, but not CB2, receptor antagonists [24]. In mice, peripheral administration of low doses of JZL184 was found to prevent the development of cisplatin-induced mechanical hyperalgesia in a CB1 receptor, but not CB2 receptor, dependent manner [26]. URB597 and JZL184 were also reported to suppress paclitaxel-induced mechanical and cold allodynia in mice [29]. These studies show that FAAH and MGL inhibitors can both prevent the development and attenuate established CINP symptoms mainly in a CB1 receptor-dependent manner.

5. Effect of Cannabinoid Agonists on Chemotherapy-Induced Neuropathic Pain

The majority of the studies (21 studies) on cannabinoids and CINP in animal models evaluated the effects of agonists via CB1 and CB2 receptors (Table 3). The use of nonselective CB1/CB2 agonists was found in 11 studies, CB1 receptor-selective agonists in 2 studies, and CB2 receptor-selective agonists in 11 studies. Some studies evaluated drugs in more

Table 1: Expression of endocannabinoids in animal models of CINP.

	CINP model		Expression of endocannabinoids		
Chemotherapy drug	Animals	CINP symptom	Tissue	Change in endocannabinoid levels relative to control	Reference
Cisplatin	Male C3H/HeN mice	Mechanical and heat hyperalgesia	Plantar paw skin	Decrease in AEA but no change in 2-AG	[25]
Cisplatin	Male SD rats	Mechanical and cold allodynia	Lumbar spinal cord	Both 2-AG and AEA increased	[24]
			Dorsal hind paw skin	2-AG decreased but not AEA	
Cisplatin	Male C3H/HeN mice	Mechanical hyperalgesia	Plantar paw skin	Both 2-AG and AEA decreased	[26]
			DRGs	Both 2-AG and AEA decreased	
			Lumbar spinal cord	Both 2-AG and AEA increased	
			Midbrain	No effect on both 2-AG and AEA	
Cisplatin	Male C3H/HeJ mice	Mechanical allodynia	Plantar paw skin	Decrease in AEA but no change in 2-AG	[27]

2-AG, 2-arachidonoylglycerol; AEA, *N*-arachidonoylethanolamine (anandamide); SD, Sprague-Dawley.

Table 2: Effects of inhibitors of enzymes that degrade endocannabinoids in animal models of CINP.

CINP model					
Chemotherapy drug	Animal	Inhibitor of enzymes that degrade endocannabinoids	Effects	Effects of CB receptor antagonists on the activity of the compound	Reference
Vincristine	Male SD rats	FAAH inhibitor ST4070	Suppressed established mechanical allodynia	No antagonists were used against vincristine	[28]
Cisplatin	Male C3H/HeN mice	FAAH inhibitor URB597	Delayed the onset and decreased the magnitude of mechanical and heat hyperalgesia	CB1 antagonist AM281 antagonised	[25]
			Suppressed established mechanical and thermal hyperalgesia	CB2 antagonist AM630 had no effect	
Cisplatin	Male SD rats	FAAH inhibitors URB597 and URB937 MGL inhibitor JZL184	Suppressed established mechanical and cold allodynia	CB1 antagonist AM251 antagonised CB2 antagonist AM630 had no effect	[24]
Cisplatin	Male C3H/HeN mice	MGL inhibitor JZL184	Prevented the development of mechanical hyperalgesia Suppressed established mechanical allodynia	CB1 receptor antagonist AM281 antagonised CB2 receptor antagonist AM630 had no effect	[26]
Paclitaxel	Male CD1 and C57BL/6J mice	URB597 and JZL184	Suppressed mechanical and cold allodynia	Antagonists were not tested	[29]

FAAH, fatty acid amide hydrolase; MGL, monoacylglycerol lipase; SD, Sprague-Dawley.

than one of the categories of selectivity for CB receptors. All the studies that stated the gender (19 out of 21) conducted on CB receptor agonists and CINP utilised male rodents (Table 3). Two studies did not state the gender of the mice used (Table 3).

Nonselective CB1/CB2 receptor agonists such as the endocannabinoids 2-AG and AEA, CP55,940, Δ^9-tetrahydrocannabinol (THC), and WIN 55,212-2 were reported to prevent the development and/or suppress established symptoms of CINP in mice and rats. The endocannabinoids 2-AG and AEA suppressed established cisplatin-induced mechanical hyperalgesia in mice in a CB1, but not CB2, receptor-dependent manner [25, 26]. The phytocannabinoid THC was found to suppress established mechanical and cold allodynia induced by either cisplatin or paclitaxel in mice [30, 31]. However, the role of CB receptors in the activity of THC against CINP was not investigated. THC failed to prevent the development of cisplatin-induced mechanical allodynia [31]. A synthetic nonselective CB receptor agonist CP55,940 suppressed paclitaxel-induced allodynia in mice, via both CB1 and CB2 receptor-dependent mechanisms, but the CB2 receptor-dependent mechanism was only observed at high doses of CP55,940 in CB1 receptor-deficient mice [32]. The nonselective CB receptor agonist used most on CINP in rodents is WIN 55,212-2. WIN 55,212-2 both prevented the development and suppressed established CINP, in a manner which was CB1 and CB2 receptor dependent [33–39]. It has both systemic and local effects; however, its local effects appear to be CB1, but not CB2, receptor dependent [38]. Several studies show that

Table 3: Effects of CB receptor agonists in animal models of CINP.

CINP model		CB receptor agonist	Effects	Effects of CB receptor antagonists on the activity of the compound	Reference
Chemotherapy drug	Animal				
Nonselective CB1/CB2 receptor agonists					
Cisplatin	Male C3H/HeN mice	2-AG	Suppressed established mechanical hyperalgesia	CB1 receptor antagonist AM281 antagonised CB2 receptor antagonist AM630 had no effect	[26]
Cisplatin	Male C3H/HeN mice	AEA	Suppressed established mechanical hyperalgesia	CB1 antagonist AM281 antagonised CB2 antagonist AM630 had no effects	[25]
Paclitaxel	CD1 and C57BL/6J mice	THC	Suppressed established mechanical and cold allodynia	No antagonists were used	[30]
Cisplatin	Male C57BL/6 mice	THC	Suppressed established mechanical allodynia Did not prevent the development of mechanical allodynia	No antagonists were used	[31]
Paclitaxel	CD1 and C57BL/6J mice	CP55,940	Suppressed established mechanical and cold allodynia	CB2 antagonist AM630 antagonised	[32]
Paclitaxel	Male Wistar rats	WIN	Suppressed established thermal hyperalgesia and mechanical allodynia	CB1 antagonist SR141716A antagonised	[33]
Vincristine	Male SD rats	WIN	Suppressed established mechanical allodynia	Both CB1 antagonist SR141716 and CB2 antagonist SR144528 antagonised	[34]
Cisplatin	Male Wistar rats	WIN	Prevented the development of mechanical allodynia	No antagonists were used	[35]
Paclitaxel	Male Wistar rats	WIN	Prevented the development of thermal hyperalgesia and mechanical allodynia	No antagonists were used	[36]
Cisplatin	Male Wistar rats	WIN	Prevented the development of mechanical allodynia	No antagonists were used	[37]
Cisplatin	Male Wistar rats	WIN	Suppressed established mechanical allodynia	Both CB1 antagonist AM251 and CB2 antagonist SR144528 antagonised	[38]
Paclitaxel	Male SD rats	WIN	Prevented the development of mechanical and cold allodynia	CB1 receptor antagonist AM251 antagonised mechanical allodynia but not cold allodynia CB2 receptor antagonist AM630 did not reliably antagonise both mechanical and cold allodynia	[39]
CB1 receptor-selective agonists					
Cisplatin	Male Wistar rats	ACEA	Suppressed established mechanical allodynia	CB1 antagonist AM251 antagonised	[38]
Paclitaxel	Male CD1 and C57BL/6J mice	GAT211 (CB1 PAM)	Suppressed mechanical and cold allodynia	CB1 receptor antagonist AM251 antagonised CB2 receptor antagonist AM630 had no effect	[29]
CB2 receptor-selective agonists					
Vincristine	Male SD rats	AM1241	Suppressed established mechanical allodynia	CB1 antagonist SR141716 had no effect CB2 antagonist SR144528 antagonised	[34]
Paclitaxel	Male SD rats	AM1241 and AM1714	Suppressed established mechanical allodynia	CB1 antagonist SR141716 had no effect CB2 antagonist SR144528 antagonised	[40]

Table 3: Continued.

CINP model		CB receptor agonist	Effects	Effects of CB receptor antagonists on the activity of the compound	Reference
Chemotherapy drug	Animal				
Cisplatin and paclitaxel	Male SD rats	AM1710	Suppressed established mechanical and cold allodynia	CB1 antagonist AM251 had no effect CB2 antagonist AM630 antagonised	[41]
Paclitaxel	Male SD rats	AM1710	Prevented the development of mechanical and cold allodynia	CB1 receptor antagonist AM251 had no effect CB2 receptor antagonist AM630 antagonised	[39]
Paclitaxel	CD1 and C57BL/6J mice	AM1710	Suppressed established mechanical and cold allodynia	CB2 antagonist AM630 antagonised	[30]
Paclitaxel	Male SD rats	MDA7	Suppressed established mechanical allodynia	No antagonists were used	[42]
Paclitaxel	Male SD rats and mice (strain not specified)	MDA7	Suppressed established mechanical allodynia	CB2 antagonist AM630 antagonised	[43]
Paclitaxel	Male SD rats	MDA7	Prevented the development of mechanical allodynia	No antagonists were used in paclitaxel-induced mechanical allodynia	[44]
Paclitaxel	Male SD rats and mice (strain not specified)	MDA19	Suppressed established mechanical allodynia	No antagonists were used	[45]
Paclitaxel	Male C57BL/6J mice	LY2828360	Suppressed established mechanical and cold allodynia	No antagonists were used	[46]
Cisplatin	Male Wistar rats	JWH133	Suppressed established mechanical allodynia	CB2 antagonist SR144528 antagonised	[38]
Paclitaxel	Male Swiss mice	BCP	Prevented the development of mechanical allodynia Suppressed established mechanical allodynia	CB1 receptor antagonist AM251 had no effect CB2 receptor antagonist AM630 antagonised	[47]

AEA, *N*-arachidonoylethanolamine (anandamide); BCP, β-caryophyllene; PAM, positive allosteric modulator; SD, Sprague-Dawley; THC, Δ^9-tetrahydrocannabinol; WIN, WIN 55,212-2.

nonselective CB receptor agonists attenuate CINP in a CB1, but not CB2, receptor-dependent manner most likely because CB1 receptors are expressed at higher levels in the nervous system than CB2 receptors, while CB2 receptors are expressed mainly in immune cells and the levels increase in the nervous system during injury. Therefore, when nonselective CB receptor agonists are used, the effects on CB1 receptors are more likely to be predominant.

A CB1 receptor-selective agonist ACEA was found to prevent the development of cisplatin-induced mechanical allodynia in rats, when administered either locally or systemically [38]. However, various problems are associated with CB1 receptor activation such as physical dependence, withdrawal adverse effects, and development of tolerance [29, 30]. A novel CB1 positive allosteric modulator (PAM), GAT211, was found to suppress paclitaxel-induced cold and mechanical allodynia in mice without producing the cardinal signs of CB1 activation, physical dependence or tolerance, which were produced by WIN 55,212-2, an orthosteric cannabinoid agonist [29].

Various CB2 receptor-selective agonists have been reported to prevent the development and/or suppress established symptoms of CINP in mice and rats. The aminoalkylindole cannabinoid AM1241 and the cannabilactones AM1710 and AM1714 were found to prevent the development and suppress established mechanical and cold allodynia induced by cisplatin, paclitaxel, or vincristine in rodents in a CB2, but not CB1, receptor-dependent manner [30, 34, 39, 40, 41]. Other CB2 receptor-selective agonists MDA7, MDA19, JWH133, and LY2828360 were reported to prevent the development and suppress established paclitaxel-induced mechanical and cold allodynia [38, 42–46]. The CB2 receptor-dependent antiallodynic effects were demonstrated by blocking the effects of MDA7 and JWH133 by CB2 receptor antagonists [38, 43], whilst the other studies did not utilise antagonists. LY2828360 suppressed paclitaxel-induced allodynia without producing tolerance [46]. β-Caryophyllene (BCP), a CB2 receptor-selective agonist found in many essential oils including clove oil and *Cannabis sativa* essential oil [48], prevented the development and attenuated established paclitaxel-induced mechanical allodynia in mice in a CB2, but not CB1, receptor-dependent manner [47]. Some of the advantages of CB2 receptor-selective agonists such as AM1710, over nonselective CB1/CB2 receptor agonists, such as WIN 55,212-2 and THC, described were the favourable therapeutic ratio because of sustained efficacy and absence of tolerance, physical withdrawal, or CB1-mediated side effects [30]. Therefore, selectively targeting CB2 receptors can produce antiallodynic effects whilst bypassing the unwanted central effects associated with CB1 receptor activation [30].

Table 4: Effects of cannabidiol in animal models of CINP.

CINP model		Effects	Effects of CB receptor antagonists on the activity of the compound	Reference
Chemotherapy drug	Animal			
Paclitaxel	Female C57Bl6 mice	Prevented the development of cold and mechanical allodynia	No antagonists were used	[49]
Paclitaxel	Female C57Bl6 mice	Prevented the development of mechanical allodynia	CB1 receptor antagonist SR141716 and CB2 receptor antagonist SR144528 had no effects 5-HT1A receptor antagonist WAY 100635 antagonised	[50]
Cisplatin	Male C57BL/6 mice	Suppressed established mechanical allodynia Did not prevent the development of mechanical allodynia	No antagonists were used	[31]

6. Effect of the Nonpsychoactive Phytocannabinoid Cannabidiol on Chemotherapy-Induced Neuropathic Pain

The effects of the nonpsychoactive phytocannabinoid cannabidiol in mice models of CINP were evaluated in 3 studies. Different from the trend noted above, the majority of these studies (two out of three) utilised female mice (Table 4).

Cannabidiol was found to prevent the development of paclitaxel-induced cold and mechanical allodynia [49, 50]. However, in another study, cannabidiol attenuated established cisplatin-induced mechanical allodynia but could not prevent its development [31]. Cannabidiol displays low affinity for CB1 and CB2 receptors but antagonises cannabinoid CB1/CB2 receptor agonists [51]. The antiallodynic effects of cannabidiol were not blocked by either CB1 or CB2 receptor antagonists but were blocked by a 5-HT1A receptor antagonist [50].

7. Effect of Other Drugs That Affect the Endocannabinoid System on Chemotherapy-Induced Neuropathic Pain

Other drugs that produce biologic activity via other mechanisms independent of the cannabinoid system have been reported to have antiallodynic and antihyperalgesic activities in animal models of CINP in a cannabinoid receptor-dependent manner [52, 53]. Fifty percent of the studies (one out of two) used female animals (Table 5).

Parvathy and Masocha reported that coadministration of indomethacin plus minocycline attenuates paclitaxel-induced thermal hyperalgesia in mice, whereas the individual drugs did not [53]. The effects of the combination were dependent on CB1 receptors; however, the role of CB2 receptors was not investigated [53]. Indomethacin reduces pain principally through inhibition of cyclooxygenase enzymes, whereas minocycline has anti-inflammatory activities and inhibits lipoxygenases and microglia activation. In addition, these two drugs have been reported to individually modulate the levels of endocannabinoids [54, 55]. Further research is needed to study whether the synergistic effect of coadminstration of indomethacin plus minocycline is via increased levels of endocannabinoids. Coadministration of indomethacin and minocycline previously been reported has more antinociceptive effects in a mouse model of arthritis than when either drug alone was administered [56]. Moreover, indomethacin and minocycline are already clinically used for managing pain and inflammation in humans with conditions such as rheumatoid arthritis [57, 58]. Thus, if confirmed useful in other models of CINP, it would be easier to translate the findings to humans than with synthetic cannabinoid agonists or modulators not yet tried in the clinics.

The role of the cannabinoid receptors in the antiallodynic effects of desipramine was evaluated in mice with paclitaxel-induced mechanical and cold allodynia [52]. Desipramine is a tricyclic antidepressant used clinically in the management of neuropathic pain including CINP [59]. Cannabinoid CB1 and CB2 receptor antagonists partially attenuated the ability of desipramine to prevent the development of paclitaxel-induced mechanical and cold allodynia in these mice [52]. This study adds an understanding of other possible mechanisms of action of desipramine in the management of CINP.

8. Concluding Remarks

The endocannabinoid system is dysregulated in animal models of CINP, most notably the reduced levels of AEA and 2-AG in the paw skin, which suggest their deficiency in the periphery but not in the CNS. These findings indicate that inhibitors of FAAH and MGL could result in an elevation of the endocannabinoids and alleviation of CINP. Indeed, FAAH and MGL inhibitors have been found to prevent or attenuate symptoms of CINP in animal models. Closely related to the changes in the expression of endocannabinoids in the periphery, a peripherally acting FAAH inhibitor URB937 alleviated established CINP in rats [24]. Further research on peripherally acting FAAH and MGL inhibitors in the management of CINP is warranted, since they would lack the CNS side effects of centrally acting drugs.

Various agonists of CB1 and CB2 receptors prevent or attenuate symptoms of CINP in animal models; however, various problems are associated with CB1 receptor activation including physical dependence, development of tolerance, and other cannabimimetic adverse effects such as

Table 5: Effects of other agents, in a CB receptor-dependent manner, in animal models of CINP.

CINP model		Molecule	Effects	Effects of CB receptor antagonists on the activity of the compound	Reference
Chemotherapy drug	Animal				
Paclitaxel	Female and male BALB/c mice	Indomethacin (NSAID) plus minocycline (semisynthetic tetracycline antibiotic)	Reduced established thermal hyperalgesia	CB1 antagonist AM251 antagonised	[53]
Paclitaxel	Male Sprague-Dawley rats	Desipramine (tricyclic antidepressant)	Prevented the development of mechanical and cold allodynia	CB1 antagonist AM251 and CB2 antagonist AM630 partially antagonised	[52]

NSAID, nonsteroidal anti-inflammatory drug.

hypothermia and catalepsy. Options to circumvent these problems that have been explored include the use of a CB1 receptor PAM or CB2 receptor-selective agonists. Both the CB1 receptor PAM and CB2 receptor-selective agonists attenuate CINP in animals with less adverse effects than nonselective CB1/CB2 receptor agonists, FAAH and MGL inhibitors. Thus, CB1 receptor PAMs or CB2 receptor-selective agonists warrant further research as they might have a better safety profile than the classical cannabinoids.

Cannabidiol, which is a major constituent of cannabis, attenuates allodynia in animal models of CINP, in part via 5-HT1A receptors but independent of the CB receptors.

Desipramine which is a TCA used clinically in the management of CINP seems to be working partially via CB1 and CB2 receptors. This information aids in the understanding of how some of the drugs currently used to manage CINP work. The study on the coadministration of minocycline and indomethacin shows that the combination attenuates CINP in animals in a CB1 receptor-dependent manner. This study opens an avenue for modulating the endocannabinoid system for managing CINP with drugs that are already being used in the clinics for other conditions.

The studies analysed suggest that targeting the endocannabinoid system for prevention and treatment of CINP is a plausible therapeutic option. Further research is needed to ascertain whether this approach has advantages compared to already existing treatment options for CINP and whether this can be translated into clinical applications.

One striking observation is that the majority of the studies on animal models of CINP analysed in this review utilised male rodents (almost 90%). Current clinical and experimental findings show that there are sex/gender differences in the manifestation and mechanisms involved in pain including CINP [60–63]. Moreover, sex/gender differences in both the expression of endocannabinoids and antinociceptive activity of cannabinoids have been reported [64, 65]. A consensus report published by members of the Sex, Gender and Pain Special Interest Group of the International Association for the Study of Pain recommended that "all pain researchers consider testing their hypotheses in both sexes, or if restricted by practical considerations, only in females" [66]. This is important because of the higher prevalence of some types of pain in females compared to males, the gender differences in response to analgesics both in experimental animals and humans, and the higher number of studies done in male than in female models of pain [66]. Taking this into consideration, it is imperative that future studies on CINP utilise more female models.

References

[1] M. Seretny, G. L. Currie, E. S. Sena et al., "Incidence, prevalence, and predictors of chemotherapy-induced peripheral neuropathy: a systematic review and meta-analysis," *Pain*, vol. 155, no. 12, pp. 2461–2470, 2014.

[2] C. C. Reyes-Gibby, P. K. Morrow, A. Buzdar, and S. Shete, "Chemotherapy-induced peripheral neuropathy as a predictor of neuropathic pain in breast cancer patients previously treated with paclitaxel," *Journal of Pain*, vol. 10, no. 11, pp. 1146–1150, 2009.

[3] A. J. Rampen, J. L. Jongen, I. van Heuvel, M. Scheltens-de Boer, P. Sonneveld, and M. J. van den Bent, "Bortezomib-induced polyneuropathy," *Netherlands Journal of Medicine*, vol. 71, pp. 128–133, 2013.

[4] P. M. Dougherty, J. P. Cata, J. V. Cordella, A. Burton, and H. R. Weng, "Taxol-induced sensory disturbance is characterized by preferential impairment of myelinated fiber function in cancer patients," *Pain*, vol. 109, no. 1, pp. 132–142, 2004.

[5] F. H. Hausheer, R. L. Schilsky, S. Bain, E. J. Berghorn, and F. Lieberman, "Diagnosis, management, and evaluation of chemotherapy-induced peripheral neuropathy," *Seminars in Oncology*, vol. 33, no. 1, pp. 15–49, 2006.

[6] S. Wolf, D. Barton, L. Kottschade, A. Grothey, and C. Loprinzi, "Chemotherapy-induced peripheral neuropathy: prevention and treatment strategies," *European Journal of Cancer*, vol. 44, no. 11, pp. 1507–1515, 2008.

[7] D. L. Hershman, C. Lacchetti, R. H. Dworkin et al., "Prevention and management of chemotherapy-induced peripheral neuropathy in survivors of adult cancers: American Society of Clinical Oncology clinical practice guideline," *Journal of Clinical Oncology*, vol. 32, no. 18, pp. 1941–1967, 2014.

[8] D. I. Abrams, "Using medical cannabis in an oncology practice," *Oncology*, vol. 30, no. 5, pp. 397–404, 2016.

[9] D. I. Abrams, "Integrating cannabis into clinical cancer care," *Current Oncology*, vol. 23, no. 2, pp. S8–S14, 2016.

[10] D. I. Abrams, C. A. Jay, S. B. Shade et al., "Cannabis in painful HIV-associated sensory neuropathy: a randomized placebo-controlled trial," *Neurology*, vol. 68, no. 7, pp. 515–521, 2007.

[11] P. F. Whiting, R. F. Wolff, S. Deshpande et al., "Cannabinoids for medical use: a systematic review and meta-analysis," *JAMA*, vol. 313, no. 24, pp. 2456–2473, 2015.

[12] M. E. Lynch, P. Cesar-Rittenberg, and A. G. Hohmann, "A double-blind, placebo-controlled, crossover pilot trial with extension using an oral mucosal cannabinoid extract for treatment of chemotherapy-induced neuropathic pain," *Journal of Pain and Symptom Management*, vol. 47, no. 1, pp. 166–173, 2014.

[13] J. Guindon and A. G. Hohmann, "The endocannabinoid system and pain," *CNS & Neurological Disorders–Drug Targets*, vol. 8, no. 6, pp. 403–421, 2009.

[14] A. Giuffrida, L. H. Parsons, T. M. Kerr, F. Rodriguez de Fonseca, M. Navarro, and D. Piomelli, "Dopamine activation of endogenous cannabinoid signaling in dorsal striatum," *Nature Neuroscience*, vol. 2, no. 4, pp. 358–363, 1999.

[15] J. Kim, M. Isokawa, C. Ledent, and B. E. Alger, "Activation of muscarinic acetylcholine receptors enhances the release of endogenous cannabinoids in the hippocampus," *Journal of Neuroscience*, vol. 22, no. 23, pp. 10182–10191, 2002.

[16] A. Luchicchi and M. Pistis, "Anandamide and 2-arachidonoylglycerol: pharmacological properties, functional features, and emerging specificities of the two major endocannabinoids," *Molecular Neurobiology*, vol. 46, no. 2, pp. 374–392, 2012.

[17] N. Varma, G. C. Carlson, C. Ledent, and B. E. Alger, "Metabotropic glutamate receptors drive the endocannabinoid system in hippocampus," *Journal of Neuroscience*, vol. 21, no. 24, p. RC188, 2001.

[18] V. Di Marzo, T. Bisogno, T. Sugiura, D. Melck, and L. De Petrocellis, "The novel endogenous cannabinoid 2-arachidonoylglycerol is inactivated by neuronal- and basophil-like cells: connections with anandamide," *Biochemical Journal*, vol. 331, no. 1, pp. 15–19, 1998.

[19] D. Piomelli, "The endocannabinoid system: a drug discovery perspective," *Current Opinion in Investigational Drugs*, vol. 6, no. 7, pp. 672–679, 2005.

[20] V. Di Marzo, "Targeting the endocannabinoid system: to enhance or reduce?," *Nature Reviews Drug Discovery*, vol. 7, no. 5, pp. 438–455, 2008.

[21] B. F. Cravatt, D. K. Giang, S. P. Mayfield, D. L. Boger, R. A. Lerner, and N. B. Gilula, "Molecular characterization of an enzyme that degrades neuromodulatory fatty-acid amides," *Nature*, vol. 384, no. 6604, pp. 83–87, 1996.

[22] T. P. Dinh, D. Carpenter, F. M. Leslie et al., "Brain monoglyceride lipase participating in endocannabinoid inactivation," *Proceedings of the National Academy of Sciences*, vol. 99, no. 16, pp. 10819–10824, 2002.

[23] S. M. Saario, J. R. Savinainen, J. T. Laitinen, T. Jarvinen, and R. Niemi, "Monoglyceride lipase-like enzymatic activity is responsible for hydrolysis of 2-arachidonoylglycerol in rat cerebellar membranes," *Biochemical Pharmacology*, vol. 67, no. 7, pp. 1381–1387, 2004.

[24] J. Guindon, Y. Lai, S. M. Takacs, H. B. Bradshaw, and A. G. Hohmann, "Alterations in endocannabinoid tone following chemotherapy-induced peripheral neuropathy: effects of endocannabinoid deactivation inhibitors targeting fatty-acid amide hydrolase and monoacylglycerol lipase in comparison to reference analgesics following cisplatin treatment," *Pharmacological Research*, vol. 67, no. 1, pp. 94–109, 2013.

[25] I. A. Khasabova, S. Khasabov, J. Paz, C. Harding-Rose, D. A. Simone, and V. S. Seybold, "Cannabinoid type-1 receptor reduces pain and neurotoxicity produced by chemotherapy," *Journal of Neuroscience*, vol. 32, no. 20, pp. 7091–7101, 2012.

[26] I. A. Khasabova, X. Yao, J. Paz et al., "JZL184 is antihyperalgesic in a murine model of cisplatin-induced peripheral neuropathy," *Pharmacological Research*, vol. 90, pp. 67–75, 2014.

[27] M. L. Uhelski, I. A. Khasabova, and D. A. Simone, "Inhibition of anandamide hydrolysis attenuates nociceptor sensitization in a murine model of chemotherapy-induced peripheral neuropathy," *Journal of Neurophysiology*, vol. 113, no. 5, pp. 1501–1510, 2015.

[28] A. Caprioli, R. Coccurello, C. Rapino et al., "The novel reversible fatty acid amide hydrolase inhibitor ST4070 increases endocannabinoid brain levels and counteracts neuropathic pain in different animal models," *Journal of Pharmacology and Experimental Therapeutics*, vol. 342, no. 1, pp. 188–195, 2012.

[29] R. A. Slivicki, Z. Xu, P. M. Kulkarni et al., "Positive allosteric modulation of cannabinoid receptor type 1 suppresses pathological pain without producing tolerance or dependence," *Biological Psychiatry*, 2017.

[30] L. Deng, J. Guindon, B. L. Cornett, A. Makriyannis, K. Mackie, and A. G. Hohmann, "Chronic cannabinoid receptor 2 activation reverses paclitaxel neuropathy without tolerance or cannabinoid receptor 1-dependent withdrawal," *Biological Psychiatry*, vol. 77, no. 5, pp. 475–487, 2015.

[31] H. M. Harris, K. J. Sufka, W. Gul, and M. A. ElSohly, "Effects of delta-9-tetrahydrocannabinol and cannabidiol on cisplatin-induced neuropathy in mice," *Planta Medica*, vol. 82, no. 13, pp. 1169–1172, 2016.

[32] L. Deng, B. L. Cornett, K. Mackie, and A. G. Hohmann, "CB1 knockout mice unveil sustained CB2-mediated antiallodynic effects of the mixed CB1/CB2 agonist CP55,940 in a mouse model of paclitaxel-induced neuropathic pain," *Molecular Pharmacology*, vol. 88, no. 1, pp. 64–74, 2015.

[33] D. Pascual, C. Goicoechea, M. Suardiaz, and M. I. Martin, "A cannabinoid agonist, WIN 55,212-2, reduces neuropathic nociception induced by paclitaxel in rats," *Pain*, vol. 118, no. 1, pp. 23–34, 2005.

[34] E. J. Rahn, A. Makriyannis, and A. G. Hohmann, "Activation of cannabinoid CB1 and CB2 receptors suppresses neuropathic nociception evoked by the chemotherapeutic agent vincristine in rats," *British Journal of Pharmacology*, vol. 152, no. 5, pp. 765–777, 2007.

[35] G. Vera, A. Chiarlone, P. A. Cabezos, D. Pascual, M. I. Martin, and R. Abalo, "WIN 55,212-2 prevents mechanical allodynia but not alterations in feeding behaviour induced by chronic cisplatin in the rat," *Life Sciences*, vol. 81, no. 6, pp. 468–479, 2007.

[36] E. Burgos, D. Gomez-Nicola, D. Pascual, M. I. Martin, M. Nieto-Sampedro, and C. Goicoechea, "Cannabinoid agonist WIN 55,212-2 prevents the development of paclitaxel-induced peripheral neuropathy in rats. Possible involvement of spinal glial cells," *European Journal of Pharmacology*, vol. 682, no. 1–3, pp. 62–72, 2012.

[37] R. Abalo, P. A. Cabezos, G. Vera, A. E. Lopez-Perez, and M. I. Martin, "Cannabinoids may worsen gastric dysmotility induced by chronic cisplatin in the rat," *Neurogastroenterology & Motility*, vol. 25, no. 5, pp. e292–e382, 2013.

[38] G. Vera, P. A. Cabezos, M. I. Martin, and R. Abalo, "Characterization of cannabinoid-induced relief of neuropathic pain in a rat model of cisplatin-induced neuropathy," *Pharmacology, Biochemistry, and Behavior*, vol. 105, pp. 205–212, 2013.

[39] E. J. Rahn, L. Deng, G. A. Thakur et al., "Prophylactic cannabinoid administration blocks the development of paclitaxel-induced neuropathic nociception during analgesic treatment and following cessation of drug delivery," *Molecular Pain*, vol. 10, p. 27, 2014.

[40] E. J. Rahn, A. M. Zvonok, G. A. Thakur, A. D. Khanolkar, A. Makriyannis, and A. G. Hohmann, "Selective activation of cannabinoid CB2 receptors suppresses neuropathic nociception induced by treatment with the chemotherapeutic agent paclitaxel in rats," *Journal of Pharmacology and Experimental Therapeutics*, vol. 327, no. 2, pp. 584–591, 2008.

[41] L. Deng, J. Guindon, V. K. Vemuri et al., "The maintenance of cisplatin- and paclitaxel-induced mechanical and cold allodynia is suppressed by cannabinoid CB(2) receptor activation and independent of CXCR4 signaling in models of chemotherapy-induced peripheral neuropathy," *Molecular Pain*, vol. 8, p. 71, 2012.

[42] M. Naguib, P. Diaz, J. J. Xu et al., "MDA7: a novel selective agonist for CB2 receptors that prevents allodynia in rat neuropathic pain models," *British Journal of Pharmacology*, vol. 155, no. 7, pp. 1104–1116, 2008.

[43] M. Naguib, J. J. Xu, P. Diaz et al., "Prevention of paclitaxel-induced neuropathy through activation of the central cannabinoid type 2 receptor system," *Anesthesia and Analgesia*, vol. 114, no. 5, pp. 1104–1120, 2012.

[44] J. J. Xu, P. Diaz, B. Bie et al., "Spinal gene expression profiling and pathways analysis of a CB2 agonist (MDA7)-targeted prevention of paclitaxel-induced neuropathy," *Neuroscience*, vol. 260, pp. 185–194, 2014.

[45] J. J. Xu, P. Diaz, F. Astruc-Diaz, S. Craig, E. Munoz, and M. Naguib, "Pharmacological characterization of a novel cannabinoid ligand, MDA19, for treatment of neuropathic pain," *Anesthesia and Analgesia*, vol. 111, no. 1, pp. 99–109, 2010.

[46] X. Lin, A. S. Dhopeshwarkar, M. Huibregtse, K. Mackie, and A. G. Hohmann, "Slowly signaling G protein-biased CB2 cannabinoid receptor agonist LY2828360 suppresses neuropathic pain with sustained efficacy and attenuates morphine tolerance and dependence," *Molecular Pharmacology*, vol. 93, no. 2, pp. 49–62, 2018.

[47] G. C. Segat, M. N. Manjavachi, D. O. Matias et al., "Anti-allodynic effect of beta-caryophyllene on paclitaxel-induced peripheral neuropathy in mice," *Neuropharmacology*, vol. 125, pp. 207–219, 2017.

[48] J. Gertsch, M. Leonti, S. Raduner et al., "Beta-caryophyllene is a dietary cannabinoid," *Proceedings of the National Academy of Sciences*, vol. 105, no. 26, pp. 9099–9104, 2008.

[49] S. J. Ward, M. D. Ramirez, H. Neelakantan, and E. A. Walker, "Cannabidiol prevents the development of cold and mechanical allodynia in paclitaxel-treated female C57Bl6 mice," *Anesthesia and Analgesia*, vol. 113, no. 4, pp. 947–950, 2011.

[50] S. J. Ward, S. D. McAllister, R. Kawamura, R. Murase, H. Neelakantan, and E. A. Walker, "Cannabidiol inhibits paclitaxel-induced neuropathic pain through 5-HT(1A) receptors without diminishing nervous system function or chemotherapy efficacy," *British Journal of Pharmacology*, vol. 171, no. 3, pp. 636–645, 2014.

[51] R. G. Pertwee, "The diverse CB1 and CB2 receptor pharmacology of three plant cannabinoids: delta9-tetrahydrocannabinol, cannabidiol and delta9-tetrahydrocannabivarin," *British Journal of Pharmacology*, vol. 153, no. 2, pp. 199–215, 2008.

[52] L. Deng, W. H. Lee, Z. Xu, A. Makriyannis, and A. G. Hohmann, "Prophylactic treatment with the tricyclic antidepressant desipramine prevents development of paclitaxel-induced neuropathic pain through activation of endogenous analgesic systems," *Pharmacological Research*, vol. 114, pp. 75–89, 2016.

[53] S. S. Parvathy and W. Masocha, "Coadministration of indomethacin and minocycline attenuates established paclitaxel-induced neuropathic thermal hyperalgesia: involvement of cannabinoid CB1 receptors," *Scientific Reports*, vol. 5, no. 1, article 10541, 2015.

[54] L. Guasti, D. Richardson, M. Jhaveri et al., "Minocycline treatment inhibits microglial activation and alters spinal levels of endocannabinoids in a rat model of neuropathic pain," *Molecular Pain*, vol. 5, p. 35, 2009.

[55] H. Guhring, M. Hamza, M. Sergejeva et al., "A role for endocannabinoids in indomethacin-induced spinal antinociception," *European Journal of Pharmacology*, vol. 454, no. 2-3, pp. 153–163, 2002.

[56] A. A. Abu-Ghefreh and W. Masocha, "Enhancement of antinociception by coadministration of minocycline and a non-steroidal anti-inflammatory drug indomethacin in naive mice and murine models of LPS-induced thermal hyperalgesia and monoarthritis," *BMC Musculoskeletal Disorders*, vol. 11, no. 1, p. 276, 2010.

[57] N. Garrido-Mesa, A. Zarzuelo, and J. Galvez, "Minocycline: far beyond an antibiotic," *British Journal of Pharmacology*, vol. 169, no. 2, pp. 337–352, 2013.

[58] S. Nalamachu and R. Wortmann, "Role of indomethacin in acute pain and inflammation management: a review of the literature," *Postgraduate Medicine*, vol. 126, no. 4, pp. 92–97, 2014.

[59] D. R. Pachman, D. L. Barton, J. C. Watson, and C. L. Loprinzi, "Chemotherapy-induced peripheral neuropathy: prevention and treatment," *Clinical Pharmacology and Therapeutics*, vol. 90, no. 3, pp. 377–387, 2011.

[60] R. B. Fillingim, C. D. King, M. C. Ribeiro-Dasilva, B. Rahim-Williams, and J. L. Riley, "Sex, gender, and pain: a review of recent clinical and experimental findings," *Journal of Pain*, vol. 10, no. 5, pp. 447–485, 2009.

[61] J. C. Mapplebeck, S. Beggs, and M. W. Salter, "Sex differences in pain: a tale of two immune cells," *Pain*, vol. 157, no. 1, pp. S2–S6, 2016.

[62] H. Naji-Esfahani, G. Vaseghi, L. Safaeian, A. A. Pilehvarian, A. Abed, and M. Rafieian-Kopaei, "Gender differences in a mouse model of chemotherapy-induced neuropathic pain," *Laboratory Animals*, vol. 50, no. 1, pp. 15–20, 2016.

[63] D. Ruau, L. Y. Liu, J. D. Clark, M. S. Angst, and A. J. Butte, "Sex differences in reported pain across 11,000 patients captured in electronic medical records," *Journal of Pain*, vol. 13, no. 3, pp. 228–234, 2012.

[64] H. B. Bradshaw, N. Rimmerman, J. F. Krey, and J. M. Walker, "Sex and hormonal cycle differences in rat brain levels of pain-related cannabimimetic lipid mediators," *American Journal of Physiology Regulatory, Integrative and Comparative Physiology*, vol. 291, no. 2, pp. R349–R358, 2006.

[65] R. M. Craft, J. A. Marusich, and J. L. Wiley, "Sex differences in cannabinoid pharmacology: a reflection of differences in the endocannabinoid system?," *Life Sciences*, vol. 92, no. 8-9, pp. 476–481, 2013.

[66] J. D. Greenspan, R. M. Craft, L. LeResche et al., "Studying sex and gender differences in pain and analgesia: a consensus report," *Pain*, vol. 132, no. 1, pp. S26–S45, 2007.

16

Working Together and Being Physically Active Are Not Enough to Advise Uniformly and Adequately Low Back Pain Patients: A Cross-Sectional Study

C. Praz,[1] J. Ducki,[1,2] M. L. Connaissa,[1,2] P. Terrier,[1] P. Vuistiner,[1] B. Léger,[1] and F. Luthi[1,3,4]

[1]*Institute for Research in Rehabilitation, Clinique Romande de Réadaptation Suvacare, Avenue Grand-Champsec 90, 1950 Sion, Switzerland*
[2]*Institute of Sports Sciences, University of Lausanne, Géopolis, Campus Dorigny, 1015 Lausanne, Switzerland*
[3]*Department for Musculoskeletal Rehabilitation, Clinique Romande de Réadaptation Suvacare, Avenue Grand-Champsec 90, 1950 Sion, Switzerland*
[4]*Department of Physical Medicine and Rehabilitation, Orthopaedic Hospital, Lausanne University Hospital, Rue du Bugnon 21, 1011 Lausanne, Switzerland*

Correspondence should be addressed to C. Praz; caroline.praz@crr-suva.ch

Academic Editor: Manfred Harth

The profession of the health-care providers (HCPs) influences their recommendations to the patients. Conversely, interdisciplinarity seeks to challenge such differences, so that the patient receives one single and consistent therapeutic message. Some studies also suggest associations between HCPs life habits and recommendations. Our hypotheses were (1) that despite interdisciplinary work, the profession remains a predictor of recommendations and (2) that HCPs who are more physically active recommend more activity. Three clinical vignettes were presented to a group of experts of low back pain (LBP) (guidelines), and 20 physicians, 22 physiotherapists, and 23 nurses to assess how they evaluate the symptoms and pathologies of LBP patients and how much work and physical activity they recommend. Physical activity was assessed with accelerometers and questionnaires. Some interprofessional differences remained present within an interdisciplinary team. The nurses were more restrictive and further away from the guidelines. The physicians were the most in line with them. The physiotherapists recommend as much physical activity, but less work activity than the physicians. The level of physical activity of the HCPs is not associated with their recommendations. To ensure a clear and unique message, educational actions may be undertaken to promote the biopsychosocial model and clarify the guidelines.

1. Introduction

Interdisciplinarity has become a key concept in health care. It allows a comprehensive approach to develop consensual guidelines and recommendations [1]. According to Mitchell et al. [2] five key principles underpin effective team-based care: shared goals, clear roles, mutual trust, effective communication, and measurable processes and outcomes. To be efficient, interdisciplinarity should ensure that the patient gets one single and consistent message through uniform recommendations from all the health-care providers (HCPs) within a team [2, 3]. However, it is still unclear to what extent individual HCPs' characteristics, such as professional background or personal believes, may prejudice the coherence of recommendations. Notably, no one has examined if the interdisciplinary work decreases the interprofessional differences of recommendations.

What is already known is that individual beliefs and life habits may affect attitude and recommendations of HCPs notably regarding low back pain (LBP) [4–10]. Likewise, two studies showed that chiropractors endorse a more biomedical approach than physiotherapists and osteopaths

[4, 11]. Another study demonstrated that physiotherapists, nurses, and physicians have different beliefs about movement and LBP [12]. Concerning life habits, HCPs with a higher level of physical activity (PA) may recommend more activity to their patients [13–17]. Lobelo and deu Qevedo also highlighted the role of the HCPs as models for patients regarding PA [18]. Despite this abundance of evidence of a large influence of individual traits and professional background on recommendations, it is still unclear whether interdisciplinary work tends to equalize recommendations among team members.

Interdisciplinarity is important in LBP care and rehabilitation [19]. LBP is indeed a very highly prevalent condition [20–24]. However, causes, prognosis, and course are often undefined, leading to important variations in clinical practice [25]. Two main treatment orientations are defined: the biomedical orientation that considers that pain is always caused by a lesion and that it may justify disability and the avoidance of activities and the today recommended biopsychosocial model that takes into account biological, psychological, and social factors and promotes early return to activity and work [5, 7, 26–29]. Despite the guidelines, it was reported that many HCPs are still too restrictive and believe that LBP requires some avoidance of activities and to remain off work [5]. Simmonds et al. showed that only 12% of the physiotherapists identify correctly the guidelines, and most of them do not agree with them regarding return to work or activity [30]. To summarize, however, interdisciplinarity is particularly important in LBP care, a high risk of divergence exist among HCPs' recommendations, which deserves further investigation.

Our main objective was to evaluate the coherence of PA recommendations to patients within an interdisciplinary team of physicians, physiotherapists, and nurses. We postulated that if the team worked coordinately, the members of the team should give similar recommendations regardless of the professional background. Conversely, in case of a strong professional group effect, the recommendations could differ despite the interdisciplinary work.

Our secondary objective was to test whether recommendations depended on PA level and personal beliefs. Specifically, the hypotheses were (1) more physically active HCPs would recommend more PA and (2) HCPs that perceived themselves as more active would recommend more PA.

2. Materials and Methods

2.1. Setting. The study included HCPs of the Clinique Romande de Réadaptation, a teaching rehabilitation centre in the French-speaking part of Switzerland. Patients with chronic LBP represent a large proportion of the musculoskeletal patients' population (about 25% of the patients, 250 cases/year). The aim of the administrated therapeutic program (4 to 5 weeks with at least 3 to 4 h of daily therapies excluding weekends) is to manage pain and to improve function, activity, and participation, including return to work (usual or adapted), using a multidisciplinary biopsychosocial approach according to the recommended practice for patients with chronic pain [31].

The rehabilitation centre strongly encourages interdisciplinary work and makes efforts to implement shared goal, clear role for each HCP, mutual trust, effective communication, and measurable processes and outcomes, as advanced by Mitchell et al. [2]. Every week, the HCPs of the different professional groups meet to discuss the cases and plan therapeutic goals according to the ICF framework (taking into account the personal and environmental factors, which could influence the recovery). Additionally, internal trainings common for all the professional groups are organized, including training about the biopsychosocial model and about fear-avoidance beliefs. These trainings take place at least twice a year, and all the HCPs should be familiar with the fear-avoidance and biopsychosocial models [32, 33].

The therapeutic team is mainly composed of physicians, nurses, and physiotherapists. Occupational therapists, education and vocational guidance professionals, and psychologists are also members of the team, but they are far less numerous and were therefore excluded from this study for statistical reasons. During the rehabilitation program, the physicians are responsible for the diagnosis, the prescription of medication and treatment, the coordination of the rehabilitation program, and the follow-up of the patients. The physiotherapists assume the therapeutic training, the functional tests, the reconditioning (strengthening and aerobic exercises), stretching, and manual therapy; they are specialized in the rehabilitation of the musculoskeletal system. The nurses are responsible for the assessment of the biopsychosocial complexity, for the training for self-administrated medication, for counseling for the management of activities of daily living, and upon request for the psychological support and assistance. Moreover, the nurses conduct patients' interviews at the beginning of the rehabilitation program, according to the INTERMED tool, to detect biopsychosocial complexity [34–36].

2.2. Participants. We invited 97 HCPs working in the centre as physicians, physiotherapists, or nurses to participate in the study. Information about the study was given during the weekly teaching team meeting of each professional group. The HCPs who were absent on the day of the meeting were excluded from the study. The participants were informed of the procedures involved in the study and gave written informed consent.

2.3. Design. We conducted a cross-sectional survey in January 2015. The study consisted of clinical vignettes and questionnaires that the HCPs have to fulfil during questionnaire sessions and objective measurements of the PA with accelerometers. The accelerometers were distributed to HCPs between November 2014 and February 2015, according to their availability. The local Research Ethics Committee granted the approval to undertake the study (CCVEM 041/14).

2.4. Primary Outcome: Severity and Recommendations. To assess the effects of the professional discipline and the level of PA performed by the HCPs on their therapeutic advices, the HCPs were asked to evaluate three hypothetical medical cases and to give their recommendations for it.

Three clinical vignettes as described by Rainville et al. [28] were used to assess the beliefs and attitudes of HCPs regarding patients with chronic LBP. The vignettes describe cases with working situation, symptoms, relevant physical findings, results of examinations, and previous treatments. All vignettes suggested LBP with a nonspecific cause. For each vignette, the HCPs were asked to answer four questions on a one to five Likert scale about (1) the severity of the symptoms (from "very mild" to "extremely severe"), (2) the severity of pathology (same scale), (3) the recommendations for the level of activity (from "no activity limitations" to "limit all physical activities") and (4) the recommendations for the work activity (from "full time" to "remain out of work"). Higher scores indicate recommendations that are more restrictive and symptom and pathology perceptions that are more severe. The three vignettes and the corresponding questions were translated into French by a professional translator. Then members of the research team who are fluent in French and English assessed and verified the translation. The outcome of the HCPs was compared with the evaluation and the recommendations of a group of respected experts in the field. This group consisted of twelve specialists of LBP: seven physicians and five physiotherapists from three different medical centres in Switzerland (teaching rehabilitation centres and university hospitals). To be considered as an expert, they had to spend more than 80% of their working time with patients with LBP for at least 10 years and to be referring physicians or physiotherapists for LBP in their institution. The experts answered the four questions about the three vignettes and their average opinion for each item is considered as a guideline to get the best treatment for patients with LBP.

2.5. Variables with Potential Effect on the Recommendations. Six different self-administrated questionnaires were completed by the HCPs to assess some variables with a potential effect on the evaluation and recommendations of the clinical vignettes.

2.5.1. Sociodemographic. Demographic data were collected which included age, gender, working discipline, working experience, training in LBP, and LBP history (present or previous).

2.5.2. Activity Pattern. The Pattern of Activity Measure (POAM-P) is usually administered to assess the activity pattern in chronic pain patients [37]. POAM-P allows the identification of three different activity patterns: "avoidance," "pacing," and "overdoing." We used the validated French version of the POAM-P [38]. Since this questionnaire has been designed for chronic pain patients, we modified the instructions asking the HCPs to imagine themselves suffering of chronic LBP. The questionnaire is composed of 30 items, 10 items for each pattern. For each item, the participants were asked to describe the extent to which the selected item describes how they would perform their activity. A Likert scale was used, ranging from zero "not at all" to four "all the time." For each pattern of behaviour, a score from 0 to 40 was obtained. A higher score indicated that the participant would be more likely to use the considered activity pattern.

2.5.3. Pain-Related Fear of Movement. The Tampa Scale for Kinesiophobia (TSK) was originally designed to evaluate the fear of movement and/or (re)injury in patients with LBP [39]. The TSK is composed of 17 items. Each item is rated on a four points Likert scale ranging from one, "strongly disagree," to four, "strongly agree." Overall score lies between 17 and 68 [40, 41]. A higher score indicates a higher level of kinesiophobia. Houben et al. adapted the questionnaire for HCPs by changing the instructions to determine to what extent HCPs believe that movement and PA are harmful for their LBP patients [4].

2.5.4. Treatment Orientation. The Health Care Providers' Pain and Impairment Relationship Scale (HC-PAIRS) is a questionnaire that estimates the attitudes and beliefs of HCPs about functional expectations for chronic LBP patients [42]. The HC-PAIRS consists of 15 statements about the functional expectations for patients with chronic back pain. Each statement is evaluated on a seven point Likert scale, from one, "totally disagree," to seven, "totally agree," on which the HCPs marked their level of agreement with that statement. By summing the results of the 15 items, we got a score from 15 to 105. Higher scores suggested that the HCP has a more biomedical approach of LBP and is more likely to agree with the fact that back pain necessitates the avoidance of activities and justifies disability. In contrast, lower scores are linked with a more biopsychosocial approach. This questionnaire was send afterward by email.

2.5.5. Anxiety and Depression Symptoms. The HCPs completed the validated French version of the Hospital Anxiety and Depression Scale (HADS) [43, 44] to measure their tendency to be anxious and depressed. This self-administrated questionnaire was originally designed for hospitalized patients but has been also validated for the general population [45]. The HADS is composed from two subscales: one for anxiety symptoms and one for depression symptoms. Each subscale includes seven items and each item is rated on a zero to three Likert scale. Therefore, the subscores for both anxiety and depression are ranging from 0 to 21. Higher scores indicate more anxious/depressive symptoms. There is evidence of a relationship between the HADS scores and the patient's pain chronification [46].

2.5.6. Intolerance of Uncertainty. The Intolerance of Uncertainty Scale (IUS) is a 27-item questionnaire used to assess the belief that uncertainty is unacceptable and leads to frustration, stress, and the inability to take action [47]. Each item is evaluated on a one to five scale from 1, "not at all characteristic of me," to 5, "entirely characteristic of me."

It results with scores between 27 and 135. Higher scores represent greater intolerance of uncertainty (IU). Simmonds et al. has demonstrated a positive association between IU and biomedical orientation [30].

2.6. Perceived and Objective Physical Activity Level. We used questionnaires and accelerometers to evaluate the PA level.

2.6.1. Self-Reported Physical Activity. To assess the HCPs' habitual PA, the Baecke habitual physical activity questionnaire [48] was completed. It is a brief questionnaire of 16 items, translated and validated in French [49]. It consists of three sections assessing, respectively, the PA at work (work index), at sport (sport index), and during leisure time, excluding sport (leisure time index). Every domain results in a separate subscore, and the overall score is calculated by averaging the three subscores. The results are given in metabolic equivalent of task (METs) [50]. This measure is subjective and represents the perceived PA of the participant.

2.6.2. Objective Physical Activity. The participants' objective PA level was assessed during a normal working week, from Tuesday to the following Sunday (six consecutive days). The PA was measured with a validated three-axis microelectromechanical system (MEMS) accelerometer, the ActiGraph wGT3X-BT (ActiGraph, Pensacola, USA). The ActigGraph recorded body accelerations continuously (sampling rate: 50 Hz). The sensor is a small and light box (19 g) attached on an elastic belt, and that should be worn on the left hip. Participants were instructed to wear the device during waking hours, from awakening to bedtime to measure their habitual PA. The accelerometer detected when and how much the HCPs were walking. The number of steps per day was calculated and considered as a marker of the HCP's PA [51].

For the analysis, the days with less than 12 h of acceleration data were discarded. We also discarded rest days, according to the working schedule of each participant. The Matlab software (Mathworks, Natick, MA, USA) was used for data analysis. An algorithm specifically recognized walking through signal amplitude and frequency pattern and computed the average number of steps per day performed by the subjects [52]. The number of steps is deduced from the duration of each walking bouts and the cadence (i.e., average number of steps per second). Total daily number of steps is the sum across all the walking bouts. The average number of daily steps per day over the week is finally computed.

2.7. Potential Bias. Different measures were taken to avoid or evaluate the bias that could interfere. Firstly, all the HCPs of the same professional group answered the questionnaires on the same day during the same weekly meeting to avoid contamination of the data by discussions and mutual influence. Secondly, we assessed social desirability that is the tendency of the respondents to answer questions in a manner that will be viewed favorably by others. Social desirability was used to evaluate to what extent it was possible to rely on the answers as a reflection of the real behaviour of the HCPs. The Marlowe–Crowne Social Desirability Scale (MC-SDS) measures the inclination to respond in a socially desirable way [53]. The MC-SDS questionnaire consisted of 33 statements to which participants were asked to answer "true" (one point) or "false" (zero point). It results in a score from 1 to 33. Scores ≥ 20 indicate a high social desirability. This questionnaire allows assessing the validity of the scores calculated for all the other self-administered questionnaires.

2.8. Data Analysis. Data were analysed using Stata 13.1 (StataCorp, College Station, TX, USA). For each variable, the means (M) and standard deviations (SD) were calculated for the three professional groups and for all the HCPs. Analysis of variance (ANOVA) followed by post hoc Scheffe multiple-comparison tests (for continuous data) and chi-squared tests (for categorical data) was performed to measure the associations between the professional groups and the different variables. In addition, η^2 was used as an effect size measure, as it can be interpreted as the proportion of variance in the dependent variable that is attributable to the professional groups. The significance level was set at $p < 0.05$.

The mean responses of the experts were considered as the guideline. For each HCP, the discrepancies between their answers and the guideline were expressed with the bias (raw difference between the answer of the HCP and the guideline) and the intraclass correlation coefficient (ICC) calculated with Shrout and Fleiss form 2.1 [54]. Bias was calculated for the average of the three questions (one for each vignette) about severity of symptoms ($bias_{sev\text{-}sympt}$), for the average of the three questions about severity of pathology ($bias_{sev\text{-}patho}$), for the average of the three questions about recommendations for daily PA ($bias_{rec\text{-}act}$), and for the average of the three questions about recommendations for work ($bias_{rec\text{-}work}$). ICC was calculated for the average of the six questions about severity (two for each vignette) (ICC_{sev}) and for the average of the six questions about the recommendations (ICC_{rec}). We did not calculate the ICC for each of the four subscales separately because the number of items was not sufficient to get statistically significant ICC values.

For the PA (objective and perceived), the Pearson correlations between the subscores on Baecke (perceived) and the number of steps per day (objective) and the evaluation of severity and the recommendations were also determined independently of the professional groups.

3. Results

3.1. Response Rate. Ninety-seven HCPs were invited to participate during their weekly team meetings. Seventy-two HCPs gave written informed consent, which results in an overall inclusion rate of 74%. Seven HCPs were excluded due to incomplete data. Finally, 65 HCPs were considered for the analysis: 20 physicians, 22 physiotherapists, and 23 nurses. The HC-PAIRS, which was sent afterward, was answered by 56 HCPs only (14 physicians, 19 physiotherapists, and 22 nurses).

3.2. Subjects' Characteristics. The main anthropometric and professional characteristics of the subjects are summarised in Table 1. The majority of the physiotherapists and nurses

Table 1: Characteristics of the professional groups (mean and SD or proportion of each group).

	Physicians ($n = 20$)	Physiotherapists ($n = 22$)	Nurses ($n = 23$)	Total sample ($n = 65$)
Age (years)	44 (10)	36 (11)	34 (11)	38 (11)
Men/women	12/8	7/15	7/16	26/39
BMI ($kg{\cdot}m^{-2}$)	25 (4)	23 (3)	22 (2)	23 (3)
Working experience (years)	17 (10)	13 (11)	10 (9)	13 (10)
Proportion of HCPs with special training for LBP	85%	73%	22%	58%
Proportion of HCPs with special training for pain	90%	45%	35%	55%
Proportion of HCPs with previous experience of LBP	60%	32%	65%	52%
Proportion of HCPs with current LBP	10%	9%	30%	17%

BMI: body mass index. HCP: health care providers. LBP: low back pain.

Table 2: Answers for the group of experts (mean and SD, $n = 12$). The severity was evaluated on a one to four Likert scale from "very mild" to "extremely severe" and the recommendations also on a one to four Likert scale from "no limitation" to "limit all PA" (level of activity) and from "full time" to "remain out of work" (level of work).

	Vignette 1	Vignette 2	Vignette 3
Severity of the symptoms	3.8 (1.0)	2.4 (0.7)	3.3 (0.5)
Severity of the pathology	2.0 (0.9)	2.0 (0.6)	2.0 (1.0)
Recommendations for the level of activity	1.9 (0.9)	1.4 (0.7)	1.5 (0.9)
Recommendations for the level of work	2.9 (0.5)	2.3 (0.8)	2.5 (1.2)

were women (68% and 70%), while only 40% of the physicians were women. However, this difference was not significant ($p = 0.09$). The physicians tend to be older than the nurses (significant Scheffé's post hoc comparison). A large majority of the physicians have a special training external to the medical centre for LBP and/or pain (85% for LBP and 90% for pain). It is less the case for physiotherapists (73% and 45%) and it is much less common for nurses (22% and 35% resp.) (significant difference between the professions ($p < 0.01$)).

Body mass index (BMI) was not significantly different among the professional disciplines. No significant interprofessional difference was found for the number of years of working experience and the prior and current LBP experience.

3.3. Responses of the Experts. The group of experts answered the four questions about the three clinical vignettes. Table 2 presents the average scores of the 12 experts.

3.4. Primary Outcome: Comparison of the Evaluation and Recommendations between Professional Groups and Discrepancies with the Experts. Overall, the total variance explained by professions was moderate (20%–30%, η^2, Table 3). The highest between-group difference was found for work recommendation ($\eta^2 = 0.3$).

The physicians evaluated the overall severity as less severe than physiotherapists and nurses. A more detailed analysis showed that the difference between the physiotherapists and the physicians was not significant for the severity of symptoms but was significant for the severity of the pathology, while the differences between the nurses and the physicians were significant for the severity of the symptoms and for the severity of the pathology.

In average, the nurses recommended less activity (daily and work activity) than the physicians and the physiotherapists. Concerning PA recommendations, nurses recommended significantly less daily PA than the physicians and the physiotherapists. Concerning work recommendations, the physicians recommended more work than the nurses and the physiotherapists.

The answers of the HCPs were compared with the experts. The bias and the ICC are presented in Table 3. Differences between professions were observed on $bias_{sev\text{-}symp}$ (physicians significantly different from nurses), on $bias_{seve\text{-}patho}$ (physicians significantly different from physiotherapists and nurses), on $bias_{rec\text{-}act}$ (nurses significantly different from physicians and physiotherapists), and on $bias_{rec\text{-}work}$ (physicians significantly different from physiotherapists and from nurses). ICC_{rec} tended to be different ($p = 0.05$) across the professional groups, while ICC_{sev} was not different ($p = 0.24$).

3.5. Variables Potentially Associated with the Recommendations. The main scores of the questionnaires are summarised in Table 4.

There were significant differences across the three professional groups for the POAM-P (avoidance score), the TSK, the HC-PAIRS, the HADS (both anxiety and depression), and the IUS.

Nurses have a greater tendency to think that they would avoid activity if they suffered from LBP. For the pacing and overdoing subscores, no significant difference was found between the three groups.

The TSK score was also significantly different between the professions ($p \leq 0.01$). The belief that movement and PA are harmful for LBP patients was more developed by nurses. They were significantly more afraid of movement and (re)injury for their patients than physicians and physiotherapists.

The HC-PAIRS score indicated significant differences between the professions in the treatment orientation ($p \leq 0.01$). The nurses had the most biomedical approach

Table 3: Mean differences between HCPs and guidelines for the average answers of the three vignettes.

	Physicians (PY), M (SD) (n = 20)	Physiotherapists (PT), M (SD) (n = 22)	Nurses (NU), M (SD) (n = 23)	Overall, M (SD) (n = 65)	F (2.62)	p	η^2	Post hoc Scheffé
$Bias_{sev\text{-}sympt}$	−0.9 (1.6)	0.2 (1.7)	1.0 (1.7)	0.1 (1.8)	6.95	<0.01*	0.2 (0.03; 0.3)	NU > PY
$Bias_{sev\text{-}patho}$	0.5 (1.4)	2.2 (1.6)	1.8 (2.0)	1.5 (1.8)	6.27	<0.01*	0.2 (0.02; 0.3)	PT, NU > PY
$Bias_{rec\text{-}act}$	1.2 (2.2)	1.9 (2.3)	4.1 (2.1)	2.5 (2.5)	10.05	<0.01*	0.2 (0.1;0.4)	NU > PT, PY
$Bias_{rec\text{-}work}$	0.2 (1.6)	1.9 (2.1)	2.6 (1.8)	1.6 (2.1)	9.30	<0.01*	0.3 (0.1;0.4)	PT, NU > PY
ICC_{sev}	0.57 (0.25)	0.50 (0.23)	0.46 (0.15)	0.51 (0.21)	1.45	0.24	0.04 (0;0.2)	—
ICC_{rec}	0.45 (0.30)	0.42 (0.27)	0.26 (0.22)	0.37 (0.27)	3.13	0.05	0.1 (0;0.2)	—

$p < 0.05$ indicates that there was a significant difference between the groups and is labelled with a*. A bias <0 means that the HCPs evaluated the symptoms or the pathology as less severe or recommended more activity or work than the experts. An ICC nearest of 1 means a higher adequacy with the group of experts. The column post hoc Scheffé indicates all the significant differences between two groups.

Table 4: Scores on the questionnaires for the three professional groups and all the subjects (mean ± SD).

Questionnaires		Physicians (PY), M (SD) (n = 20)	Physiotherapists (PT), M (SD) (n = 22)	Nurses (NU), M (SD) (n = 23)	Overall, M (SD) (n = 65)	p	F	η^2	Post hoc Scheffé
POAM-P	Avoidance	17 (9)	18 (7)	22 (6)	19 (8)	(2.62) 3.30	0.04*	0.1 (0;0.2)	—
	Pacing	24 (10)	26 (9)	22 (8)	24 (9)	(2.62) 0.66	0.52	0.02 (0;0.1)	—
	Overdoing	26 (7)	24 (6)	24 (7)	24 (7)	(2.62) 1.03	0.37	0.03 (0;0.1)	—
TSK		31 (6)	34 (7)	40 (5)	35 (7)	(2.62) 12.99	<0.01*	0.3 (0.1;0.4)	NU > PY, PT
HC-PAIRS		52 (7) (n = 14)	57 (8) (n = 19)	65 (9) (n = 22)	59 (10) (n = 56)	(2.51) 11.98	<0.01*	0.3 (0.1;0.5)	NU > PY, PT
HADS	Anxiety	6 (2)	5 (2)	8 (3)	6 (2)	(2.62) 4.35	0.02*	0.1 (0.002; 0.3)	NU > PT
	Depression	2 (2)	2 (2)	4 (2)	3 (2)	(2.62) 4.20	0.02*	0.1 (0.004; 0.3)	NU > PT
IUS		45 (12)	42 (8)	52 (14)	47 (12)	(2.62) 3.71	0.03*	0.1 (0;0.2)	NU > PY
MC-SDS		19 (5)	19 (4)	20 (4)	20 (4)	(2.62) 0.38	0.68	0.01 (0;0.1)	—

p value < 0.05 is labelled with a* which indicates that there was a significant difference between the three professional groups. The column post hoc Scheffé indicates all the significant differences between two groups.

(65 (9)), whereas the physicians the less biomedical approach (52 (7)); the physiotherapists were in between. The HC-PAIRS scores of nurses were significantly higher than those of the physicians and the physiotherapists.

HADS scores were significantly different between the professional groups ($p = 0.02$ for both anxiety and depression). Nurses showed the most anxious and depressive symptoms while the opposite was observed for the physiotherapists.

For the IU, the mean score was 47 (12) with a significant difference between the professional groups ($p = 0.03$). The nurses tended to be the most intolerant to uncertainty (51 (14)), significantly more than physicians. The scores of the physiotherapists were once again in between.

3.6. *Secondary Outcomes: Perceived and Objective Physical Activity Level*

3.6.1. Self-Reported Physical Activity. The HCPs' mean activity level assessed with the Baecke questionnaire (Table 5) was 3.1 ± 0.4 METs, which is considered as moderate (from 3 to 4.9 METs [50], physician's subscore for the work index was the only one classified as low (2.2 (0.4)). Physician's score was significantly lower than the score of the physiotherapists and the nurses. Nurses had the lowest sport and leisure time indexes when compared to physiotherapists and physicians, respectively.

Independently of the professional group, the work index was significantly correlated with the global evaluation of severity of symptoms and pathology ($r = 0.34$, $p < 0.01$) and with the recommendations for work and daily activity ($r = 0.47$, $p < 0.01$). The HCPs who considered themselves as less active at work are those who considered the severity as lower and who recommended more activity.

3.6.2. Objective Physical Activity. Table 5 compares the number of steps per working day of the different professional groups. According to Tudor-Locke et al., 10,000 steps per day is a reasonable target for a healthy lifestyle for adults [51]. On average, the HCPs did not reach the target (7,812 (2,699)). The difference between the groups was significant ($p < 0.01$). The physiotherapists were the most

Table 5: Perceived PA and objective PA for the three professional groups and all the HCPs (mean ± SD): scores on the Baecke and number of steps per day during working days and days off.

	Physicians (PY), M (SD) $n = 20$	Physiotherapists (PT), M (SD) $n = 22$	Nurses (NU), M (SD) $n = 23$	Overall, M (SD) $n = 65$	F (2.62)	p	η^2	Post hoc Scheffé
Work index	2.2 (0.4)	3.4 (0.3)	3.6 (0.6)	3.1 (0.8)	51.67	<0.01*	0.6 (0.5;0.7)	PT, NU > PY
Sport index	3.3 (0.7)	3.5 (0.5)	2.9 (0.7)	3.2 (0.7)	5.34	0.01*	0.1 (0.01; 0.3)	PT > NU
Leisure activity index	3.3 (0.4)	3.1 (0.6)	2.9 (0.5)	3.1 (0.5)	4.23	0.02*	0.1 (0;0.3)	PY > NU
Baecke overall	2.9 (0.3)	3.3 (0.3)	3.1 (0.3)	3.1 (0.4)	9.73	<0.01*	0.2 (0;0.4)	PT > PY, NU
Steps/day (working day)	6,153 (1,884)	8,951 (2,885)	8,197 (2,313)	7,812 (2,699)	13.60	<0.01*	0.3 (0.1;0.4)	PT, NU > PY

p value <0.05 is labelled with a* which indicates that there was a significant difference between the three professional groups. The column post hoc Scheffé indicates all the significant differences between two groups.

active during working days. The physicians walked significantly less than physiotherapists and nurses.

Independently of the professional group, no significant relationship was found between the number of steps per day and the evaluation and recommendations for the clinical vignettes.

3.7. Social Desirability. The mean score on MC-SDS was 19.2 ± 4.3 with no significant difference between the professional groups (Table 4). The cut-off score that define a high social desirability is set at 20. 32 subjects (49%) reached scores over the cut-off.

4. Discussion

4.1. Key Results (Primary Outcome). We aimed at investigating the influence of the profession on the recommendations given to the LBP patients within an interdisciplinary team. Our results suggest that despite interdisciplinary team working, each profession keeps its own beliefs and attitudes. Physicians thus considered symptoms and pathology as less severe than the other professions and were more in line with guidelines. Conversely, nurses diverged substantially from guidelines. In fact, they recommended more limitation of work and PA. Physiotherapists ranged generally between the two other groups; their recommendations for PA were similar to physicians' recommendations, whereas their recommendations for work were closer to those of the nurses.

4.2. Interpretations of the Interprofessional Difference. We observed a strong influence of professional background on recommendations and beliefs. HCPs that were less in accordance with the guidelines and gave more restrictive PA and work recommendations (i.e., nurses) had the following characteristics: (1) they had a more biomedical approach; (2) they were more likely to behave with an "avoidance" pattern; (3) they were more kinesiophobic and (4) intolerant to uncertainty, and (5) they had more anxious and depressive symptoms.

Generally, our results are consistent with previous studies. Houben and colleagues have noted an association between the TSK score, the HC-PAIRS score, and the recommendations for the clinical vignettes [4, 10]. Likewise, an association between the subscore "avoidance" (POAM-P) and the TSK score has been observed, but only for patients so far [37]. Simmonds et al. have shown that the greatest IU is associated with a more biomedical approach and more developed anxious symptoms [30, 55, 56]. All of these factors seem to influence each other and to have an effect on the recommendations.

The nurses diverged substantially from the experts (Table 3). They tended to recommend less activity than other HCPs. Nurses' beliefs (Table 4) confirmed a trend toward more fear of movement and a more biomedical approach. Paradoxically, in our institution, nurses follow regular training on the biopsychosocial model and play an important role to determine patients' biopsychosocial complexity. Differences between nurses' recommendations and the guidelines are especially concerning because their role is of prime importance in health care [57]. Unfortunately, their recommendations and believes were often neglected so far. The lack of basic training and knowledge may be a reason for the discrepancy with the guidelines. Dermody et al. showed that young nurses perceived that they lack knowledge and training to safely mobilize hospitalized patients [58]. In our sample, the nurses were the HCPs, who have less formalized professional training on LBP and chronic pain in general (Table 1). This may be related to our clinic or more likely to the Swiss health care system, which has only recently developed such special trainings available for nurses (e.g., certificate of advanced studies). Accordingly, nurses should benefit from more training about chronic pain during their basic training and afterward.

The physiotherapists were often between nurses and physicians regarding attitudes and beliefs. Concerning recommendations, the relevant differences with the physicians were for the severity of pathology, and the recommendations for work, physiotherapists were more restrictive than physicians. This may be because the physicians are especially trained to diagnose pathologies and to certificate medical leave [59]. Conversely, the physiotherapists' training on LBP and chronic pain is often more focused on biomedical approach (e.g., manual therapy) than on exercise therapy and on the biopsychosocial approach although the biopsychosocial approach is also part of their training and profession. Moreover Simmonds et al. demonstrated that only 12% of the physiotherapists identified correctly the guidelines, while Mikhail et al. showed that even when they were aware of recommendations, they did not necessarily implement them [30, 60].

The physicians were more in line with the experts. Thus, they evaluated the symptoms and the pathology as less severe than the other professions and recommended a higher level of activity and work. A possible explanation could be that physicians are generally well trained in pain and LBP management (Table 1). In addition, physicians exhibit greater specialization in the return to work process. Physicians' educational background in rehabilitation medicine favors a biopsychosocial orientation [61]. The physicians spend also less time with the patients (about once a week) than physiotherapists (several times a week) and nurses (extended period every day). Thus, the physiotherapists and especially the nurses may consider they have a supportive role to play, which may lead them to be less pushy and rigorous.

These results highlight the necessity to improve the educational background of HCPs that play a key role with the patients.

4.3. Additional Results (Secondary Outcome): Perceived and Objective Physical Activity Level. The hypothesis that more active HCPs would recommend more PA for their patients is not supported by the results. On the contrary, we observed that the less active HCPs (i.e., physicians) recommend more PA. Physician's worktime is mostly dedicated to patients' examination and administrative work, which is not conductive for a high PA level. Likewise, physiotherapists' engagement in physical therapies makes them the most active professional group, but they do not recommend the most PA. So it is probably an effect of the profession rather than a real association between low PA level and more activity is recommended. Furthermore, Baecke's work index was negatively correlated with the recommendations. In other words, concerning PA recommendations, professional background seems dominate over personal PA practice. Previous studies suggested a possible effect of the perceived PA on the recommendations [18]. By using both subjective and objective PA measures, we cannot confirm that physically active HCPs are more likely to provide PA counseling to their patients and can indeed be PA role models.

4.4. Strengths of the Study. The originality of our study resides in the inclusion of a group of experts to establish valid answers according to the guidelines. The main advantage was that the experts gave their opinion about practical cases that can be directly compared with those of the HCPs.

The assessment of both perceived and objective PA is another strength of the study; in this way, the different facets of PA that may affect the recommendations were measured.

Through the MC-SDS questionnaire, we take into account social desirability. The MC-SDS scores are moderate. Therefore, the other questionnaires probably reflect the real beliefs and attitudes of the HCPs. Importantly, the MC-SDS scores were not significantly different among the three professional groups. Between-group comparisons were thus not biased.

4.5. Limitations of the Study. A limitation of our study is that we did not observe the actual HCP's professional practice and behaviour. We only relied on their subjective opinion facing hypothetical cases (vignettes) and situations (questionnaires).

The limited sample size is also a limitation. As we want to compare all HCP working within the same team, it is rather difficult to include larger sample size.

Another limitation may come from the selection of the experts. The fact that the experts were either physicians or physiotherapists may limit the interpretation of the differences observed between the nurses and the others professional groups.

The use of the number of steps to assess PA is also limitation because it neglects sport activities, in particular cycling, strength training, or swimming. Additionally, it would be interesting to assess the PA during days off to have a more global view of the PA with more leisure time.

Finally, our study was conducted in a teaching centre, whose characteristics might not be comparable to other settings. Further studies are necessary to verify the external validity of our findings.

5. Conclusion and Perspectives

Our main finding is that, despite working together and sharing similar regular teaching meetings, HCPs deliver recommendations that substantially differ according to their professions. With that in mind, efforts should be made to harmonize the beliefs, attitudes, and recommendations. These efforts should be especially directed to the nurses and physiotherapists whose approach of pain and treatments is more biomedical and further from the guidelines. In our opinion, a better anchoring of the biopsychosocial model must be obtained through a focused training of the new HCPs and dedicated information to medical centres. The importance of training was highlighted by Kennedy et al. who showed that the beliefs of students in medicine and physiotherapy are closer to the guideline at the end of their studies compared to the beginning [12]. Furthermore, even a short training about the biopsychosocial model may already change the treatment orientation of physiotherapists [6, 8, 12, 62]. In our centre, HCPs follows regular theoretical trainings about the biopsychosocial and fear-avoidance models. It may be more profitable to integrate practical training, with discussions of real cases or vignettes. These trainings should also preferably mix the professions to encourage the HCPs to discuss the cases and the recommendations together. Additionally, it would be interesting thereafter to test whether such trainings are translated into the real-life practice and may improve patients' outcomes.

Acknowledgments

This study was supported by a gift from the Loterie Romande. The authors would like to thank the head and the staff of the Clinique romande de réadaptation for their support and participation, the LBP experts of the Hôpitaux Universitaires de Genève (HUG), the Centre Hospitalier Universitaire Vaudois, and the Rehaklink Bellikon, and Roger Hilifiker for his editing work on the manuscript.

References

[1] B. C. Choi and A. W. Pak, "Multidisciplinarity, interdisciplinarity and transdisciplinarity in health research, services, education and policy: 1. Definitions, objectives, and evidence of effectiveness," *Clinical and Investigative Medicine Medecine Clinique et Experimentale*, vol. 29, no. 6, pp. 351–364, 2006.

[2] P. Mitchell, M. Wynia, R. Golden et al., *Core Principles & Values of Effective Team-Based Health Care*, Institute of Medicine, Washington, DC, 2012.

[3] B. C. Choi and A. W. Pak, "Multidisciplinarity, interdisciplinarity, and transdisciplinarity in health research, services, education and policy: 2. Promotors, barriers, and strategies of enhancement," *Clinical and Investigative Medicine Medecine Clinique et Experimentale*, vol. 30, no. 6, pp. E224–E232, 2007.

[4] R. M. A. Houben, R. W. J. G. Ostelo, J. W. S. Vlaeyen, P. M. J. C. Wolters, M. Peters, and S. G. M. Stomp-van Berg, "Health care providers' orientations towards common low back pain predict perceived harmfulness of physical activities and recommendations regarding return to normal activity," *European Journal of Pain*, vol. 9, pp. 173–183, 2005.

[5] A. Bishop, N. E. Foster, E. Thomas, and E. M. Hay, "How does the self-reported clinical management of patients with low back pain relate to the attitudes and beliefs of health care practitioners? A survey of UK general practitioners and physiotherapists," *Pain*, vol. 135, no. 1, pp. 187–195, 2008.

[6] C. M. Jacobs, B. J. Guildford, W. Travers, M. Davies, and L. M. McCracken, "Brief psychologically informed physiotherapy training is associated with changes in physiotherapists' attitudes and beliefs towards working with people with chronic pain," *British Journal of Pain*, vol. 10, no. 1, pp. 38–45, 2016.

[7] T. Gardner, K. Refshauge, L. Smith, J. McAuley, M. Hubscher, and S. Goodall, "Physiotherapists' beliefs and attitudes influence clinical practice in chronic low back pain: a systematic review of quantitative and qualitative studies," *Journal of Physiotherapy*, vol. 63, no. 3, pp. 132–143, 2017.

[8] A. M. Briggs, H. Slater, A. J. Smith, G. F. Parkin-Smith, K. Watkins, and J. Chua, "Low back pain-related beliefs and likely practice behaviours among final-year cross-discipline health students," *European Journal of Pain*, vol. 17, no. 5, pp. 766–775, 2013.

[9] M.-A. L. E. Laekeman, H. Sitter, and H. D. Basler, "The pain attitudes and beliefs scale for physiotherapists: psychometric properties of the German version," *Clinical Rehabilitation*, vol. 22, no. 6, pp. 564–575, 2008.

[10] R. M. Houben, J. W. Vlaeyen, M. Peters, R. W. Ostelo, P. M. Wolters, and S. G. Stomp-van den Berg, "Health care providers' attitudes and beliefs towards common low back pain: factor structure and psychometric properties of the HC-PAIRS," *Clinical Journal of Pain*, vol. 20, no. 1, pp. 37–44, 2004.

[11] T. Pincus, N. E. Foster, S. Vogel, R. Santos, A. Breen, and M. Underwood, "Attitudes to back pain amongst musculoskeletal practitioners: a comparison of professional groups and practice settings using the ABS-mp," *Manual Therapy*, vol. 12, no. 2, pp. 167–175, 2007.

[12] N. Kennedy, J. Healy, and K. O'Sullivan, "The beliefs of third-level healthcare students towards low-back pain," *Pain Research and Treatment*, vol. 2014, Article ID 675915, 5 pages, 2014.

[13] E. Frank, "Physician health and patient care," *Journal of the American Medical Association*, vol. 291, no. 5, p. 637, 2004.

[14] A. M. Araya, S. F. Leal, G. P. Huerta, A. N. Fernandez, O. G. Fernandez, and E. J. Millones, "[The influence of smoking habits of Chilean physicians on the use of the structured medical advice about smoking]," *Revista Medica De Chile*, vol. 140, pp. 347–352, 2012.

[15] Y. Dresner, E. Frank, T. Baevsky, E. Rotman, and S. Vinker, "Screening practices of Israeli doctors' and their patients," *Preventive Medicine*, vol. 50, no. 5-6, pp. 300–303, 2010.

[16] S. N. Bleich, S. Bandara, W. L. Bennett, L. A. Cooper, and K. A. Gudzune, "Impact of non-physician health professionals' BMI on obesity care and beliefs," *Obesity*, vol. 22, no. 12, pp. 2476–2480, 2014.

[17] S. N. Bleich, W. L. Bennett, K. A. Gudzune, and L. A. Cooper, "Impact of physician BMI on obesity care and beliefs," *Obesity*, vol. 20, no. 5, pp. 999–1005, 2012.

[18] F. Lobelo and I. G. deu Qevedo, "The evidence in support of physicians and health care providers as physical activity role models," *American Journal of Lifestyle Medicine*, vol. 10, no. 1, pp. 36–52, 2014.

[19] T. J. Marin, D. Van Eerd, E. Irvin et al., "Multidisciplinary biopsychosocial rehabilitation for subacute low back pain," *Cochrane Database of Systematic Reviews*, vol. 6, article CD002193, 2017.

[20] A. M. Briggs and R. Buchbinder, "Back pain: a national health priority area in Australia?," *Medical Journal of Australia*, vol. 190, no. 9, pp. 499–502, 2009.

[21] J. W. Frymoyer and W. L. Cats-Baril, "An overview of the incidences and costs of low back pain," *Orthopedic Clinics of North America*, vol. 22, no. 2, pp. 263–271, 1991.

[22] J. W. Frymoyer, "Back pain and sciatica," *New England Journal of Medicine*, vol. 318, no. 5, pp. 291–300, 1988.

[23] B. F. Walker, "The prevalence of low back pain: a systematic review of the literature from 1966 to 1998," *Journal of Spinal Disorders*, vol. 13, no. 3, pp. 205–217, 2000.

[24] S. Wieser, B. Horisberger, S. Schmidhauser et al., "Cost of low back pain in Switzerland in 2005," *European Journal of Health Economics*, vol. 12, no. 5, pp. 455–467, 2011.

[25] C. da, C. L. Menezes, C. G. Maher et al., "The prognosis of acute and persistent low-back pain: a meta-analysis," *Canadian Medical Association Journal*, vol. 184, no. 11, pp. E613–E624, 2012.

[26] T. Derghazarian and M. J. Simmonds, "Management of low back pain by physical therapists in Quebec: how are we doing?," *Physiotherapy Canada Physiotherapie Canada*, vol. 63, no. 4, pp. 464–473, 2011.

[27] R. J. Gatchel, Y. B. Peng, M. L. Peters, P. N. Fuchs, and D. C. Turk, "The biopsychosocial approach to chronic pain: scientific advances and future directions," *Psychological Bulletin*, vol. 133, no. 4, pp. 581–624, 2007.

[28] J. Rainville, N. Carlson, P. Polatin, R. J. Gatchel, and A. Indahl, "Exploration of physicians' recommendations for activities in

chronic low back pain," *Spine*, vol. 25, no. 17, pp. 2210–2220, 2000.
[29] A. Delitto, S. Z. George, L. R. Van Dillen et al., "Orthopaedic section of the American physical therapy a low back pain," *Journal of Orthopaedic and Sports Physical Therapy*, vol. 42, no. 4, pp. A1–A57, 2012.
[30] M. J. Simmonds, T. Derghazarian, and J. W. Vlaeyen, "Physiotherapists' knowledge, attitudes, and intolerance of uncertainty influence decision making in low back pain," *Clinical Journal of Pain*, vol. 28, no. 6, pp. 467–474, 2012.
[31] S. J. Kamper, A. T. Apeldoorn, A. Chiarotto et al., "Multidisciplinary biopsychosocial rehabilitation for chronic low back pain: cochrane systematic review and meta-analysis," *BMJ*, vol. 350, no. 5, p. h444, 2015.
[32] J. Lethem, P. D. Slade, J. D. Troup, and G. Bentley, "Outline of a fear-avoidance model of exaggerated pain perception–I," *Behaviour Research and Therapy*, vol. 21, no. 4, pp. 401–408, 1983.
[33] J. W. Vlaeyen and S. J. Linton, "Fear-avoidance and its consequences in chronic musculoskeletal pain: a state of the art," *Pain*, vol. 85, no. 3, pp. 317–332, 2000.
[34] F. J. Huyse, J. S. Lyons, F. C. Stiefel et al., ""INTERMED": a method to assess health service needs. I. Development and reliability," *General Hospital Psychiatry*, vol. 21, no. 1, pp. 39–48, 1999.
[35] F. C. Stiefel, P. de Jonge, F. J. Huyse et al., ""INTERMED": a method to assess health service needs. II. Results on its validity and clinical use," *General Hospital Psychiatry*, vol. 21, no. 1, pp. 49–56, 1999.
[36] F. C. Stiefel, P. de Jonge, F. J. Huyse et al., "INTERMED—an assessment and classification system for case complexity. Results in patients with low back pain," *Spine*, vol. 24, no. 4, pp. 378–384, 1999.
[37] D. Cane, W. R. Nielson, M. McCarthy, and D. Mazmanian, "Pain-related activity patterns: measurement, interrelationships, and associations with psychosocial functioning," *Clinical Journal of Pain*, vol. 29, no. 5, pp. 435–442, 2013.
[38] C. Benaim, B. Leger, P. Vuistiner, and F. Luthi, "Validation of the French version of the "Patterns of Activity Measure" in patients with chronic musculoskeletal pain," *Pain Research & Management*, vol. 2017, Article ID 6570394, 7 pages, 2017.
[39] R. P. Miller, S. Kori, and D. Todd, "The Tampa Scale: a measure of kinesiophobia,"Clinical Journal of Pain, vol. 7, no. 1, p. 51, 1991.
[40] J. W. Vlaeyen, A. M. Kole-Snijders, A. M. Rotteveel, R. Ruesink, and P. H. Heuts, "The role of fear of movement/(re)injury in pain disability," *Journal of Occupational Rehabilitation*, vol. 5, no. 4, pp. 235–252, 1995.
[41] J. W. Vlaeyen, A. M. Kole-Snijders, R. G. Boeren, and H. van Eek, "Fear of movement/(re)injury in chronic low back pain and its relation to behavioral performance," *Pain*, vol. 62, no. 3, pp. 363–372, 1995.
[42] J. Rainville, D. Bagnall, and L. Phalen, "Health care providers' attitudes and beliefs about functional impairments and chronic back pain," *Clinical Journal of Pain*, vol. 11, no. 4, pp. 287–295, 1995.
[43] A. S. Zigmond and R. P. Snaith, "The hospital anxiety and depression scale," *Acta Psychiatrica Scandinavica*, vol. 67, no. 6, pp. 361–370, 1983.
[44] J. P. Lepine, M. Godchau, P. Brun, and T. Lemperiere, "[Evaluation of anxiety and depression among patients hospitalized on an internal medicine service]," *Annales Medico-Psychologiques*, vol. 143, no. 2, pp. 175–189, 1985.
[45] J. R. Crawford, J. D. Henry, C. Crombie, and E. P. Taylor, "Normative data for the HADS from a large non-clinical sample," *British Journal of Clinical Psychology*, vol. 40, no. 4, pp. 429–434, 2001.
[46] H. P. Kindermans, J. Roelofs, M. E. Goossens, I. P. Huijnen, J. A. Verbunt, and J. W. Vlaeyen, "Activity patterns in chronic pain: underlying dimensions and associations with disability and depressed mood," *Journal of Pain*, vol. 12, no. 10, pp. 1049–1058, 2011.
[47] M. H. Freeston, J. Rhéaume, H. Letarte, M. J. Dugas, and R. Ladouceur, "Why do people worry?," *Personality and Individual Differences*, vol. 17, no. 6, pp. 791–802, 1994.
[48] J. A. Baecke, J. Burema, and J. E. Frijters, "A short questionnaire for the measurement of habitual physical activity in epidemiological studies," *American Journal of Clinical Nutrition*, vol. 36, no. 5, pp. 936–942, 1982.
[49] A. X. Bigard, F. Duforez, P. Portero, and C. Y. Guezennec, "Assessment of physical activity by questionnaire: validity of the Baecke questionnaire," *Science & Sports*, vol. 7, no. 4, pp. 215–221, 1992.
[50] B. E. Ainsworth, W. L. Haskell, A. S. Leon et al., "Compendium of physical activities: classification of energy costs of human physical activities," *Medicine and Science in Sports and Exercise*, vol. 25, no. 1, pp. 71–80, 1993.
[51] C. Tudor-Locke, C. L. Craig, W. J. Brown et al., "How many steps/day are enough? For adults," *International Journal of Behavioral Nutrition and Physical Activity*, vol. 8, no. 1, p. 79, 2011.
[52] P. Terrier, J. Le Carre, M. L. Connaissa, B. Leger, and F. Luthi, "Monitoring of gait quality in patients with chronic pain of lower limbs," *IEEE Transactions on Neural Systems and Rehabilitation Engineering*, vol. 25, no. 10, pp. 1843–1852, 2017.
[53] D. P. Crowne and D. Marlowe, "A new scale of social desirability independent of psychopathology," *Journal of Consulting Psychology*, vol. 24, no. 4, pp. 349–354, 1960.
[54] J. P. Weir, "Quantifying test-retest reliability using the intraclass correlation coefficient and the SEM," *Journal of Strength & Conditioning Research*, vol. 19, no. 1, pp. 231–240, 2005.
[55] H. J. Tan, L. S. Marks, M. A. Hoyt et al., "The relationship between intolerance of uncertainty and anxiety in men on active surveillance for prostate cancer," *Journal of urology*, vol. 195, no. 6, pp. 1724–1730, 2016.
[56] A. Counsell, M. Furtado, C. Iorio et al., "Intolerance of uncertainty, social anxiety, and generalized anxiety: differences by diagnosis and symptoms," *Psychiatry Research*, vol. 252, pp. 63–69, 2017.
[57] S. W. Salmond and M. Echevarria, "Healthcare transformation and changing roles for nursing," *Orthopedic Nursing*, vol. 36, no. 1, pp. 12–25, 2017.
[58] G. Dermody and C. R. Kovach, "Nurses' experience with and perception of barriers to promoting mobility in hospitalized older adults: a descriptive study," *Journal of Gerontological Nursing*, vol. 43, no. 11, pp. 22–29, 2017.
[59] R. Horppu, K. P. Martimo, E. Viikari-Juntura, T. Lallukka, and E. MacEachen, "Occupational physicians' reasoning about recommending early return to work with work modifications," *PLoS One*, vol. 11, no. 7, Article ID e0158588, 2016.
[60] C. Mikhail, N. Korner-Bitensky, M. Rossignol, and J. P. Dumas, "Physical therapists' use of interventions with high evidence of effectiveness in the management of a hypothetical typical patient with acute low back pain," *Physical Therapy*, vol. 85, no. 11, pp. 1151–1167, 2005.
[61] Swiss Medical Association, "Program of training in physical and rehabilitation medicine in Switzerland," 2017, https://www.fmh.ch/files/pdf16/physikalische_medizin_version_internet_f.pdf.

17

Transforaminal Epiduroscopic Basivertebral Nerve Laser Ablation for Chronic Low Back Pain Associated with Modic Changes: A Preliminary Open-Label Study

Hyeun Sung Kim,[1] Nitin Adsul,[1] Farid Yudoyono,[2] Byapak Paudel,[1] Ki Joon Kim,[1] Sung Ho Choi,[1] Jeong Hoon Kim,[1] Sung Kyun Chung,[1] Jeong-Hoon Choi,[1] Jee-Soo Jang,[1] Il-Tae Jang,[3] and Seong-Hoon Oh[4]

[1]*Department of Neurosurgery, Nanoori Suwon Hospital, Suwon, Republic of Korea*
[2]*Department of Neurosurgery, Hasan Sadikin Hospital, College of Medicine, Universitas Padjadjaran, Bandung, Jawa Barat, Indonesia*
[3]*Department of Neurosurgery, Nanoori Hospital, Seoul, Republic of Korea*
[4]*Department of Neurosurgery, Nanoori Incheon Hospital, Incheon, Republic of Korea*

Correspondence should be addressed to Nitin Adsul; no1.nitinadsul@gmail.com

Academic Editor: Filippo Brighina

Background. Chronic low back pain (CLBP) arising from degenerative disc disease continues to be a challenging clinical and diagnostic problem whether treated with nonsurgical, pain intervention, or motion-preserving stabilization and arthrodesis. *Methods*. Fourteen patients with CLBP, greater than 6 months, unresponsive to at least 4 months of conservative care were enrolled. All patients were treated successfully following screening using MRI findings of Modic type I or II changes and positive confirmatory provocative discography to determine the affected levels. All patients underwent ablation of the basivertebral nerve (BVN) using 1414 nm Nd:YAG laser-assisted energy guided in a transforaminal epiduroscopic approach. Macnab's criteria and visual analog scale (VAS) score were collected retrospectively at each follow-up interval. *Results*. The mean age was 46 ± 9.95 years. The mean symptoms duration was 21.21 ± 21.87 months. The mean follow-up was 15.3 ± 2.67 months. The preoperative VAS score of 7.79 ± 0.97 changed to 1.92 ± 1.38, postoperatively ($P < 0.01$). As per Macnab's criteria, seven patients (50%) had excellent, six patients (42.85%) had good, and one patient (7.14%) had fair outcomes. *Conclusion*. The transforaminal epiduroscopic basivertebral nerve laser ablation (TEBLA) appears to be a promising option in carefully selected patients with CLBP associated with the Modic changes.

1. Introduction

Chronic low back pain (CLBP) is a serious medico-social problem and a cause of disability. According to the United States National Center for Health Statistics reports, 14% of new hospital visits are patients with chronic low back pain. The expense of treating low back pain is over $100 billion per year [1–3]. In cases with difficulty in identifying the cause of CLBP, magnetic resonance imaging (MRI) can clearly identify pathologies of CLBP. However, the importance of all these pathologies is still controversial [3]. de Roos and coworkers [4] first introduced evidence of the degenerative vertebral endplate and subchondral bone marrow changes due to an inflammatory process of the endplate on MRI. Modic changes were identified in 19%–59% of patients with lumbar degenerative disk disease (DDD) and prolonged back pain. In most cases, nocturnal pain is characteristic, and it causes most commonly localized constant pain [5–8].

The Modic change is closely associated with low back pain [9]. A recent study showed that, in nonspecific low back pain (LBP), the prevalence of any type of Modic change was 46%, as opposed to 6% in the general population [10–13]. Most individuals with Modic changes of more than 90% on MRI will have back pain within one year [8, 13, 14].

Although a few number of patients need surgical interventions, most of them get better spontaneously with conservative management without much worsening in the middle age. Treatment of CLBP associated with Modic changes has not been established yet. We have treated this condition with the transforaminal epiduroscopic approach (Figure 1) with laser targeting to the basivertebral nerve (BVN) with a good outcome. We want to share its efficacy and safety.

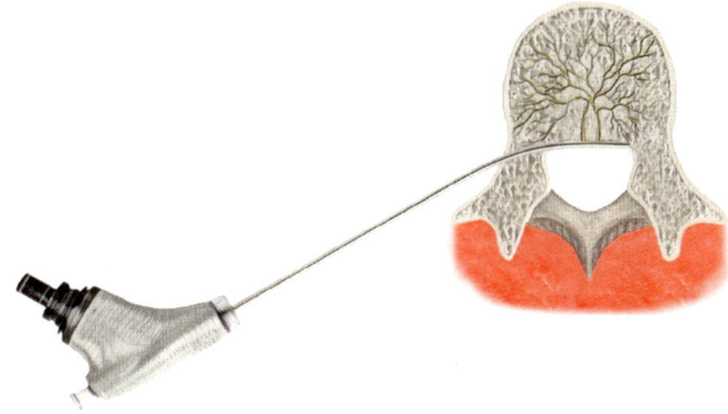

FIGURE 1: Transforaminal epiduroscopic basivertebral nerve laser ablation (TEBLA) procedure illustration.

2. Methods

Patients with isolated CLBP and type 1 or type 2 Modic changes on MRI for more than 6 months' duration that was nonresponsive to at least 3 months of conservative care were analyzed in this single-center retrospective observational study to evaluate the preliminary safety and effectiveness of BVN ablation for the treatment of CLBP with Modic changes.

No specific course of conservative care was mandated before enrollment. Exclusion criteria included were Modic changes without CLBP, spondylolisthesis, scoliosis, history of spinal infection, and prior spinal malignancy. Patients who had radicular symptoms were also excluded. The study was also limited to the L2, L3, L4, L5, and S1 vertebrae. Patients with the identified pathology at more cephalad levels were excluded. Determination of the treatment level(s) was made by clear evidence of Modic type 1 or type 2 changes on MRI and by provocative discography.

Treatment was limited to two or three contiguous vertebral bodies representing one or two motion segments, respectively. A detailed history and physical examination were performed on each patient to exclude origins of pain such as sacroiliac joint, hip, myofascial, genitourinary, gastrointestinal, or gynecologic sources.

We performed 3 steps of provocation tests to check the Modic changes as the source of pain as follows: (1) preoperative provocative discography, (2) intraoperative laser provocation into the basivertebral nerve of the vertebral body with Modic changes, and (3) intraoperative relief of pain assessment by laser reprovocation of the same painful area after completion of the laser ablation procedure.

TABLE 1: Patient characteristics of TEBLA.

Characteristic	Value
Patients (n)	14
Sex (n)	Women = 8/men = 6
Age (years)	46 ± 9.95 (31–63)
Symptoms duration (months)	21.21 ± 21.87 (4–84)
Follow-up duration (months)	15.3 ± 2.67 (12–20)
Surgical level	
L2-3	3
L3-4	2
L4-5	1
L4-5-S1	1
L5-S1	7
Number of complications	0
Macnab criteria	
Excellent	7 (50%)
Good	6 (43%)
Fair	1 (7%)
Poor	0

2.1. Surgical Technique. Fluoroscopic guidance during procedures in the anteroposterior and lateral projection was essential to ensure a precise skin entry point. Anesthesia was limited to 1% local lidocaine 7–10 cc with epinephrine mixed with 1.6% lidocaine 2-3 cc, 3–5 minutes after the 1st injection. In the provocation steps, the main painful point was commonly located in the upper endplate of the lower vertebral body. The needle was inserted into the suprapedicular notch [15] to get access to the vertebral endplate with the Modic change through the epidural space near to the upper endplate of the lower vertebral body. A guide wire was inserted through the needle into the suprapedicular notch. After withdrawing the needle, a tapered cannulated obturator was slid over the guide wire and advanced into the epidural space. A beveled working cannula was introduced over the obturator, and the obturator was removed. Semirigid epiduroscope, NeedleView CH (Lutronic®, Ilsan, South Korea) (Figure 1), was introduced through the working cannula. For laser ablation, a side-firing Nd : YAG laser cable included in the TELA (transforaminal epiduroscopic laser ablation) system (Lutronic®, Ilsan, South Korea) with a wavelength of 1414 nm operating in the 0.75–12 watt range was used. However, for our patients, we used a range of 4.5~6 W. This laser system is capable of thermovibration and can ablate an approximately spherical region of 10 mm diameter (5 mm radius). The laser cable was guided to the predetermined target (BVN terminus) near the Modic change area under fluoroscopic imaging. Each vertebral endplate having a painful Modic change was treated giving a laser locally at the BVN terminus by a 1414 nm Nd : YAG laser system (Figure 1). Self-reported outcome instruments were used to assess the patient's condition preoperatively and at each follow-up. VAS score and Macnab's criteria were

Table 2: Clinical outcomes.

Score	Preoperative‡	Postoperative‡	P value*	3-month postoperative‡	P value*	Final follow-up‡	Value*
VAS score	7.79 ± 0.98	1.93 ± 1.39	<0.0001	2.21 ± 0.89	<0.0001	2.36 ± 1.01	<0.0001

*For statistical analysis, the paired t-test was used. P value <0.05 was considered significant. ‡All values are expressed as mean ± standard deviation.

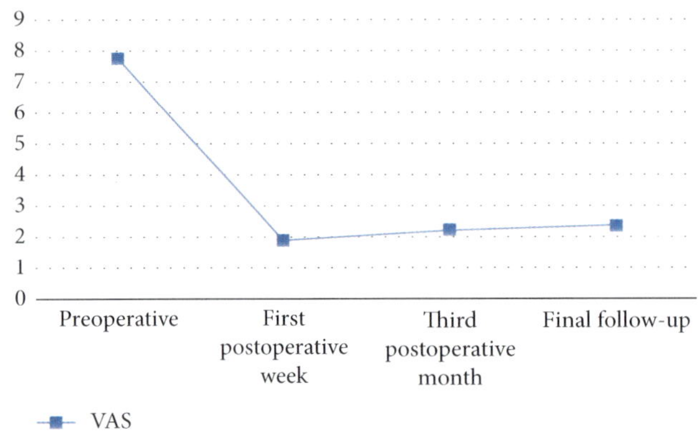

Figure 2: Graphs showing changes in the visual analog scale (VAS) score.

Table 3: Individual patient details with the pain response.

Number	Age	Sex	Symptom duration (months)	Level	VAS score				ODI				Macnab's criteria
					Pre-op	Post-op (1 week)	Post-op (3 months)	Final follow-up	Pre-op	Post-op (1 week)	Post-op (3 months)	Final follow-up	Post-op (1 week)
1	45	F	15	L5-S1	7	1	2	2	46	24	22	24	Good
2	56	M	8	L5-S1	7	1	1	1	52	18	19	18	Excellent
3	41	M	7	L3-4	8	2	2	2	64	24	22	24	Excellent
4	50	F	6	L2-3	8	1	2	1	58	22	26	24	Excellent
5	44	F	24	L5-S1	8	2	2	3	61	24	26	28	Excellent
6	62	M	28	L2-3	8	1	2	2	65	18	20	22	Excellent
7	37	F	6	L3-4	9	1	2	3	68	20	22	25	Good
8	35	F	24	L5-S1	8	1	3	2	58	22	26	24	Excellent
9	55	F	84	L5-S1	8	2	2	3	56	24	23	27	Good
10	31	F	24	L5-S1	8	1	2	2	63	18	21	22	Excellent
11	63	M	48	L2-3	6	6	5	5	54	48	42	42	Fair
12	41	M	5	L5-S1	10	3	2	3	72	28	24	24	Good
13	38	F	14	L4-5	7	3	2	2	55	28	25	25	Good
14	46	M	4	L4-5-S1	7	2	2	2	58	23	23	24	Good

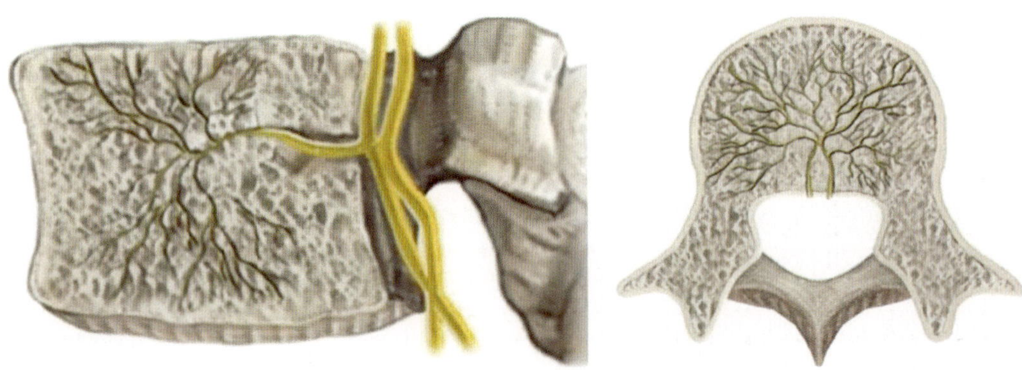

(a) (b)

Figure 3: Anatomy of the basivertebral nerve. (a) Sagittal view. (b) Axial view.

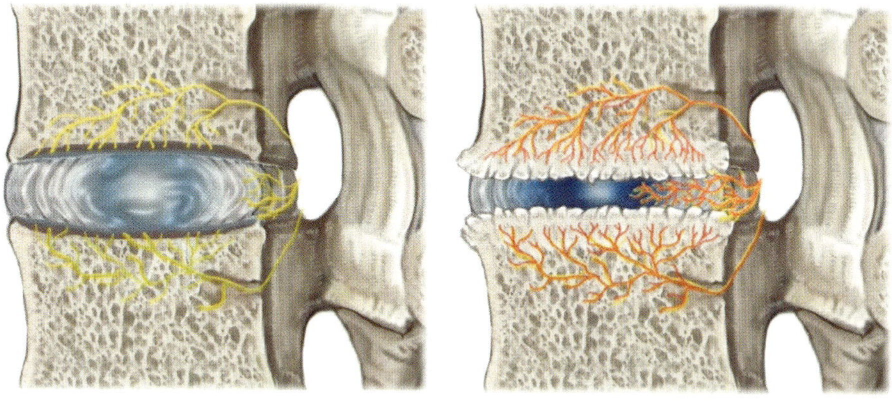

FIGURE 4: (a) Anatomy of BVN with a sinuvertebral nerve in the normal disc. (b) Pathological disc.

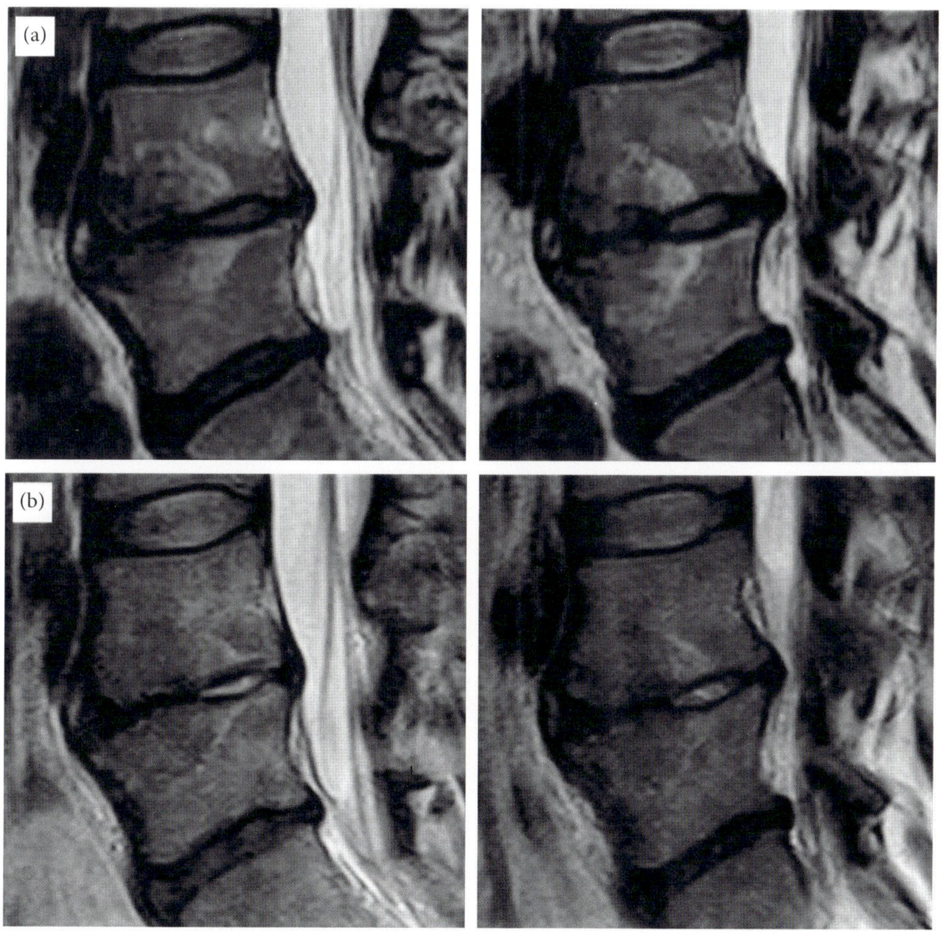

FIGURE 5: Magnetic resonance imaging (MRI) of a 35-year-old female patient who had suffered severe back pain and bilateral referred leg pain for more than 2 years. This patient's symptom improved significantly after TEBLA at the L4-5 level. The preoperative VAS score of 8 decreased to 1 postoperatively. (a) Preoperative T2WI lumbar magnetic resonance imaging (MRI) sagittal views with Modic Type 1 changes. (b) Postoperative T2WI lumbar MRI sagittal views showing resolution of the Modic reaction.

used in this study. Neurologic examination and adverse event screening and reporting were also performed at each follow-up.

The clinical outcomes were evaluated using descriptive statistical analysis. We conducted Student's paired t-test to evaluate the significant difference in the preoperative and postoperative clinical outcome parameter, that is, VAS score. The significance level was considered at 0.05. The statistical software used for the study was SPSS version 20.0 (IBM Corp., Armonk, New York, USA).

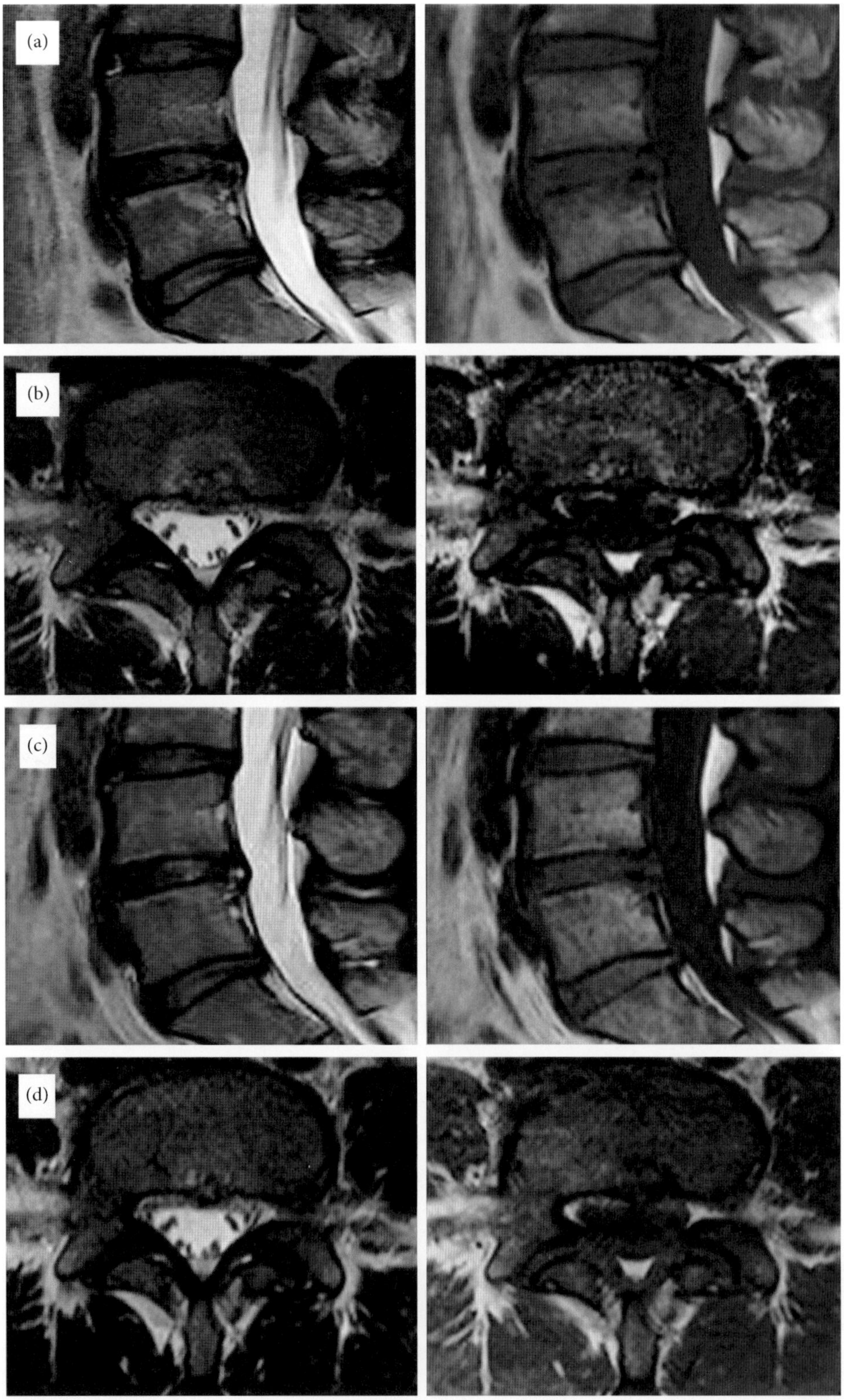

Figure 6: Magnetic resonance imaging (MRI) of a 31-year-old female patient who had suffered severe back pain and bilateral referred leg pain for more than 2 years. This patient's symptom improved significantly after TEBLA at the L4-L5 level. The preoperative VAS score of 8 decreased to 1 postoperatively. Preoperative T1WI and T2WI lumbar magnetic resonance imaging (MRI) sagittal (a) and axial (b) views with Modic type 1 changes. Postoperative T1WI and T2WI lumbar MRI sagittal (c) and axial (d) views showing resolution of the Modic reaction.

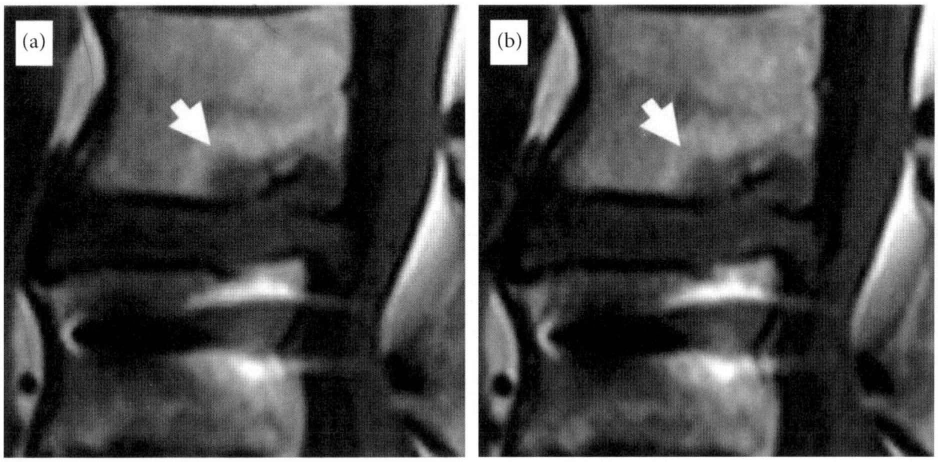

Figure 7: Magnetic resonance imaging (MRI) of a 65-year-old male patient who had fusion surgery previously and was suffering from back pain and buttock pain for more than 28 months. The preoperative VAS score of 7 decreased to 1 postoperatively. (a) Preoperative T1WI lumbar magnetic resonance imaging (MRI) sagittal view with Modic type 1 changes. (b) T1WI lumbar MRI taken after 6 months of the TEBLA sagittal view showing resolution of the Modic reaction (white arrow).

3. Results

A total of 14 consecutive patients were analyzed. The mean age was 46 ± 9.95 (range: 31–63) years. There were six men and eight women; in all patients, MRI findings correlated with clinical findings. The mean symptoms duration was 21.21 ± 21.87 (range: 4–84) months. The mean follow-up was 15.3 ± 2.67 months (range: 12–20 months). Pfirmann's disc degeneration grade was grade IV in 8 (57.14%) patients and grade V in 6 (42.85%) patients. Eight and six patients had Modic type 1 and type 2 changes, respectively (Table 1). The preoperative VAS score was 7.79 ± 0.98 (range: 6–10), and the postoperative VAS score improved to 1.93 ± 1.39 (range: 1–6). The improvement was significant at $P < 0.0001$ (Table 2). Significant improvement was maintained at the third month and at final follow-up with VAS scores of 2.21 ± 0.89 (range: 1–5; $P < 0.0001$) and 2.36 ± 1.01 (range: 1–5; $P < 0.0001$), respectively (Figure 2). As per Macnab's criteria, seven patients (50%) had excellent, six patients (42.85%) had good, and one patient (7.14%) had fair outcomes (Table 3).

There were no occurrences of infections, discitis, paresis, dural tears, vascular injuries, or systemic complications until the latest follow-up. Furthermore, the patient's VAS scores for back pain and Macnab's criteria were maintained at the final follow-up compared with postoperative scores. All patients maintained their functional neurologic status throughout the entire study follow-up. There were no device- or procedure-related serious adverse events in this study.

4. Discussion

The Modic change caused by disc degenerative processes involving damage and microfractures to the vertebral endplates results in the development of edema and inflammation of the adjacent vertebrae [5, 11]. Factors associated with endplate damage following degenerative disc disease, ingrowth of new vessels, and collection of inflammatory agents may be important characteristics in the generation of pain [5, 6, 11, 16]. In the normal state, bony endplates have a rich supply of small free nerve endings; degeneration and inflammation will likely trigger the inflammatory pain [13] (Figures 3 and 4).

Modic change is associated with chronic back pain [8]. While previous studies concluded that, among Modic changes, type 1 changes are the strongest and most crucial element in the disc degenerative process in relation to LBP, they also demonstrated that DDD with Modic changes was much more frequently associated with clinical symptoms [6, 11, 16]. Our patients also had mainly Modic type 1 changes, but some patients with Modic type 2 changes were also symptomatic in provocative discography; so they were also treated with TEBLA.

A study by Becker and coworkers reported that the primary innervation for the vertebral body is by the BVN that enters the bone of the vertebral body via the midline of the posterior cortex. The large, usually paired, neurovascular foramina are located equidistant from each endplate. These nerves accompany the basivertebral artery and vein [17] (Figure 3). Previous studies also reported on the innervation within the bone marrow with the presence of immunoreactive neural tissue in rat vertebral bodies and histologically identified intraosseous nerves and neurovascular bundles.

Basivertebral nerve sensitization causes CLBP. Substance P, a peptide neurotransmitter of the tachykinin family, is found within the basivertebral nerve, and there is very strong evidence that this nerve has the potential for transmitting pain signals [16, 18–20]. Ablation of this nerve was our target. A recent study also supports ablation of the basivertebral nerve for CLBP associated with Modic changes. They used radiofrequency through the transpedicular and extrapedicular approach and obtained significant improvement in ODI [17]. Our study differs from this study. We used the transforaminal epiduroscopic approach (Figure 1) with three steps of provocation. We used a laser instead of radiofrequency. Some of the representative cases are illustrated in Figures 5–7.

The major limitation of this study is the lack of a comparative control group. Similar to any other retrospective studies, limitations associated with our study include retrospective clinical outcome assessments and small sample size since very few patients actually require surgical intervention. Nevertheless, after TEBLA, we got 93% good-to-excellent results according to Macnab's criteria, and the preoperative VAS score of 7.79 ± 0.97 decreased to 1.92 ± 1.38 at the latest follow-up ($P < 0.0001$). This result is encouraging and the procedure was safe.

5. Conclusion

The TEBLA appears to be a promising option in carefully selected patients with chronic low back pain associated with the Modic changes. The treatment improved patients' self-reported outcomes, and the improvement was largely maintained through more than 12 months of the follow-up period.

Acknowledgments

The authors would like to acknowledge scientific team members Ms. Jae Eun Park and Mr. Kyeong Rae Kim for providing assistance in acquiring full-text articles and managing digital works.

References

[1] Y.-g. Zhang, T.-m. Guo, X. Guo, and S.-x. Wu, "Clinical diagnosis for discogenic low back pain," *International Journal of Biological Sciences*, vol. 5, no. 7, pp. 647–658, 2009.

[2] B.-G. Peng, "Pathophysiology, diagnosis, and treatment of discogenic low back pain," *World Journal of Orthopedics*, vol. 4, no. 2, p. 42, 2013.

[3] J. Tonosu, H. Inanami, H. Oka et al., "Diagnosing discogenic low back pain associated with degenerative disc disease using a medical interview," *PLoS One*, vol. 11, Article ID e0166031, 2016.

[4] A. de Roos, H. Kressel, C. Spritzer, and M. Dalinka, "MR imaging of marrow changes adjacent to end plates in degenerative lumbar disk disease," *American Journal of Roentgenology*, vol. 149, no. 3, pp. 531–534, 1987.

[5] H. B. Albert, P. Kjaer, T. S. Jensen, J. S. Sorensen, T. Bendix, and C. Manniche, "Modic changes, possible causes and relation to low back pain," *Medical Hypotheses*, vol. 70, no. 2, pp. 361–368, 2008.

[6] R. Rahme and R. Moussa, "The modic vertebral endplate and marrow changes: pathologic significance and relation to low back pain and segmental instability of the lumbar spine," *American Journal of Neuroradiology*, vol. 29, no. 5, pp. 838–842, 2008.

[7] C. Manniche, "Vertebral endplate (modic) changes and the treatment of back pain using antibiotics," *Clinical Practice*, vol. 11, no. 6, pp. 585–590, 2014.

[8] R. K. Jensen, P. Kent, and M. Hancock, "Do MRI findings identify patients with chronic low back pain and Modic changes who respond best to rest or exercise: a subgroup analysis of a randomised controlled trial," *Chiropractic and Manual Therapies*, vol. 23, no. 1, p. 26, 2015.

[9] F. P. Mok, D. Samartzis, J. Karppinen, D. Y. Fong, K. D. Luk, and K. M. Cheung, "Modic changes of the lumbar spine: prevalence, risk factors, and association with disc degeneration and low back pain in a large-scale population-based cohort," *Spine Journal*, vol. 16, no. 1, pp. 32–41, 2016.

[10] I. Braithwaite, J. White, A. Saifuddin, P. Renton, and B. Taylor, "Vertebral end-plate (Modic) changes on lumbar spine MRI: correlation with pain reproduction at lumbar discography," *European Spine Journal*, vol. 7, no. 5, pp. 363–368, 1998.

[11] H. B. Albert, J. S. Sorensen, B. S. Christensen, and C. Manniche, "Antibiotic treatment in patients with chronic low back pain and vertebral bone edema (Modic type 1 changes): a double-blind randomized clinical controlled trial of efficacy," *European Spine Journal*, vol. 22, no. 4, pp. 697–707, 2013.

[12] L. Sheng-yun, S. Letu, C. Jian et al., "Comparison of modic changes in the lumbar and cervical spine, in 3167 patients with and without spinal pain," *PLoS One*, vol. 9, Article ID e114993, 2014.

[13] C Manniche and A Jordan, "10 years of research: from ignoring Modic changes to considerations regarding treatment and prevention of low-grade disc infections," *Future Science OA*, vol. 2, no. 2, article FSO117, 2016.

[14] O. Eser, C. Gomleksiz, M. Sasani et al., "Dynamic stabilisation in the treatment of degenerative disc disease with modic changes," *Advances in Orthopedics*, vol. 2013, pp. 1–6, 2013.

[15] H. S. Kim, C. I. Ju, S. W. Kim, and J. G. Kim, "Endoscopic transforaminal suprapedicular approach in high grade inferior migrated lumbar disc herniation," *Journal of Korean Neurosurgical Society*, vol. 45, no. 2, pp. 67–73, 2009.

[16] M. Heggeness, S. Becker, A. Hadjipavlou et al., "Ablation of the basivertebral nerve for the treatment of back pain: a pilot clinical study," *Spine Journal*, vol. 11, no. 10, pp. S65–S66, 2011.

[17] S. Becker, A. Hadjipavlou, and M. H. Heggeness, "Ablation of the basivertebral nerve for treatment of back pain: a clinical study," *Spine Journal*, vol. 17, no. 2, pp. 218–223, 2017.

[18] C. Hirsh, "The anatomical basis for low back pain: studies on the presence of sensory nerve endings in ligamentous, capsular and intervertebral disc structures in the human lumbar spine," *Acta Orthopaedica Scandinavica*, vol. 33, no. 1–4, pp. 1–17, 1963.

[19] M. D. Antonacci, D. R. Mody, and M. H. Heggeness, "Innervation of the human vertebral body: a histologic study," *Journal of Spinal Disorders*, vol. 11, no. 6, pp. 526–531, 1998.

[20] C. Fras, P. Kravetz, D. R. Mody, and M. H. Heggeness, "Substance P-containing nerves within the human vertebral body: an immunohistochemical study of the basivertebral nerve," *Spine Journal*, vol. 3, no. 1, pp. 63–67, 2003.

18

Perioperative Immunosuppression and Risk of Cancer Progression: The Impact of Opioids on Pain Management

Renata Zajączkowska,[1] Wojciech Leppert,[2] Joanna Mika,[3] Magdalena Kocot-Kępska,[4] Jarosław Woroń,[1] Anna Wrzosek,[1] and Jerzy Wordliczek[1]

[1]*Department of Interdisciplinary Intensive Care, Jagiellonian University Medical College, Kraków, Poland*
[2]*Department of Palliative Medicine, Poznan University of Medical Sciences, Poznan, Poland*
[3]*Department of Pain Pharmacology, Institute of Pharmacology, Polish Academy of Sciences, Kraków, Poland*
[4]*Department of Pain Research and Treatment, Jagiellonian University Medical College, Kraków, Poland*

Correspondence should be addressed to Anna Wrzosek; awrzosek@su.krakow.pl

Academic Editor: Massimiliano Valeriani

Opioids comprise an important group of drugs used in cancer pain pharmacotherapy. In recent years, more and more studies have emerged indicating the potentially immunosuppressive effects of opioid analgesics and their serious consequences, including the risk of cancer progression. The identification of these risks has prompted a search for other effective, and most importantly, safer methods of perioperative analgesic management. Regional analgesia techniques, which allow for a significant reduction in opioid dosing and thus diminish the risk of immunosuppression associated with these drugs, seem to offer substantial hope in this respect. A number of studies available in the literature assess the effects of regional analgesia techniques on cancer progression; however, it is often difficult to interpret their results owing to several perioperative factors (such as surgical trauma, inadequate pain and stress relief, and hypothermia) which are also attributed immunosuppressive effects and tend to be implicated in increased risk of cancer progression. Further research is needed to verify the available data on both the potential adverse effects of opioids and the possible protective effects of regional analgesia techniques on cancer patients.

1. Introduction

Cancer pain poses a serious clinical and epidemiological problem. It may be the first symptom of the disease, occurs during its diagnosis and treatment, and accompanies patients at the advanced stages of the disease. It is estimated that, regardless of the stage, at least one-half of cancer patients experience pain, but their proportion is significantly higher as the disease progresses. The World Health Organisation (WHO) reports that over 5.5 million patients worldwide do not receive or receive inadequate treatment for cancer-related pain. The above data, due to the lack of worldwide registers, are based on epidemiological estimates [1]. A meta-analysis published in 2016, which included 117 reports of pain in cancer patients, showed that the goal of effective pain management still remains far from being achieved: pain was experienced by 39.3% of patients after radical cancer treatment, by 55% of patients during cancer treatment, and by 66.4% at the advanced stage of cancer treatment. 38% of patients experienced moderate to severe pain (NRS > 5) [2].

Apart from the unimaginable suffering and the humanitarian aspect of the problem, the consequences of insufficiently treated pain, both acute and chronic, can also be disastrous from a purely medical point of view. This is particularly important in cancer patients as more and more data indicate a correlation between severe pain and increased risk of cancer progression and a shorter time to the appearance of metastatic lesions [3]. Research shows that ineffective pain and stress treatment adversely affects the body's defence systems, including cellular immunity and the functioning of the natural killer (NK) cells. Andersen et al.

demonstrated that the stress associated with the diagnosis and surgical treatment of breast cancer in women impaired their immune cell response, including NK cell toxicity and T-cell responses. Stress levels significantly predicted lower NK cell lysis, diminished response of NK cells to recombinant interferon gamma, and decreased proliferative response of peripheral blood lymphocytes to plant lectins and to a monoclonal antibody directed against the T-cell receptor [4].

Experimental and clinical studies demonstrate the importance of effective pain management also in terms of cancer progression. Page et al. found a longer time interval to lung metastasis in a group of experimental animals (rats in the experimental model of breast adenocarcinoma) with effective analgesia (intrathecal or systemic opioids) compared with a group of animals not subject to analgesic treatment [5]. Lillemoe et al. in their randomised prospective study (RCT), which included a group of patients with advanced pancreatic cancer, concluded that alcohol-induced visceral neurolysis (neurolytic splanchnicectomy) performed in one of the two groups of patients provided not only pain relief but also longer survival time, compared with the group of patients given saline instead of alcohol. There was no improvement in overall survival (OS) compared with the control group of patients who underwent the same procedure but who did not experience pain prior to its onset [6].

Opioids are being used by the anaesthesiologists not only to treat acute pain in the perioperative period but also to control chronic cancer pain. Studies conducted over the recent years have given results indicating the potentially immunosuppressive effects of opioids and their serious consequences, including the risk of cancer progression. This is a very important and complex problem both in perioperative period and in chronic pain treatment course. Morphine has immunosuppressant properties which can promote cancer, but on the other hand suppressing of pain alleviates the surgical stress and thus might be protective against tumour metastases.

2. Opioids and Their Receptors

Pharmacotherapy constitutes the basic pain treatment method in cancer patients. For moderate to severe pain in cancer patients, the mainstay of the therapy is opioid analgesics (weak or strong ones, depending on pain severity). These drugs exert their clinical effects by influencing individual opioid receptors, which are currently classified into three groups: MOP (μ, mu), DOP (σ, delta), and KOP (κ, kappa). Opioids can also affect other receptors, especially NOPs (nonclassical nociceptin/orphanin FQ receptor, N/OFQ). In everyday practice, depending on the type of pain (receptor: somatic and visceral or neuropathic), the clinical condition of the patient, the coexisting diseases, and capacities of organs crucial for drug metabolism and excretion (liver and kidneys), different opioids are used, including morphine, oxycodone, hydromorphone, fentanyl, buprenorphine, tapentadol, methadone, tramadol, codeine; the last two are being classified as the so-called "weak" opioids.

Owing to the steadily increasing use of opioids, their potential side effects are being studied in more depth. In recent years, a number of studies have suggested immunosuppressive effects of opioid analgesics and their potential serious consequences, including an increased risk of cancer progression in patients treated with these drugs [3].

Classically, three opioid receptor types (μ, σ, and κ) have been identified on the central and peripheral nervous system neurons. Moreover, based on the analysis of mRNA, receptor protein, or opioid binding capacity of cells or their opioid response, it has been confirmed that opioid receptors are also present on other cells, including cancer cells [7]. Interestingly, it has been shown that, by influencing the proliferation and apoptosis processes, opioids can regulate the growth and activity of a number of cells, including the cancer cells [8]. This may result in an increased risk of cancer progression. However, the test results are ambiguous as they depend on the type of cell tested, the dosage, the time of administration, and the type of opioid used. The question remains whether the direct effect of opioids on cancer cells observed in experimental studies translates into comparable effects in vivo and how opioids ultimately affect the immune system status of cancer patients.

3. Potential Mechanisms of Opioid-Induced Immunosuppression

The immune system plays a key role in cancer defence. Its important components include NK (natural killer cells), T cells, mast cells, macrophages and mediators, including cytokines (interleukins and chemokines). It turns out that acute and chronic administration of exogenous opioids affects both the cellular and humoral components of the immune response. Exogenous opioids affect several of the components of the immune system, including lymphocyte proliferation, their phagocytic activity, NK cell activity, cytokine expression, and antibody production [9]. Several mechanisms responsible for immunosuppression associated with the use of opioids in cancer patients have been identified. They can be divided into central and peripheral ones and are schematically presented in Figure 1.

The importance of central mechanisms is demonstrated by the fact that opioids that easily penetrate the blood-brain barrier have a stronger immunosuppressive effect compared with those that do not pass through it—the latter demonstrates this effect only after central administration [10]. Moreover, it turned out that MOP knockout mice did not show any immune-modulating effect after central administration of morphine in experimental studies. This confirms the view that central immune modulatory effects of opioids are mediated by the MOP receptor [11]. A central site for opiate action in the induction of immunosuppression appears to be the periaqueductal gray matter (PAG) which also subserves a variety of diverse autonomic functions. Microinjections of morphine into the PAG result in a rapid suppression of natural killer (NK) cell activity [12].

The peripheral mechanisms most likely involve the activation of MOP opioid receptors located on immunocompetent cells [13]. Opioid receptors have been identified

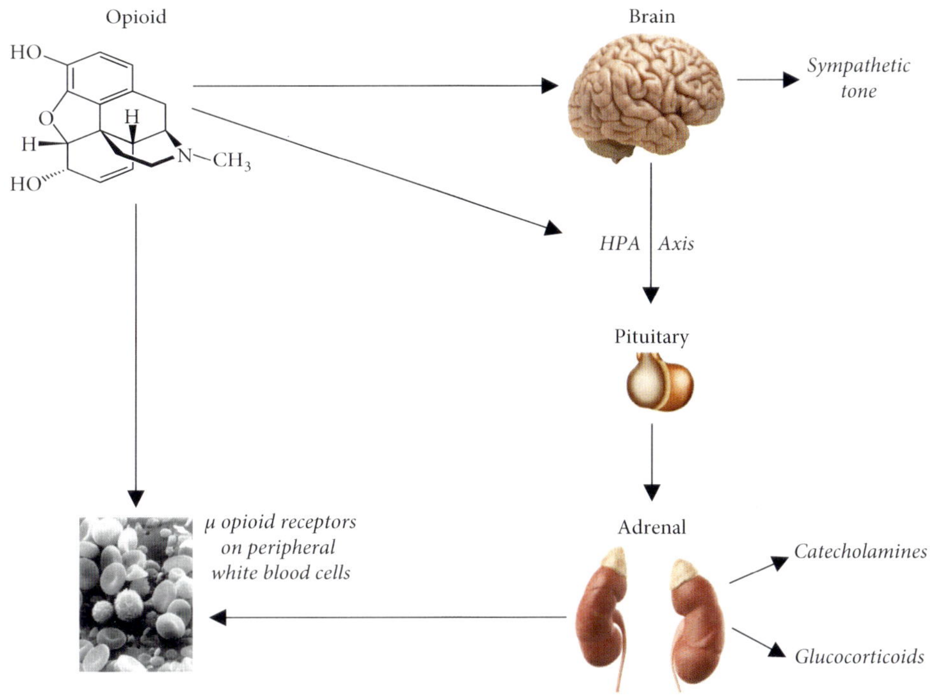

FIGURE 1: Potential mechanisms of immunosuppressive effects of opioids [13].

on the surface of several types of immune system cells, including multinuclear leukocytes, macrophages, T cells, and splenocytes [9]. Opioids added directly to certain types of immune cells in vitro change the protein expression profile [14] and their function: they reduce macrophage chemotaxis and phagocytosis and weaken B-cell proliferation and antibody production [15]. In contrary to exogenous opioids, data on endogenous opioids are not clear, and however there are some studies suggesting the immunostimulating effect. Mathews et al. showed an increase in NK cells activity in response to beta-endorphin, which was reversible by naloxone [16].

A number of potential mechanisms of opioid-induced immunosuppression have been identified in experimental studies. It turns out that these drugs may reduce the number of macrophages available to fight infections [17] and weaken leucocyte migration as well as and peritoneal macrophage phagocytosis [18]. They may also interfere with respiratory burst activity, chemotaxis and superoxide production from neutrophils and macrophages [19], and immune cell recruitment to the wound site, which, in turn, may lead to impaired wound healing [20]. Studies show that opioids may also impair leucocyte endothelial adhesion by weakening intracellular adhesion molecules [21] and intensifying the apoptosis of macrophages [22] and T cells [23], which results in the impairment of the host defence barrier.

A number of mechanisms via which opioids impair adaptive immunity have also been studied. It turns out that these drugs may impair the T-cell viability and their proliferative response [9], T-helper cell function, and macrophage activity [9]. Moreover, opioids may also adversely affect humoral immunity by impairing primary antibody response (B cells) [24] and B-cell mitogenic response to bacterial liposaccharides (LPS) [25].

Another potential opioid-induced immunosuppression pathway is the hypothalamic-pituitary-adrenal (HPA) axis: the corticotrophin releasing hormone (CRH) stimulates the anterior part of the pituitary gland to produce adrenocorticotrophic hormone (ACTH), which, in turn, activates the adrenal cortex to produce glucocorticoids. The latter influences various components of the innate and adaptive immune system, suppresses cellular immunity, and contributes to the tolerance of various antigens by altering T- and B-cell function [26]. The effects of opioids on the HPA axis and its components (ACTH and glucocorticoids) are complex, species dependent, and time dependent and vary after acute and chronic administration [26]. Studies show that, in humans, acute administration of opioids results in a reduction or no change in ACTH or glucocorticoid levels [27]. On the contrary, chronic opioid administration may suppress the HPA, which may lead to adrenal insufficiency [10, 27]. Case reports have documented adrenal insufficiency after oral [28] or transdermal [29] opioid application. Additionally, chronic opioid injections are usually accompanied by disturbances in the daily rhythm of ACTH and cortisol secretion [27].

Studies have shown that opioids also affect the sympathetic system and by activating it, may cause immunosuppression. It is manifested, among others, by depressed NK cell activity and suppressed peripheral blood lymphocyte proliferation [30]. Felten et al. examined and described the contribution of the sympathetic system to the alteration of opioid-induced immune function and concluded that the phenomenon is caused by the rich sympathetic innervation of lymph nodes [31]. Other studies also validate this mechanism by indicating that the immune status is changed by opioids following sympathetic activation results from the rich adrenergic innervation of the spleen, lymph nodes, and bone marrow [30]. Moreover, both α and β adrenergic receptors have been identified in experimental studies on lymphocytes and macrophages in rodents [32].

Not all opioid drugs share the same immune profile. Some opioids seem to have no effects on immune function, whereas others tend to be immunosuppressive. This is probably due to the combination of direct effects on immunocytes and indirect effects in vivo that involve centrally mediated mechanisms as well as the systemic production and release of immunomodulatory mediators. Studies suggest that morphine has the highest immunosuppressive potential, fentanyl ranks medium, while buprenorphine and tramadol show the lowest or no immunosuppressive effect [33]. Morphine, codeine, and fentanyl suppress NK cell activity [3]. Hydromorphone and oxycodone, unlike morphine and fentanyl, do not impair the immunological functions, although they are more potent opioids than morphine [34]. Buprenorphine, which is a partial MOP opioid receptor agonist, has no immunosuppressive effect and does not impair the activity of NK cells and, hence from the immunological point of view, it is the safest opioid [35].

A list of opioids broken down by the degree of the immunosuppressive effect they induce is given in Table 1.

Table 1: Opioids and their immunosuppressive effects [33–35].

Strong immune modulation	Weak or no immune modulation
Morphine	Buprenorphine (the least or no effect)
Fentanyl	Oxycodone
Sufentanyl	Hydromorphone
Codeine	Tramadol

4. How Can Surgery and Perioperative Opioids Contribute to Cancer Progression?

Several possible mechanisms which are jointly responsible for cancer progression in the perioperative period have been identified. Numerous studies have confirmed that surgical manipulation, tumour dissection, and resection cause cancer cells to migrate to the cardiovascular system and their subsequent spread throughout the body [36]. Additionally, surgical intervention activates and intensifies the proliferation of neoplastic cells, inhibits their apoptosis [37], and stimulates their mobility, invasiveness, and adhesion—features considered very important in terms of the capacity of neoplastic cells to reach distant organs and metastasize [38]. It also promotes angiogenesis and networking of blood vessels, which offer cancer cells a kind of pathway to the host cardiovascular system and then further to the metastatic sites. The mechanism of neoplastic neoangiogenesis involves the vascular endothelial growth factor (VEGF), whereas other mediators, such as matrix metalloproteinases (MMPs), intensify adhesion and aid cancer cells in settling in distant organs [39].

The findings also suggest that the choice of the surgical technique also appears to be important. Less invasive options, including laparoscopic ones, demonstrate a less intense immunosuppressive effect compared with laparotomy [40]. Other factors of proven significance in increasing the risk of cancer progression are perioperative blood loss and blood product transfusions, especially kept in long-term storage [41], and hypothermia, which leads to intensified glucocorticosteroid secretion as well as impaired cellular and humoral immune response [42].

Stress and pain, unfortunately often experienced by patients in the perioperative period, also constitute important factors. They lead to stress hormone bursts and impair cellular immunity, including NK cell activity [43, 44]. The most important known factors responsible for cancer progression in the perioperative period are listed in Table 2.

Numerous studies suggest that opioids may promote cancer progression. The main mechanisms responsible for this adverse effect include the stimulation of angiogenesis and immunosuppression. Opioids, by activating MOP (μ) opioid receptors located on vascular endothelial cells, activate and promote angiogenesis and networking of new blood vessels, which play an important role in the transfer of cancer cells from the primary lesion site to the host cardiovascular system and further to the metastatic lesion sites. This mechanism involves, among other things, the vascular endothelial growth factor (VEGF) [33, 45]. Studies by Lennon et al. have confirmed that opioids stimulate the migration and proliferation of endothelial cells, including vascular endothelial cells via the vascular endothelial growth factor (VEGF) [46]. This mechanism involves the MOP (μ) receptor, since the administration of methylnaltrexone, which is a peripheral antagonist of the MOP receptor, reduces angiogenesis. Moreover, methylnaltrexone administered in combination with bevacizumab, which is an anti-VEGF monoclonal antibody, shows synergy in the inhibition of VEGF-induced angiogenesis [47]. Gupta et al. have shown that breast cancer cells implanted into mice grow and multiply much faster and show intensive neovascularization after the experimental animals have been exposed to morphine [48].

Opioids may lead to progressive immunosuppression via many of the mechanisms described in the previous part of the article. Studies show that fentanyl, an opioid frequently used intraoperatively, blocks the cytotoxic effect of NK cells in the postoperative period, whereas sufentanyl and alfentanyl, apart from their effect on NK cells, further weaken mitogen-induced lymphocyte multiplication [49]. Figure 2 shows the most important mechanisms of opioid-induced cancer progression.

5. Perioperative Setting: Possible Benefits of Regional Analgesia and Multimodal Analgesia

The increasing awareness of the immunosuppressive properties of opioids has prompted sustained efforts in search of other effective, but most importantly, safer methods of perioperative analgesic management. Regional

Table 2: Perioperative factors affecting cancer progression.

I. *Surgical factors*
1. Cancer cells enter the cardiovascular system during surgical procedures, including tumour resection, and subsequently spread across the body [36].
2. Surgical procedures activate and intensify the proliferation of cancer cells, stimulate their mobility and invasiveness, and increase their capacity for adhesion [37, 38].
3. Surgical factors inhibit the apoptosis of cancer cells [37].
4. Angiogenesis and the network of newly created blood vessels constitute a kind of "pathway" for the transfer of cancer cells to the host cardiovascular and further to metastatic lesion sites [39].
5. The selection of the surgical technique: less invasive techniques, including laparoscopic ones, have a less intense immunosuppressive effect compared with open techniques [40].
II. *The transfusion of blood and blood products*, especially those kept in long-term storage [41].
III. *Hypothermia* leads to glucocorticosteroid burst and impaired immune cellular and humoral response [42].
IV. *Stress and pain*, often experienced by patients during the perioperative period, cause stress hormone bursts and impair cellular immunity, including the activity of NK cells [43, 44].
VI. *Anaesthetic management*: type of anaesthesia used (general and regional), choice of drugs, especially opioids [50–55].

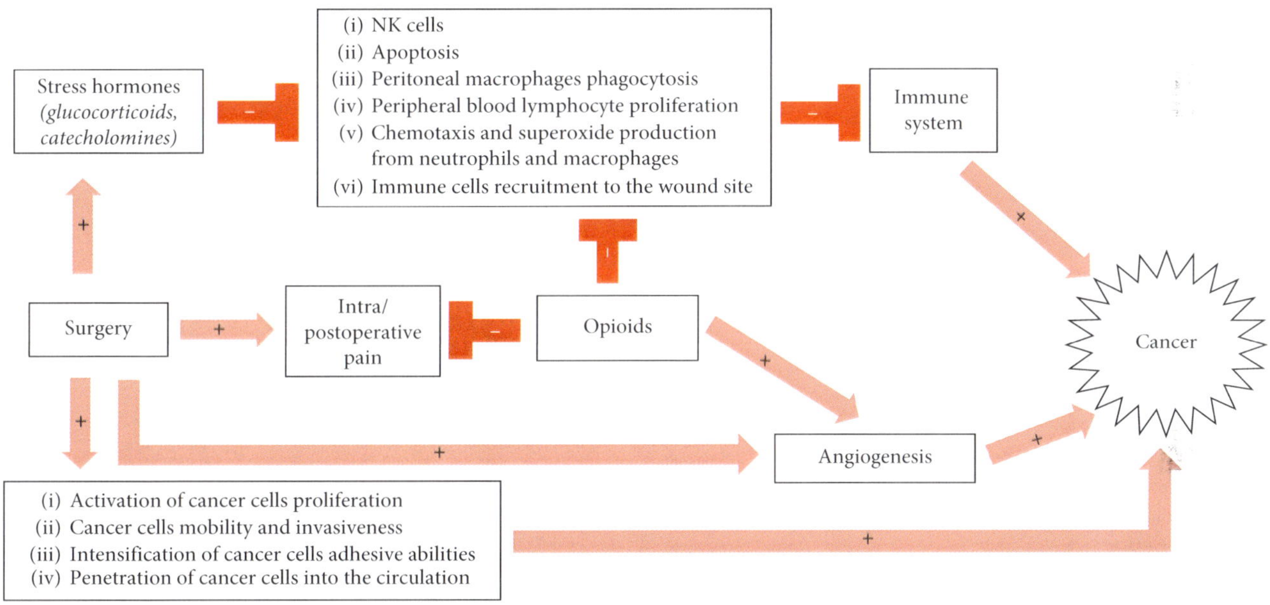

Figure 2: Perioperative immunosuppression mechanisms [16–23].

analgesia techniques raise hopes in this respect. Their beneficial mechanism of action is complex: on the one hand, they provide effective analgesia, thus minimising the adverse effects of pain on the body of the operated patient and reducing the necessary doses of systemic analgesics (including opioids), which translates into improved safety of the therapy in terms of opioid-induced immunosuppression and potential risk of cancer progression. On the other hand, these techniques minimize the adverse effects of the surgical procedure itself by attenuating of the metabolic, neuroendocrine, and cytokine stress response to surgery and reducing the potential immunosuppressive and prognostic impact of stress and surgical trauma.

A number of studies have assessed the impact of regional analgesia techniques on cancer progression. The interpretation of their findings is difficult, since the surgical injury itself, ineffective pain treatment, and perioperative stress all exhibit immunosuppressive effects and increase cancer progression risk. Moreover, most studies assess the impact of regional analgesia techniques on patients who have additionally received general anaesthesia for surgery, yet, as is well known, numerous anaesthetics administered either intravenously or inhalationally also produce immunosuppressive effects. However, it does not alter the fact that the appropriately chosen and performed regional anaesthesia techniques (for a specific patient and surgical procedure) very effectively relieve pain and effectively block the surgical trauma-induced neuroendocrine response of the body and thus better preserves the patient's immune status. In a study done by Koltun et al., it has been seen that patients receiving epidural anaesthesia during colectomy had lower plasma levels of epinephrine and cortisol, compared to patients receiving general anaesthesia, and also the NK cell activity was better preserved in patients receiving regional anaesthesia [50].

Most of the studies in question assess the influence of central blocks (including continuous epidural anaesthesia) in prostate [51] and colorectal cancer surgery patients

[52, 53]. The effects of the paraspinal block in breast cancer patients undergoing mastectomy were also assessed [54]. The findings of the studies are not unequivocal: some of them suggest a positive influence of regional anaesthesia techniques on immunological parameters (assessed differently in individual studies, e.g., VEGF, TGF-β, and IL-1β) and on the reduction of the risk of cancer progression, including prolonged overall survival time in patients in whom these techniques were used, whereas other studies fail to confirm these results [53, 55].

The currently recommended optimal approach to pain management is the multimodal analgesia approach, which involves combining analgesics and anaesthetic techniques with different mechanisms of action in order to take advantage of their synergistic effects. One of the components of multimodal analgesia are regional anaesthesia techniques: continuous epidural anaesthesia, paraspinal blocks, plexus blocks, and interfascial blocks which are increasingly often used in everyday clinical practice, thanks to the recent developments in ultrasonography. In the event of contraindications to regional anaesthesia techniques, combination pharmacotherapy involving nonopioid drugs and coanalgesics is a recommended analgesic management method (e.g., with intravenous lidocaine, magnesium, dexamethasone, ketamine, and dexmedetomidine). Such an approach, thanks to the combination of drugs with different mechanisms of action, ensures satisfactory analgesia at lower opioid doses, which is an important aspect of safety of the latter group of drugs referred to a number of times in this paper. Experimental studies show that NSAIDs administered together with opioids reduce immunosuppression associated with the use of the latter [54]. However, it should be remembered that the use of NSAIDs is subject to a number of restrictions due to the risk of gastrointestinal and renal damage, increased cardiovascular risk, and increased risk of bleeding secondary to the antiplatelet effect of nonselective NSAIDs. However, these drugs are worth considering as therapeutic options in cancer patients (taking into account the contraindications to their use), especially due to the NSAIDs' preventive effect on certain types of cancer and the possible anticancer effect of this group of drugs [56].

It should also be emphasized that the development of effective therapeutic strategies requires a better understanding of cellular mechanisms underlying the pathogenesis of pain. Progress in pain research points to an important role of microglial cells in the development of pain. The inhibition of spinal microglia has been shown to attenuate postoperative pain as well as morphine-induced antinociceptive tolerance [57]. Targeting microglial signaling might lead to more effective treatments for pain partly via improving the analgesic efficacy of opioids [58–60].

6. Conclusions

Insufficiently treated pain and stress associated with cancer adversely affect the body's defence mechanisms, including cellular immunity, natural killer (NK) cell function, and humoral response. Experimental and clinical studies also show the importance of effective pain management for checking cancer progression. Apart from the basic humanitarian aspect, these data provide an argument for the need to effectively alleviate stress and suffering in cancer patients. The question of how to do it optimally and in the safest possible way is still relevant, given the substantial evidence concerning the potentially adverse opioid effects to have emerged in recent studies (including immunosuppression, increased risk of infection, and cancer progression).

It should be clearly emphasized that the findings of research on the latter issue are ambiguous and as such should be treated with great caution. They must not be interpreted as an argument against using opioids in pain management in cancer patients. Effective pain treatment, alleviation of suffering associated with cancer, and improvement in the quality of life should always be a priority, while the awareness of potential risks should prompt the use of regional analgesia techniques, using local analgesics and possibly coanalgesics. Where it is impossible, recommendations include combined systemic pharmacotherapy comprising nonopioid analgesics and coanalgesics, some of which (including lidocaine and NSAIDs) also exhibit proven oncologically beneficial effects. Such an approach contributes to the optimization of analgesic management, and thus to obtaining the best analgesic effects at lower opioid doses, which, in turn, reduces the frequency and intensity of adverse effects associated with their use. Further research is needed to verify the currently available data on both the potential adverse effects of opioids and the possible protective effects of regional analgesia techniques on cancer patients.

Acknowledgments

The study was supported by the scientific grant of Foundation of Pain Medicine, Poland.

References

[1] E. L. Krakauer, R. Wenk, R. Buitrago, P. Jenkins, and W. J. Scholten, "Opioid inaccessibility and its human consequences: reports from the field," *Journal of Pain and Palliative Care Pharmacotherapy*, vol. 24, no. 2, pp. 239–243, 2010.

[2] M. H. Van den Beuken-van Everdingen, L. M. J. Hochstenbach, E. A. J. Joosten et al., "Update on prevalence of pain in patients with cancer: systematic review and meta-analysis," *Journal of Pain and Symptom Management*, vol. 51, no. 6, pp. 1070–1090, 2016.

[3] J. R. Meserve, A. D. Kaye, A. Prabhakar, and R. D. Urman, "The role of analgesics in cancer propagation," *Best Practice and Research Clinical Anaesthesiology*, vol. 28, no. 2, pp. 139–151, 2014.

[4] B. L. Andersen, W. B. Farrar, D. Golden-Kreutz et al., "Stress and immune responses after surgical treatment for regional

breast cancer," *Journal of the National Cancer Institute*, vol. 90, no. 1, pp. 30–36, 1998.

[5] G. G. Page, W. P. Blakely, and S. Ben-Eliyahu, "Evidence that postoperative pain is a mediator of the tumor-promoting effects of surgery in rats," *Pain*, vol. 90, no. 1, pp. 191–199, 2001.

[6] K. D. Lillemoe, J. L. Cameron, H. S. Kaufman, C. J. Yeo, H. A. Pitt, and P. K. Sauter, "Chemical splanchnicectomy in patients with unresectable pancreatic cancer. A prospective randomized trial," *Annals of Surgery*, vol. 217, no. 5, pp. 447–455, 1993.

[7] G. Nylund, A. Pettersson, C. Bengtsson, A. Khorram-Manesh, S. Nordgren, and D. S. Delbro, "Functional expression of μ-opioid receptors in the human colon cancer cell line, HT-29, and their localization in human colon," *Digestive Diseases and Sciences*, vol. 53, no. 2, pp. 461–466, 2008.

[8] B. Afsharimani, P. Cabot, and M. O. Parat, "Morphine and tumor growth and metastasis," *Cancer and Metastasis Reviews*, vol. 30, no. 2, pp. 225–238, 2011.

[9] R. Vallejo, O. de Leon-Casasola, and R. Benyamin, "Opioid therapy and immunosuppression: a review," *American Journal of Therapeutics*, vol. 11, no. 5, pp. 354–365, 2004.

[10] M. Hernandez, L. Flores, and B. Bayer, "Immunosuppression by morphine is mediated by central pathways," *Journal of Pharmacology and Experimental Therapeutics*, vol. 267, no. 3, pp. 1336–1341, 1993.

[11] C. Gaveriaux-Ruff, H. W. Matthes, J. Peluso, and B. L. Kiefer, "Abolition of morphine-immunosuppression in mice lacking the μ-opioid receptor gene," *Proceedings of the National Academy of Sciences*, vol. 95, no. 11, pp. 6326–6330, 1998.

[12] R. J. Weber and A. Pert, "The periaqueductal gray matter mediates opiate-induced immunosuppression," *Science*, vol. 245, no. 4914, pp. 188–190, 1989.

[13] M. Al-Hashimi, S. W. M. Scott, J. P. Thompson, and D. G. Lambert, "Opioids and immune modulation: more questions than answers," *British Journal of Anaesthesia*, vol. 111, no. 1, pp. 80–88, 2013.

[14] G. B. Stefano, J. D. Burrill, S. Labur, J. Blake, and P. Cadet, "Regulation of various genes in human leukocytes acutely exposed to morphine: expression microarray analysis," *Medical Science Monitor*, vol. 11, no. 5, pp. 35–42, 2005.

[15] T. K. Eisenstein and M. E. Hilburger, "Opioid modulation of immune responses: effects on phagocyte and lymphoid cell populations," *Journal of Neuroimmunology*, vol. 83, no. 1-2, pp. 36–44, 1998.

[16] P. M. Mathews, C. J. Froelich, W. L. Sibbitt, and A. D. Bankhurst, "Enhancement of natural cytotoxicity by beta-endorphin," *Journal of Immunology*, vol. 130, no. 4, pp. 1658–1662, 1983.

[17] S. Roy, J. Wang, J. Kelschenbech, L. Koodie, and J. Martin, "Modulation of immune function by morphine: implications for susceptibility to infection," *Journal of Neuroimmune Pharmacology*, vol. 1, no. 1, pp. 77–89, 2006.

[18] A. M. Casellas, H. Guardiola, and F. L. Renaud, "Inhibition by opioids of phagocytosis in peritoneal macrophages," *Neuropeptides*, vol. 18, no. 1, pp. 35–40, 1991.

[19] I. D. Welters, A. Menzebach, Y. Goumon et al., "Morphine suppresses complement receptor expression, phagocytosis, and respiratory burst in neutrophils by nitric oxide and μ 3 opiate receptor-dependent mechanisms," *Journal of Neuroimmunology*, vol. 111, no. 1-2, pp. 139–145, 2000.

[20] J. L. Martin, L. Koodie, A. G. Krishnan et al., "Chronic morphine administration delays wound healing by inhibiting immune cells recruitment to the wound site," *American Journal of Pathology*, vol. 176, no. 2, pp. 786–799, 2010.

[21] T. J. Min, J. H. Kim, K. H. Noh, T. W. Kim, and W. Y. Kim, "Morphine post-conditioning attenuates ICAM-1 expression on endothelial cells," *Journal of Korean Medical Science*, vol. 26, no. 2, pp. 290–296, 2011.

[22] L. Frenklakh, R. S. Bhat, M. Bhaskaran, S. Sharma, M. Sharma, and A. Dinda, "Morphine-induced degradation of the host defence barrier role of intestinal mucosal injury," *Digestive Diseases and Sciences*, vol. 51, no. 2, pp. 318–325, 2006.

[23] J. Wang, R. A. Barke, R. Charboneau, H. H. Loh, and S. Roy, "Morphine negatively regulates interferon-gamma promoter activity in activated murine T cells through two distinct cyclic AMP-dependent pathways," *Journal of Biological Chemistry*, vol. 278, no. 39, pp. 37622–37631, 2003.

[24] J. L. Bussiere, M. W. Adler, T. J. Rogers, and T. K. Eisenstein, "Cytokine reversal of morphine-induced suppression of the antibody response," *Journal of Pharmacology and Experimental Therapeutics*, vol. 264, no. 2, pp. 591–597, 1993.

[25] H. N. Bhargava, P. T. Thomas, S. Thorat, and R. V. House, "Effects of morphine tolerance and abstinence on cellular immune function," *Brain Research*, vol. 642, no. 1-2, pp. 1–10, 1994.

[26] D. Franchimont, "Overview of the actions of glucocorticoids on the immune response: a good model to characterize new pathways of immunosuppression for new treatment strategies," *Annals of the New York Academy of Sciences*, vol. 1024, no. 1, pp. 124–137, 2004.

[27] C. Vuong, S. H. M. V. Uum, L. E. O'Dell, K. Lutfy, and T. C. Friedman, "The effects of opioids and opioid analogues on animal and human endocrine systems," *Endocrine Reviews*, vol. 31, no. 1, pp. 98–132, 2010.

[28] K. Müssig, D. Knaus-Dittmann, H. Schmidt, K. Mörike, and H. U. Häring, "Secondary adrenal failure and secondary amenorrhoea following hydromorphone treatment," *Clinical Endocrinology*, vol. 66, pp. 604-605, 2007.

[29] K. M. Oltmanns, H. L. Fehm, and A. Peters, "Chronic fentanyl application induces adrenocortical insufficiency," *Journal of Internal Medicine*, vol. 257, no. 5, pp. 478–480, 2005.

[30] D. M. Holl, J. L. Suo, and R. J. Weber, "Opioid mediated effects on the immune system sympathetic nervous system involvement," *Journal of Neuroimmunology*, vol. 83, no. 1-2, pp. 29–35, 1998.

[31] D. L. Felten, S. Y. Felten, S. L. Carlson, J. A. Olschowka, and S. Livnat, "Nordarenergic and peptidergic innervation of lymphoid tissue," *Journal of Immunology*, vol. 135, no. 2, pp. 755–765, 1985.

[32] K. Fecho, K. A. Maslonek, L. A. Dykstra, and D. T. Lysle, "Alterations of immune status induced by the sympathetic nervous system: immunomodulatory effects of DMPP alone and in combination with morphine," *Brain, Behavior, and Immunity*, vol. 7, no. 3, pp. 253–270, 1993.

[33] J. L. Bonilla-Garcia, M. Cortinas-Saenz, and E. del Pozo-Gavilan, "Opioids and immunosuppression in oncological postoperative patients," *Revista da Associação Médica Brasileira*, vol. 63, no. 9, pp. 753–763, 2017.

[34] P. Sacerdote, B. Manfredi, P. Mantegazza et al., "Antinociceptive and immunosuppressive effects of opiate drugs: a structure-related activity study," *British Journal of Pharmacology*, vol. 121, no. 4, pp. 834–840, 1997.

[35] S. Franchi, A. E. Panerai, and P. Sacerdote, "Buprenorphine ameliorates the effect of surgery on hypothalamus-pituitary-adrenal axis, natural killer cell activity and metastatic colonisation in rats in comparison with morphine or fentanyl treatment," *Brain, Behavior, and Immunity*, vol. 21, no. 6, pp. 767–774, 2007.

[36] P. Eschwege, F. Dumas, P. Blanchet et al., "Haematogenous dissemination of prostatic epithelial cells during radical prostatectomy," *The Lancet*, vol. 346, no. 8989, pp. 1528–1530, 1995.
[37] I. Kirman, V. Cekic, N. Poltaratskaia et al., "Plasma from patients undergoing major open surgery stimulates *in vitro* tumor growth: lower insulin-like growth factor binding protein 3 levels may, in part, account for this change," *Surgery*, vol. 132, no. 2, pp. 186–192, 2002.
[38] I. Kirman, S. Jain, V. Cekic et al., "Altered plasma matrix metalloproteinase-9/tissue inhibitor of matrix [corrected] metalloproteinase-1 concentration during the early postoperative period in patients with colorectal cancer," *Surgical Endoscopy*, vol. 20, no. 3, pp. 482–486, 2006.
[39] M. N. Svendsen, K. Werther, H. J. Nielsen, and P. E. Kristjansen, "VEGF and tumour angiogenesis. Impact of surgery, wound healing, inflammation and blood transfusion," *Scandinavian Journal of Gastroenterology*, vol. 37, no. 4, pp. 373–379, 2002.
[40] A. M. Lacy, J. C. Garcia-Valdecasas, S. Delgado et al., "Laparoscopy-assisted colectomy versus open colectomy for treatment of non-metastatic colon cancer: a randomized trial," *The Lancet*, vol. 359, no. 9325, pp. 2224–2229, 2002.
[41] S. Atzil, M. Arad, A. Glasner et al., "Blood transfusion promotes cancer progression: a critical role for aged erythrocytes," *Anesthesiology*, vol. 109, no. 6, pp. 989–997, 2008.
[42] S. Ben-Eliyahu, G. Shakhar, E. Rosenne, Y. Levinson, and B. Beilin, "Hypothermia in barbiturate-anesthetized rats suppresses natural killer cell activity and compromises resistance to tumor metastasis: a role for adrenergic mechanisms," *Anesthesiology*, vol. 91, no. 3, pp. 732–740, 1999.
[43] S. Ben-Eliyahu, G. G. Page, R. Yirmiya, and G. Shakhar, "Evidence that stress and surgical interventions promote tumor development by suppressing natural killer cell activity," *International Journal of Cancer*, vol. 80, no. 6, pp. 880–888, 1999.
[44] J. W. Lee, M. M. Shahzad, Y. G. Lin et al., "Surgical stress promotes tumor growth in ovarian carcinoma," *Clinical Cancer Research*, vol. 15, no. 8, pp. 2695–2702, 2009.
[45] K. Gupta, "Iatrogenic angiogenesis," in *Morphine and Metastasis*, M. Parat, Ed., p. 63, Netherlands, 2013.
[46] F. E. Lennon, T. Mirzapoiazova, B. Mambetsariev et al., "Overexpression of the mu-opioid receptor in human non-small cell lung cancer promotes Akt and mTOR activation, tumor growth, and metastasis," *Anesthesiology*, vol. 116, no. 4, pp. 857–867, 2012.
[47] P. A. Singleton, J. G. Garcia, and J. Moss, "Synergistic effects of methylnaltrexone with 5-fluorouracil and bevacizumab on inhibition of vascular endothelial growth factor-induced angiogenesis," *Molecular Cancer Therapeutics*, vol. 7, no. 6, pp. 1669–1679, 2008.
[48] K. Gupta, S. Kshirsagar, L. Chang et al., "Morphine stimulates angiogenesis by activating proangiogenic and survival-promoting signaling and promotes breast tumor growth," *Cancer Research*, vol. 62, no. 15, pp. 4491–4498, 2002.
[49] Y. Shavit, S. Ben-Eliyahu, A. Zeidel, and B. Beilin, "Effect of fentanyl on natural killer cell activity and on resistance to tumour metastasis in rats. Dose and timing study," *Neuroimmunomodulation*, vol. 11, no. 4, pp. 255–260, 2004.
[50] W. A. Koltun, M. M. Bloomer, A. F. Tilberq et al., "Awake epidural anaesthesia is associated with improved natural killer cell cytotoxicity and a reduced stress response," *American Journal of Surgery*, vol. 171, no. 1, pp. 68–72, 1996.
[51] B. Biki, E. Mascha, D. C. Moriarty, J. M. Fitzpatrick, D. I. Sessler, and D. J. Buggy, "Anesthetic technique for radical prostatectomy surgery affects cancer recurrence: a retrospective analysis," *Anesthesiology*, vol. 109, no. 2, pp. 180–187, 2008.
[52] R. Christopherson, K. E. James, M. Tableman, P. Marshall, and F. E. Johnson, "Long-term survival after colon cancer surgery: a variation associated with choice of anesthesia," *Anesthesia and Analgesia*, vol. 107, no. 1, pp. 325–332, 2008.
[53] A. Gottschalk, J. G. Ford, C. C. Regelin et al., "Association between epidural analgesia and cancer recurrence after colorectal cancer surgery," *Anesthesiology*, vol. 113, no. 1, pp. 27–34, 2010.
[54] A. K. Exadaktylos, D. J. Buggy, D. C. Moriarty, E. Mascha, and D. I. Sessler, "Can anesthetic technique for primary breast cancer surgery affect recurrence or metastasis?," *Anesthesiology*, vol. 105, no. 4, pp. 660–664, 2006.
[55] B. C. Tsui, S. Rashiq, D. Schopflocher et al., "Epidural anesthesia and cancer recurrence rates after radical prostatectomy," *Canadian Journal of Anaesthesia*, vol. 57, no. 2, pp. 107–112, 2010.
[56] M. Farooqui, Y. Li, T. Rogers et al., "COX-2 inhibitor celecoxib prevents chronic morphine-induced promotion of angiogenesis, tumour growth, metastasis, and mortality, without compromising analgesia," *British Journal of Cancer*, vol. 97, no. 11, pp. 1523–1531, 2007.
[57] J. Mika, A. Wawrzczak-Bargiela, M. Osikowicz, W. Makuch, and B. Przewlocka, "Attenuation of morphine tolerance by minocycline and pentoxifylline in naive and neuropathic mice," *Brain, Behavior, and Immunity*, vol. 23, no. 1, pp. 75–84, 2009.
[58] Y. R. Wen, P. H. Tan, J. K. Cheng, Y. C. Liu, and R. R. Ji, "Microglia: a promising target for treating neuropathic and postoperative pain, and morphine tolerance," *Journal of the Formosan Medical Association*, vol. 110, no. 8, pp. 487–494, 2011.
[59] J. Mika, "Modulation of microglia can attenuate neuropathic pain symptoms and enhance morphine effectiveness," *Pharmacological Reports*, vol. 60, no. 3, pp. 297–307, 2008.
[60] J. Mika, M. Zychowska, K. Popiolek-Barczyk, E. Rojewska, and B. Przewlocka, "Importance of glial activation in neuropathic pain," *European Journal of Pharmacology*, vol. 716, no. 1–3, pp. 106–119, 2013.

19

Pain Intensity Is Not Always Associated with Poorer Health Status: Exploring the Moderating Role of Spouse Personality

Carlos Suso-Ribera,[1] Michael J. L. Sullivan,[2] and Santiago Suso-Vergara[3]

[1]*Department of Basic and Clinical Psychology and Psychobiology, Jaume I University, Castellón de la Plana, Spain*
[2]*Department of Psychology, McGill University, Montreal, Canada*
[3]*Department of Traumatology, Clinic Hospital, Barcelona, Spain*

Correspondence should be addressed to Carlos Suso-Ribera; susor@uji.es

Academic Editor: Giustino Varrassi

Background. Past decades have seen a surge of studies investigating the role of spouses in chronic illness. The present study explored an interpersonal model of health-related quality of life in chronic pain settings. Spouse personality was tested as a moderator of pain intensity-to-health associations in patients with chronic pain. *Methods.* This is a cross-sectional study. Participants were 185 noncancer chronic pain patients and their spouses. Patients were mostly females (58.4%). Mean age was approximately 56 years for patients and spouses. Patients completed a measure of pain intensity, health-related quality of life, and personality. Spouses also reported on their personality characteristics. Spouse personality was used as the moderator in the relationship between patients' pain intensity and health status. Patient personality was used as a covariate in the moderation analyses. *Results.* Spouse neuroticism moderated the relationship between pain intensity and physical health status, while spouse introversion moderated the pain-to-mental health association. *Conclusions.* Results support the idea that the relationship between a chronic stressor, namely, chronic pain, and health-related quality of life may be complex and contextually determined by spousal characteristics. Clinical implications are discussed in the context of couples.

1. Introduction

Chronic pain is a common and disabling disease [1–3]. Similar to other chronic illnesses [4, 5], spouses of pain patients have been argued to play an important role in the disease due to their caregiving role [6]. In chronic pain, spouse responses to patients' pain behavior have been the focus of most research [7], while the influence of spouse personality characteristics has been mostly overlooked. This is surprising because personality traits have been consistently associated with mental and physical health status across healthy and sick populations, including chronic pain [8, 9].

Personality can be defined as relatively stable ways in which people think, feel, and behave [10]. The five-factor model of personality (FFM), which describes personality in terms of five dimensions (neuroticism, extraversion, agreeableness, openness to experience, and conscientiousness), is currently the dominant framework for personality. In the FFM, neuroticism is understood as a tendency to be emotionally unstable and to experience negative emotions (i.e., anxiety, depression, and anger). Neuroticism is considered a risk factor for health as it has been associated with poorer physical functioning, increased worry about symptoms, and greater mental distress. Conversely, extraversion and conscientiousness tend to be associated with better health outcomes, including physical functioning and mental well-being. Extraverts tend to be optimistic, physically active, and socially competent, while conscientiousness is associated with high self-discipline, dutifulness, and low risk taking. Agreeableness and openness, which are the socio-affective and intellect dimensions, respectively, have the less consistent and weakest associations with health outcomes [9, 11, 12].

Consistent with the literature on neuroticism, when spouse interaction styles are characterized by negative emotionality (i.e., preoccupied and fearful or angry and critical), patients tend to report increased mental distress. By contrast, the relationship between these negative responses and pain intensity and physical disability levels is weaker and inconsistent, and the role of arguably positive spouse behaviors, such as solicitous and validating responses, is still inconclusive [13–17]. One limitation of existent research is that spouse factors are argued to have a direct effect on patient outcomes. However, it is also possible that spouse characteristics influence patients' status by moderating (i.e., reducing or aggravating) the impact that pain has on health [7]. This is consistent with the Transactional Model Of Health, which emphasizes that challenges of the painful condition occur in a social (family) context and argues that spouse factors can improve or exacerbate stressors [18].

There is, indeed, some support for this contextual (i.e., moderating) role of spouse personality in the context of couples. For instance, a study showed that spouse neuroticism influenced the associations between everyday problems and affect and physical symptoms in older couples [19]. In another investigation, the relationship between patient personality and patient psychological health differed as a function of spouse personality [20]. What these studies suggest is that the relationship between stressors (i.e., everyday problems and certain personality styles) and patient health can be influenced by spouse characteristics. The extent to which spouse personality can also be an important contextual factor in the presence of a chronic stressor, such as pain, remains unexplored.

The present study aims at testing whether the negative influence of patient pain (stressor) on patient health-related quality of life (outcome) is moderated by psychological factors in the spouse (e.g., spouse personality; contextual factor). Research has consistently shown that health-related quality of life decreases with pain [21, 22]. Based on previous research showing that neuroticism, introversion, and low conscientiousness are also associated with poor health status [9], we expect that the aforementioned spouse psychological characteristics will impose low health-related quality of life in pain patients irrespective of pain levels (i.e., the burden of pain is increased).

2. Methods

2.1. Design, Participants, and Settings. This observational study was conducted at the Pain Clinic of the Valld'Hebron Hospital in Barcelona, which is a tertiary care pain clinic. This clinic was selected because it was the home institution of the corresponding author, C. S. R., when the study was conducted. Also, past research by our team has revealed that patient characteristics at this clinic are comparable to those of other tertiary pain clinics [23], so the results obtained might be applicable to a considerable number of pain clinics.

Eligibility criteria included (i) having a diagnosis of chronic noncancer pain (>3 months of duration), (ii) having an appointment at the Pain Clinic of the Valld'Hebron Hospital between January 2014 and December 2015, and (iii) being married at the time of assessment. Consecutive sampling was used for recruitment, which started in January 2014 and finished in December 2015. One month prior to the patients' appointment at the Pain Clinic, the lead researcher, C. S. R., explored the eligibility criterion of having a diagnosis of chronic pain in the electronic medical records and ICD-9 code 338.2. Patients meeting this criterion were called to explore the eligibility criterion of marital status. If they were married and willing to participate in the study, two letters were sent to the patient's home, one for the patient and the other for the spouse. For both, each letter included a description of the goals, procedures, and possible risks of participating in the study, together with the contact information of the lead researcher, C. S. R., the informed consent form, and the questionnaires.

Couples were asked to complete the forms separately and were given an envelope that had to be sealed and returned to the physician the day of the patient's first visit to the Pain Clinic. All participants provided their written consent to participate in the study and did not receive any economic compensation for their participation.

The Ethics Committee of the Vall d'Hebron Hospital in Barcelona approved the current study.

2.2. Measures

2.2.1. Spouse Personality. The NEO five-factor Inventory (NEO-FFI) [10] evaluates five dimensions of adult personality, namely, neuroticism, extraversion, openness to experience, agreeableness, and conscientiousness. Of these, only neuroticism, extraversion, and conscientiousness appear to be consistently associated with health outcomes in chronic pain settings [8, 9, 12]. However, because this is a novel approach to the role of personality in chronic pain, the moderating role of openness and agreeableness will also be investigated.

In the NEO-FFI participants rate their degree of agreement on a 5-point Likert scale (0 = *totally disagree*; 4 = *completely agree*). Each of the five personality dimensions is composed of 12 items, so scores for each dimension range from 0 to 48. The internal reliability of the personality dimensions in our study ($0.64 < \alpha < 0.84$) was comparable to previous findings ($0.66 < \alpha < 0.81$) [10, 24].

2.2.2. Patient Pain Intensity. Current pain intensity was assessed with a Numerical Rating Scale, which has become a standard in the measurement of pain [25] and is widely recommended due to its compliance rate, responsiveness, and ease of use [26]. Participants in our study rated their pain from 0 = *no pain* to 10 = *worst possible pain.*

2.2.3. Patient Health-Related Quality of Life. Physical and mental components of quality of life were assessed with the Short Form-36 Health Survey [27], which has become one of the most widely used instruments for the assessment of health-related quality of life [28]. Physical aspects include the ability to perform daily activities (Physical Functioning) and work-related activities (Role Physical), plus the average intensity of pain in the last four weeks (Bodily Pain). Some elements correlate to physical and mental health, such as the perception of present and future health (General Health), the evaluation of personal energy (Vitality), and the interference of health problems in their interpersonal life (Social Functioning). The remaining components, namely, the role of emotions on functioning (Role Emotional) and psychological well-being (Mental Health), mainly reflect psychological aspects of health [21]. A composite score can be obtained for physical and mental health using the aforementioned subscales. The use of these composite scores is often recommended for methodological reasons [29]. However, the use of the physical composite in the present study would be problematic because it contains a pain subscale, which would contaminate the relationship between the dependent variable (i.e., health) and the independent variable (i.e., pain intensity). Thus, physical health was measured by means of the Physical Functioning scale. The Mental Composite Score is not contaminated by the presence of pain intensity ratings, so it was used to assess overall mental health to reduce the number of statistical tests. Scales and composite scores in the Short Form-36 have a 0–100 range. High scores represent better functioning. The internal consistency in our study ($0.86 < \alpha < 0.95$), which is calculated for the 8 subscales, was consistent with previous findings ($0.78 < \alpha < 0.94$) [30].

2.2.4. Covariates. Patient age, sex, pain duration, educational level, and personality were used as covariates due to their relationship with patient health status [8, 31]. Patient education was coded as 0 = "less than 12 years of education" and 1 = "more than 12 years of education." Patient personality was assessed with the NEO-FFI, the same measure that was used to evaluate spouse personality.

2.3. Statistical Analyses. The moderating effect of spouse personality on the relationship between pain and health-related quality of life in the patient was tested using multiple linear regressions. In the regressions, patient sex, age, and personality were included as covariates in the first block. Patient pain intensity was entered next. The third and the forth blocks included spouse personality and the interaction term (patient pain intensity ∗ spouse personality), respectively. Multiple regression diagnostics included an analysis of multicollinearity (i.e., two predictors are linear combinations of one another) and a test of unusual and influential data (i.e., whether certain observations are responsible for the results).

All analyses were computed using SPSS version 22 [32].

3. Results

3.1. Sample Characteristics. From January 2014 to December 2015, 515 phone calls were made. In total, 203 patients met the eligibility criteria, so a letter was sent to these patients and their spouses. Eighteen patients did not return the protocol (either them or the spouse lost interest in the study). The final sample comprised 185 chronic pain patients and their spouses (91.1% response rate). All couples were heterosexual. Patients had an average age of 56.55 years ($SD = 13.59$) and were mostly females (58.4%). The mean age for spouses was 56.66 years ($SD = 13.85$) and 41.6% were females. Approximately 94% of participants were born in Spain. Academic degree was similar for both samples, with approximately half of the participants having achieved more than 12 years of education (47.3% of patients and 50.3% of spouses). Patients had been suffering pain for an average of 6.55 years ($SD = 8.57$). Pain was mostly located in the back (58.8%) and neck (11.1%).

Means and standard deviations of study variables are presented in Table 1. Mean pain intensity was 7.71 ($SD = 1.56$) with a range of 3 to 10. The sample would be characterized as experiencing moderate to severe pain [33]. Scores for patients' physical and mental health status were comparable (between +1 *SD* and −1 *SD*) to those of previous investigations assessing similar pain populations [34–36]. Compared with population norms, mean values on physical and mental composite scores were, respectively, 2 *SD* and 1 *SD* below the mean of the general population in Spain [37]. Pain patients in this sample were significantly more physically disabled and psychologically distressed than the general population. Mean scores for spouse and patient personality were comparable (within 1 *SD*) with previously reported scores in the general population in Spain [24, 38].

3.2. Moderation Analyses. Before performing the moderation analyses, all predictors were centered. Patient openness and agreeableness were not used as covariates due to their weak associations with patient health-related quality of life and to reduce multicollinearity problems.

Spouse neuroticism moderated the association between patients' pain intensity and patient Physical Functioning (Table 2), while spouse extraversion moderated the pain-to-mental health relationship (Table 3). In a moderation analysis, this should be interpreted as revealing that the contribution of the independent variable (i.e., patients' pain intensity) on the dependent variable (i.e., physical and mental health) varies among different levels of the moderator (i.e., spouse neuroticism and extraversion).For example, the positive interaction coefficient between spouse neuroticism and patient pain intensity in the prediction of physical functioning ($\beta = 0.19$, $p = 0.009$, 95% CI = 0.08, 0.54) means that patient pain intensity is less intensely associated with physical functioning at higher levels of spouse neuroticism. On the contrary, the negative coefficient in the interaction between extraversion and pain intensity in the prediction of mental health ($\beta = -0.17$, $p = 0.014$, 95% CI = −0.30, −0.03) reveals that patient pain intensity is less intensely associated with mental health at low levels of spouse extraversion. No moderation effect was found for spouse openness to experience, agreeableness, and conscientiousness.

Post hoc analyses were then performed to explore if the simple slopes were significant and in the expected direction. Simple slopes are often calculated at one standard deviation

Table 1: Means and standard deviations of patient and spouse characteristics.

	Patient	Spouse
Age	56.82 (13.60)	56.66 (13.85)
Pain duration (years)	6.56 (8.57)	
Personality		
Neuroticism	20.05 (8.45)	24.19 (7.05)
Extraversion	26.99 (7.54)	31.79 (5.53)
Conscientiousness	32.43 (6.87)	24.54 (8.96)
Openness	31.86 (6.84)	26.26 (8.08)
Agreeableness	30.88 (6.20)	22.74 (7.41)
Pain and health status		
Pain intensity	7.71 (1.56)	
Physical Functioning	34.80 (23.65)	
Mental Composite Score	39.04 (12.44)	

from the sample mean, but its use has been argued to be arbitrary and sample specific, which might limit the generalizability of the findings (i.e., what is high in one sample might be moderate or low in another sample) [39]. Thus, we plotted the moderation using the Spanish population norms for low (percentile 30) and high (percentile 65) neuroticism and extraversion, which are 16 and 23 for neuroticism and 28 and 35 for extraversion [40]. As reflected in Figure 1, the relationship between patient pain intensity and patient physical functioning at daily activities was strongest when spouse neuroticism was low ($\beta = -0.47$, $t = -4.22$, $p < 0.001$; 95% CI = −14.08, −5.03) or moderate ($\beta = -0.55$, $t = -4.67$, $p < 0.001$; 95% CI = −12.31, −4.90), as opposed to high ($\beta = -0.33$, $t = -2.82$, $p = 0.006$; 95% CI = −7.17, −1.23).

The post hoc probing with extraversion as a moderator (Figure 2) showed similar results to those obtained for neuroticism. Specifically, pain intensity was not significantly associated with mental health for participants with an introverted (low in extraversion) spouse ($\beta = -0.15$, $t = -1.5$, $p = 0.115$; 95% CI = −2.38, 0.26). On the contrary, pain intensity was significantly related to mental health when the spouse extraversion was either high ($\beta = -0.34$, $t = -2.43$, $p = 0.019$; 95% CI = −6.58, −0.61) or moderate ($\beta = -0.53$, $t = -3.22$, $p = 0.003$; 95% CI = −8.46, −1.87).

Multiple regression diagnostics revealed no problems of model fit to the data. Specifically, the variance inflation factor, which reveals to what extent the variance is inflated due to multicollinearity, was lower than 2 for all predictors. To test the existence of influential cases, we assessed how the regression coefficients changed by excluding an observation by means of the standardized DFBETA, with a particular interest in the interaction coefficient. All values were smaller than 1, suggesting that none of the observations substantially influenced the model [41].

4. Discussion

The present investigation aimed at exploring the moderating role of spouse personality in the relationship between pain intensity and health-related quality of life in patients with chronic pain. Based on previous research showing pain intensity and certain personality dispositions (i.e., neuroticism, introversion, and low conscientiousness) associated with poor health outcomes [4, 9], we expected that spouse neuroticism, introversion, and low conscientiousness would add to the burden of pain by imposing poor health across pain levels. Our results partially support our hypothesis. On the one hand, the predicted moderation occurred for spouse neuroticism and extraversion. On the other hand, these findings were not replicated for conscientiousness, and the moderation of neuroticism and extraversion only occurred for physical and mental components of health-related quality of life, respectively.

Research has repeatedly shown that experiencing pain impacts negatively on the physical and mental health status of individuals [42–45]. In our study, this was replicated when spouse neuroticism and introversion were low or moderate (i.e., health-related quality of life decreased with pain). However, pain intensity was weakly or non-significantly associated with health outcomes when spouse neuroticism or spouse introversion were high, indicating similar levels of (low) functioning irrespective of the intensity of the stressor (pain) and suggesting that spouse personality adds to the burden of pain on health-related quality of life, especially at lower levels of pain intensity. A mechanism by which spouse personality might influence pain-health associations is proposed in accordance with the Transactional Model Of Health [18], although this remains speculative and further conclusions cannot be drawn from the present study results.

The Transactional Model Of Health and more recent discussions on interpersonal models of health in chronic pain [7, 18] propose that spouse appraisal might enhance similar cognitive patterns in patients, ultimately explaining patient behavior and health-related quality of life. Individuals scoring high in neuroticism tend to be fearful and preoccupied and report poor mental and physical health status [46–48]. Similarly, spouses' worry and negativity towards the patient's pain behavior has been associated with impaired physical and mental health of pain patients [17, 49]. According to the Transactional Model of Health, the moderating effect of spouse neuroticism revealed in the present investigation would be explained by means of modeling mechanism by which spouse preoccupation and worry would enhance similar affective and cognitive reactions in patient. These affective states are known to lead to maladaptive behaviors (i.e., avoidance of movement and disuse of painful body parts due to fear) and, ultimately, to impaired physical status [50], which would be consistent with our findings.

In our study, pain-to-health associations in the patient also varied as a function of spouse extraversion. Specifically, patients whose spouses presented low levels of extraversion (i.e., introversion) showed poor mental health irrespective of the intensity of their pain. Research in chronic pain has indicated that optimism, social interactions, and physical activities are key factors associated with the mental well-being of pain patients [23, 51–53]. However, evidence suggests that individuals low in extraversion are not very physically active, pessimistic, and have little interest for social interactions [9, 54]. Again, though this is only a hypothesis, a possible mechanism explaining these results is

Table 2: Moderation analysis of neuroticism in the relationship between pain intensity and Physical Functioning.

Block	Independent variables	β	95% CI	t	p	R^2	F	p
	Patient age	−0.22	−0.62, −0.13	−3.01	0.003			
	Patient sex	<0.01	−6.24, 6.40	0.02	0.981			
	Pain duration	−0.08	−0.70, 0.17	−1.21	0.229			
1	Educational level	0.03	−4.93, 8.14	0.49	0.628	0.104	4.05	<0.001
	Patient N	−0.01	−0.43, 0.37	−0.13	0.899			
	Patient E	0.15	0.03, 0.87	2.12	0.035			
	Patient C	0.06	−0.28, 0.66	0.80	0.424			
2	Patient pain intensity	−0.45	−8.94, −4.73	−6.41	<0.001	0.138	30.25	<0.001
3	Spouse N	−0.01	−0.35, 0.39	0.12	0.907	<0.001	<0.01	0.969
4	Spouse N * patient pain	0.19	0.08, 0.54	2.65	0.009	0.021	7.01	0.009

Note. R^2 is adjusted. R^2 and F refer to changes in each block. Reported beta values are standardized and correspond to the final model. N, neuroticism; E, extraversion; C, conscientiousness.

Table 3: Moderation analysis of extraversion in the pain-mental health relationship.

Block	Independent variables	β	95% CI	t	p	R^2	F	p
	Patient age	0.08	−0.05, 0.20	1.17	0.244			
	Patient sex	−0.06	−4.67, 1.60	−0.97	0.334			
	Pain duration	−0.06	−0.33, 0.11	−0.95	0.341			
1	Educational level	0.10	−0.89, 5.79	1.45	0.150	0.265	10.50	<0.001
	Patient N	−0.36	−0.70, −0.30	−4.86	<0.001			
	Patient E	0.11	−0.04, 0.38	1.58	0.116			
	Patient C	0.10	−0.07, 0.41	1.39	0.166			
2	Patient pain intensity	−0.25	−3.03, −0.90	−3.65	<0.001	0.030	8.37	0.004
3	Spouse E	0.02	−0.18, 0.24	0.29	0.770	<0.001	<0.01	0.995
4	Spouse E * patient pain	−0.17	−0.30, −0.03	−2.47	0.014	0.016	6.10	0.014

Note. R^2 is adjusted. R^2 and F refer to changes in each block. Reported beta values are standardized and correspond to the final model. N, neuroticism; E, extraversion; C, conscientiousness.

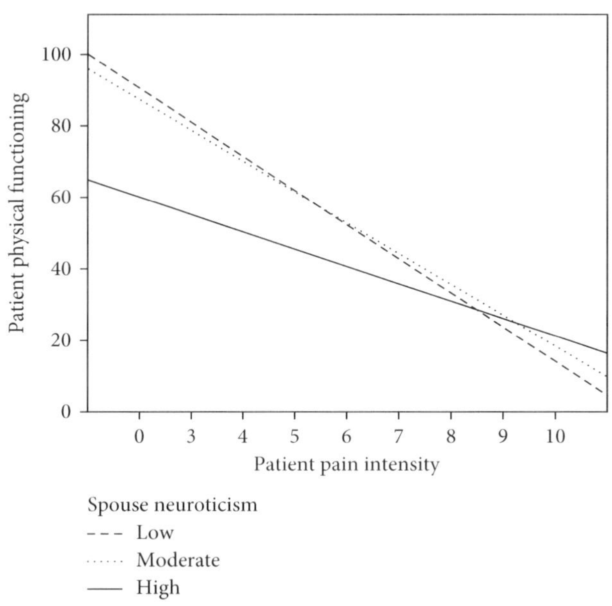

Figure 1: Neuroticism as a moderator of the relationship between pain intensity and Physical Functioning.

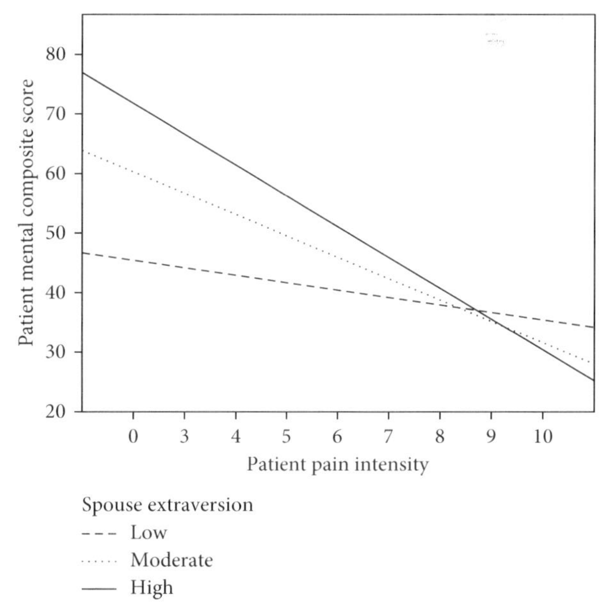

Figure 2: Extraversion as a moderator of the pain intensity to mental health relationship.

provided in accordance with the Transactional Model of Health. Specifically, it is possible that introverted spouses may add to the patients' mental burden when experiencing lower levels of pain by stimulating pessimistic thoughts about the disease and failing to promote the use of beneficial coping efforts, such as social interactions and physical activity.

Regarding the other personality dimensions, our study revealed that spouse openness to experience, agreeableness, and conscientiousness did not moderate the pain-health relationship in the pain patient. Research has previously shown that the contribution of openness and agreeableness to well-being is small when compared with that of neuroticism, extraversion, and conscientiousness [9, 55, 56]. The fact that conscientiousness did not emerge as a significant moderator of the pain-health relation is surprising in light of the role of this personality dimension in health settings [11]. However, its role in chronic pain settings has been argued to be modest [57–59], so its contribution might not be generalizable to all populations.

In our study, spouse neuroticism moderated pain-to-physical health associations, while the moderation of extraversion occurred for mental health. Extraversion is frequently associated with better physical and mental health in the general population [9]. However, its relation with physical health in pain settings appears to be less clear [57, 60], which might explain the results in our study. It is less clear why neuroticism of the spouse only correlated to physical and not to mental health. Most studies show a negative association between neuroticism and mental health [8, 57], so one would also expect a moderating effect neuroticism on pain-to-mental health associations. In fact, there is previous evidence to suggest that the relationship between a stressor (i.e., everyday problems) and both affective and physical problems are moderated by spouse neuroticism [19]. While the present study replicated this moderating effect of spouse neuroticism on physical health status, this was not the case for mental well-being.

The study of spouse personality, the inclusion of important covariates of patient health (i.e., patient personality and demographic factors), and the analysis of moderation are some of the strengths of the present investigation. Previous research had explored the association between spouse behaviors (i.e., response styles) and several outcomes in the patient, including pain intensity reports and physical and mental health status [16, 61, 62]. However, the role of spouse personality, as well as the moderating effect of spouse characteristics remained unexplored. The present study adds to the existent literature by showing that a possible mechanism by which spouse factors (i.e., personality) might contribute to patient health is by exacerbating or attenuating its relationship with pain intensity. Also importantly, moderation occurred even after controlling for patient demographic and personality characteristics.

The present study is not without limitations. Although some mechanisms explaining the moderation effects were proposed, they should be considered as hypotheses and need further investigation. Also, the effect sizes of the moderator were low. Although this is frequent in moderation studies, the power of the associations should not be overestimated. Additionally, some factors that might be important for the mental well-being of couples, such as length and quality of marriage, were not assessed in this investigation. In fact, while being married was a key eligibility factor in the study, the quality of the relationship, even without marriage, might be an interesting factor to be considered in the present study, as well as in future, similar investigations. Finally, there are methodological limitations in this study too. For example, the design used prevents us from drawing any causal relationship from our findings and do not allow us to determine the direction of the associations. Also, the exclusion of unmarried couples inevitably affects the generalizability of findings.

5. Conclusions

While acknowledging the aforementioned shortcomings, our study might be important for applied settings: first, because patient and spouse characteristics in this study (patient health status and pain intensity and patient and spouse personality) were comparable to those of previous investigations, thus supporting the generalizability of the results; also, because the results revealed that the relationship between a chronic stressor (i.e., chronic pain) and health status may be complex. Specifically, our results suggest that this relationship may be influenced by contextual variables (i.e., spouse personality), as suggested in previous research [63, 64]. Therefore, it would be interesting to see whether a reduction of situational demands (i.e., pain intensity) before couple-oriented interventions maximizes the positive effects of treatments.

Abbreviations

FFM: Five-factor model
NEO-FFI: NEO five-factor inventory.

Ethical Approval

The Ethics Committee of the Valld'Hebron Hospital in Barcelona approved the current study.

Authors' Contributions

CSR and SSV designed the study. CSR collected the data. MS and CSR agreed on the analyses needed and CSR performed them. MS and SSV commented on the results and helped in their interpretation. CSR elaborated the first draft, which was then revised by MS and SSV. All authors read and approved the final manuscript.

Acknowledgments

We would like to thank the staff members at the Pain Clinic of the Valld'Hebron for their support during recruitment. Preparation of this manuscript was supported by Grant FPU-AP2010-5585 from the Ministerio de Educación y Cultura (Spanish Government).

References

[1] S. Arvidsson, B. Arvidsson, B. Fridlund, and S. Bergman, "Health predicting factors in a general population over an eight-year period in subjects with and without chronic musculoskeletal pain," *Health and Quality of Life Outcomes*, vol. 6, no. 1, p. 98, 2008.

[2] D. Schopflocher, P. Taenzer, and R. Jovey, "The prevalence of chronic pain in Canada," *Pain Research and Management*, vol. 16, no. 6, pp. 445–450, 2011.

[3] H. Breivik, B. Collett, V. Ventafridda, R. Cohen, and D. Gallacher, "Survey of chronic pain in Europe: prevalence, impact on daily life, and treatment," *European Journal of Pain*, vol. 10, no. 4, p. 287, 2006.

[4] M. Pinquart and S. Sörensen, "Spouses, adult children, and children-in-law as caregivers of older adults: a meta-analytic comparison," *Psychology and Aging*, vol. 26, no. 1, pp. 1–14, 2011.

[5] J. Lim and B. Zebrack, "Caring for family members with chronic physical illness: a critical review of caregiver literature," *Health and Quality of Life Outcomes*, vol. 2, no. 1, p. 50, 2004.

[6] F. Akbari, M. Dehghani, A. Khatibi, and T. Vervoort, "Incorporating family function into chronic pain disability: the role of catastrophizing," *Pain Research and Management*, vol. 2016, Article ID 6838596, 9 pages, 2016.

[7] M. T. Leonard, A. Cano, and A. B. Johansen, "Chronic pain in a couples context: a review and integration of theoretical models and empirical evidence," *Journal of Pain*, vol. 7, no. 6, pp. 377–390, 2006.

[8] C. Suso-Ribera and D. Gallardo-Pujol, "Personality and health in chronic pain: have we failed to appreciate a relationship?," *Personality and Individual Differences*, vol. 96, pp. 7–11, 2016.

[9] D. J. Ozer and V. Benet-Martínez, "Personality and the prediction of consequential outcomes," *Annual Review of Psychology*, vol. 57, no. 1, pp. 401–421, 2006.

[10] P. T. Costa and R. R. McCrae, *Revised NEO Personality Inventory (NEO-PI-R) and the NEO Five-Factor Inventory (NEO-FFI) Professional Manual*, Psychological Assessment Resources, Odessa, FL, USA, 1992.

[11] T. Bogg and B. W. Roberts, "Conscientiousness and health-related behaviors: a meta-analysis of the leading behavioral contributors to mortality," *Psychological Bulletin*, vol. 130, no. 6, pp. 887–919, 2004.

[12] C. A. Magee, P. C. L. Heaven, and L. M. Miller, "Personality change predicts self-reported mental and physical health," *Journal of Personality*, vol. 81, no. 3, pp. 324–334, 2013.

[13] C. Ballús-Creus, M. V. Rangel, A. Peñarroya, J. Pérez, and J. Leff, "Expressed emotion among relatives of chronic pain patients, the interaction between relatives' behaviours and patients' pain experience," *International Journal of Social Psychiatry*, vol. 60, no. 2, pp. 197–205, 2014.

[14] J. W. Burns, K. M. Peterson, D. A. Smith et al., "Temporal associations between spouse criticism/hostility and pain among patients with chronic pain: a within-couple daily diary study," *Pain*, vol. 154, no. 12, pp. 2715–2721, 2013.

[15] A. Cano, M. Gillis, W. Heinz, M. Geisser, and H. Foran, "Marital functioning, chronic pain, and psychological distress," *Pain*, vol. 107, no. 1, pp. 99–106, 2004.

[16] A. Cano, "Pain catastrophizing and social support in married individuals with chronic pain: the moderating role of pain duration," *Pain*, vol. 110, no. 3, pp. 656–664, 2004.

[17] K. A. Raichle, J. M. Romano, and M. P. Jensen, "Partner responses to patient pain and well behaviors and their relationship to patient pain behavior, functioning, and depression," *Pain*, vol. 152, no. 1, pp. 82–88, 2011.

[18] R. D. Kerns and L. H. Weiss, "Family influences on the course of chronic illness: a cognitive-behavioral transactional model," *Annals of Behavioral Medicine*, vol. 16, pp. 116–121, 1994.

[19] J. C. Lay and C. A. Hoppmann, "Spousal neuroticism moderates everyday problem-wellbeing associations in older couples," *Health Psychology*, vol. 33, no. 8, pp. 803–812, 2014.

[20] E. C. Karademas and I. Tsaousis, "The relationship of patient and spouse personality to cardiac patients' health: two observational studies of mediation and moderation," *Annals of Behavioral Medicine*, vol. 47, no. 1, pp. 79–91, 2014.

[21] S. Bergman, L. T. H. Jacobsson, P. Herrström, and I. F. Petersson, "Health status as measured by SF-36 reflects changes and predicts outcome in chronic musculoskeletal pain: a 3-year follow up study in the general population," *Pain*, vol. 108, no. 1, pp. 115–123, 2004.

[22] P. Langley, G. Müller-Schwefe, A. Nicolaou, H. Liedgens, J. Pergolizzi, and G. Varrassi, "The societal impact of pain in the European Union: health-related quality of life and healthcare resource utilization," *Journal of Medical Economics*, vol. 13, no. 3, pp. 571–581, 2010.

[23] C. Suso-Ribera, L. Camacho-Guerrero, L. M. L. M. McCracken, A. Maydeu-Olivares, and D. Gallardo-Pujol, "Social problem solving in chronic pain: an integrative model of coping predicts mental health in chronic pain patients," *Journal of Health Psychology*, vol. 21, no. 6, pp. 1015–1025, 2016.

[24] M. D. Solé i Fontova, *Validació i estandarització espanyola del NEO-PI-R, NEO-FFI, NEO-FFI-R i escales de Schinka, en mostres universitèries i població general*, Universitat de Lleida, Lleida, Spain, 2014, http://www.tdx.cat/handle/10803/8294.

[25] C. Brunelli, E. Zecca, C. Martini et al., "Comparison of numerical and verbal rating scales to measure pain exacerbations in patients with chronic cancer pain," *Health and Quality of Life Outcomes*, vol. 8, no. 1, p. 42, 2010.

[26] M. J. Hjermstad, P. M. Fayers, D. F. Haugen et al., "Studies comparing numerical rating scales, verbal rating scales, and visual analogue scales for assessment of pain intensity in adults: a systematic literature review," *Journal of Pain and Symptom Management*, vol. 41, no. 6, pp. 1073–1093, 2011.

[27] J. Ware and C. Sherbourne, "The MOS 36-item short-form health survey (SF-36). I. Conceptual framework and item selection," *Medical Care*, vol. 30, no. 6, pp. 473–483, 1992.

[28] D. Armstrong, R. Lilford, J. Ogden, and S. Wessely, "Health-related quality of life and the transformation of symptoms," *Sociology of Health & Illness*, vol. 29, no. 4, pp. 570–583, 2007.

[29] J. Ware, M. Kosinski, M. Bayliss, C. McHorney, W. Rogers, and A. Raczek, "Comparison of methods for the scoring and statistical analysis of SF-36 health profile and summary measures: summary of results from the Medical Outcomes Study," *Medical Care*, vol. 33, no. 4, pp. AS264–AS279, 1995.

[30] J. Alonso, E. Regidor, G. Barrio et al., "Valores poblacionales de referencia de la versión Española del cuestionario de salud SF-36," *Medicina Clínica*, vol. 111, no. 11, pp. 410–416, 1998.

[31] S. J. Park, D. M. Yoon, K. B. Yoon, J. A. Moon, and S. H. Kim, "Factors associated with higher reported pain levels in patients with chronic musculoskeletal pain: a cross-sectional, correlational analysis," *PLoS One*, vol. 11, no. 9, Article ID e0163132, 2016.

[32] IBM Corp., *IBM SPSS Statistics for Windows, Version 22.0*, IBM Corp., Armonk, NY, USA, 2013.

[33] M. P. Jensen, D. G. Smith, D. M. Ehde, and L. R. Robinsin, "Pain site and the effects of amputation pain: further clarification of the meaning of mild, moderate, and severe pain," *Pain*, vol. 91, no. 3, pp. 317–322, 2001.

[34] P. Keeley, F. Creed, B. Tomenson, C. Todd, G. Borglin, and C. Dickens, "Psychosocial predictors of health-related quality of life and health service utilisation in people with chronic low back pain," *Pain*, vol. 135, no. 1, pp. 142–150, 2008.

[35] A. E. Rippentrop, E. M. Altmaier, J. J. Chen, E. M. Found, and V. J. Keffala, "The relationship between religion/spirituality and physical health, mental health, and pain in a chronic pain population," *Pain*, vol. 116, no. 3, pp. 311–321, 2005.

[36] J. L. Wetherell, N. Afari, T. Rutledge et al., "A randomized, controlled trial of acceptance and commitment therapy and cognitive-behavioral therapy for chronic pain," *Pain*, vol. 152, no. 9, pp. 2098–2107, 2011.

[37] G. Vilagut, J. María Valderas, M. Ferrer, O. Garin, E. López-García, and J. Alonso, "Interpretación de los cuestionarios de salud SF-36 y SF-12 en España: componentes físico y mental [Interpretation of the SF-36 and the SF-12 in Spain: physical and mental components]," *Medicina Clínica*, vol. 130, no. 19, pp. 726–735, 2008.

[38] T. J. D'Zurilla, A. M. Nezu, and A. Maydeu-Olivares, *Social Problem-Solving Inventory—Revised (SPSI-R): Technical Manual*, Multi-Health Systems, North Tonawanda, NY, USA, 2002.

[39] J. F. Dawson, "Moderation in management research: what, why, when, and how," *Journal of Business and Psychology*, vol. 29, no. 1, pp. 1–19, 2014.

[40] D. Manga, F. Ramos, and C. Morán, "The Spanish norms of the NEO five-factor inventory: new data and analyses for its improvement," *International Journal of Psychology and Psychological Therapy*, vol. 4, pp. 639–648, 2004.

[41] J. Steven, *Applied Multivariate Statistics for the Social Sciences*, Taylor & Francis, Hillsdale, NJ, USA, 4th edition, 2003.

[42] S. Chan, T. Hadjistavropoulos, R. N. Carleton, and H. Hadjistavropoulos, "Predicting adjustment to chronic pain in older adults," *Canadian Journal of Behavioural Science/ Revue canadienne des sciences du comportement*, vol. 44, no. 3, pp. 192–199, 2012.

[43] G. K. Lee, J. Chronister, and M. Bishop, "The effects of psychosocial factors on quality of life among individuals with chronic pain," *Rehabilitation Counseling Bulletin*, vol. 51, no. 3, pp. 177–189, 2008.

[44] J. L. McParland and C. Knussen, "Just world beliefs moderate the relationship of pain intensity and disability with psychological distress in chronic pain support group members," *European Journal of Pain*, vol. 14, no. 1, pp. 71–76, 2010.

[45] P. Zis, A. Daskalaki, I. Bountouni, P. Sykioti, G. Varrassi, and A. Paladini, "Depression and chronic pain in the elderly: links and management challenges," *Clinical Interventions in Aging*, vol. 12, pp. 709–720, 2017.

[46] P. T. Costa and R. R. McCrae, "Neuroticism, somatic complaints, and disease : is the bark worse than the bite?," *Journal of Personality*, vol. 55, no. 2, pp. 299–316, 1987.

[47] M. R. Esteve and L. Camacho, "Anxiety sensitivity, body vigilance and fear of pain," *Behaviour Research and Therapy*, vol. 46, no. 6, pp. 715–727, 2008.

[48] L. Goubert, G. Crombez, and S. Van Damme, "The role of neuroticism, pain catastrophizing and pain-related fear in vigilance to pain: a structural equations approach," *Pain*, vol. 107, no. 3, pp. 234–241, 2004.

[49] L. P. Forsythe, J. M. Romano, M. P. Jensen, and B. E. Thorn, "Attachment style is associated with perceived spouse responses and pain-related outcomes," *Rehabilitation Psychology*, vol. 57, no. 4, pp. 290–300, 2012.

[50] M. Leeuw, M. E. J. B. Goossens, S. J. Linton, G. Crombez, K. Boersma, and J. W. S. Vlaeyen, "The fear-avoidance model of musculoskeletal pain: current state of scientific evidence," *Journal of Behavioral Medicine*, vol. 30, no. 1, pp. 77–94, 2007.

[51] A. W. M. Evers, F. W. Kraaimaat, R. Geenen, J. W. G. Jacobs, and J. W. J. Bijlsma, "Pain coping and social support as predictors of long-term functional disability and pain in early rheumatoid arthritis," *Behaviour Research and Therapy*, vol. 41, no. 11, pp. 1295–1310, 2003.

[52] L. R. Miller and A. Cano, "Comorbid chronic pain and depression: who is at risk?," *Journal of Pain*, vol. 10, no. 6, pp. 619–627, 2009.

[53] L. A. Seibert, J. D. Miller, L. R. Pryor, D. E. Reidy, and A. Zeichner, "Personality and laboratory-based aggression: comparing the predictive power of the Five-Factor Model, BIS/BAS, and impulsivity across context," *Journal of Research in Personality*, vol. 44, no. 1, pp. 13–21, 2010.

[54] R. E. Rhodes and N. E. I. Smith, "Personality correlates of physical activity: a review and meta-analysis," *British Journal of Sports Medicine*, vol. 40, no. 12, pp. 958–965, 2006.

[55] B. W. Roberts, N. R. Kuncel, R. Shiner, A. Caspi, and L. R. Goldberg, "The power of personality: the comparative validity of personality traits, socioeconomic status, and cognitive ability for predicting important life outcomes," *Perspectives on Psychological Science*, vol. 2, no. 4, pp. 313–345, 2007.

[56] U. Schimmack, S. Oishi, R. M. Furr, and D. C. Funder, "Personality and life satisfaction: a facet-level analysis," *Personality and Social Psychology Bulletin*, vol. 30, no. 8, pp. 1062–1075, 2004.

[57] M. P. Martínez, A. I. Sánchez, E. Miró, A. Medina, and M. J. Lami, "The relationship between the fear-avoidance model of pain and personality traits in fibromyalgia patients," *Journal of Clinical Psychology in Medical Settings*, vol. 18, no. 4, pp. 380–391, 2011.

[58] S. R. Nitch and K. B. Boone, "Normal personality correlates of chronic pain subgroups," *Journal of Clinical Psychology in Medical Settings*, vol. 11, no. 3, pp. 203–209, 2004.

[59] J. E. Schmidt, W. M. Hooten, and C. R. Carlson, "Utility of the NEO-FFI in multi-dimensional assessment of orofacial pain conditions," *Journal of Behavioral Medicine*, vol. 34, no. 3, pp. 170–181, 2011.

[60] G. Affleck, H. Tennen, S. Urrows, and P. Higgins, "Neuroticism and the pain-mood relation in rheumatoid arthritis: Insights from a prospective daily study," *Journal of Consulting and Clinical Psychology*, vol. 60, no. 1, pp. 119–126, 1992.

[61] M. E. Geisser, A. Cano, and M. T. Leonard, "Factors associated with marital satisfaction and mood among spouses of persons with chronic back pain," *Journal of Pain*, vol. 6, no. 8, pp. 518–525, 2005.

[62] R. K. Papas, M. E. Robinson, and J. L. Riley, "Perceived spouse responsiveness to chronic pain: three empirical subgroups," *Journal of Pain*, vol. 2, no. 5, pp. 262–269, 2001.

20

A Concurrent Cognitive Task Does Not Perturb Quiet Standing in Fibromyalgia and Chronic Fatigue Syndrome

Omid Rasouli,[1,2] **Egil A. Fors**,[2] **Ottar Vasseljen**,[2] **and Ann-Katrin Stensdotter**[1]

[1]*Department of Neuromedicine and Movement Science, Faculty of Medicine and Health Sciences, Norwegian University of Science and Technology (NTNU), Trondheim, Norway*
[2]*Department of Public Health and Nursing, Faculty of Medicine and Health Sciences, Norwegian University of Science and Technology (NTNU), Trondheim, Norway*

Correspondence should be addressed to Ann-Katrin Stensdotter; ann-katrin.stensdotter@ntnu.no

Academic Editor: Frauke Nees

Background and Objectives. Cognitive complaints are common in fibromyalgia (FM) and chronic fatigue syndrome (CFS). Fatigue as well as pain may require greater effort to perform cognitive tasks, thereby increasing the load on processing in the central nervous system and interfering with motor control. *Methods.* The effect of a concurrent arithmetic cognitive task on postural control during quiet standing was investigated in 75 women (aged 19–49 years) and compared between FM, CFS, and matched controls ($n = 25$/group). Quiet standing on a force plate was performed for 60 s/condition, with and without a concurrent cognitive task. The center of pressure data was decomposed into a slow component and a fast component representing postural sway and adjusting ankle torque. *Results.* Compared to controls, CFS and FM displayed lower frequency in the slow component ($p < 0.001$), and CFS displayed greater amplitude in the slow ($p = 0.038$ and $p = 0.018$) and fast ($p = 0.045$) components. There were no interactions indicating different responses to the added cognitive task between any of the three groups. *Conclusion.* Patients displayed insufficient postural control across both conditions, while the concurrent cognitive task did not perturb quiet standing. Fatigue but not pain correlated with postural control variables.

1. Introduction

Executive function generally requires concerted cognitive and motor ability. In patients suffering pain and fatigue, there is evidence of cognitive difficulties as well as motor control deficits [1, 2], and patients often complain about increased effort and difficulty performing cognitive tasks [3, 4]. Cognitive dysfunctions, including working memory impairment, attention deficit, and less efficient information-processing capacity, are core symptoms reporting pain and fatigue conditions, specifically in chronic fatigue syndrome (CFS) and in fibromyalgia (FM). These patients are often more troubled by cognitive difficulties than by other symptoms [5]. Neuroimaging has demonstrated functional and structural alterations in the central nervous system (CNS) and a pattern of increased neural recruitment during cognitive tasks in both CFS [6] and FM [7]. Increased effort in these patients to perform is reported after physical as well as mental exertion, and is seen as lingering postexertional fatigue [8, 9]. Whether a greater mental effort and increased neural recruitment during cognitive tasks may interfere with motor control remains to be shown.

Possible consequences of pain and fatigue on motor function are often forgotten but need to be recognized. Cognitive neuroscience has shown that pain and fatigue are overlapping symptoms between different conditions and diagnoses and may be an effect of chronification with changes in similar regulatory mechanisms in the central nervous system (CNS), particularly in domains not under voluntary control [10]. This may affect certain aspects of motor performance, as sensory motor learning requires ability to maintain and update internal models. This is a prerequisite for prediction of action, necessary to allow a series of events to be contained without the need of voluntary control [11]. Perception of pain and fatigue may interfere with this process as deficits in balance and postural steadiness have been demonstrated in patients with FM as well as in CFS [12, 13] with similar deficits found in dynamic postural control at gait initiation [14].

Notably, brain-body-environment interactions and perception-action links are common basis for behavior without representational separation between domains [15]. Deficits in either domain may thus affect performance when executed concurrently due to sharing of neural networks between cortical areas [16]. Attention and sensory integration are essential to produce appropriate motor output such as balance control [17]. In some populations, particularly the fragile elderly, the risk of falling increases with the addition of a concurrent task such as talking while walking [18], and execution of multiple tasks is a major risk factor for falls [19]. Notably, there is some evidence suggesting premature aging of brain areas in both FM and CFS [20, 21], which may affect the execution of multiple tasks in persons with these diagnoses.

The addition of a cognitive task while maintaining postural control in quiet standing is thus expected to increase the load on central processing and therefore affects the ability to sustain postural equilibrium. In healthy persons, the controlling strategy appears to tighten to maintain postural equilibrium when a cognitive component is added. As an effect, postural sway may decrease [22]. In contrast, elderly with risk of falling display increased rather than decreased postural sway [23].

A dual task paradigm is generally used to study the interference between postural control and cognitive loading [17], and was therefore considered appropriate to investigate motor responses during quiet standing in FM and CFS. To find whether patients with FM and CFS would respond either similarly to healthy young individuals with reduced postural sway [24] or similar to elderly with increased postural sway [23] and greater regulatory force [25], both the controlled and the controlling parameters need to be assessed [26]. That is, on the level of performance and on the level of control of posture. A means to asses this is via structural data analyses by decomposition of ground reaction forces registered by a force platform. In addition to measures in the time domain that describe the magnitude of these components, additional measurements in the frequency domain are necessary to define the control strategies [27, 28]. Impaired postural control and the effect of added cost of a concurrent task may be expressed as deviations in both components in both the time and frequency domains.

Given the evidence that pain as well as fatigue affects motor and cognitive ability and findings of reduced postural stability, cognitive complaints, problems with sensory integration, and signs of premature aging in patients with FM and in patients with CFS, it was hypothesized that a cognitive task would cause an increased load on central processing in both patient groups. This would cause reduced drive for maintaining satisfactory postural control. Hence, postural sway was expected to increase, similar to in elderly [25].

2. Methods

A cross-sectional case-control study was designed to investigate the effect of a concurrent cognitive task on postural control parameters during quiet standing. Seventy-five females, aged 19–49 years, participated in this study (Table 1). The number of participants was estimated based on a previous study, using a similar protocol, on schizophrenic patients with 30 participants divided into two groups [29]. In the present study with three groups and less severe conditions, the number of participants was increased to 25 in each group. Inclusion criteria were young to middle aged females, as diagnoses of CFS and FM are predominant in women within this age span. Patients diagnosed with both FM and CFS were excluded. Eighty-seven patients were found eligible for participation, and those interested were referred by their attending physician and included consecutively during a period of 20 months. Thirty-two declined and data from four were excluded due to unsatisfactory quality. One patient with FM did not complete the test due to pain. Data were used from 25 patients diagnosed with CFS according to the Centers for Disease Control and Prevention criteria [30] and 25 patients diagnosed with FM according to the American College of Rheumatology (ACR) 1990 criteria [31]. Diagnoses were determined in collaboration between a rheumatologist, psychiatrist, and neurologist at the National Competence Centre for Complex Symptom Disorders. Condition severity was determined by the Fibromyalgia Impact Questionnaire (FIQ) and the Chalder Fatigue Scale. Twenty-five healthy control (HC) persons recruited from students and staff of the hospital and university constituted an age- and gender-matched control group with no history of chronic pain or fatigue. Exclusion criteria for all were diagnosed psychiatric disorder, clinical depression, neurological condition, musculoskeletal disorder, vestibular deficits, or uncorrected reduced vision potentially interfering with postural control. Verbal and written information was given, and written informed consent was obtained from each participant. The study was registered in Clinical Trials (NCT01686074) and approved by the Regional Ethical Committee for Medical and Health Research Ethics (2012/679/REK midt) and conducted according to the Declaration of Helsinki.

2.1. Data Acquisition. Participants performed two different trials of quiet standing with open eyes on a firm surface: a baseline condition without a concurrent cognitive task and an experimental condition with a concurrent cognitive task. The concurrent task consisted of counting backward aloud from 150 in steps of 7, designed to ensure actual execution of the cognitive task and minimize verbalization to prevent rhythmic counting and breathing, potentially influencing quiet standing performance [32]. Three-dimensional (3D) ground reaction forces were registered at 100 Hz with a Kistler force plate (9260AA6; Kistler Instruments AG, Switzerland).

Each test was performed once, for 60 seconds [33], without shoes, feet parallel, and arms folded across the chest.

TABLE 1: Characteristics of the participants in each group.

Variables	HC (N = 25)	CFS (N = 25)	FM (N = 25)
Age (years)	34.4 (7.9)	34.0 (8.9)	38.6 (8.0)
Weight (kg)	68.0 (9.8)	71.6 (12.9)	75.4 (14.3)
Height (cm)	167.2 (7.1)	169.1 (5.4)	168.5 (6.0)
BMI (kg/m^2)	24.3 (3.5)	25.2 (5.1)	26.5 (4.5)
Education (years)	16.1 (2.3)**	13.4 (2.5)**	13.5 (2.2)**
Pain level[a]	0.08 (0.28)*,**	1 (1.16)*	3.7 (1.8)**
Fatigue level[a]	0.6 (0.8)**	3 (1.8)**	3.2 (2.2)**
Chalder score	5.8 (5.7)*,**	25.4 (3.8)**	21.1 (5)*
FIQ	—	—	56.9 (13)

Data are presented as means (SD). HC: healthy control; CFS: chronic fatigue syndrome; FM: fibromyalgia; FIQ: Fibromyalgia Impact Questionnaire. [a]Level of pain and fatigue on the day of testing registered upon arrival to the lab. *Significance level 0.05; **significance level 0.01.

Feet width was individually standardized as the distance equal to half the shoulder width between the acromial processes and marked on the platform to ensure the same foot position for both conditions. All participants started with the baseline condition to ensure equal potential learning and/or fatigue effect. Instructions were to step onto the platform, stand still and relaxed without moving the head or extremities, or talk except articulating the numbers. A red cross (21 × 21 cm), 4 m away at eye level, served as a visual reference point for postural control. To establish a steady, quiet stance, the participant was informed that the test was commenced 10 s before the recording started and that it was finished 3 s after the data collection was completed. One-minute seated rest was provided between the conditions.

2.2. Data Analysis. Fifty-eight seconds of data were used from each trial, excluding one second at the start and end of the recording to avoid potential electronic noise from the start and stop key. Data were analyzed in MATLAB (R2014a; MathWorks Inc., Natick, MA). The preprocessed center of pressure (CoP) signals (2nd order Butterworth, 8 Hz, low pass, zero lag) was decomposed into a slow component and a fast component according to the concept of instant equilibrium forces [26]. Instants of equilibrium points in the signal, when the total horizontal force equals zero, were identified, and the CoP positions at these instants were determined and interpolated by a cubic spline function for estimation of the trajectory of the slow component. The slow component is ascribed to the movement of the center of mass (CoM) of the body, that is, postural sway. Deviation of CoP from the approximated trajectory of the slow component was determined as an estimation of the trajectory of the fast component. The fast component can be attributed to the torque created by the movement of the ankle joint to control postural sway [26].

Amplitude and frequency parameters were computed for the slow and fast components. Amplitudes were calculated by computing the 95% confidence ellipse area (mm^2), defined from the first two principal components of each of the slow and fast components [34]. The two radii of the ellipses were defined by the mediolateral (ML) and anteroposterior (AP) directions. The frequency content of the slow and fast components in the ML and AP directions were estimated by the Fourier analysis of the characteristics of the power spectral density using Welch's periodogram method [34].

2.3. Statistical Analysis. The statistics were performed using the SPSS statistical software (Version 22; IBM Corporation, USA). Normal distribution was verified with P-P plots, and histograms were inspected for control of skewness and kurtosis. A mixed-design analysis of variance (ANOVA) was used to analyze the effect of group, condition, and interaction (group × condition), with group (n = 3; HC, CFS, and FM) as the between-subjects factor and condition (n = 2; baseline and experimental) as the within-subjects factor. Sphericity was determined according to Mauchly's test. Wilks' lambda was used for multivariate exact statistics for between-subjects effects. Pairwise comparisons with Bonferroni corrections were performed to identify significant differences between groups and between conditions. Pearson correlations were used to investigate the influence of pain, fatigue, and education on postural control variables in the patient groups. Age, weight, and BMI did not differ between the three groups (Table 1), and there were no correlations between these variables and the outcome variables. Therefore, they were not included as covariates. Partial eta-squared ($\eta^2 p$) was used for effect size. The alpha level was set at $p < 0.05$.

3. Results

Overall, there were no statistical differences between CFS and FM, and both groups displayed generally similar and greater amplitudes and lower frequencies for the slow component as well as the fast component compared to HC, across both conditions (Figures 1 and 2; Table 2). Differences in strategy for postural control as an effect of the added concurrent cognitive task could not be inferred from single variables as there were no significant interactions between group and condition on any variable. Table 2 shows the results of the main effects and post hoc comparisons. Across patient groups, there were some scattered correlations between fatigue variables with postural control, but no correlations with pain variables.

3.1. The Slow Component. The analysis showed that *amplitude (AP and ML)* differed between groups: $F_{2;71} = 3.96$, $p = 0.023$, $\eta^2 p = 0.100$ (Figure 1). Significant main effects of the group were found for amplitude in both the AP ($p = 0.044$) and the ML ($p = 0.020$) directions. Post hoc analyses showed greater amplitude for CFS compared to HC in the AP ($p = 0.038$) and the ML ($p = 0.018$) directions, but no differences were found between FM and HC (Figure 1; Table 2).

The analysis showed that *frequency* differed between groups: $F_{2;71} = 7.03$, $p = 0.002$, $\eta^2 p = 0.162$ (Figure 1). Significant main effects of the group were found for frequency in both AP ($p < 0.001$) and ML ($p < 0.001$) directions. Post hoc comparisons showed similar and lower frequency for both FM and CFS compared to HC in both the AP and the ML directions ($p < 0.001$ for all) (Figure 1; Table 2).

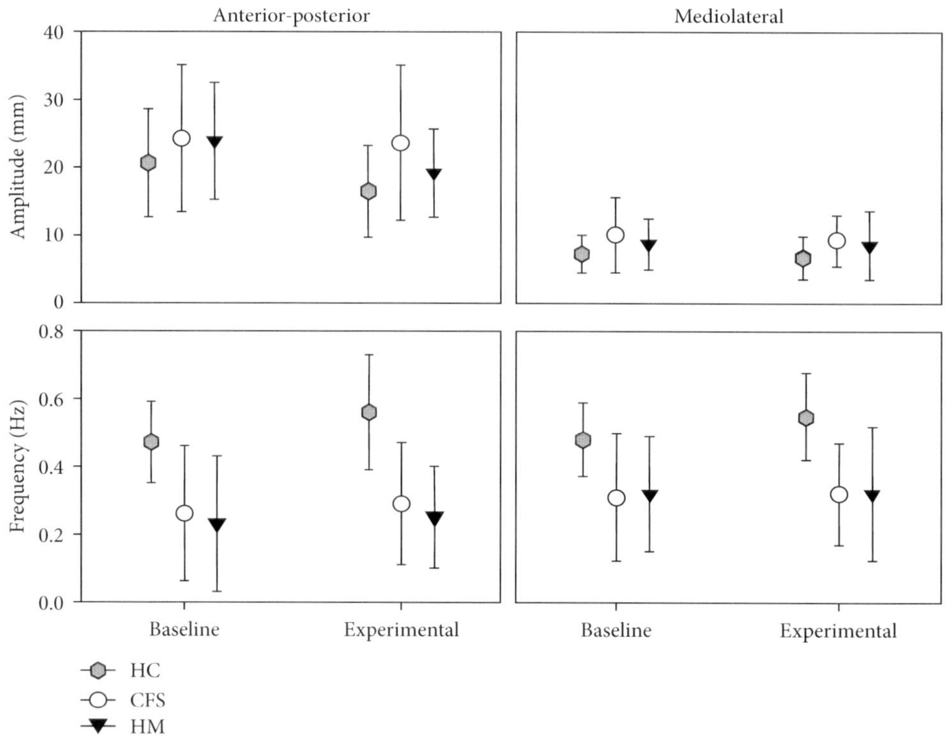

FIGURE 1: Estimated group means (standard error) of the slow component derived from the center of pressure data representing postural sway during quiet standing in both anteroposterior and mediolateral directions. Baseline and experimental conditions with the concurrent cognitive task are shown.

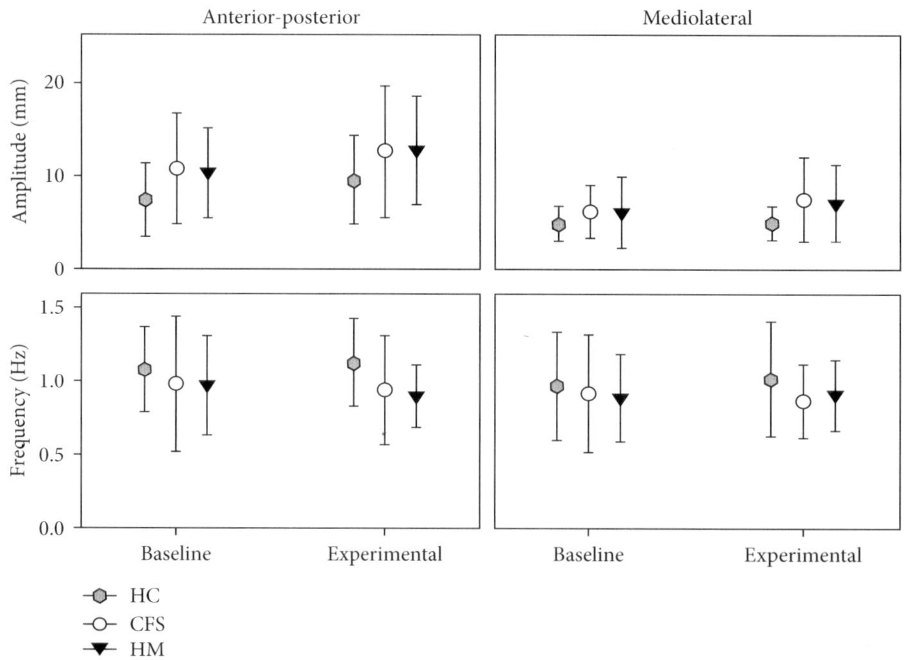

FIGURE 2: Estimated group means (standard error) of the fast component derived from the center of pressure data representing adjusting ankle torque during quiet standing in both directions. Baseline and experimental conditions with the concurrent cognitive task are shown.

As an effect of condition, the amplitude in the AP direction decreased ($p = 0.006$) with the experimental task, whereas the frequency increased in both the AP ($p = 0.02$) and the ML ($p = 0.030$) directions.

3.2. The Fast Component. The analysis showed that *amplitude (AP and ML)* differed between groups: $F_{2;71} = 4.38$, $p = 0.016$, $\eta^2 p = 0.110$ (Figure 2). There was a significant main effect of the group for amplitude in the AP ($p = 0.033$) and

Table 2: The results of repeated-measures ANOVA for each variable.

	Variable	Group * condition	Condition	Group	Post hoc
Area	CoP	$F(2, 81) = 0.45$	$F(1, 81) = 0.76$	$F(2, 81) = 6.16^{**}$	HC-CFS**, HC-FM*
	Postural sway	$F(2, 81) = 0.20$	$F(1, 81) = 4.32^{*}$	$F(2, 81) = 5.08^{**}$	HC-CFS**
	Adjusting ankle torque	$F(2, 81) = 2.41$	$F(1, 81) = 15.93^{**}$	$F(2, 81) = 5.97^{**}$	HC-FM**
Postural sway	Amp-AP	$F(2, 81) = 0.84$	$F(1, 81) = 6.92^{*}$	$F(2, 81) = 4.36^{*}$	HC-CFS*
	Amp-ML	$F(2, 81) = 0.41$	$F(1, 81) = 0.71$	$F(2, 81) = 4.90^{*}$	HC-CFS*
	F-AP	$F(2, 81) = 1.61$	$F(1, 81) = 13.08^{**}$	$F(2, 81) = 22.08^{**}$	HC-CFS**, HC-FM**
	F-ML	$F(2, 81) = 1.24$	$F(1, 81) = 5.67^{*}$	$F(2, 81) = 16.01^{**}$	HC-CFS**, HC-FM**
Adjusting ankle torque	Amp-AP	$F(2, 81) = 1.07$	$F(1, 81) = 12.38^{**}$	$F(2, 81) = 4.89^{*}$	HC-FM*
	Amp-ML	$F(2, 81) = 0.70$	$F(1, 81) = 4.79^{*}$	$F(2, 81) = 4.99^{**}$	HC-CFS*, HC-FM*
	F-AP	$F(2, 81) = 0.82$	$F(1, 81) = 0.53$	$F(2, 81) = 2.51$	—
	F-ML	$F(2, 81) = 0.77$	$F(1, 81) = 0.01$	$F(2, 81) = 1.55$	—

CoP: center of pressure; Amp: amplitude (mm); F: frequency (Hz); AP: anteroposterior; ML: mediolateral; conditions: baseline and experimental conditions with the concurrent cognitive task; HC: healthy control; CFS: chronic fatigue syndrome; FM: fibromyalgia; $^{*}p < 0.05$; $^{**}p < 0.010$.

the ML ($p = 0.031$) directions. Post hoc analysis showed a greater amplitude only in the ML direction and only for CFS ($p = 0.045$) compared to HC (Figure 2; Table 2). A multivariate analysis for the AP and ML directions showed that *frequency* did not differ between groups: $F_{2:71} = 0.20, p = 0.820, \eta^2 p = 0.006$.

As an effect of condition, the amplitude increased only in the AP direction ($p = 0.005$) as a response to the experimental task, whereas the frequency did not change significantly (Figure 2; Table 2).

3.3. Correlations. Across patient groups, the frequency in the AP direction in the slow component increased with fatigue before the test across both conditions (baseline $r = 0.306, p = 0.030$; experimental $r = 0.329, p = 0.020$). In the experimental condition, the frequency in the AP direction in the slow component also increased with fatigue after the test ($r = 0.332, p = 0.019$) and with Chalder's fatigue score ($r = 0.350, p = 0.001$). In the experimental condition, Chalder's fatigue score also correlated positively with the frequency in the ML direction in the slow component ($r = 0.318, p = 0.024$). At baseline, the amplitude in the AP direction in the fast component correlated with fatigue before the test (baseline $r = 0.405, p = 0.003$). Pain variables, including FIQ, and education did not correlate with postural control.

4. Discussion

This study is, to our knowledge, the first that collectively evaluated the effect of a concurrent cognitive task on postural control in quiet standing in patients with FM and CFS compared to controls. The study comprised both the fast and the slow components derived from CoP measurements, defining the controlling variable (attributed to adjusting ankle torque) and the controlled variable (ascribed to postural sway), respectively. The results supported our hypothesis only in part, showing unsatisfactory postural control in both patient groups, characterized by larger amplitudes and lower frequencies for the slow and fast component in both the anteroposterior and mediolateral directions during both conditions, with and without a concurrent cognitive task. There were no significant differences between the patient groups, but the CFS group performed in general worse than the FM group when compared to controls. We found no interactions that supported different patterns of postural control strategies in response to the added cognitive task in any of the patient groups compared to controls. As seen in Figures 1 and 2, the profiles of the responses are similar for all groups.

Both patient groups displayed larger amplitude in the slow component, which represents the movement of the body's CoM, thus indicating larger postural sway. This suggests worse performance in patients. Both patient groups also displayed larger amplitudes in the fast component, which is attributed to lateral forces that controls the position and movement of CoM. This suggests a deficit in control where the ankle torque is too large relative to the frequency. Notably, the frequency of the fast component was similar across all three groups. In theory, if the torque is too large relative to the frequency, it will cause greater postural sway as CoM is pushed too far in one direction before a counteracting force is created [29]. Alternatively, larger postural sway may be due to that the timing of the adjusting ankle torque was not sufficiently synchronized to correct the drift of CoM at the right moment. This assumption fits with the Drift-and-Act Hypothesis, which proposes that postural control includes a sequence of drift-and-act episodes where the body deviates from the vertical line until the sensory information has been processed in the CNS and a corrective action is initiated [35].

Our hypothesis that the amplitude of the slow component would increase and amplitude and frequency in the fast component decrease in patients as an effect of the concurrent cognitive task, indicating larger postural sway and reduced drive to maintain adequate postural control, was not supported. Even though patients in general displayed larger amplitudes relative to the frequency in the fast component, and larger amplitudes and lower frequencies in the slow component, the intrinsic patterns at baseline and in the experimental task followed a similar profile in all groups. This implies that the nature of the response to an added cognitive task was not different in patients compared to controls. Similar responses in healthy subjects to added cognitive loading during quiet standing were presented in previous studies, showing reduced CoP area [36] and sway amplitude [37] and increased sway frequency [32]. CoP is a measure of the migration of the total reaction force across the support surface and postural sway is the parameter that the system needs to control. In addition to measures used in these previous studies mentioned above, the present study also assessed the fast component in the CoP signal, which is interpreted as the lateral and controlling force that can be attributed to ankle torque [26]. Increased amplitude in the fast component confirmed the assumption of upgraded control with a concurrent cognitive task in quiet standing, proposed by Dault et al. [32]. This furthermore supports the assumption that arousal and postural control are related and that a concurrent cognitive task can increase arousal and attention compared to only quiet standing without an additional task, thus upgrading the control [38].

Performing a concurrent cognitive task in quiet standing increases the load on central processing [37], and was expected to negatively affect postural control in the patients. Although the amplitude of the slow component was generally larger in patients, it decreased while performing the concurrent cognitive task, which reflects a normal response to an added or increased cognitive load [37]. This normal response in patients may be explained by that the level of difficulty for either the cognitive or the postural task was too low to challenge control. Other explanations may be that patients were, despite their diagnoses, in relatively good shape and participated on a good day. We noted several cancellations due to feeling too unwell to come to the lab, and one patient who was unable to finish the test due to pain. Thus, a more challenging test may, or may not, trigger responses similar to in elderly with risk of falling, that is, larger amplitude in the slow component and reduced amplitude and/or frequency in the fast component. That the cognitive task did not cause increased amplitude in the fast component may also be explained by the "posture first principle" [39] as attention is typically aimed toward postural control at the cost of other tasks, to secure stability, provided a sufficient level of control.

The generally worse performance in patients compared to controls may be explained by several factors. Deficits in the sensory motor processing [40] and neurological symptoms such as muscle weakness and poor balance [41] have been reported in both FM and CFS. Evidence of the accelerated age-related decrease in white and gray matter in the CNS has been shown in both patient groups [20, 21], suggesting reduced ability in central processing comparable to elderly persons, including cognitive dysfunction that links to postural instability [42]. Reduced attentional and cognitive capacity as a result of pain and fatigue may contribute to explain the generally reduced postural control displayed in patients in the present study [43]. Multiple factors could potentially contribute to explain the reduced control of standing posture, more specifically, delayed triggering of a corrective action, and a slow action process [1, 44].

In the present study, we could however not find any correlations between pain, before or after the test or for FIQ, with any of the postural control variables. Fatigue before and after the test as well as the Chalder Fatigue Scale did in contrast correlate with several, but apparently scattered, postural control variables. Two correlations were found at baseline, while four were found in the experimental condition. Of those, two were for the same variable, frequency for the slow component in the AP direction, which suggests that the correlations were not totally random. It was however counter intuitive that the correlations with fatigue were positive for frequency, as frequency was generally lower in patients. Higher frequency and larger amplitude do however add up to higher velocity, and velocity is shown to be the most important cue that the system uses for control of posture rather than position or acceleration [45]. For a full explanation of the nature of postural control deficits, several different measurements may have to be considered.

Post hoc comparisons revealed larger and other differences for postural control in patients with CFS than in patients with FM when compared to controls. This finding was in line with shown correlations between fatigue and postural control. Notably, there is up to 70% diagnostic overlap between CFS and FM [46], indicating that fatigue is common also in FM. Note that education did not correlate with postural control variables in the present study. Thus, fatigue rather than pain or cognition may explain demonstrated deficits in postural control.

Although the response to the concurrent cognitive task in patients did not indicate reduced control as expected, the number of correlations between fatigue and postural control variables increased. Importantly, there is a link between mental fatigue and cognition, at least in CFS [3]. Previous studies seem to point to different cognitive deficits in these patient groups that may depend on fatigue. Slow information processing has been demonstrated in patients with CFS, while patients with FM display impaired ability of attention [5]. A review of the current research on neuropsychological functioning in CFS shows that slowed processing speed, impaired working memory, and poor retention of information are the most prominent features of cognitive dysfunction [47]. Note, however, that more recent research in cognitive neuroscience claim that overlapping symptoms between these conditions may be an effect of chronification with changes in similar regulatory mechanisms in the CNS [10]. Essentially, described discrepancies between cognitive difficulties in FM and CFS may thus owe to different study methods in different studies rather than true differences in underlying deficits. Recent studies support the findings of motor and cognitive affection both in patients with CFS [1] and FM [2], but hitherto no specific or unique patterns of cerebral changes have been found that distinguish these conditions from each other.

Future research on the effect on postural control of concurrent tasks should increase the level of task difficulty to challenge capacity in the patients. Future research should also study the interrelationship in central processing between pain and fatigue with cognition and motor control.

The present results should be interpreted with reservation to the following limitations: we did not assess the cognitive functioning, and medications were not controlled beyond the use of analgesics for pain. Verbalization and respiratory pattern, as potential interference with postural sway, was not monitored. Although the cognitive task was designed to minimize verbalization, to prevent rhythmic counting and thereby rhythmic breathing, the frequency of verbalization was not standardized or controlled for. A relatively small sample size may limit external validity due to the great heterogeneity of symptoms in both CFS and FM.

5. Conclusion

The intrinsic patterns at baseline and in the experimental condition followed a similar profile in all groups, without any interactions that supported different postural control strategies in response to the concurrent cognitive task in patients. Both patient groups did however display insufficient postural control compared to control persons, generally characterized by larger amplitude and lower frequency in the slow component representing postural sway, and larger amplitude in the fast component attributed to adjusting ankle torque. It is proposed that a mismatch between the magnitude and frequency of the controlling ankle torque induced greater postural sway in patients. The CFS group displayed greater differences than the FM group compared to controls, suggesting a somewhat worse general performance. Correlations between fatigue and postural control but not between pain and postural control indicate that fatigue is the explaining factor for reduced postural control in both groups. There were no statistical differences between patient groups.

Acknowledgments

This project was internally funded by NTNU. The authors gratefully thank all the participants, the National Competence Centre for Complex Symptom Disorders, and the Norwegian Fibromyalgia Association for their cooperation. Their sincere appreciation goes to Håvard Lorås for assistance with data analyses.

References

[1] D. Neu, O. Mairesse, X. Montana et al., "Dimensions of pure chronic fatigue: psychophysical, cognitive and biological correlates in the chronic fatigue syndrome," *European Journal of Applied Physiology*, vol. 114, no. 9, pp. 1841–1851, 2014.

[2] J. Oncu, F. Basoglu, and B. Kuran, "A comparison of impact of fatigue on cognitive, physical, and psychosocial status in patients with fibromyalgia and rheumatoid arthritis," *Rheumatology International*, vol. 33, no. 12, pp. 3031–3037, 2013.

[3] L. Capuron, L. Welberg, C. Heim et al., "Cognitive dysfunction relates to subjective report of mental fatigue in patients with chronic fatigue syndrome," *Neuropsychopharmacology*, vol. 31, no. 8, pp. 1777–1784, 2006.

[4] O. Gelonch, M. Garolera, J. Valls, L. Rosselló, and J. Pifarré, "Cognitive complaints in women with fibromyalgia: are they due to depression or to objective cognitive dysfunction?," *Journal of Clinical and Experimental Neuropsychology*, vol. 39, no. 10, pp. 1013–1025, 2017.

[5] J. M. Glass, "Cognitive dysfunction in fibromyalgia and chronic fatigue syndrome: new trends and future directions," *Current Rheumatology Reports*, vol. 8, no. 6, pp. 425–429, 2006.

[6] J. Boissoneault, J. Letzen, S. Lai et al., "Abnormal resting state functional connectivity in patients with chronic fatigue syndrome: an arterial spin-labeling fMRI study," *Magnetic Resonance Imaging*, vol. 34, no. 4, pp. 603–608, 2015.

[7] E. Ichesco, T. Puiu, J. P. Hampson et al., "Altered fMRI resting-state connectivity in individuals with fibromyalgia on acute pain stimulation," *European Journal of Pain*, vol. 20, no. 7, pp. 1079–1089, 2016.

[8] E. Cvejic, C. X. Sandler, A. Keech, B. K. Barry, A. R. Lloyd, and U. Vollmer-Conna, "Autonomic nervous system function, activity patterns, and sleep after physical or cognitive challenge in people with chronic fatigue syndrome," *Journal of Psychosomatic Research*, vol. 103, pp. 91–94, 2017.

[9] A. R. Light, C. J. Vierck, and K. C. Light, "Myalgia and fatigue: translation from mouse sensory neurons to fibromyalgia and chronic fatigue syndromes," in *Translational Pain Research: From Mouse to Man*, L. Kruger and A. R. Light, Eds., CRC Press, Boca Raton, FL, USA, 2010.

[10] M. Ingvar, "Learning mechanisms in pain chronification–teachings from placebo research," *Pain*, vol. 156, no. 1, pp. S18–S23, 2015.

[11] D. M. Wolpert, J. Diedrichsen, and J. R. Flanagan, "Principles of sensorimotor learning," *Nature Reviews Neuroscience*, vol. 12, no. 12, pp. 739–751, 2011.

[12] I. D. Costa, A. Gamundí, J. G. Vivas Miranda, L. G. Souza França, C. N. De Santana, and P. Montoya, "Altered functional performance in patients with fibromyalgia," *Frontiers in Human Neuroscience*, vol. 11, p. 14, 2017.

[13] R. Ash-Bernal, C. Wall, A. L. Komaroff et al., "Vestibular function test anomalies in patients with chronic fatigue syndrome," *Acta Oto-Laryngologica*, vol. 115, no. 1, pp. 9–17, 1995.

[14] O. Rasouli, A. K. Stensdotter, and A. L. Van der Meer, "TauG-guidance of dynamic balance control during gait initiation in patients with chronic fatigue syndrome and fibromyalgia," *Clinical Biomechanics*, vol. 37, pp. 147–152, 2016.

[15] L. W. Barsalou, "Grounded cognition," *Annual Review of Psychology*, vol. 59, no. 1, pp. 617–645, 2008.

[16] R. K. Y. Chong, B. Mills, L. Dailey, E. Lane, S. Smith, and K. H. Lee, "Specific interference between a cognitive task and sensory organization for stance balance control in healthy young adults: visuospatial effects," *Neuropsychologia*, vol. 48, no. 9, pp. 2709–2718, 2010.

[17] E. V. Fraizer and S. Mitra, "Methodological and interpretive issues in posture-cognition dual-tasking in upright stance," *Gait and Posture*, vol. 27, no. 2, pp. 271–279, 2008.

[18] O. Beauchet, C. Annweiler, V. Dubost et al., "Stops walking when talking: a predictor of falls in older adults?," *European Journal of Neurology*, vol. 16, no. 7, pp. 786–795, 2009.

[19] A. Zijlstra, T. Ufkes, D. A. Skelton, L. Lundin-Olsson, and W. Zijlstra, "Do dual tasks have an added value over single tasks for balance assessment in fall prevention programs? A mini-review," *Gerontology*, vol. 54, no. 1, pp. 40–49, 2008.

[20] A. Kuchinad, P. Schweinhardt, D. A. Seminowicz, P. B. Wood, B. A. Chizh, and M. C. Bushnell, "Accelerated brain gray matter loss in fibromyalgia patients: premature aging of the brain?," *Journal of Neuroscience*, vol. 27, no. 15, pp. 4004–4007, 2007.

[21] B. K. Puri, P. M. Jakeman, M. Agour et al., "Regional grey and white matter volumetric changes in myalgic encephalomyelitis (chronic fatigue syndrome): a voxel-based morphometry 3 T MRI study," *British Journal of Radiology*, vol. 85, no. 1015, pp. e270–e273, 2012.

[22] M. C. Dault, A. C. H. Geurts, T. W. Mulder, and J. Duysens, "Postural control and cognitive task performance in healthy participants while balancing on different support-surface configurations," *Gait and Posture*, vol. 14, no. 3, pp. 248–255, 2001.

[23] H. G. Kang and L. A. Lipsitz, "Stiffness control of balance during quiet standing and dual task in older adults: the MOBILIZE Boston Study," *Journal of Neurophysiology*, vol. 104, no. 6, pp. 3510–3517, 2010.

[24] M. C. Dault, J. S. Frank, and F. Allard, "Influence of a visuo-spatial, verbal and central executive working memory task on postural control," *Gait and Posture*, vol. 14, no. 2, pp. 110–116, 2001.

[25] K. Masani, A. H. Vette, M. Kouzaki, H. Kanehisa, T. Fukunaga, and M. R. Popovic, "Larger center of pressure minus center of gravity in the elderly induces larger body acceleration during quiet standing," *Neuroscience Letters*, vol. 422, no. 3, pp. 202–206, 2007.

[26] V. M. Zatsiorsky and M. Duarte, "Rambling and trembling in quiet standing," *Motor Control*, vol. 4, no. 2, pp. 185–200, 2000.

[27] A. K. Stensdotter, H. W. Lorås, J. Christian Fløvig, and M. Djupsjöbacka, "Postural control in quiet standing in patients with psychotic disorders," *Gait and Posture*, vol. 38, no. 4, pp. 918–922, 2013.

[28] L. E. Cofre Lizama, M. Pijnappels, N. Peter Reeves, S. M. Verschueren, and J. H. van Dieën, "Centre of pressure or centre of mass feedback in mediolateral balance assessment," *Journal of Biomechanics*, vol. 48, no. 3, pp. 539–543, 2015.

[29] A. K. Stensdotter, A. K. Wanvik, and H. W. Loras, "Postural control in quiet standing with a concurrent cognitive task in psychotic conditions," *Journal of Motor Behavior*, vol. 45, no. 4, pp. 279–287, 2013.

[30] K. Fukuda, "The chronic fatigue syndrome: a comprehensive approach to its definition and study. International Chronic Fatigue Syndrome Study Group," *Annals of Internal Medicine*, vol. 121, no. 12, pp. 953–959, 1994.

[31] F. Wolfe, H. A. Smythe, M. B. Yunus et al., "The american college of rheumatology 1990 criteria for the classification of fibromyalgia. Report of the Multicenter Criteria Committee," *Arthritis and Rheumatism*, vol. 33, no. 2, pp. 160–172, 1990.

[32] M. C. Dault, L. Yardley, and J. S. Frank, "Does articulation contribute to modifications of postural control during dual-task paradigms?," *Cognitive Brain Research*, vol. 16, no. 3, pp. 434–440, 2003.

[33] K. Slomka, G. Juras, G. Sobota, and B. Bacik, "The reliability of a rambling-trembling analysis of center of pressure measures," *Gait and Posture*, vol. 37, no. 2, pp. 210–213, 2013.

[34] M. Duarte and S. M. Freitas, "Revision of posturography based on force plate for balance evaluation," *Revista Brasileira de Fisioterapia*, vol. 14, no. 3, pp. 183–192, 2010.

[35] J. Milton, J. L. Cabrera, T. Ohira et al., "The time-delayed inverted pendulum: implications for human balance control," *Chaos: An Interdisciplinary Journal of Nonlinear Science*, vol. 19, no. 2, article 026110, 2009.

[36] N. Vuillerme and G. Nafati, "How attentional focus on body sway affects postural control during quiet standing," *Psychological Research*, vol. 71, no. 2, pp. 192–200, 2007.

[37] G. Andersson, J. Hagman, R. Talianzadeh, A. Svedberg, and H. C. Larsen, "Effect of cognitive load on postural control," *Brain Research Bulletin*, vol. 58, no. 1, pp. 135–139, 2002.

[38] B. E. Maki and W. E. McIlroy, "Influence of arousal and attention on the control of postural sway," *Journal of Vestibular Research*, vol. 6, no. 1, pp. 53–59, 1996.

[39] A. ShumwayCook, M. Woollacott, K. A. Kerns, and M. Baldwin, "The effects of two types of cognitive tasks on postural stability in older adults with and without a history of falls," *Journals of Gerontology Series A-Biological Sciences and Medical Sciences*, vol. 52, no. 4, pp. M232–M240, 1997.

[40] C. S. McCabe, H. Cohen, and D. R. Blake, "Somaesthetic disturbances in fibromyalgia are exaggerated by sensory motor conflict: implications for chronicity of the disease?," *Rheumatology*, vol. 46, no. 10, pp. 1587–1592, 2007.

[41] N. F. Watson, D. Buchwald, J. Goldberg, C. Noonan, and R. G. Ellenbogen, "Neurologic signs and symptoms in fibromyalgia," *Arthritis and Rheumatism*, vol. 60, no. 9, pp. 2839–2844, 2009.

[42] F. B. Horak, "Postural orientation and equilibrium: what do we need to know about neural control of balance to prevent falls?," *Age and Ageing*, vol. 35, no. 2, pp. ii7–ii11, 2006.

[43] K. D. Jones, F. B. Horak, K. Winters-Stone, J. M. Irvine, and R. M. Bennett, "Fibromyalgia is associated with impaired balance and falls," *Journal of Clinical Rheumatology*, vol. 15, no. 1, pp. 16–21, 2009.

[44] O. Rasouli, E. Fors, P. Borchgrevink, F. Öhberg, and A. N. Stensdotter, "Gross and fine motor function in fibromyalgia and chronic fatigue syndrome," *Journal of Pain Research*, vol. 10, pp. 303–309, 2017.

[45] J. Jeka, T. Kiemel, R. Creath, F. Horak, and R. Peterka, "Controlling human upright posture: velocity information is more accurate than position or acceleration," *Journal of Neurophysiology*, vol. 92, no. 4, pp. 2368–2379, 2004.

[46] D. Buchwald and D. Garrity, "Comparison of patients with chronic fatigue syndrome, fibromyalgia, and multiple chemical sensitivities," *Archives of Internal Medicine*, vol. 154, no. 18, pp. 2049–2053, 1994.

[47] V. Michiels and R. Cluydts, "Neuropsychological functioning in chronic fatigue syndrome: a review," *Acta Psychiatrica Scandinavica*, vol. 103, no. 2, pp. 84–93, 2001.

Impaired Autophagy of GABAergic Interneurons in Neuropathic Pain

Yuhua Yin,[1,2] Min-Hee Yi,[3] and Dong Woon Kim[1,2]

[1]*Department of Medical Science, Chungnam National University School of Medicine, Daejeon 35015, Republic of Korea*
[2]*Department of Anatomy and Cell Biology, Brain Research Institute, Chungnam National University School of Medicine, Daejeon 35015, Republic of Korea*
[3]*Department of Neurology, Mayo Clinic, Rochester, MN 55905, USA*

Correspondence should be addressed to Dong Woon Kim; visnu528@cnu.ac.kr

Academic Editor: Parisa Gazerani

Neuropathic pain (NP) is caused by lesions of the peripheral fibers and central neurons in the somatosensory nervous system and affects 7–10% of the general population. Although the distinct cause of neuropathic pain has been investigated in primary afferent neurons over the years, pain modulation by central sensitization remains controversial. NP is believed to be driven by cell type-specific spinal synaptic plasticity in the dorsal horn. Upon intense afferent stimulation, spinothalamic tract neurons are potentiated, whereas GABAergic interneurons are inhibited leading to long-term depression. Growing evidences suggest that the inhibition of GABAergic neurons plays pivotal roles in the manifestation of neuropathic and inflammatory pain states. Downregulation of GABA transmission and impairment of GABAergic interneurons in the dorsal horn are critical consequences after spinal cord and peripheral nerve injuries. These impairments in GABAergic interneurons may be associated with dysfunctional autophagy, resulting in neuropathic pain. Here, we review an emerging number of investigations that suggest a pivotal role of impaired autophagy of GABAergic interneurons in NP. We discuss relevant research spurring the development of new targets and therapeutic agents of NP and emphasize the need for a multidisciplinary approach to manage NP in the future.

1. Introduction

More than 20 million individuals have neuropathic pain (NP) worldwide and suffer from highly acute diseases, greater healthcare costs, and lower quality of life [1–3]. In some cases, the most severe NP leads to increased episodes of depression and suicide [4–6]. The etiology of NP is broad and classified into central nervous system (CNS), peripheral nervous system, and complex neuropathic disorders, including complex regional pain syndrome types I (reflex sympathetic dystrophy) and II. Complex regional pain syndrome refers to a chronic pain condition characterized by progressively worsening spontaneous regional pain in the absence or presence of peripheral nerve damage. The traditional treatments for chronic pain, such as medications, massage therapy, acupuncture, electrical stimulation, nerve blocks, and surgery, cause severe side effects and fail to reduce or eliminate NP [7]. Further research is needed to understand the mechanisms underlying NP to allow for the design of individual and rational treatment strategies but also for the development of optimal therapeutic drugs.

Changes in the properties of neurons in the CNS can result in central sensitization. Even normal inputs that usually evoke innocuous sensations can lead to pain hypersensitivity due to the changes in the sensory response [8]. Moreover, there is evidence that central sensitization refers to subsequent peripheral nerve injury (PNI) or neuropathy [9]. In the past, many researchers believed that NP following PNI was due to the changes in the CNS and peripheral nervous system (PNS) neurons and their functions. Accordingly, many studies have focused on spinal dorsal neurons to elucidate the mechanism of NP. These studies have suggested that NP is a consequence of the aberrant response of the sensory neurons in the dorsal horn to the PNS inputs, anatomical reorganization of the pain pathway, as well as attenuated microglial activation and inhibitory processes [10]. A number of mechanisms have been suggested for central sensitization, among which there is strongest evidence for the dysfunction of GABAergic interneurons and their role in modifying synaptic transmission of pain signaling pathways in response to PNI [11–13].

Under normal circumstances, inhibitory interneurons continuously release GABA to decrease the excitability of lamina I output neurons and modulate pain transmission. However, this inhibition can be lost after an injury, resulting in hyperalgesia [10, 14]. This may occur as a result of changes in loss of GABAergic function or apoptosis. Additionally, disinhibition may enable nonnociceptive myelinated $A\beta$ primary afferents to engage the pain transmission circuitry, leading to a perception of pain in patients in response to normally innocuous stimuli. It remains highly controversial to link the changes of cell types and cell death in the spinal dorsal horn with NP. It was reported that partial PNI leads to neuronal cell death in the dorsal horn [15]. Spinal cord injury-induced GABAergic interneuron cell death and their decreased number in the dorsal horn diminishes GABAergic tone and NP [14]. However, it has also been reported that the number of GABAergic interneurons and the synaptic boutons at $GABA_A$ synapses, as well as the expression levels of intracellular GAD65, GAD67, GABA, GABA transporters 1 and 3, and $GABA_A$ and $GABA_B$ receptors can all remain unaltered [16–20].

The differences in these reports may be reconciled when considering time-dependent changes due to autophagy. Autophagy, a cellular self-digestion pathway involved in protein and organelle degradation, is known to be highly involved in various human diseases and physiology. Autophagy regulates cell homeostasis with a dual role in cell protection and cell death. However, some roles of autophagy are related to NP. We will discuss the importance of GABAergic neurons in NP and their regulation by autophagy in this review.

1.1. GABAergic Neuron Dysfunction in NP. Lamina II of the dorsal horn (substantia gelatinosa) is a major target of nociceptive primary afferents. Although excitatory and inhibitory interneurons show considerable heterogeneity, a morphological study reported that the islet cells are inhibitory, the radial and large vertical cells are excitatory, and some neurons with a morphological appearance of vertical cells are GABAergic [21]. It is estimated that approximately 30% of lamina II neurons are GABAergic, especially with enriched glycine. The rest appear to be glutamatergic and have high expression of vesicular glutamate transporter 2 [22–24].

GABAergic inhibition has been suggested to play a pivotal role in the manifestation of NP and inflammatory pain states [15], and GABAergic interneurons are densely innervated in lamina I giant project neurons [25]. As a result, NP occurs during pharmacological inhibition of spinal $GABA_A$ and $GABA_B$ receptor-mediated inhibitory transmission [26–28]. Furthermore, $GABA_A$ receptor-mediated postsynaptic currents were observed to be inhibited after substantially reducing the primary afferents in the substantia gelatinosa of the spinal dorsal horn [15]. Moreover, $GABA_B$ receptor-mediated inhibition was lost after spinal nerve injury, particularly in the central terminals of primary afferents, leading to allodynia or spontaneous pain behavior [18, 29].

Endoplasmic reticulum (ER) stress was shown to be related to cellular reactive oxygen species (ROS) production, followed by an impaired autophagic flux. This cascade of events contributes to central sensitization of GABAergic interneuron dysfunction [30–33]. In particular, ROS are involved in long-term depression of GABAergic interneurons in mice [11]. Scavenging ROS enhance GABA current, and applying hydrogen peroxide inhibits GABA current, indicating that GABA release is redox sensitive [12]. L4 and L5 bilateral dorsal rhizotomy increases extracellular concentrations of excitatory amino acids in the dorsal horn and reduces the sensory glutamate-induced decreases in the expression of GABA-synthesizing enzymes and presynaptic inhibition [34, 35]. Taken together, both autophagic impairment and ER stress contribute to dysfunction of dorsal horn GABAergic neurons in patients with NP. Therefore, regulating GABAergic neurons and inhibiting their function in the superficial dorsal horn of the spinal cord [15] are attractive therapeutic strategies developed to treat NP.

1.2. Autophagic Impairment in NP. There are several mechanisms of programmed cell death, including apoptosis and autophagy. Apoptosis involves a cooperation among caspases, whereas autophagic cell death involves (but not necessarily by) autophagic vacuolization [36]. Most previous studies focused only on apoptosis, but the study by Berliocchi et al. introduced the role of disrupted autophagy in an NP model using spinal nerve ligation (SNL) [37]. LC3II and Beclin 1 protein levels were found to be elevated after SNL. We also first reported that LC3 and Beclin 1 levels were significantly increased in the L4-5 spinal cord segment ipsilateral to the injured side in rats after SNL compared with the sham group [20]. In addition, the levels of LC3 and Beclin 1 were also significantly increased in GABAergic interneurons of the spinal dorsal horn following PNI [20]. Taken together, these studies suggest that autophagy is involved in the induction and maintenance of NP. Furthermore, a disturbance in autophagy renders GABAergic interneurons vulnerable to PNI or NP stimuli.

1.3. Inhibition of Autophagic Induction by 3-Methyladenine (3-MA) Reduces NP Behavior. Autophagy is an evolutionarily conserved catabolic process that involves degradation of cytoplasmic components. Autophagy involves multiple proteins and signaling pathways that can be divided into four distinct steps: (1) induction, (2) assembly and formation of autophagosomes, (3) docking and fusion with lysosomal membranes, and (4) degradation [38]. Autophagic flux is defined as a measure of autophagic degradation activity [39]. Therapeutic strategies that inhibit autophagy-induced cell death have the potential to identify novel and effective targeted treatments for NP.

3-methyladenine (3-MA) inhibits the induction of autophagy by blocking the formation of autophagosomes and inhibiting class III phosphatidylinositol 3-kinases [20, 40]. We injected 3-MA intrathecally to investigate whether inhibition of autophagic dysfunction would result in effective relief of NP. 3-MA treatment was found to significantly reduce mechanical allodynia in a time-dependent manner during postoperative observations before decreasing to baseline on day 14 (Figure 1) [20]. These results suggest that autophagy is a central regulator in the pathogenesis of NP.

1.4. Inhibition of Autophagic Flux by Chloroquine Reduces NP Behavior. Berliocchi et al. suggested that autophagy is modulated differently depending on the experimental pain model by demonstrating LC3I, Beclin 1, and p62 levels modulated differently for chronic constriction injury (CCI) versus spared nerve injury [41]. As described above, p62/SQSTM1 is an autophagic substrate and a key LC3-binding protein, which serves as a link between LC3 and ubiquitinated proteins [42]. p62 and p62-bound polyubiquitinated proteins become incorporated into the completed autophagosome and are degraded in autolysosomes. Because of the correlation between modulation of autophagy and p62 levels, this substrate is considered a useful proxy for autophagic degradation [42–44], and p62 levels are often increased when autophagy is impaired [43]. We previously demonstrated the increased accumulation of p62 on the ipsilateral side of CCI-induced mice compared with their contralateral side, suggesting that CCI leads to a blockage of the final degradative steps of autophagy [45].

We also reported that a high tissue content of omega-3 polyunsaturated fatty acids (PUFAs) attenuates formalin-induced pain sensitivity, microglial activation, inducible nitric oxide synthase expression, and phosphorylation of NR2B [46]. In addition, we also showed higher levels of LC3II and Beclin 1 but lower levels of p62 in fat-1 mice, suggesting that polyunsaturated fatty acid enrichment enhances the induction and flux of autophagy. In that experiment, we demonstrated that brain-derived neurotrophic factor (BDNF) is expressed at higher levels in fat-1 mice, suggesting that BDNF and its associated proteins Akt and CREB, may be therapeutic targets for NP, because BDNF might be a neuroprotective factor by potentially upregulating autophagic flux activity.

Finally, we investigated blocking autophagy using chloroquine. Chloroquine reverses autophagy by accumulating in the lysosomes and disturbing vacuolar H^+ ATPase. This leads to a lysosomal acidification and results in autophagy inhibition [47]. Intrathecal injection of chloroquine into wild-type mice induces a significant reduction in the threshold of mechanical sensitivity [45]. Intrathecal chloroquine injection into naïve mice induces spinal accumulation of LC3 and p62, in parallel with significant mechanical hypersensitivity, thus confirming inhibition of autophagosome clearance and suggesting the participation of autophagy in spinal mechanisms of pain processing. Taken together, the analysis of LC3, Beclin 1, and p62 indicates that impaired autophagy in CCI-induced NP may result from blocking the late phase, rather than the induction phase of autophagic flux.

2. Mitophagy Impairment in NP

ROS are a major source of mitochondrial dysfunction and can induce mutations in mitochondrial DNA that result in protein deficiencies, restricted self-repair ability, and increase vulnerability of cells to ROS attack [48, 49]. Indeed, ROS induces oxidative stress, which damages mitochondrial proteins and lipids [50, 51]. In particular, mitochondrial oxidative damage is usually caused by aging and is the most important risk factor in most cases of mitochondrial dysfunction [52]. As a result, mitophagy counteracts against excessive intracellular ROS and blocks ROS sources, which are important in the therapeutic management of NP [53].

Mitophagy is the selective autophagic degradation of mitochondria that occurs when mitochondria become defective following a damage or stress [54, 55], such as hypoxia, nutrient starvation, energy depletion, and other pharmacological or viral stimuli [56]. Increased generation of mitochondrial ROS detected in L5 dorsal horn neurons of SNL-induced neuropathic rats in dorsal horn neurons [57]. PINK1 is a neuroprotective protein involved in the activation of mitophagy by selectively accumulating in depolarized mitochondria and promoting PARK2/Parkin translocation [58]. We examined the expression of PINK1 in the spinal cord and found the number of immunoreactive cells and PINK1 protein expression were both increased significantly on the ipsilateral and contralateral sides of the spinal dorsal horn in wild-type mice. However, no such significant differences were observed in toll-like receptor 4 (TLR4) knockout mice [45]. PINK1 is expressed in neurons in the spinal dorsal horn, but not in astrocytes or microglia [45]. Thus, we demonstrated that mitophagy may play a role in NP-related processes, but further studies are needed to clarify the function of mitophagy in NP, especially in GABAergic interneurons.

3. Impaired ER Stress in NP

ER stress is caused by disruption of the structure and function of the ER [59]. The unfolded protein response (UPR) can be induced by a variety of cellular stresses, such as glucose deprivation, depletion of ER Ca^{2+} stores, exposure to free radicals, and accumulation of unfolded or misfolded proteins [60, 61]. UPR is mediated by three ER stress receptors: PKR-like ER kinase, inositol-requiring enzyme 1, and activating transcription factor-6. Both ER stress and the resulting UPR are part of the cellular homeostasis program that balance the protein turnover and synthesis [62, 63]. However, if this equilibrium is disrupted, ER stress can activate programmed cell death pathways. Accordingly, activated ER stress pathways have been observed

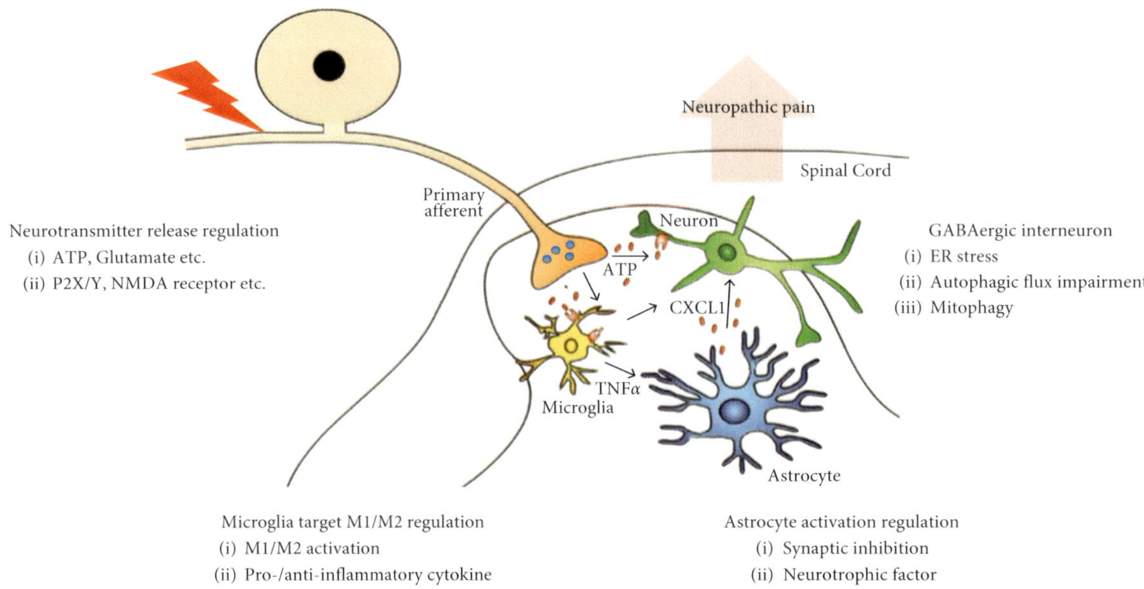

Figure 1: Therapeutic strategy to regulate GABAergic interneurons in spinal central sensitization. There is growing evidence that impaired autophagy and ER stress contribute to dysfunction of dorsal horn GABAergic neurons. Autophagosome accumulation and impairment of autophagic flux in GABAergic neurons make them susceptible to peripheral nerve injury or other pain stimuli. Therefore, there are several ways to control GABA neurons to control the spinal central sensitization that contributes to neuropathic pain. (1) Functional recovery of GABAergic interneurons, (2) neurotransmitter release regulation, (3) microglia targeted M1/2 polarization regulation, and (4) astrocyte targeted regulation.

in various disease pathogenesis, such as those of diabetes, cancers [64, 65], Alzheimer's disease, Parkinson's disease, amyotrophic lateral sclerosis, and prion diseases [60, 66]. We also reported that the causes of ER stress in NP are related to autophagy and that autophagy was activated in an SNL-induced NP model [33].

As a common cytoprotective mechanism, autophagy controls homeostasis in various ways, such as protein and organelle turnover [67, 68]. Moreover, autophagy is associated with the ER at various molecular levels, and ER stress induces autophagy in mammalian cells via several canonical UPR pathways [69, 70]. We previously found that impaired ER stress in an SNL model and after ATF6 siRNA treatment significantly reduced NP-associated behaviors [33], indicating that ER stress is involved in the induction and maintenance of NP. Furthermore, we suggested that a disruption of the UPR pathway may render the neurons to become sensitive to PNI or NP stimuli. Further elucidation of the mechanisms of ER stress on GABAergic interneurons in the spinal cord during NP will be critical to guide the future development of novel pharmacological NP treatments.

4. Nonneuronal Cell Regulation of NP

In parallel with the progress achieved regarding these neuronal mechanisms, there has been an increased appreciation of the importance of nonneuronal cells, particularly glial cells such as microglia and astrocytes, to also play an important role in chronic pain. Over the past decade, there has been a dramatic increase in the number of pain research studies investigating the role of glia, which we briefly summarize in the following.

4.1. Activation of Spinal Microglia and NP. Microglia are resident macrophages of the spinal cord and brain. Although microglia comprise 5–12% of the cells in the CNS [71], abundant evidence supports their role in pathological pain [72–74]. Microglia are activated in the pathophysiological condition that occurs after PNI. [75] Once activated, microglia show morphological changes [76], increased expression of microglial markers, e.g., IBA1, MHC II, and CD 11b [76–78], increased numbers (proliferation) [79–81], and increased phagocytosis [82]. TLR4 was previously reported to be primarily expressed in microglia; it was found that neuronal TLR4 regulates the proliferation of neural precursor cells during axonal growth, adult neurogenesis, and neuronal plasticity [83]. We reported previously that neuronal cells, and not astrocytes or microglia, of the CCI-induced NP spinal dorsal horn had impaired autophagy [45]. Our data showed that chloroquine treatment in TLR4 knockout mice attenuated the pain threshold in CCI-induced mechanical allodynia compared with TLR4 wild-type mice. Therefore, it is reasonable to conclude that the proinflammatory cytokines release in microglia, and the impaired autophagy in neurons synergistically contribute to pain sensory hypersensitivity via TLR4, suggesting TLR4-mediated microglial activation may be indirectly coupled to autophagy.

4.2. Activation of Spinal Astrocytes. Increasing number of studies has shown that astrocytes are important in the development of chronic pain by regulating the extracellular concentrations of GABA released from neurons and glia by controlling its uptake [84–86]. Ischemia or hypoxia and gangliosides activate the autophagic/lysosomal pathway in astrocytes under oxidative stress [87]. Those authors reported that inhibiting this key system is protective. However, there have been no reports of activated autophagy in astrocytes of the spinal dorsal horn following NP or of autophagic impairment as an effective alternative treatment for NP. A tonic form of synaptic inhibition occurs in discrete regions of the CNS and has an important role in controlling neuronal excitability [88]. GABA in astrocytes is the major source of tonic inhibition in the cerebellum [89]. Although it is known that PNI alters astrocyte activity [90], it is unknown how astrocytes function as GABAergic and GABAceptive cells following PNI. Taken together, astrocytic GABA may actively participate in disinhibition of the neuronal networks in the spinal dorsal horn to regulate pain.

5. Conclusions

An accumulating body of literature has provided compelling evidence for the importance of neurons and glial cells in NP. The mechanisms regarding GABAergic interneuron dysfunction remain to be further elucidated. In this review, autophagic impairment of GABAergic interneurons in the spinal dorsal horn was identified as a new regulator of spinal neuronal circuits (Figure 1). We propose that impaired autophagy plays a critical role in spinal hypersensitivity, to which reduced GABAergic interneuronal activity is a key contributor in NP. This concept provides insight into the pathogenesis of NP and suggests potential strategies for developing new treatments for NP.

Acknowledgments

This research was supported by the Brain Research Program through the National Research Foundation of Korea (NRF) funded by the Ministry of Science, ICT and Future Planning (NRF-2016M3C7A1905074 and 2016R1A2B4009409). We are grateful to Prof. Yonghyun Kim (University of Alabama) for kind advice.

References

[1] B. H. McCarberg and R. Billington, "Consequences of neuropathic pain: quality-of-life issues and associated costs," *American Journal of Managed Care*, vol. 12, no. 9, pp. S263–S268, 2006.

[2] A. B. O'Connor, "Neuropathic pain: quality-of-life impact, costs and cost effectiveness of therapy," *Pharmacoeconomics*, vol. 27, no. 2, pp. 95–112, 2009.

[3] B. H. Smith, N. Torrance, M. I. Bennett, and A. J. Lee, "Health and quality of life associated with chronic pain of predominantly neuropathic origin in the community," *Clinical Journal of Pain*, vol. 23, no. 2, pp. 143–149, 2007.

[4] R. Alakhverdian and D. Koev, "Fibrinogen-fibrin degradation products in diabetes mellitus," *Vŭtreshni Bolesti*, vol. 26, no. 6, pp. 72–75, 1987.

[5] T. D. Hall, S. Shah, B. Ng et al., "Changes in mood, depression and suicidal ideation after commencing pregabalin for neuropathic pain," *Australian Family Physician*, vol. 43, no. 10, pp. 705–708, 2014.

[6] M. Risse and G. Weiler, "Histologic distribution pattern of thymus hemorrhages in sudden infant death," *Beiträge zur gerichtlichen Medizin*, vol. 46, pp. 351–355, 1988.

[7] T. Hashimoto, "Communication by personal computer," *Josanpu Zasshi*, vol. 42, no. 7, pp. 578–581, 1988.

[8] S. W. Snyder and M. S. Cardwell, "Neuromuscular blockade with magnesium sulfate and nifedipine," *American Journal of Obstetrics and Gynecology*, vol. 161, no. 1, pp. 35-36, 1989.

[9] D. Bridges, S. W. Thompson, and A. S. Rice, "Mechanisms of neuropathic pain," *British Journal of Anaesthesia*, vol. 87, no. 1, pp. 12–26, 2001.

[10] A. I. Basbaum, D. M. Bautista, G. Scherrer, and D. Julius, "Cellular and molecular mechanisms of pain," *Cell*, vol. 139, no. 2, pp. 267–284, 2009.

[11] A. Bittar, J. Jun, J. H. La, J. Wang, J. W. Leem, and J. M. Chung, "Reactive oxygen species affect spinal cell type-specific synaptic plasticity in a model of neuropathic pain," *Pain*, vol. 158, no. 11, pp. 2137–2146, 2017.

[12] D. W. Hogg, M. E. Pamenter, D. J. Dukoff, and L. T. Buck, "Decreases in mitochondrial reactive oxygen species initiate GABA(A) receptor-mediated electrical suppression in anoxia-tolerant turtle neurons," *Journal of Physiology*, vol. 593, no. 10, pp. 2311–2326, 2015.

[13] Y. H. Kim, S. K. Back, A. J. Davies et al., "TRPV1 in GABAergic interneurons mediates neuropathic mechanical allodynia and disinhibition of the nociceptive circuitry in the spinal cord," *Neuron*, vol. 74, no. 4, pp. 640–647, 2012.

[14] J. G. Meisner, A. D. Marsh, and D. R. Marsh, "Loss of GABAergic interneurons in laminae I-III of the spinal cord dorsal horn contributes to reduced GABAergic tone and neuropathic pain after spinal cord injury," *Journal of Neurotrauma*, vol. 27, no. 4, pp. 729–737, 2010.

[15] K. A. Moore, T. Kohno, L. A. Karchewski, J. Scholz, H. Baba, and C. J. Woolf, "Partial peripheral nerve injury promotes a selective loss of GABAergic inhibition in the superficial dorsal horn of the spinal cord," *Journal of Neuroscience*, vol. 22, no. 15, pp. 6724–6731, 2002.

[16] M. J. Janssen, R. P. Yasuda, and S. Vicini, "GABA(A) receptor beta3 subunit expression regulates tonic current in developing striatopallidal medium spiny neurons," *Frontiers in Cellular Neuroscience*, vol. 5, p. 15, 2011.

[17] G. Miletic and V. Miletic, "Loose ligation of the sciatic nerve is associated with TrkB receptor-dependent decreases in KCC2 protein levels in the ipsilateral spinal dorsal horn," *Pain*, vol. 137, no. 3, pp. 532–539, 2008.

[18] E. Polgar and A. J. Todd, "Tactile allodynia can occur in the spared nerve injury model in the rat without selective loss of GABA or GABA(A) receptors from synapses in laminae I-II of the ipsilateral spinal dorsal horn," *Neuroscience*, vol. 156, no. 1, pp. 193–202, 2008.

[19] C. Sommer, A. Fahrner, and M. Kiessling, "Postischemic neuroprotection in the ischemia-tolerant state gerbil hippocampus is associated with increased ligand binding to inhibitory GABA(A) receptors," *Acta Neuropathologica*, vol. 105, no. 3, pp. 197–202, 2003.

[20] E. Zhang, M. H. Yi, Y. Ko et al., "Expression of LC3 and beclin 1 in the spinal dorsal horn following spinal nerve ligation-induced neuropathic pain," *Brain Research*, vol. 1519, pp. 31–39, 2013.

[21] T. Yasaka, S. Y. Tiong, D. I. Hughes, J. S. Riddell, and A. J. Todd, "Populations of inhibitory and excitatory interneurons in lamina II of the adult rat spinal dorsal horn revealed by a combined electrophysiological and anatomical approach," *Pain*, vol. 151, no. 2, pp. 475–488, 2010.

[22] M. Mackie, D. I. Hughes, D. J. Maxwell, N. J. Tillakaratne, and A. J. Todd, "Distribution and colocalisation of glutamate decarboxylase isoforms in the rat spinal cord," *Neuroscience*, vol. 119, no. 2, pp. 461–472, 2003.

[23] D. J. Maxwell, M. D. Belle, O. Cheunsuang, A. Stewart, and R. Morris, "Morphology of inhibitory and excitatory interneurons in superficial laminae of the rat dorsal horn," *Journal of Physiology*, vol. 584, no. 2, pp. 521–533, 2007.

[24] A. J. Todd, D. I. Hughes, E. Polgar et al., "The expression of vesicular glutamate transporters VGLUT1 and VGLUT2 in neurochemically defined axonal populations in the rat spinal cord with emphasis on the dorsal horn," *European Journal of Neuroscience*, vol. 17, no. 1, pp. 13–27, 2003.

[25] E. Polgar, T. C. Sardella, M. Watanabe, and A. J. Todd, "Quantitative study of NPY-expressing GABAergic neurons and axons in rat spinal dorsal horn," *Journal of Comparative Neurology*, vol. 519, no. 6, pp. 1007–1023, 2011.

[26] S. P. Janssen, M. Truin, M. Van Kleef, and E. A. Joosten, "Differential GABAergic disinhibition during the development of painful peripheral neuropathy," *Neuroscience*, vol. 184, pp. 183–194, 2011.

[27] J. Lee, S. K. Back, E. J. Lim et al., "Are spinal GABAergic elements related to the manifestation of neuropathic pain in rat?," *Korean Journal of Physiology and Pharmacology*, vol. 14, no. 2, pp. 59–69, 2010.

[28] T. P. Malan, H. P. Mata, and F. Porreca, "Spinal GABA(A) and GABA(B) receptor pharmacology in a rat model of neuropathic pain," *Anesthesiology*, vol. 96, no. 5, pp. 1161–1167, 2002.

[29] M. P. Engle, M. Gassman, K. T. Sykes, B. Bettler, and D. L. Hammond, "Spinal nerve ligation does not alter the expression or function of GABA(B) receptors in spinal cord and dorsal root ganglia of the rat," *Neuroscience*, vol. 138, no. 4, pp. 1277–1287, 2006.

[30] S. S. Cao and R. J. Kaufman, "Endoplasmic reticulum stress and oxidative stress in cell fate decision and human disease," *Antioxidants and Redox Signaling*, vol. 21, no. 3, pp. 396–413, 2014.

[31] Y. Ge, Y. Jiao, P. Li et al., "Coregulation of endoplasmic reticulum stress and oxidative stress in neuropathic pain and disinhibition of the spinal nociceptive circuitry," *Pain*, vol. 159, no. 5, pp. 894–906, 2018.

[32] H. K. Kim, S. K. Park, J. L. Zhou et al., "Reactive oxygen species (ROS) play an important role in a rat model of neuropathic pain," *Pain*, vol. 111, no. 1-2, pp. 116–124, 2004.

[33] E. Zhang, M. H. Yi, N. Shin et al., "Endoplasmic reticulum stress impairment in the spinal dorsal horn of a neuropathic pain model," *Scientific Reports*, vol. 5, no. 1, article 11555, 2015.

[34] M. Mende, E. V. Fletcher, J. L. Belluardo et al., "Sensory-derived glutamate regulates presynaptic inhibitory terminals in mouse spinal cord," *Neuron*, vol. 90, no. 6, pp. 1189–1202, 2016.

[35] B. A. Rooney, E. D. Crown, C. E. Hulsebosch, and D. J. McAdoo, "Preemptive analgesia with lidocaine prevents failed back surgery syndrome," *Experimental Neurology*, vol. 204, no. 2, pp. 589–596, 2007.

[36] L. Galluzzi, I. Vitale, S. A. Aaronson et al., "Molecular mechanisms of cell death: recommendations of the nomenclature committee on cell death 2018," *Cell Death and Differentiation*, vol. 25, no. 3, pp. 486–541, 2018.

[37] L. Berliocchi, R. Russo, M. Maiaru, A. Levato, G. Bagetta, and M. T. Corasaniti, "Autophagy impairment in a mouse model of neuropathic pain," *Molecular Pain*, vol. 7, p. 83, 2011.

[38] C. W. Wang and D. J. Klionsky, "The molecular mechanism of autophagy," *Molecular Medicine*, vol. 9, no. 3-4, pp. 65–76, 2003.

[39] B. Loos, A. du Toit, and J. H. Hofmeyr, "Defining and measuring autophagosome flux-concept and reality," *Autophagy*, vol. 10, no. 11, pp. 2087–2096, 2014.

[40] Y. T. Wu, H. L. Tan, G. Shui et al., "Dual role of 3-methyladenine in modulation of autophagy via different temporal patterns of inhibition on class I and III phosphoinositide 3-kinase," *Journal of Biological Chemistry*, vol. 285, no. 14, pp. 10850–10861, 2010.

[41] L. Berliocchi, M. Maiaru, G. P. Varano et al., "Spinal autophagy is differently modulated in distinct mouse models of neuropathic pain," *Molecular Pain*, vol. 11, p. 3, 2015.

[42] G. Bjorkoy, T. Lamark, A. Brech et al., "p62/SQSTM1 forms protein aggregates degraded by autophagy and has a protective effect on huntingtin-induced cell death," *Journal of Cell Biology*, vol. 171, no. 4, pp. 603–614, 2005.

[43] M. Komatsu, S. Waguri, M. Koike et al., "Homeostatic levels of p62 control cytoplasmic inclusion body formation in autophagy-deficient mice," *Cell*, vol. 131, no. 6, pp. 1149–1163, 2007.

[44] S. Pankiv, T. H. Clausen, T. Lamark et al., "p62/SQSTM1 binds directly to Atg8/LC3 to facilitate degradation of ubiquitinated protein aggregates by autophagy," *Journal of Biological Chemistry*, vol. 282, no. 33, pp. 24131–24145, 2007.

[45] Y. Piao, D. H. Gwon, D. W. Kang et al., "TLR4-mediated autophagic impairment contributes to neuropathic pain in chronic constriction injury mice," *Molecular Brain*, vol. 11, no. 1, p. 11, 2018.

[46] E. Zhang, J. J. Kim, N. Shin et al., "High omega-3 polyunsaturated fatty acids in fat-1 mice reduce inflammatory pain," *Journal of Medicinal Food*, vol. 20, no. 6, pp. 535–541, 2017.

[47] A. Nalbandian, K. J. Llewellyn, C. Nguyen, P. G. Yazdi, and V. E. Kimonis, "Rapamycin and chloroquine: the in vitro and in vivo effects of autophagy-modifying drugs show promising results in valosin containing protein multisystem proteinopathy," *Plos One*, vol. 10, no. 4, Article ID e0122888, 2015.

[48] I. Shokolenko, N. Venediktova, A. Bochkareva, G. L. Wilson, and M. F. Alexeyev, "Oxidative stress induces degradation of mitochondrial DNA," *Nucleic Acids Research*, vol. 37, no. 8, pp. 2539–2548, 2009.

[49] J. F. Turrens, "Mitochondrial formation of reactive oxygen species," *Journal of Physiology*, vol. 552, no. 2, pp. 335–344, 2003.

[50] S. Koirala, Q. Guo, R. Kalia et al., "Interchangeable adaptors regulate mitochondrial dynamin assembly for membrane scission," *Proceedings of the National Academy of Sciences*, vol. 110, no. 15, pp. E1342–E1351, 2013.

[51] B. Uttara, A. V. Singh, P. Zamboni, and R. T. Mahajan, "Oxidative stress and neurodegenerative diseases: a review of upstream and downstream antioxidant therapeutic options," *Current Neuropharmacology*, vol. 7, no. 1, pp. 65–74, 2009.

[52] B. A. Payne and P. F. Chinnery, "Mitochondrial dysfunction in aging: much progress but many unresolved questions," *Biochimica et Biophysica Acta*, vol. 1847, no. 11, pp. 1347–1353, 2015.

[53] M. A. Arruda, P. Barcellos-de-Souza, A. L. Sampaio, A. G. Rossi, A. V. Graca-Souza, and C. Barja-Fidalgo, "NADPH oxidase-derived ROS: key modulators of heme-induced mitochondrial stability in human neutrophils," *Experimental Cell Research*, vol. 312, no. 19, pp. 3939–3948, 2006.

[54] I. Kim, S. Rodriguez-Enriquez, and J. J. Lemasters, "Selective degradation of mitochondria by mitophagy," *Archives of Biochemistry and Biophysics*, vol. 462, no. 2, pp. 245–253, 2007.

[55] J. Lee, S. Giordano, and J. Zhang, "Autophagy, mitochondria and oxidative stress: cross-talk and redox signalling," *Biochemical Journal*, vol. 441, no. 2, pp. 523–540, 2012.

[56] S. Mai, B. Muster, J. Bereiter-Hahn, and M. Jendrach, "Autophagy proteins LC3B, ATG5 and ATG12 participate in quality control after mitochondrial damage and influence lifespan," *Autophagy*, vol. 8, no. 1, pp. 47–62, 2012.

[57] E. S. Park, X. Gao, J. M. Chung, and K. Chung, "Levels of mitochondrial reactive oxygen species increase in rat neuropathic spinal dorsal horn neurons," *Neuroscience Letters*, vol. 391, no. 3, pp. 108–111, 2006.

[58] V. Gelmetti, P. De Rosa, L. Torosantucci et al., "PINK1 and BECN1 relocalize at mitochondria-associated membranes during mitophagy and promote ER-mitochondria tethering and autophagosome formation," *Autophagy*, vol. 13, no. 4, pp. 654–669, 2017.

[59] D. Lindholm, H. Wootz, and L. Korhonen, "ER stress and neurodegenerative diseases," *Cell Death and Differentiation*, vol. 13, no. 3, pp. 385–392, 2006.

[60] K. M. Doyle, D. Kennedy, A. M. Gorman, S. Gupta, S. J. Healy, and A. Samali, "Unfolded proteins and endoplasmic reticulum stress in neurodegenerative disorders," *Journal of Cellular and Molecular Medicine*, vol. 15, no. 10, pp. 2025–2039, 2011.

[61] J. D. Malhotra and R. J. Kaufman, "The endoplasmic reticulum and the unfolded protein response," *Seminars in Cell and Developmental Biology*, vol. 18, no. 6, pp. 716–731, 2007.

[62] G. S. Hotamisligil, "Endoplasmic reticulum stress and the inflammatory basis of metabolic disease," *Cell*, vol. 140, no. 6, pp. 900–917, 2010.

[63] Y. Kozutsumi, M. Segal, K. Normington, M. J. Gething, and J. Sambrook, "The presence of malfolded proteins in the endoplasmic reticulum signals the induction of glucose-regulated proteins," *Nature*, vol. 332, no. 6163, pp. 462–464, 1988.

[64] J. H. Lin, P. Walter, and T. S. Yen, "Endoplasmic reticulum stress in disease pathogenesis," *Annual Review of Pathology: Mechanisms of Disease*, vol. 3, no. 1, pp. 399–425, 2008.

[65] S. Wang and R. J. Kaufman, "The impact of the unfolded protein response on human disease," *Journal of Cell Biology*, vol. 197, no. 7, pp. 857–867, 2012.

[66] R. A. Stetler, Y. Gan, W. Zhang et al., "Heat shock proteins: cellular and molecular mechanisms in the central nervous system," *Progress in Neurobiology*, vol. 92, no. 2, pp. 184–211, 2010.

[67] B. Levine and G. Kroemer, "Autophagy in the pathogenesis of disease," *Cell*, vol. 132, no. 1, pp. 27–42, 2008.

[68] T. Yorimitsu and D. J. Klionsky, "Autophagy: molecular machinery for self-eating," *Cell Death and Differentiation*, vol. 12, no. 2, pp. 1542–1552, 2005.

[69] H. O. Rashid, R. K. Yadav, H. R. Kim, and H. J. Chae, "ER stress: autophagy induction, inhibition and selection," *Autophagy*, vol. 11, no. 11, pp. 1956–1977, 2015.

[70] R. Sano and J. C. Reed, "ER stress-induced cell death mechanisms," *Biochimica et Biophysica Acta (BBA)-Molecular Cell Research*, vol. 1833, no. 12, pp. 3460–3470, 2013.

[71] L. J. Lawson, V. H. Perry, P. Dri, and S. Gordon, "Heterogeneity in the distribution and morphology of microglia in the normal adult mouse brain," *Neuroscience*, vol. 39, no. 1, pp. 151–170, 1990.

[72] P. M. Grace, M. R. Hutchinson, S. F. Maier, and L. R. Watkins, "Pathological pain and the neuroimmune interface," *Nature Reviews Immunology*, vol. 14, no. 4, pp. 217–231, 2014.

[73] R. R. Ji, T. Berta, and M. Nedergaard, "Glia and pain: is chronic pain a gliopathy?," *Pain*, vol. 154, no. 1, pp. S10–S28, 2013.

[74] R. R. Ji, A. Chamessian, and Y. Q. Zhang, "Pain regulation by non-neuronal cells and inflammation," *Science*, vol. 354, no. 6312, pp. 572–577, 2016.

[75] M. Tsuda, K. Inoue, and M. W. Salter, "Neuropathic pain and spinal microglia: a big problem from molecules in "small" glia," *Trends in Neurosciences*, vol. 28, no. 2, pp. 101–107, 2005.

[76] N. P. Eriksson, J. K. Persson, M. Svensson, J. Arvidsson, C. Molander, and H. Aldskogius, "A quantitative analysis of the microglial cell reaction in central primary sensory projection territories following peripheral nerve injury in the adult rat," *Experimental Brain Research*, vol. 96, no. 1, pp. 19–27, 1993.

[77] D. E. Coyle, "Partial peripheral nerve injury leads to activation of astroglia and microglia which parallels the development of allodynic behavior," *Glia*, vol. 23, no. 1, pp. 75–83, 1998.

[78] L. Liu, E. Tornqvist, P. Mattsson et al., "Complement and clusterin in the spinal cord dorsal horn and gracile nucleus following sciatic nerve injury in the adult rat," *Neuroscience*, vol. 68, no. 1, pp. 167–179, 1995.

[79] R. W. Colburn, J. A. DeLeo, A. J. Rickman, M. P. Yeager, P. Kwon, and W. F. Hickey, "Dissociation of microglial activation and neuropathic pain behaviors following peripheral nerve injury in the rat," *Journal of Neuroimmunology*, vol. 79, no. 2, pp. 163–175, 1997.

[80] N. Gu, J. Peng, M. Murugan et al., "Spinal microgliosis due to resident microglial proliferation is required for pain hypersensitivity after peripheral nerve injury," *Cell Reports*, vol. 16, no. 3, pp. 605–614, 2016.

[81] Y. Yao, S. Echeverry, X. Q. Shi et al., "Dynamics of spinal microglia repopulation following an acute depletion," *Scientific Reports*, vol. 6, no. 1, article 22839, 2016.

[82] J. Gehrmann and R. B. Banati, "Microglial turnover in the injured CNS: activated microglia undergo delayed DNA fragmentation following peripheral nerve injury," *Journal of Neuropathology and Experimental Neurology*, vol. 54, no. 5, pp. 680–688, 1995.

[83] E. Okun, K. J. Griffioen, and M. P. Mattson, "Toll-like receptor signaling in neural plasticity and disease," *Trends in Neurosciences*, vol. 34, no. 5, pp. 269–281, 2011.

[84] J. Y. Chatton, L. Pellerin, and P. J. Magistretti, "GABA uptake into astrocytes is not associated with significant metabolic cost: implications for brain imaging of inhibitory transmission," *Proceedings of the National Academy of Sciences*, vol. 100, no. 21, pp. 12456–12461, 2003.

[85] A. Schousboe, A. Sarup, O. M. Larsson, and H. S. White, "GABA transporters as drug targets for modulation of GABAergic activity," *Biochemical Pharmacology*, vol. 68, no. 8, pp. 1557–1563, 2004.

[86] B. E. Yoon, J. Woo, and C. J. Lee, "Astrocytes as GABA-ergic and GABA-ceptive cells," *Neurochemical Research*, vol. 37, no. 11, pp. 2474–2479, 2012.

[87] S. J. Lee, K. S. Cho, and J. Y. Koh, "Oxidative injury triggers autophagy in astrocytes: the role of endogenous zinc," *Glia*, vol. 57, no. 12, pp. 1351–1361, 2009.
[88] M. Farrant and Z. Nusser, "Variations on an inhibitory theme: phasic and tonic activation of GABA(A) receptors," *Nature Reviews Neuroscience*, vol. 6, no. 3, pp. 215–229, 2005.
[89] S. Lee, B. E. Yoon, K. Berglund et al., "Channel-mediated tonic GABA release from glia," *Science*, vol. 330, no. 6005, pp. 790–796, 2010.
[90] W. Wang, W. Wang, X. Mei et al., "Crosstalk between spinal astrocytes and neurons in nerve injury-induced neuropathic pain," *PLoS One*, vol. 4, no. 9, Article ID e6973, 2009.

22

DC/TMD Examiner Protocol: Longitudinal Evaluation on Interexaminer Reliability

Marit Slåttelid Skeie,[1] Paula Frid,[2] Manal Mustafa,[3] Jörg Aßmus,[4] and Annika Rosén[5]

[1]*Department of Clinical Dentistry, Pediatric Dentistry, The Faculty of Medicine, University of Bergen, Bergen, Norway*
[2]*Department of Otorhinolaryngology, Division of Oral and Maxillofacial Surgery, University Hospital North Norway and Public Dental Service Competence Centre of North Norway and Department of Clinical Medicine, Faculty of Health Sciences, The Arctic University of Norway, Tromsø, Norway*
[3]*Oral Health Centre of Expertise in Western Norway, Hordaland, Norway*
[4]*Centre for Clinical Research, Haukeland University Hospital, 5021 Bergen, Norway*
[5]*Department of Clinical Dentistry, Division of Oral and Maxillofacial Surgery, The Faculty of Medicine, University of Bergen, Bergen, Norway*

Correspondence should be addressed to Marit Slåttelid Skeie; marit.skeie@uib.no

Academic Editor: Parisa Gazerani

Objectives. The objectives of this study were to assess the interexaminer agreement between one "reference" (gold standard) and each of two examiners, using the DC/TMD examination method, Axis I and to evaluate whether a recalibration changed reliability values. *Methods.* Participants (4 healthy and 12 TMD patients) in 2013 underwent a clinical examination according to DC/TMDs, Axis I. In 2014, additionally 16 participants (4 healthy and 12 TMD patients) were recruited. Two trainee examiners (one more experienced) and one "reference examiner" (gold standard) at both sessions assessed the participants. Calibration preparation (2013): The clinical protocol was sent to the trainee examiners with a request that its verbal commands should be learned by heart. An eight-hour-course was provided on the day preceding the examination session day. Recalibration preparation (2014): The same examiners in advance to this year's examination session were also asked to recapture the protocol's instructions (verbal commands to be learned by heart) and go through the information from the 2013 course and encouraged to contact by e-mail in case of unclear subjects. At a meeting prior to the examination session, they were also given the opportunities to ask questions. The interexaminer agreements in 2013 and 2014 between the "reference" and each examiner were analysed using Bland–Altman plots, intraclass correlation coefficient, Cohen's kappa, and consistency values. *Results.* For the majority of the gathered data, no clear change of agreement between 2013 and 2014 could be observed, and only one muscle zone in 2014 could show any clear difference in agreement between the examiners. *Conclusions.* No clear and consistent difference in the level of agreement between the two examiners could be observed, although one was more experienced than the other. Likewise, for most components of the DC/TMD tool, recalibration of examiners did not change the reliability findings.

1. Introduction

The temporomandibular disorders (TMDs) and orofacial pain affect around 10–15% of adults [1]. The annual incidence of first-onset TMDs, based on a prospective study, has been reported to be almost 4% [2], meaning that of 100 TMD-free people enrolled, nearly four persons per year will develop the disorder. In the Scandinavian countries, studies have documented pain-related TMDs among adolescents to be 4–7% [3–5], and according to the DC/TMD criteria and examination protocol, to be as high as 12% [4]. Although the disorder may impact the patient's quality of life negatively [6], not all patients receive sufficient and appropriate treatment through the dental health care system [7]. Whether the low provision of treatment is due to under- or misdiagnoses has to be further investigated. What is certain is that the many different diagnostic systems for identifying TMDs contribute to difficulties in agreeing on consistent diagnosis.

The most internationally used diagnostic tools during the last two decades have been the Research Diagnostic Criteria for TMD (RDC/TMD) [8] and the TMD classification according to the American Academy of Orofacial Pain [9], but in 2014, a new diagnostic classification system, the Diagnostic Criteria for Temporomandibular Disorders (DC/TMD), was launched, developed from RDC/TMD [10]. Some of the reasons for updating the RDC/TMDs were that its application was found impractical for use in clinical settings, there was a need to update definitions of TMD subtypes [11, 12], and there was a need for instructions with clear stipulation of specifications in the examination procedures [13]. The goal behind this was to agree on a diagnostic tool for wide use in clinical and research settings [14]. The DC/TMD system has also increasingly gained ground.

The DC/TMDs includes two components, Axis I and Axis II. The Axis I protocol is used for screening and differentiation of the most common pain-related TMDs and also for intra-articular disorders. For TMJ intra-articular disorders, Axis I is appropriate for screening purposes, but not for a definitive diagnosis. To reach a diagnosis, different types of imaging are often needed, such as magnetic resonance imaging (MRI) or computed tomography (CT/CBCT). The Axis II protocol is used to assess jaw physical functioning and to screen behavioural and additional psychosocial status [14].

An important prerequisite, emphasized by the World Health Organization in all oral health survey final reports, is to focus on reliability in the examination process [15]. Without training and calibration, experienced clinicians show low measurement reliability [16]. There are several studies evaluating the reliability and validity of different TMD diagnostic tools [16–23]. In this literature, training and also recalibration have been considered important for improving interexaminer reliability [17]. As far as we know, only a few studies have focused on the reliability of the clinical use of Axis I of the DC/TMDs. Schiffman and Ohrbach [14] have reported Axis I diagnostic criteria for temporomandibular pain-related disorders to have acceptable validity, but the most common pain-related TMJ intra-articular disorders, to be appropriate for screening purposes only. Furthermore, Leskinen et al., who reported on a Finnish version of Axis I DC/TMD clinical diagnoses, have demonstrated sufficiently high reliability for pain-related TMD diagnoses [24]. Graue and colleagues, who estimated the prevalence among Norwegian adolescents using DC/TMDs, also found acceptable clinical interexaminer results [4].

Hitherto, we have found no study using DC/TMDs that focuses on whether recalibration has an effect on reliability. An effect of a prior DC/TMD training course for examiners on reliability, however, has been investigated by Brazilian researchers. They found that the diagnostic reliability of formal DC/TMD training and calibration vs. DC/TMD self-instruction, gave similar values, except for subgroups of myalgia [25].

Arriving at reliable diagnoses is critical and for a relatively new diagnostic tool like DC/TMDs, more research should be given priority. The objective of this study was therefore to assess the interexaminer agreement between one "reference examiner" (gold standard) and each of two trainee examiners, using the DC/TMD examination method, Axis I and to evaluate whether a recalibration changed reliability values.

2. Materials and Methods

The null hypothesis to be tested was that there was no difference in reliability values at Time point 1 and Time point 2.

The study protocol was sent to the Regional Committee for Medical Research Ethics in Aarhus, Denmark, for approval. According to the committee's evaluation, the work was accepted as a type of reliability study since identification data, such as participants' names and unique personal identification numbers, were not obtained. In advance of the study, all study participants signed an informed consent.

The study was performed at the Section of Clinical Oral Physiology, Department of Dentistry, Aarhus University, Denmark. The reason why the researchers chose Denmark and not Norway when they conducted the study was due to the fact that in 2013, no course in DC/TMDs was available in Norway. Two independent exercises in DC/TMDs were conducted in 2013 (Sept. 3-4, 2013: Time point 1) and 2014 (June 19, 2014: Time point 2). The examiners (MSS and PF), one (PF) more experienced in diagnosis/treatment of TMDs patients than the other, were tested in comparison to a "reference examiner" (gold standard). This person was an instructor and teacher at the Section of Clinical Oral Physiology, trained in the consortium guidelines, and also the contact person for the DC/TMD course. In 2013, the early edition of the protocol "Diagnostic Criteria for TMDs, Clinical Protocol and Assessment Instruments" [13] was sent in the English version to the examiners two weeks preceding the examination session. The purpose was that the examiners would be able to learn and memorize the verbal commands previous to an eight-hour training and calibration course. Then, the protocol was implemented in a total of 16 participants including a 1 : 4 ratio of healthy/symptomatic individuals. The healthy participants originated from the patient catchment area of Aarhus University while those with a mix of muscular and joint problems were recruited among the TMD patients at the Section's clinic. In 2014, the same examiners before the examination session was conducted were encouraged to recapture the instructions and verbal commands that had been taught the year before and clarify any information related to the examination protocol. This could be done by e-mail contact or at a prior 45-minute session at the day of the clinical examination. Also, this year there were 16 participants. In both years, the same assessment procedures and parameters were used [13]. It was ensured that recorders assisted the examiners to complete the DC/TMDs examination form and that the examiners were blind to the participant's previous examinations or medical-dental history.

2.1. The Examination Procedure. The time requirement at both sessions was set to 20 minutes per examination. Four examination rounds were organised during a day, each round with four participants, which also allowed for regular breaks between the time sections. An in advance "Order of Examination Sheet" was conducted, both to assure examiner rotation in order to avoid examiner sequence could influence the results and to ensure that each participant was examined by each examiner. If this had not been taken into account, bias could have occurred as participants at the end of the series of examinations might have presented a more tensed or more stressed musculature. During the examinations, the participants who were offered a fee for participating sat comfortably upright in chairs that could be adjusted for height. The examiners stood to the right of the participants, facing them, but position changes were allowed if needed.

2.2. Measurements. The sequence of the examination process was as follows: firstly, information about pain and headache location during the last 30 days was requested, recorded as 0 (No: no pain) and 1 (Yes: pain). The subsequent registered measurements of the mandible were opening pattern, opening movements (pain-free opening, maximum-unassisted opening, and maximum-assisted opening), lateral (right lateral and left lateral) and protrusive movements, TMJ noises during opening, closing, lateral and protrusive movements, and joint locking. Pain during palpation of the TMJ and on supplemental muscles was the last measure. For accurate muscle palpation prior to the palpation examinations, finger pressure was calibrated by an appropriate force-measuring device (Palpeter®, Dentrade, Köln, Germany); 1 kg finger pressure for the masseter muscle (three horizontal zones: origin, body, and insertion of the masseter) and temporalis muscle (three vertical zones: anterior, middle, and posterior as well as around the lateral joint pole); 0.5 kg finger pressure for the lateral joint pole and for supplemental muscles. The palpation pressure was held for two seconds to determine pain and for five seconds to record a referred pain, two seconds for muscle palpation and finally, five seconds for lateral joint pole and around lateral joint pole.

2.3. Statistical Methods. A set of reliability coefficients for the clinical measurements were used. Interexaminer agreements between the "reference" and each of the two examiners (MSS and PF) of the clinical continuous data were assessed by applying Bland–Altman plots with limits of agreement (LoA) and intraclass correlation coefficients (ICC). For clinical categorical data with "Yes" and "No" responses, pain based on muscle palpation and joint sounds, kappa statistic (unweighted Cohen's kappa), and percent agreement with the "reference" were calculated. Comparison of percent agreement with the "reference" between Examiner 1 and Examiner 2 was done separately for 2013 and 2014, using McNemar's test in order to take into account that both examiners evaluated the same set of patients. Comparison of percent agreement between 2013 and 2014 was done using chi-squared tests since the patient samples in 2013 and 2014 were independent. The level of statistical significance was set to 5 percent. All analyses were undertaken with SPSS 24 (IBM Corp., Armonk, NY), and the graphics were derived using Matlab 9.0 (The MathWorks Inc., Natick, MA) to evaluate the interexaminer agreement.

3. Results

3.1. Measurement of Mandibular Range of Motion. Comparisons of the two trainee examiners (MSS and PF) in measuring the mandibular range of motion with the "reference" in 2013 and in 2014 are presented in Figure 1 (pain-free opening, maximum-unassisted opening, and maximum-assisted opening). Comparisons in respect of lateral and protrusive movements are presented in Figure 2 (right lateral, left lateral, and protrusion). Observation agreement of examiners vs. "reference" within a three-millimeter range was more frequent in the opening movements of maximum-unassisted opening and of maximum-assisted opening than in the opening movement of pain-free opening. The acceptable three-millimeter deviation was revealed by both examiners for maximum-unassisted opening, maximum-assisted opening, right lateral, left lateral and, protrusion both in 2013 and 2014. Table 1 presents interexaminer reliabilities using ICC values (average measures) and shows that the level of ICC for all measurements based on comparison between each examiner with "reference," was above 0.75 except for left lateral measurement (ICC: 0.60). For opening movements, the ICC values in 2013 and 2014 were almost identical for both trainee examiners. As for lateral at both sites and protrusive movements, the reliability scores varied depending on whether they were lower, at the same level, or higher in 2014 than in 2013. No clear and consistent change of the agreement from 2013 to 2014 could therefore be registered. Between the examiners, sometimes Examiner 1 had the higher ICC values; other times it was Examiner 2. Due to this variation between the examiners in reporting the highest reliability scores when compared to "reference," no clear difference in agreement between them could be observed.

3.2. Measurements Based on Muscle Palpation. Table 2 is descriptive and presents by Cohen's kappa scores and consistency values of the achieved interexaminer agreement between the "reference" and each of the two examiners for registering pain upon muscle palpation (Yes/No). The majority of the present percent agreement scores achieved did not significantly change from 2013 to 2014 (Supplemental Table 1). However, the percent agreement achieved when each examiner was compared to the "reference" showed statistical difference from 2013 to 2014 in two muscle zones (Examiner 1: body of m. masseter and Examiner 2: posterior zone of m. temporalis). Supplemental Table 1 shows that Examiner 1 experienced higher value (p value: 0.049), and Examiner 2 experienced lower value (p value: 0.042). Between the examiners, only in 2014, for palpation of m. masseter origin zone, statistical difference (p value: 0.022) in percent agreement could be shown (Examiner 1 had the highest reliability value). Additionally for Examiner 1, percent agreement for TMJ sounds in the form of clicking during closing movement significantly improved (p value: 0.039) from 2013 to 2014 (Supplemental Table 1).

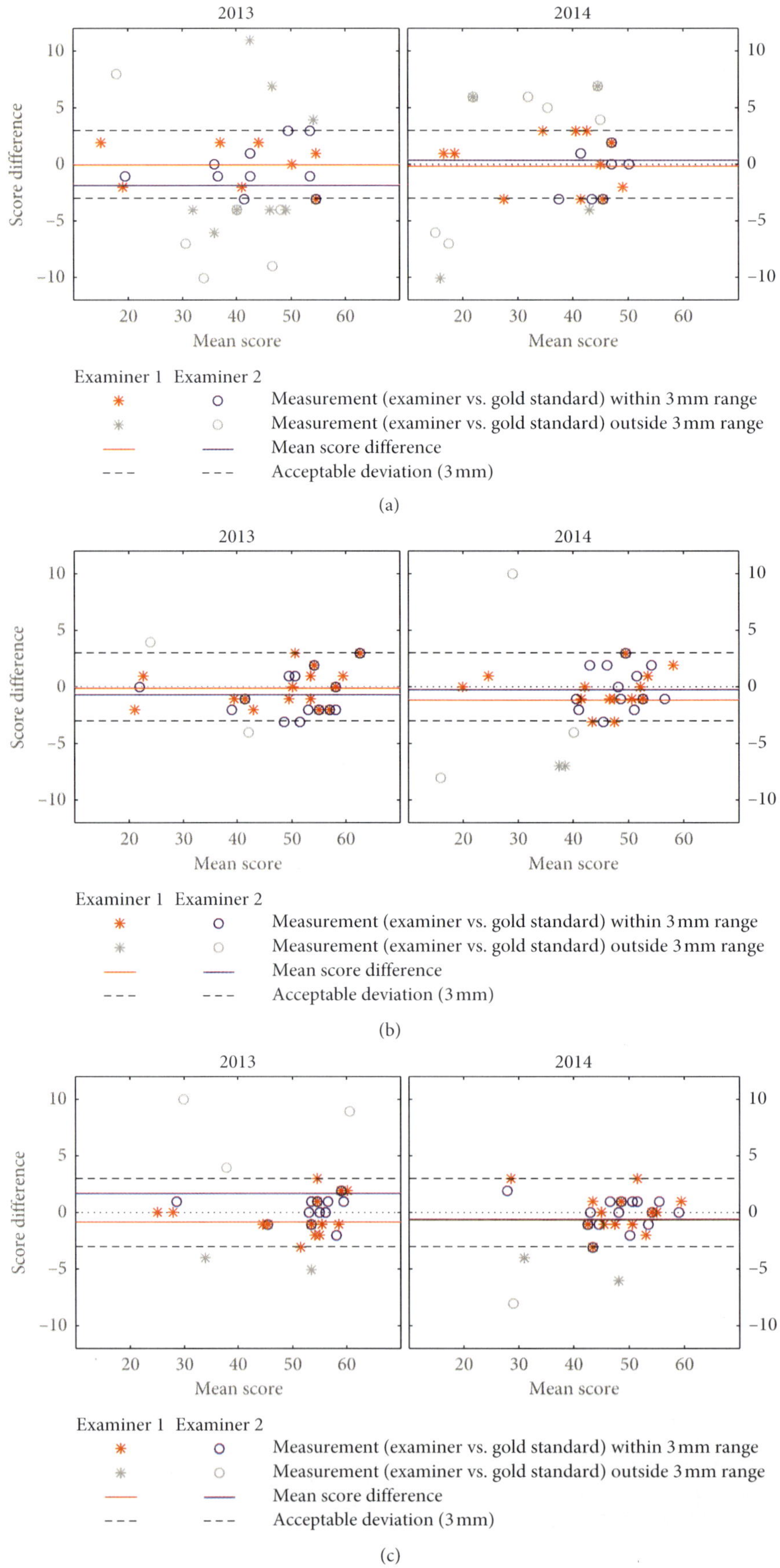

FIGURE 1: Opening movements ((a) pain-free opening, (b) maximum-unassisted opening, and (c) maximum-assisted opening). Bland–Altman plot for two examiners (raters) versus the "reference" (gold standard) at each time points (2013 and 2014). Mean scores in mm.

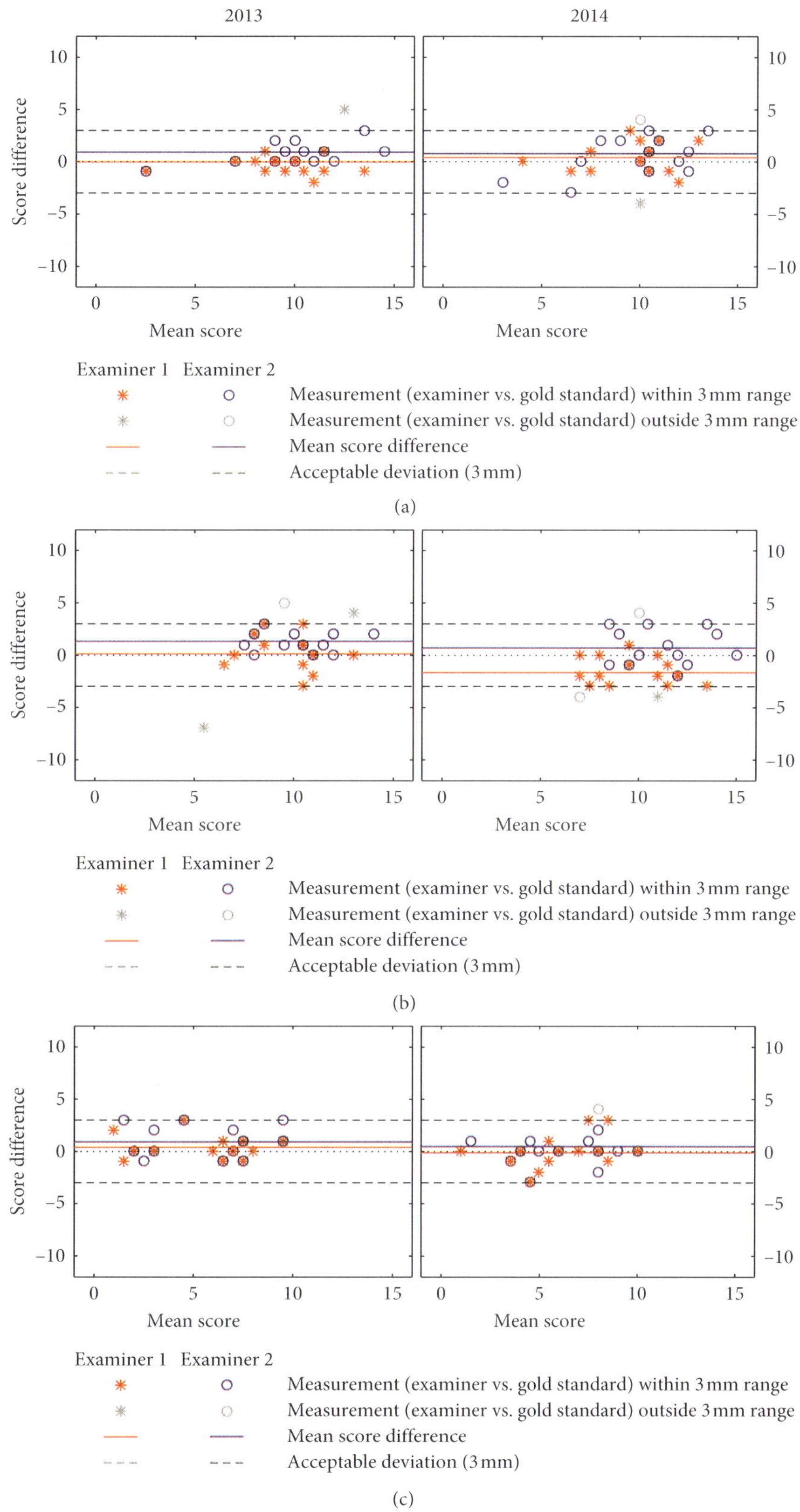

FIGURE 2: Lateral and protrusive movements ((a) right lateral, (b) left lateral, and (c) protrusion) at both sites for Bland–Altman plot for two examiners (raters) versus the "reference" (gold standard) at each time point (2013 and 2014). Mean scores in mm.

Table 1: Reliability (intraclass correlation coefficients (ICC)) for opening, lateral, and protrusive movements (mm). ICC calculations based on ICC values between the "reference" and Examiner 1 and the "reference" and Examiner 2 (average measurements). For ICC interpretation, https://www.ncbi.nlm.nih.gov/pmc/articles/PMC4913118/.

	2013		2014	
	Examiner 1	Examiner 2	Examiner 1	Examiner 2
Opening movements				
Pain-free opening	0.96 (0.89, 0.99)	0.96 (0.88, 0.99)	0.97 (0.91, 0.99)	0.96 (0.88, 0.99)
Maximum-unassisted opening	0.99 (0.99, 0.99)	0.99 (0.98, 0.99)	0.98 (0.95, 0.99)	0.96 (0.90, 0.99)
Maximum-assisted opening	0.99 (0.97, 0.99)	0.97 (0.92, 0.99)	0.98 (0.94, 0.99)	0.98 (0.94, 0.99)
Lateral at both sites and protrusive movements				
Right lateral	0.91 (0.73, 0.97)	0.96 (0.90, 0.99)	0.81 (0.46, 0.93)	0.87 (0.63, 0.95)
Left lateral	0.60 (-0.16, 0.86)	0.88 (0.65, 0.96)	0.80 (0.68, 0.96)	0.77 (0.33, 0.92)
Protrusion	0.96 (0.88, 0.99)	0.92 (0.76, 0.97)	0.90 (0.70, 0.96)	0.85 (0.56, 0.95)

Table 2: Cohen's kappa (K) and examiner agreement (% agreement values in parentheses) for reporting pain (Yes/No) and for reporting TMJ noises during opening and closing movements (Yes/No) between the "reference" and Examiner 1 and the "reference" and Examiner 2. N = number of observations.

	2013				2014			
	Examiner 1		Examiner 2		Examiner 1		Examiner 2	
	N	K (% agreement)	N	K (% agreement)	N	K (% agreement)	N	K (% agreement)
M. temporalis[1]								
Posterior	24	0.78 (91.7)	27	0.81 (92.6)	32	0.40 (78.1)	32	0.30 (71.9)
Middle	23	0.56 (78.3)	26	0.33 (65.4)	31	0.48 (74.2)	32	0.57 (81.3)
Anterior	21	0.35 (66.7)	27	0.70 (85.2)	32	0.68 (84.4)	32	0.56 (78.1)
M. masseter[2]								
Origin	24	0.50 (75.0)	26	0.34 (65.4)	31	0.69 (80.6)	31	0.27 (64.5)
Body	22	0.31 (68.3)	25	0.66 (88.0)	30	0.74 (90.0)	32	0.67 (84.3)
Insertion	20	0.50 (75.0)	26	0.57 (76.9)	30	0.67 (83.3)	32	0.87 (93.8)
TMJ sounds								
Open/close[3]								
Click								
Open	32	0.48 (75.0)	32	0.54 (78.1)	32	0.62 (90.6)	32	0.72 (93.8)
Close	32	0.69 (87.5)	32	0.72 (87.5)	32	1.00 (100.0)	32	0.72 (96.9)
Crepitus								
Open	32	(100.0)	32	(100.0)	32	(100.0)	32	(100.0)
Close	32	(100.0)	32	(93.8)	32	(96.9)	32	(96.9)
Lateral/protrusive[4]								
Click	32	0.66 (84.4)	32	0.62 (81.3)	32	0.53 (87.5%)	32	0.53 (87.5)
Crepitus	32	(100.0)	32	(100.0)	32	(90.6)	32	(90.6)

[1]Three vertical zones together (both sides). [2]Three horizontal zones together (both sides). [3]Opening and closing movements (both sides). [4]Lateral and protrusive movements (both sides). For interpretation of the kappa statistic, https://www.ncbi.nlm.nih.gov/pmc/articles/PMC3900052/.

Crepitus was infrequently observed. The "reference" did not register crepitus during the Opening movement in 2013, consistent with the other examiners (100% agreement). In 2014, however, the "reference" registered one crepitus during the Closing movement, not registered by the trainee examiners. Two cases of crepitus during lateral and protrusive movements registered by the "reference" were not noticed by the trainee examiners. On the contrary, both trainee examiners recorded crepitus in the same participant, but this was not observed by the "reference."

4. Discussion

This is the first study, as far as we know, that analyses the reliability of repeat measuring of components in the recently introduced DC/TMD diagnostic tool. Publications in the literature so far have been about whether DC/TMDs can be considered a valid screener for detecting TMDs, and whether it is a valid diagnostic criterion for different TMD subgroups [10, 24]. Due to the fact that reliability studies focusing on this new DC/TMD tool are so far few, this type of research should be appreciated.

The present study assesses the interexaminer reliability between the "reference" and each of the examiners in the DC/TMDs, and Axis I examination method failed to demonstrate any consistently clear change after recalibration; e.g., improvement as reported when the RDC/TMD was chosen as a diagnostic tool [17]. Only sporadical statistical differences were registered. Therefore, for the majority of the clinical measures, the null hypothesis could not be rejected.

The level of ICC for all but one mandibular movement was above 0.75, which was considered excellent [26]. The one registration below 0.75 of the left-lateral movement in 2013

(ICC: 0.60) was categorised as good. Interestingly, both examiners had their lowest ICC values when assessing the left-lateral movement. One explanation might be that, while standing to the right in front of the participant, it may be easier to register the movement to the right than to the left. The highest ICC values reported when the examiners were compared with the "reference" were for maximum-assisted or maximum-unassisted opening movements; this in line with other authors [18, 27].

A common method for detecting muscle tenderness is manual palpation [28]. Low agreement among examiners when examining the origin of the masseter has been reported as being a particular problem [28], a zone which also in this study showed some poor reliability values. Using standardization of palpation pressure, in spite of what was expected, did not contribute to a high level of reliability. One explanation for the relatively low reliability values for some zones of muscles might be that as many as 75% of recruited patients were TMD patients. Perhaps, applying the Palpeter standardization instrument directly on the muscle sites would have given higher reliability results.

The examiner agreement concerning the detection of click noises was consistent with a previous study of John and Zwijnenburg [18]. Examiner 1 could also show significant improvement in clicking during closing movement from 2013 to 2014. In spite of the high TMD prevalence among participants, crepitation was infrequent. The "reference" only found it once in 2014, and the examiners did not catch it. Therefore, the present extremely high percentage of agreement among the examiners with respect to crepitus most probably would have been lower if more participants had displayed it. The use of Cohen's kappa in measuring crepitus could not be used because of difficulties in interpreting the result. The underlying cause was the combination of extremely low prevalence of one of the decisions and a low sample size.

Leher et al. [20] have argued that examiner calibration rather than professional experience is the most important factor for reliable measurements of TMD symptoms. In this study, it seemed that prior experience was of lesser importance. However, the importance of clinical experience in deciding appropriate TMD diagnosis and how to treat it (outside the scope of this article) should be mentioned. Despite the ability to register clinical findings correctly, these must be combined with the appropriate imaging and other diagnostic tools to allow a correct diagnosis and treatment plan. Salloch and coworkers [29] have recently stressed the importance of the physician's expertise to find appropriate diagnoses and treatment plans for each patient in oncologic decision-making. Registration of pathology in the TMJ, including jaw movements, muscle palpation, and TMJ noises, may be seen either independently or in combination with TMDs such as myalgia, disc derangement, or inflammatory joint diseases. Therefore, it is essential that the examiner has clinical experience to make the appropriate diagnosis and treatment plan for each patient. Similar reliability between the examiners in measuring jaw movements, muscle palpation, and TMJ sounds does not always imply proper diagnosis and treatment of different TMDs but a more complex issue requiring clinical experience and knowledge of the examiner.

Self-instruction for examiners in DC/TMDs, according to Vilanova et al. [25], has been reported to be as effective as an examiner course. Explanations for this finding may be that the instructions for DC/TMD examinations are clear and easily memorised. This could also explain why the majority of the reliability coefficients in the present study did not change after recalibration such as when RCD/TMDs were applied [17].

4.1. Limitations. The instructions used in the DC/TMD protocol for the participants were provided in English, a possible source of misunderstanding as the first language of participants was Danish. However, none of the participants showed any sign of failure to understand the instructions. The reason for using the English language was that a back-translated version was not yet available. Another limitation was the relatively small sample size resulting in low power for statistical tests and that the examiners sometimes had problems recording all ($n = 32$) muscle palpation sites, especially in 2013. An explanation for better managing of the time schedule in 2014 could be that the examiners were more experienced.

5. Conclusion

No clear and consistent difference in the level of agreement between the two examiners could be observed, although one was more experienced than the other. Likewise, for most components of the DC/TMD tool, recalibration of examiners did not change the reliability findings.

The present findings underline that DC/TMDs are simple and well defined, having operational definitions with clear presentations. However, these findings should be further investigated in longitudinal clinical cohort studies using the DC/TMD protocol.

Acknowledgments

We would like to acknowledge all the participants in the study and the staff at the Section of Clinical Oral Physiology, Department of Dentistry, Aarhus University, especially Professor Peter Svensson and Assistant Professor Karina Bendixen, who made this study possible.

References

[1] National Institute of Dental and Craniofacial Research, Facial Pain, 2018, http://www.nidcr.nih.gov/DataStatistics/FindDataByTopic/FacialPain/.

[2] G. D. Slade, R. B. Fillingim, A. E. Sanders et al., "Summary of findings from the OPPERA prospective cohort study of incidence of first-onset temporomandibular disorder: implications and future directions," *Journal of Pain*, vol. 14, no. 12, pp. T116–T124, 2013.

[3] I. M. Nilsson, T. List, and M. Drangsholt, "Prevalence of temporomandibular pain and subsequent dental treatment in Swedish adolescents," *Journal of Orofacial Pain*, vol. 19, pp. 144–150, 2005.
[4] A. M. Graue, A. Jokstad, J. Assmus, and M. S. Skeie, "Prevalence among adolescents in Bergen, Western Norway, of temporomandibular disorders according to the DC/TMD criteria and examination protocol," *Acta Odontologica Scandinavica*, vol. 74, no. 6, pp. 449–455, 2016.
[5] V. Östensjo, K. Moen, T. Storesund, and A. Rosen, "Prevalence of painful temporomandibular disorders and correlation to lifestyle factors among adolescents in Norway," *Pain Research and Management*, vol. 2017, Article ID 2164825, 10 pages, 2017.
[6] S. S. Shueb, D. R. Nixdorf, M. T. John, B. F. Alonso, and J. Durham, "What is the impact of acute and chronic orofacial pain on quality of life?," *Journal of Dentistry*, vol. 43, no. 10, pp. 1203–1210, 2015.
[7] I. Nilsson, "Reliability, validity, incidence and impact of temporomandibular pain disorders in adolescents," Dissertation, University of Malmö, Malmö, Sweden, 2007.
[8] S. F. Dworkin and L. LeResche, "Research diagnostic criteria for temporomandibular disorders: review, criteria, examinations and specifications, critique," *Journal of craniomandibular disorders*, vol. 6, pp. 301–355, 1992.
[9] R. De Leeuw and G. Klasser, *Orofacial Pain: Guidelines for Assessment, Diagnosis, and Management*, American Academy of Orofacial Pain, New York, NY, USA, 6th edition, 2016.
[10] E. Schiffman, R. Ohrbach, E. Truelove et al., "Diagnostic criteria for temporomandibular disorders (DC/TMD) for clinical and research applications: recommendations of the International RDC/TMD Consortium Network∗ and Orofacial Pain Special Interest Group†," *Journal of Oral & Facial Pain and Headache*, vol. 28, no. 1, pp. 6–27, 2014.
[11] M. H. Steenks and A. de Wijer, "Validity of the research diagnostic criteria for temporomandibular disorders axis I in clinical and research settings," *Journal of Orofacial Pain*, vol. 23, pp. 9–16, 2009.
[12] T. List and C. S. Greene, "Moving forward with the RDC/TMD," *Journal of Oral Rehabilitation*, vol. 37, no. 10, pp. 731–733, 2010.
[13] E. Schiffman, R. Ohrbach, E. Truelove et al., "Diagnostic Criteria for Temporomandibular Disorders (DC/TMD) for Clinical and Research Applications: Recommendations of the International RDC/TMD Consortium Network and Orofacial Pain Special Interest Group. Version 02 June 2013," *Journal of Orofacial Pain*, 2013, In press.
[14] E. Schiffman and R. Ohrbach, "Executive summary of the diagnostic criteria for temporomandibular disorders for clinical and research applications," *Journal of the American Dental Association*, vol. 147, no. 6, pp. 438–445, 2016.
[15] World Health Organization, *Oral Health surveys—Basic Methods*, World Health Organization, Geneva, Switzerland, 5th edition, 2013.
[16] S. F. Dworkin, L. LeResche, T. DeRouen, and M. Von Korff, "Assessing clinical signs of temporomandibular disorders: reliability of clinical examiners," *Journal of Prosthetic Dentistry*, vol. 63, no. 5, pp. 574–579, 1990.
[17] T. List, M. T. John, S. F. Dworkin, and P. Svensson, "Recalibration improves inter-examiner reliability of TMD examination," *Acta Odontologica Scandinavica*, vol. 64, no. 3, pp. 146–152, 2006.
[18] M. T. John and A. J. Zwijnenburg, "Interobserver variability in assessment of signs of TMD," *International Journal of Prosthodontics*, vol. 14, pp. 265–270, 2001.
[19] M. T. John, S. F. Dworkin, and L. A. Mancl, "Reliability of clinical temporomandibular disorder diagnoses," *Pain*, vol. 118, no. 1, pp. 61–69, 2005.
[20] A. Leher, K. Graf, J. M. PhoDuc, and P. Rammelsberg, "Is there a difference in the reliable measurement of temporomandibular disorder signs between experienced and inexperienced examiners?," *Journal of Orofacial Pain*, vol. 19, pp. 58–64, 2005.
[21] M. Schmitter, B. Ohlmann, M. T. John, C. Hirsch, and P. Rammelsberg, "Research diagnostic criteria for temporomandibular disorders: a calibration and reliability study," *Cranio*, vol. 23, no. 3, pp. 212–218, 2005.
[22] J. P. Goulet, G. T. Clark, and V. F. Flack, "Reproducibility of examiner performance for muscle and joint palpation in the temporomandibular system following training and calibration," *Community Dentistry and Oral Epidemiology*, vol. 21, no. 2, pp. 72–77, 1993.
[23] J. P. Goulet, G. T. Clark, V. F. Flack, and C. Liu, "The reproducibility of muscle and joint tenderness detection methods and maximum mandibular movement measurement for the temporomandibular system," *Journal of Orofacial Pain*, vol. 12, pp. 17–26, 1998.
[24] J. Leskinen, T. Suvinen, T. Teerijoki-Oksa et al., "Diagnostic criteria for temporomandibular disorders (DC/TMD): interexaminer reliability of the Finnish version of Axis I clinical diagnoses," *Journal of Oral Rehabilitation*, vol. 44, no. 7, pp. 493–499, 2017.
[25] L. S. Vilanova, R. C. Garcia, T. List, and P. Alstergren, "Diagnostic criteria for temporomandibular disorders: self-instruction or formal training and calibration?," *Journal of Headache and Pain*, vol. 16, no. 1, p. 505, 2015.
[26] V. Cicchetti, "Guidelines, criteria, and rules of thumb for evaluating normed and standardized assessment instruments in psychology," *Psychological Assessment*, vol. 6, no. 4, pp. 284–290, 1994.
[27] A. J. Hassel, P. Rammelsberg, and M. Schmitter, "Inter-examiner reliability in the clinical examination of temporomandibular disorders: influence of age," *Community Dentistry and Oral Epidemiology*, vol. 34, no. 1, pp. 41–46, 2006.
[28] P. C. Conti, C. N. dos Santos, and J. R. Lauris, "Interexaminer agreement for muscle palpation procedures: the efficacy of a calibration program," *Cranio*, vol. 20, no. 4, pp. 289–294, 2002.
[29] S. Salloch, I. Otte, A. Reinacher-Schick, and J. Vollmann, "What does physicians' clinical expertise contribute to oncologic decision-making? A qualitative interview study," *Journal of Evaluation in Clinical Practice*, vol. 24, no. 1, pp. 180–186, 2017.

23

Pilot Trial of the Reboot Online Program: An Internet-Delivered, Multidisciplinary Pain Management Program for Chronic Pain

Regina Schultz,[1] **Jessica Smith**,[2] **Jill M. Newby**,[2,3] **Tania Gardner**,[1]
Christine T. Shiner,[1,4] **Gavin Andrews**,[2] **and Steven G. Faux**[1,4]

[1]*Department of Pain Medicine, St Vincent's Hospital, Sydney, NSW, Australia*
[2]*Clinical Research Unit for Anxiety and Depression (CRUfAD), School of Psychiatry, St Vincent's Hospital, University of New South Wales, Sydney, NSW, Australia*
[3]*School of Psychology, University of New South Wales, Sydney, Australia*
[4]*St Vincent's Clinical School, University of New South Wales, Sydney, Australia*

Correspondence should be addressed to Regina Schultz; regina.schultz@health.nsw.gov.au

Academic Editor: Gerrit Hirschfeld

Objectives. Chronic pain causes significant disability and psychological distress, but barriers often prevent people with pain from engaging in traditional face-to-face pain management programs. Accessible, feasible, and effective alternative treatment options are needed. *Methods.* A prospective, feasibility pilot study was conducted to trial a novel, multidisciplinary online pain management program: the "Reboot Online" program. Twenty participants experiencing pain of at least three months duration were recruited. All participants were enrolled in the "Reboot Online" program, consisting of eight online lessons completed over 16 weeks. Lessons incorporated multidisciplinary input from medical pain specialists, physiotherapists, and psychologists. Participants were assessed at pretreatment, posttreatment, and follow-up using a suite of outcome measures examining pain, disability, catastrophising, self-efficacy, mood, and psychological distress. *Results.* 13 participants completed the program (65% adherence). Following treatment, the participants had significantly improved scores on measures of pain-related disability, self-efficacy, catastrophising thoughts, acceptance of pain, symptoms of depression, and general psychological distress. These findings were retained at three months posttreatment. Participants also reported high levels of acceptability and satisfaction with the program. *Discussion.* This study provides pilot evidence for the feasibility, acceptability, and effectiveness of an online, multidisciplinary pain program: "Reboot Online." Future investigations will focus on conducting a randomised controlled trial of this innovative and promising treatment for chronic pain. This trial is registered with ACTRN12615000660583.

1. Introduction

Chronic pain is a multifaceted health problem with considerable burden at the individual and global level [1–3]. Multidisciplinary pain management programs (MDPPs) are the accepted best practice for chronic pain management [4, 5]. These are face-to-face treatment programs, designed to reduce disability and suffering and typically delivered in a group-based setting by a multidisciplinary pain team. These programs generally require participants to engage in face-to-face sessions of moderate (30–60 hrs) to high (>60 hours) intensity [6] and are mostly based in urban outpatient treatment facilities. This common delivery method typically restricts access for those living in rural areas, those with work and family commitments, and/or those with disabilities which prevent travel and/or face-to-face contact. Often, access to MDPPs can be further restricted by long waiting times for specialist services and the stigma surrounding chronic pain. A viable and effective Internet-based pain management program could improve access to evidence-based multidisciplinary treatment for people with chronic pain who cannot access face-to-face services.

In recent years, a strong evidence base has developed for the efficacy of Internet-based psychological treatments, especially those based on cognitive behavioural therapy (CBT) principles, to treat a wide range of mental health conditions including depression and anxiety disorders [7–9]. Moreover, several Internet-based treatment programs for chronic pain have been developed, with burgeoning evidence indicating efficacy in reducing disability, mood disturbance, and improving perceived self-efficacy [10–14]. However, the efficacy of these programs is variable due to methodological inconsistencies in the literature, including different outcome measures, key program content, types of control groups used, and clinician involvement [15]. A few meta-analyses and systematic reviews have been completed thus far and report varying effect sizes. Bender et al. [16] reported significant improvement on measures of pain intensity, depression, anxiety, and functional measures for participants who completed online pain management programs compared to controls; however, it is difficult to compare these results with other reviews because this paper did not report effect sizes. Another systematic review reported effect sizes ranging from small to large for pain intensity measures (0.20–0.85); however, most were in the small to moderate range with only one (out of 19) reporting a large effect size [15]. A consequent systematic review duplicated the small to moderate effect sizes for pain intensity scores (−0.35 to −0.16), measures of catastrophising (range −0.32 to −0.26), depression (range −0.18 to −0.14), and functional interference (−0.35 to −0.16; [14]). Therefore, given the typically small to moderate effect sizes reported of Internet-based pain management programs, it is warranted to explore the viability of developing a novel program to improve treatment efficacy.

Clinical practice guidelines for chronic pain management promote a multidisciplinary approach which includes a self-management framework with cognitive behavioural techniques, graded activities and exposure, methods to improve acceptance and cognitive flexibility, skills training, education, and notably physical exercise [5, 17–19]. In addition, the literature suggests that although no specific exercise is most beneficial, a graded approach to physical exercise is a key component of chronic pain management in reducing disability, especially for low back pain [20, 21]. Strategies which include an individualised approach, refresher sessions, or the addition of audio or video tapes can improve exercise adherence [20].

Review of the content of the existing Internet-based pain management programs shows the programs include some of these components, in different configurations, but none include all. More specifically, none provided a structured physical exercise section. Therefore, given the demonstrated relative efficacy of existing online pain management programs, the "Reboot Online" program was developed to provide a comprehensive multidisciplinary approach with all the components, with particular attention to incorporating a physical exercise component. Thus, the "Reboot Online" program, to our knowledge, is the only online pain program which includes a full multidisciplinary approach, incorporating psychoeducation, psychological skills, and a tailored graduated physical activity program. Another advantage is that the program can be monitored and used to supplement treatment plans by any member of the multidisciplinary pain team including doctors, physiotherapists, social workers, psychologists, or practice nurses. Consequently, the "Reboot Online" program provides a complete multidisciplinary approach.

The "Reboot Online" program was developed via a unique collaboration between clinical experts in chronic pain management (Department of Pain Medicine, St Vincent's Hospital, Sydney, Australia) and leading researchers in the development of Internet-based CBT (iCBT) programs (Clinical Research Unit for Anxiety and Depression, University of NSW, St Vincent's Hospital, Sydney, Australia; CRUfAD). It is closely modelled on the Reboot Pain Management program, a face-to-face MDPP developed at St Vincent's Hospital, Sydney, Australia. This group-based MDPP runs for 6 hours per day, one day per week, for 10 weeks and is located on-site at St Vincent's Hospital, Sydney. Preliminary data suggest that this program is effective in improving measures of pain, pain disability, and psychological measures of distress [22]. In addition, the "Reboot Online" program was modelled on existing iCBT programs successfully developed at CRUfAD to treat anxiety and depression [8, 23, 24].

This paper describes a pilot study conducted to explore the feasibility, acceptability, and outcomes of the novel "Reboot Online" program for chronic pain.

2. Materials and Methods

2.1. Participants. Participants with self-identified pain were recruited via hospital and Facebook advertisements and the "Virtual Clinic" website (www.virtulclinic.org.au), an online research portal of CRUfAD. Inclusion criteria were as follows: aged ≥18 years; self-reported experience of pain for ≥3 months; resident of Australia; and prepared to provide participant and general practitioner contact details. In addition, participants were required to have a phone, a computer with Internet access, be on stable doses of medications for at least three months, and have had their pain assessed by a physician within the last three months. Exclusion criteria included: an inability to communicate in English; a current diagnosis of psychosis, bipolar disorder, substance abuse or dependence; or being actively suicidal. Participants with a pain-related surgical intervention/treatment scheduled in the next six months or participants who had completed a multidisciplinary pain management program within the prior six months were also excluded.

Potential participants applied online, and screening was conducted in two phases, first via an online questionnaire [25] and subsequently via a structured phone interview for those who passed online screening (Figure 1). Phone interviews were conducted by a trained clinician to confirm the diagnosis of chronic pain and assess for the presence of a major depressive disorder. Eligible participants who met all inclusion and no exclusion criteria following both screening processes were invited to participate in the trial. All provided informed electronic consent prior to commencing the program. A letter was also sent to each participant's GP/pain

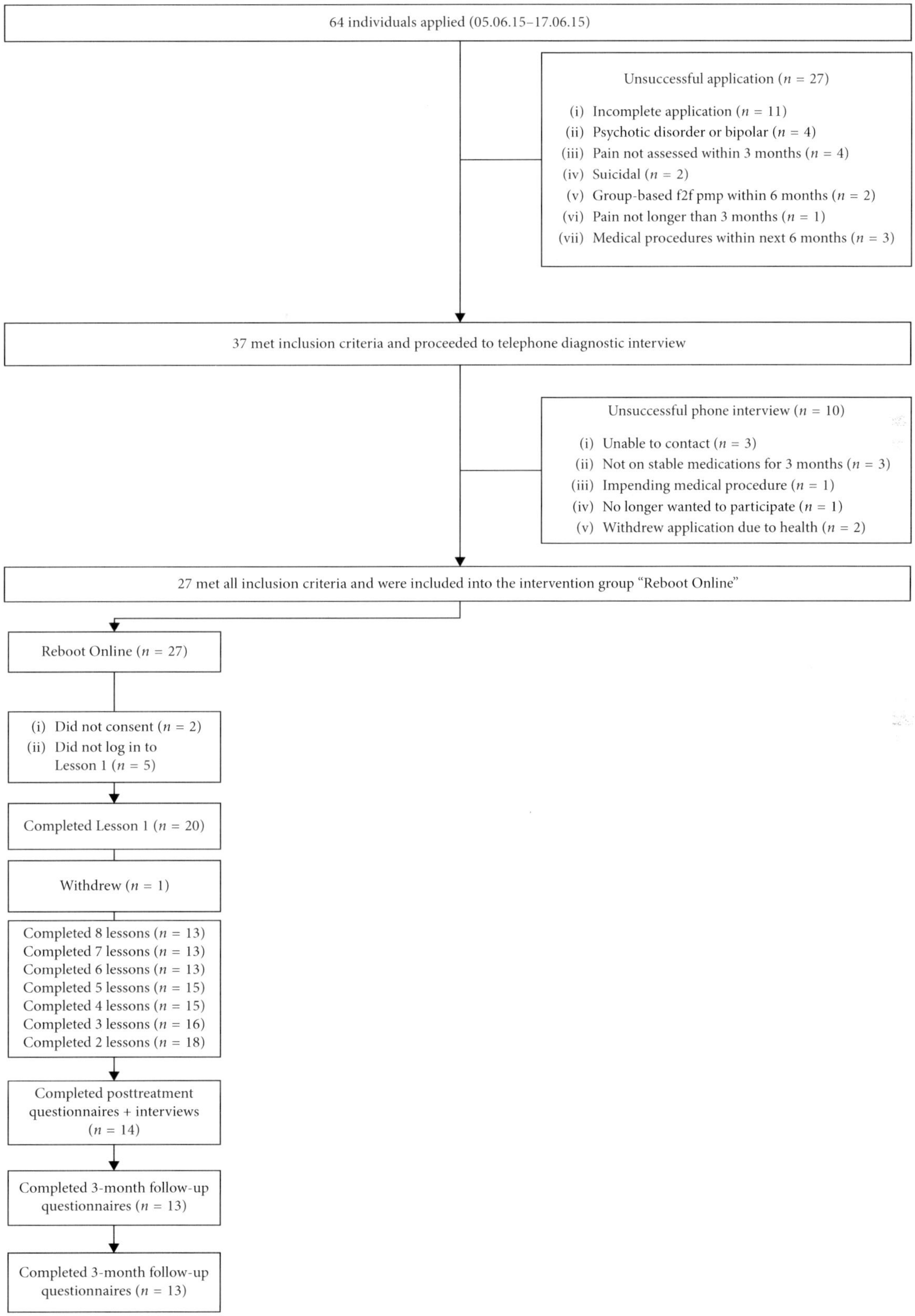

FIGURE 1: Participant flow for recruitment and adherence.

physician informing them of the participant's enrolment into the trial.

Sixty-four applicants were screened, 27 met all inclusion criteria, and 20 eligible participants were enrolled into the study (Figure 1). Baseline data from all 20 participants are included in the analyses, while posttreatment and follow-up data are available for 14 and 13 participants, respectively. This study was approved by the Human Research Ethics Committee of St Vincent's Hospital Sydney, Australia (HREC/15/SVH/32), and conducted in accordance with the Declaration of Helsinki. The trial was prospectively registered on the Australian and New Zealand Clinical Trials Registry (ACTRN12615000660583).

2.2. Treatment Program. The "Reboot Online" program consists of eight online lessons, to be completed over 16 weeks by the participant. The course was accessed via the Virtual Clinic website, with the release of content staged throughout the course duration (one new lesson released every two weeks). Lesson content is centred around an illustrated storyline that depicts a fictional character with chronic pain. Each lesson follows this character as they engage with multidisciplinary treatment to learn about and manage their chronic pain. Lesson content was focussed on (1) an introduction to the chronic pain model, (2) goal setting and acceptance, (3) movement, pacing, and daily activity scheduling, (4) monitoring and recognising unhelpful thoughts, (5) mood and pain and working with unhelpful thoughts, (6) stress and sleep management, (7) communication and relationships, and (8) managing flare-ups. With each nominated lesson, the participant has access to a downloadable lesson summary with practical homework exercises, related educational videos, a Tai Chi video, relaxation audio files, and an "at home" exercise program. Participants were only able to progress to the next lesson if they had accessed each component of the current lesson.

The core course material incorporates content developed with multidisciplinary expertise from medical, psychiatric, occupational therapy, physiotherapy, and psychology pain specialists. Unique to this program is the inclusion of a graded exercise program, accessed through the "movement station" and tailored to the needs of each participant. This incorporates four key components, namely, strength, stability, flexibility, and cardiofitness. For the strength, stability, and flexibility components, a prescribed exercise program including video demonstrations was selected, at one of four intensity levels. Progression of exercise was self-determined by the participant, although guidelines were provided that outlined the suggested competency level required in each exercise before progression. For the cardiofitness component, participants self-selected an appropriate activity to complete. Progression through to the next lesson was conditional on the participant accessing the movement station. A graded Tai Chi (Yang style) program incorporating demonstration videos and instructions was similarly provided to participants at the beginning of the program, to be completed over the course duration. Four relaxation audio files and instructions on how to practise relaxation and the benefits of relaxation for chronic pain management were included in the online material.

To supplement the core course material, participants had access to nine educational videos providing information on related topics including nutrition, common pain medications, the role of medical imaging in pain management, the nature of chronic pain, activities of daily living, and ergonomics. Viewing was encouraged, but not compulsory.

Participants were informed that during the course of the program, they had email access to a multidisciplinary team including a psychiatrist, pain specialist (medical), clinical psychologist, and physiotherapist from the trial team, who were available to respond to participant questions and concerns. Participants also received email and/or phone contact from an allied health technician (JS) until they completed lesson 2.

Of note, a participatory design process was used to include consumer feedback into the design of the "Reboot Online" program. Specifically, a focus group of service users ($n = 9$) was convened to provide feedback on the format, language, content, and structure of the program. The service users were provided with Lesson 1 from the program approximately one month before the pilot trial was launched to ensure sufficient time to incorporate appropriate changes into the program design.

2.3. Outcome Measures. Participants were formally assessed via a suite of measures at four time points: pretreatment, midtreatment, posttreatment and at three-month follow-up. Data from three time points (pretreatment, posttreatment, and follow-up) will be the focus of the current paper. As per the Virtual Clinic guidelines, prior to the start of each lesson, participants were required to complete the Kessler 10-item Psychological Distress Scale (K10) [26] to monitor any increase in psychological distress; participants were contacted if their scores significantly deteriorated.

2.3.1. Primary Outcome Measures. The two primary outcomes of interest were as follows:

(i) The Pain Self-Efficacy Questionnaire (PESQ) [27–30], a 17-item self-report questionnaire designed to assess the participant's confidence to perform activities while experiencing pain.

(ii) The Brief Pain Inventory (BPI) [31, 32], a 9-item questionnaire designed to measure the severity of pain and the interference of pain on daily function.

2.3.2. Secondary Outcome Measures

(i) The Pain Catastrophising Scale (PCS) [33, 34], a 13-item self-report measure of catastrophic thoughts related to chronic pain.

(ii) Tampa Scale of Kinesiophobia (TSK) [35, 36], a 17-item checklist which measures fear and avoidance of movement.

(iii) Pain Disability Index (PDI) [37, 38], which measures the impact of pain on the participant's confidence to perform activities while experiencing pain.

(iv) Chronic Pain Acceptance Questionnaire (CPAQ) [39, 40], which examines the participant's acceptance of chronic pain.

(v) The Depression Anxiety and Stress Scale-21 (DASS-21) [41, 42], a measure of the negative emotional states of depression, anxiety, and stress via the frequency of associated symptoms. Depression, anxiety, and stress subscores were used for analyses.

(vi) The Kessler 10-item Psychological Stress Scale (K10) [26, 43], a self-reported measure of overall psychological distress.

(vii) The Patient Health Questionnaire-9 (PHQ-9) [25], for symptoms of depression.

Given the feasibility nature of this study, data on acceptability of the program were also collected, via the following measures:

(i) Time spent reading lessons, reported by each participant as a measure of engagement with the program.

(ii) Treatment satisfaction, via completion of an 18-item satisfaction questionnaire posttreatment. Each item was scored on a 0 to 5 Likert scale.

(iii) Adherence rates, for completion of each lesson and the overall program.

2.4. Statistical Analyses. Linear mixed models were used to investigate changes in primary and secondary outcome measures from pretreatment to posttreatment, and pretreatment to 3-month follow-up. A MIXED procedure with a random intercept for subject was used, as in iCBT previous studies [44]. Mixed models are capable of estimating parameters for repeated measures studies with missing data via maximum likelihood estimation, thus were appropriate for this study [45]. For each outcome, time was treated as a categorical variable, and an identity covariance structure was specified to model the covariance structure of the random intercept. Initial model building focussed on the selection of the most appropriate covariance structure for the residual correlation matrix. Model fit indices and inspection of the variance-covariance matrix supported the selection of the identity covariance structure for each of the outcome measures. Effect sizes (Hedges g, adjusted for sample size) were calculated to determine the size of the within-group reduction between pretreatment to posttreatment, and pretreatment to 3-month follow-up. All analyses were implemented in SPSS v24, and differences where considered significant when $p < 0.05$.

3. Results

3.1. Participant Demography. 20 participants were enrolled in the "Reboot Online" program, of whom 19 were female (95%) and mean age was 47.5 years. 35% of participants ($n = 7$) reported to reside in a major city, 30% in outer regional areas ($n = 6$), 20% in remote areas ($n = 4$), and 15% in inner regional zones ($n = 3$). The majority of participants were not in paid employment (75%; $n = 15$); 30% were registered as disabled ($n = 6$), 20% were retired ($n = 4$), 15% were at-home parents ($n = 3$), and 10% were seeking work ($n = 2$). The remaining 25% were in full-time or part-time employment.

The majority of participants had experienced pain for longer than 5 years (65%) and had never participated in a MDPP before (80%). All but one participant ($n = 19$, 95%) reported that their pain was always present, they did not have an active compensation claim, and that their pain affected the number of hours they were able to work. Half the participants ($n = 10$) reported that their main pain started from no obvious cause, with the remaining describing their pain arising from illness (25%, $n = 5$), injury (15%; $n = 3$), and other causes (10%; $n = 2$). Apart from pain, the sample was relatively healthy, with nearly all participants denying a previous diagnosis of lung disease ($n = 20$), cancer, heart, stomach or kidney disease ($n = 19$), stroke, diabetes or blood diseases ($n = 18$), or high blood pressure ($n = 17$). In terms of psychological disorders, just over half the sample described a previous self-reported diagnosis of depression (55%; $n = 11$) and 25% ($n = 5$) reported a diagnosis of post-traumatic stress disorder (see Table 1 for detailed descriptive data).

3.2. Adherence and Engagement. All 20 participants completed lesson 1, 18 completed lesson 2, 16 completed lesson 3, 15 completed lessons 4 and 5, and 13 completed all 8 lessons. This represents a 65% completion rate for the program in its entirety. Participants spent an average of 39–80 minutes completing each lesson and 89–156 minutes practising the relevant skills. However, this included large intersubject variability, with self-reported time spent reading the lessons ranging from 10 to 240 minutes and between 0 and 1200 minutes for practising the skills. During the three-month follow-up period, the participants reported that they spent on average 10.6 hours (637.5 minutes) practising skills they had learnt in the program. Regarding clinician contact, the allied health technician (JS) spent an average of 40.5 minutes ($SD = 33.46$, range 6–121) emailing and calling each participant during the treatment course (including the follow-up period), and this included relaying responses to individual participant's queries from the multidisciplinary team.

3.3. Primary and Secondary Outcomes at Posttreatment. Table 2 describes the summary statistics, estimated marginal means, and the linear mixed model results for the primary and secondary outcomes at pre- and posttreatment and follow-up. For the primary outcome measures, a statistically significant change was observed between pre- and posttreatment for the PSEQ and for the BPI interference scale, with large effect sizes observed for both (Table 2 and Figure 2). Among secondary measures, significant differences were observed on the CPAQ, PCS, K10, and the depression

Table 1: Participant demographic and pain characteristics.

	Number (20 in total)
Age	
Mean	47.45 years
Range	24–75 years
Sex	
Male	1
Female	19
Highest level of education	
Postgraduate	1
Undergraduate	8
Year 12	4
TAFE	2
Other certificate	4
No qualification	1
Employment Status	
Full time	3
Part time	2
Registered sick	6
Retired	4
At-home parent	3
Unemployed	2
Place of residence	
Major city	7
Inner regional area	3
Outer regional area	6
Remote area	4
Duration of chronic pain	
1-2 years	4
2–5 years	3
>5 years	13

subscale of the DASS-21. Large effect sizes were observed for nearly all secondary outcome measures (range $g = 0.82$ to 1.46), except the TSK, DASS-A, and DASS-S score which showed moderate effect sizes ($g = 0.54$–0.66; Table 2).

3.4. Primary and Secondary Outcomes at Three-Month Follow-Up. The primary and most of the secondary outcome measures, demonstrated a statistically significant difference between the pretreatment and 3-month follow-up scores (Table 2). The large effect sizes were retained at 3-month follow-up; the primary outcome measures demonstrated large effect sizes ($g = 1.24$ to 1.53), and large effect sizes were also observed for all the secondary outcome measures (range $g = 1.01$ to 1.30), except the TSK, DASS-A, and DASS-D scores which retained a moderate effect size (range $g = 0.66$–0.76).

3.5. Participant Satisfaction. Overall, participants were satisfied with the program, 8 reported to be "very satisfied" and 5 "mostly satisfied". The majority reported that their confidence to manage their pain had improved ("significantly increased," $n = 7$; "increased," $n = 5$; "no change," $n = 2$). Moreover, nearly all the participants rated their confidence in the program teaching them pain management techniques was at least 7/10, with 8 participants rating their confidence as 10/10. When asked to rate the quality of their contact with the clinical team, all participants rated this as either excellent ($n = 10$) or good ($n = 3$). Similarly, the participants rated the quality of the materials in the program as either excellent ($n = 7$) or good ($n = 6$).

Regarding individual components of the program, the lessons, lesson summaries, and relaxation recordings were rated by all participants as either extremely important or important. Most other components were also rated as extremely important or important, with only a few participants rating the movement station ($n = 2$), the resources section ($n = 1$), automatic emails ($n = 1$), and clinical support from the team ($n = 1$) as not very important. Participant feedback identified some areas for improvement to the program. Specifically, approximately half the participants ($n = 7$) thought there was not enough time to complete the program and only six participants described themselves as relating well to the fictional online character. This feedback will be incorporated into future modification of the program.

4. Discussion

To our knowledge, "Reboot Online" represents the first comprehensive, Internet-based, multidisciplinary treatment program for chronic pain management. The structure and content of this program have been closely modelled on established face-to-face treatment programs for chronic pain, making it the first online resource to mirror face-to-face services and translate them to an Internet-based platform. The findings of the current pilot study show that following completion of the "Reboot Online" program, participants' scores significantly improved on measures assessing their ability to manage and accept their chronic pain. In addition, there was a significant reduction in scores on measures examining perceived level of disability, interference from pain, and catastrophic thoughts relating to pain. An accompanying reduction in symptoms of general psychological distress and depression were also observed. These findings were evident immediately after completion of the program and were largely retained at three months. In comparison to the typically small to moderate effect sizes previously reported in the literature [14, 15], the current results demonstrate large effect sizes on the majority of measures posttreatment (range: 0.81–1.46) and moderate effect sizes on the remaining (range: 0.54–0.66). Even compared to more efficacious Internet-based pain programs, the current results are at least comparable and on some measures more favourable [12]. This suggests that the comprehensive multidisciplinary approach delivered by "Reboot Online" is a feasible treatment option. Most notably, effect sizes even increased at follow-up for some measures, and this differs from established interventions where improvement often decays over time [46], suggesting that this novel intervention may represent not only a feasible, but also sustainable treatment approach for the ongoing management of chronic pain.

Our data demonstrate that there was a high level of engagement with the program, with participants spending an average of at least 30 minutes reading the lessons and nearly 1.5 hours applying and utilising newly acquired skills

Table 2: Estimated marginal means at pre-, mid-, and posttreatment and three months following "Reboot Online."

	Pretreatment	Midtreatment	Posttreatment	3-month follow-up	Pre- to posttreatment			Pretreatment to follow-up		
	Mean (SD), $n = 20$	Mean (SD), $n = 15$	Mean (SD), $n = 14$	Mean (SD), $n = 13$	F (df)	Effect size: Hedges g	95% CI	F (df)	Effect size: Hedges g	95% CI
PSEQ	22.95 (13.77)	31.80 (13.79)	36.79 (13.77)	40.00 (13.77)	$F(3, 58) = 13.84^{*}$	−1.00	−1.72 to −0.28	$F(3, 58) = 17.05^{**}$	−1.24	−2.00 to −0.48
BPI-interference	7.26 (2.06)	5.27 (2.05)	4.25 (2.06)	4.11 (2.06)	$F(3, 58) = 3.02^{**}$	1.46	0.69–2.23	$F(3, 58) = 3.15\#$	1.53	0.74 to 2.32
BPI-severity	5.75 (1.76)	4.71 (1.75)	4.27 (1.75)	3.69 (1.76)	$F(3, 58) = 1.48$	0.84	0.13–1.55	$F(3, 58) = 2.06^{*}$	1.17	0.42 to 1.92
PCS	24.50 (8.45)	19.00 (8.48)	13.33 (8.19)	13.55 (8.83)	$F(3, 57) = 11.17^{**}$	1.34	0.59–2.09	$F(3, 57) = 10.96^{**}$	1.27	0.51 to 2.03
TSK	40.05 (8.90)	35.47 (8.87)	34.14 (8.91)	34.18 (8.89)	$F(3, 56) = 5.91$	0.66	−0.04–1.36	$F(3, 56) = 5.87$	0.66	−0.06 to 1.38
PDI	43.60 (15.21)	3.72 (15.22)	31.21 (15.19)	27.55 (15.87)	$F(3, 56) = 12.39$	0.82	0.11–1.53	$F(3, 56) = 16.06^{*}$	1.03	0.29 to 1.77
CPAQ	51.95 (14.04)	63.73 (14.02)	69.50 (14.03)	70.18 (14.03)	$F(3, 56) = 17.55^{**}$	−1.25	−1.99 to −0.51	$F(3, 56) = 18.23^{**}$	−1.30	−2.07 to −0.53
DASS-D	17.10 (7.92)	11.87 (7.90)	8.57 (7.89)	8.91 (8.24)	$F(3, 56) = 8.53^{*}$	1.08	0.35–1.81	$F(3, 56) = 8.19^{*}$	1.01	0.27 to 1.75
DASS-A	11.10 (7.74)	9.47 (7.75)	6.29 (7.75)	5.09 (7.75)	$F(3, 56) = 4.81$	0.62	−0.08–1.32	$F(3, 56) = 6.01$	0.76	0.04 to 1.48
DASS-S	17.30 (9.21)	15.73 (9.22)	12.29 (9.24)	10.18 (9.63)	$F(3, 56) = 5.01$	0.54	−0.15–1.23	$F(3, 56) = 7.12$	0.76	0.04 to 1.48
K10	26.80 (6.57)	21.20 (6.58)	20.50 (6.59)	19.80 (6.93)	$F(3, 55) = 6.30^{*}$	0.96	0.24–1.68	$F(3, 55) = 7.00^{*}$	1.04	0.30 to 1.78
PHQ-9	12.10 (4.70)	9.40 (4.69)	8.29 (4.71)	7.18 (4.92)	$F(3, 56) = 3.81$	0.81	0.10–1.52	$F(3, 56) = 4.92^{*}$	1.02	0.28 to 1.76

$^{*}p < 0.05$; $^{**}p < 0.01$; $\#p < 0.001$.

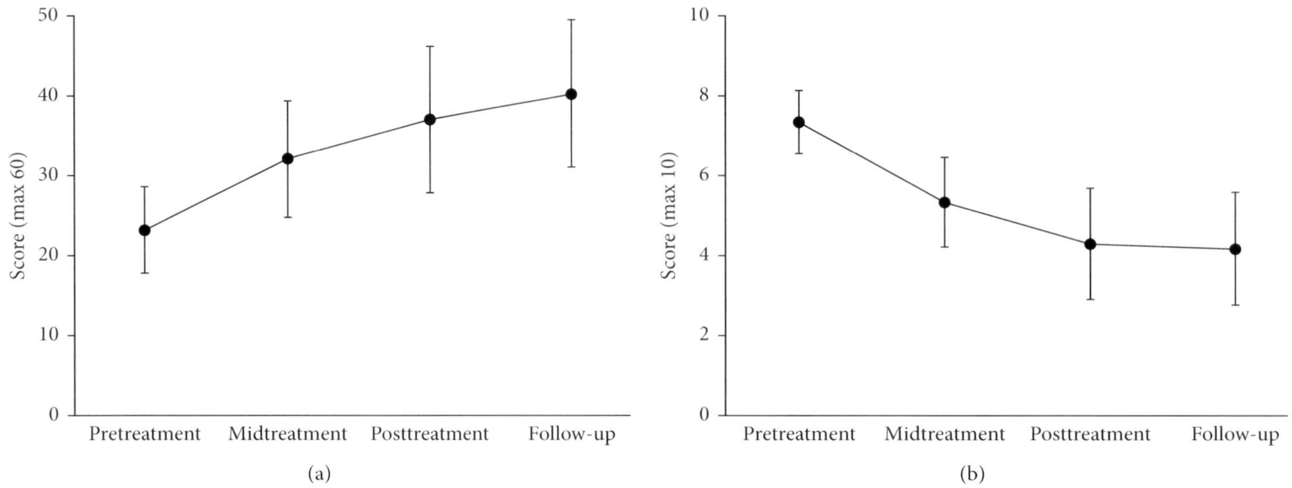

Figure 2: Participant improvement on primary outcome measures. (a) The Pain Self-efficacy Questionnaire (PSEQ), where higher scores indicate greater self-efficacy. (b) The Brief Pain Inventory (BPI)-Interference Score, where lower scores indicate less pain interference. Data are presented as mean and 95% confidence intervals.

in their everyday life. This suggests that the program was engaging for its target population and that it assisted people to incorporate pain management strategies into their lifestyle. Generally, participants found the different multidisciplinary aspects of the program to be useful and important and reported that their confidence to use pain management techniques and to manage their pain improved following the program. The moderate adherence rate suggests that not all participants could sustain their engagement with the program; however, the overall high satisfaction rate, which is comparable to similar online pain management programs [12], suggests that "Reboot Online" was an acceptable and well-received intervention.

The demographic characteristics of the current sample are similar in terms of the average age and duration of pain compared with reported participant demographics from online pain management programs and face-to-face multidisciplinary pain management clinics [14, 47, 48]. The baseline scores of the current sample on several questionnaires (DASS-D; DASS-A; DASS-S; PHQ-9; PSEQ; TSK) were comparable to those reported by participants accessing Australian and Canadian face-to-face multidisciplinary pain clinics [47, 48]. However, the current sample differed to the existing literature regarding the percentage of employed participants, with more participants actively employed in the previously reported literature (range: 30.4%–67%), compared to the current sample (25%) [47, 48]. In addition, the gender distribution was not comparable, with previous literature typically reporting fewer female participants (range: 57.4%–71.1%) than the current sample (95%); however, given the small sample size, caution should be used in making conclusions about the influence of the gender distribution on the present results [47, 48]. Therefore, the demographic characteristics and baseline scores on several of the primary and secondary outcome measures are comparable to participants accessing other online pain programs and face-to-face multidisciplinary pain clinics.

4.1. Methodological Considerations. There are some limitations of the current study, most notably the adherence rate was reasonable but not high; 35% of the initial participants did not complete all the lessons. This is comparable to the mean withdrawal rate (27.4%) reported in a systematic review of Internet-based pain management programs (range: 5.7% to 58.9%), with more than half reporting baseline differences between those who completed and withdrew from the studies [16]. However, the duration of "Reboot Online" (16 weeks), is longer compared to other online pain programs (8 weeks) [12] and given the added requirement for participants to access the graded exercise program for each lesson, the adherence rate is notable compared to programs with less onerous time and commitment requirements. Also, many of the participants who completed the trial reported that they did not relate well with the fictional character at the centre of the program. It is difficult to determine why some participants did not complete the lessons or engage well with this character. Perhaps this was because there is limited capacity to individually tailor the program content, skills, and techniques provided in an online format, as compared to face-to-face programs.

Given the small sample size, definitive conclusions about program efficacy cannot be drawn from this pilot study, rather, it should be used to inform the design of a larger, more rigorous clinical trial. The small sample and substantial missing data may have also led to an overestimation of treatment effects. Being exploratory in nature, this pilot study also examined a wide variety of outcome variables. While this may limit statistical power, here it was an important scoping exercise to determine the most pertinent measures to include in future analyses.

For each lesson, it was compulsory for the participant to access the movement station; however, limitations in the software application meant that information on how many times or how long the participants watched the exercise videos could not be recorded. Thus, there is not a clear indication of the participants' engagement with the graded exercise program. Furthermore, no direct measure of physical activity was included in the present study, due to a lack of consensus on a "gold-standard" measure, in addition to the logistical challenge of obtaining physical activity data from subjects who are engaging remotely in an online program. Given that the comprehensive multidisciplinary approach adopted by the "Reboot Online" program is novel and particularly the inclusion of a graduated exercise program, this may be of interest in future studies.

"Reboot Online" is likely to appeal to a broad section of the chronic pain population because the delivery method of the course is sufficiently convenient for those unable to attend a hospital or a face-to-face pain management centre due to family, work, health, or transport issues. Evidence for the optimal management of chronic pain supports treatment by a multidisciplinary pain team [5, 19]; however, these are rarely located in rural and remote areas in Australia. An online program represents a novel mode of service delivery, especially for those unable to face-to-face programs, thus improving equity of access to state-of-the-art multidisciplinary treatment. This is supported by the demographic profile of the current sample, with the majority of participants not residing within a major city. Finally, many people suffering from chronic nonmalignant pain have a need for education and comprehension of the problem as indicated in the Australian national pain strategy [49]. While existing online resources such as the Australian Agency for Clinical Innovation (ACI) Pain Network website may offer readers access to information [50], the "Reboot Online" MDPP can also offer effective treatment to those who have gained an understanding of their problem and the opportunity to learn relevant skills to manage their pain. The program will also benefit a range of clinicians because the design of the program allows it to be monitored by any member of the multidisciplinary pain team including doctors, physiotherapists, social workers, psychologists, or practice nurses. In addition, solo practitioners such as GPs, individual psychologists, or physiotherapists could use the program to supplement their treatment plan for patients.

5. Conclusions

The results of this pilot trial demonstrate that the novel "Reboot Online" program is a feasible and acceptable treatment program for the chronic pain population. Preliminary data suggest that this Internet-delivered MDPP may reduce pain-related disability, catastrophic thinking, reported degree of pain interference, and improve self-efficacy and chronic pain acceptance. Moreover, it may improve symptoms of depression and general psychological distress. There is some suggestion that these improvements are sustainable, being largely retained at 3-month follow-up. Given the increased time and commitment requirements of "Reboot Online" compared to other online pain management programs, the adherence rate is reasonable. This combined with the preliminary positive findings from the current pilot study suggest that "Reboot Online," a comprehensive MDT online pain management program with a graded exercise component, warrants further investigation with a randomised controlled trial.

Disclosure

This research was performed as part of employment of the authors at St Vincent's Hospital Sydney (Regina Schultz, Tania Gardner, Christine T. Shiner, and Steven G. Faux) and the Clinical Research Unit for Anxiety and Depression (Jessica Smith, Jill Newby, and Gavin Andrews).

Acknowledgments

This research was supported by funding from the Motor Accidents Authority, NSW Government (now the State Insurance Regulatory Authority). Dr. Newby was supported by a Fellowship from the National Health and Medical Research Council of Australia (Grant number 1037787).

References

[1] N. Maniadakis and A. Gray, "The economic burden of back pain in the UK," *Pain*, vol. 84, no. 1, pp. 95–103, 2000.

[2] O. van Hecke, N. Torrance, and B. H. Smith, "Chronic pain epidemiology and its clinical relevance," *British Journal of Anaesthesia*, vol. 111, no. 1, pp. 13–18, 2013.

[3] T. Vos, A. D. Flaxman, M. Naghavi et al., "Years lived with disability (YLDs) for 1160 sequelae of 289 diseases and injuries 1990-2010: a systematic analysis for the Global Burden of Disease Study 2010," *The Lancet*, vol. 380, no. 9859, pp. 2163–2196, 2012.

[4] J. M. Disorbio, D. Bruns, and G. Barolat, "Assessment and treatment of chronic pain," *Practical Pain Management*, vol. 6, no. 2, pp. 1–7, 2006.

[5] NICE, *Low Back Pain And Sciatica in Over 16s: Assessment and Management*, NICE, Manchester, UK, 2016, https://www.nice.org.uk/guidance/ng59.

[6] ACI Pain Management Network, *Pain Management Programs–Which Patient for Which Program?*, ACI, Chatswood, NSW, Australia, 2013.

[7] G. Andrews, P. Cuijpers, M. G. Craske, P. McEvoy, and N. Titov, "Computer therapy for the anxiety and depressive disorders is effective, acceptable and practical health care: a meta-analysis," *PLoS One*, vol. 5, no. 10, Article ID e13196, 2010.

[8] J. M. Newby, A. Mackenzie, A. D. Williams et al., "Internet cognitive behavioural therapy for mixed anxiety and depression: a randomized controlled trial and evidence of effectiveness in primary care," *Psychological Medicine*, vol. 43, no. 12, pp. 2635–2648, 2013.

[9] A. D. Williams and G. Andrews, "The effectiveness of internet cognitive behavioural therapy (iCBT) for depression in primary care: a quality assurance study," *PLoS One*, vol. 8, no. 2, Article ID e57447, 2013.

[10] R. L. H. Berman, M. A. Iris, R. Bode, and C. Drengenberg, "The effectiveness of an online mind-body intervention for older adults with chronic pain," *Journal of Pain*, vol. 10, no. 1, pp. 68–79, 2009.
[11] M. Buhrman, A. Fredriksson, G. Edström et al., "Guided Internet-delivered cognitive behavioural therapy for chronic pain patients who have residual symptoms after rehabilitation treatment: randomized controlled trial," *European Journal of Pain*, vol. 17, no. 5, pp. 753–765, 2013.
[12] B. F. Dear, N. Titov, K. N. Perry et al., "The pain course: a randomised controlled trial of a clinician-guided Internet-delivered cognitive behaviour therapy program for managing chronic pain and emotional well-being," *Pain*, vol. 154, no. 6, pp. 942–950, 2013.
[13] K. R. Lorig, P. L. Ritter, D. D. Laurent, and K. Plant, "The internet-based arthritis self-management program: a one-year randomized trial for patients with arthritis or fibromyalgia," *Arthritis Rheum*, vol. 59, no. 7, pp. 1009–1017, 2008.
[14] M. A. P. Vugts, M. C. W. Joosen, J. E. van der Geer, A. M. E. E. Zedlitz, and H. J. M. Vrijhoef, "The effectiveness of various computer-based interventions for patients with chronic pain or functional somatic syndromes: a systematic review and meta-analysis," *PLoS One*, vol. 13, no. 5, Article ID e0196467, 2018.
[15] A. A. Heapy, D. M. Higgins, D. Cervone, L. Wandner, B. T. Fenton, and R. D. Kerns, "A systematic review of technology-assisted self-management interventions for chronic pain," *Clinical Journal of Pain*, vol. 31, no. 6, pp. 470–492, 2015.
[16] J. L. Bender, A. Radhakrishnan, C. Diorio, M. Englesakis, and A. R. Jadad, "Can pain be managed through the internet? a systematic review of randomized controlled trials," *Pain*, vol. 152, no. 8, pp. 1740–1750, 2011.
[17] R. Chou, J. D. Loeser, D. K. Owens et al., "Interventional therapies, surgery, and interdisciplinary rehabilitation for low back pain: an evidence-based clinical practice guideline from the American Pain Society," *Spine*, vol. 34, no. 10, pp. 1066–1077, 2009.
[18] The British Pain Society, *Guidelines for Pain Management Programmes for Adults An Evidence-Based Review Prepared on Behalf of the British Pain Society*, London, UK, 2013, http://www.britishpainsociety.org.
[19] Scottish Intercollegiate Guidelines Network, *Management of Chronic Pain*, SIGN, Edinburgh, UK, 2013.
[20] J. L. Jordan, M. A. Holden, E. E. J. Mason, and N. E. Foster, "Interventions to improve adherence to exercise for chronic musculoskeletal pain in adults," *Cochrane Database of Systematic Reviews*, vol. 1, article CD005956, 2010.
[21] P. Savigny, P. Watson, M. Underwood et al., *Low Back Pain: Early Management of Persistent Non-Specific Low Back Pain*, National Collaborating Centre for Primary Care and Royal College of General Practitioners, London, UK, 2009.
[22] R. Schultz, M. Lau, S. Faux et al., "The reboot program–a new less intensive outpatient pain management program: preliminary evidence," in *Proceedings of Australian Pain Society Annual Conference*, Melbourne, VIC, Australia, April 2012.
[23] J. M. Newby, L. Robins, K. Wilhelm et al., "Web-based cognitive behavior therapy for depression in people with diabetes mellitus: a randomized controlled trial," *Journal of Medical Internet Research*, vol. 19, no. 15, p. e157, 2017.
[24] A. E. J. Mahoney, A. Mackenzie, A. D. Williams, J. Smith, and G. Andrews, "Internet cognitive behavioural treatment for obsessive compulsive disorder: a randomised controlled trial," *Behaviour Research and Therapy*, vol. 63, pp. 99–106, 2014.
[25] K. Kroenke, R. Spitzer, and J. Williams, "The PHQ-9: validity of a brief depression severity measure," *Journal of General Internal Medicine*, vol. 16, no. 9, pp. 606–613, 2001.
[26] R. Kessler, G. Andrews, L. J. Colpe et al., "Short screening scales to monitor population prevalences and trends in non-specific psychological distress," *Psychological Medicine*, vol. 32, no. 6, pp. 959–976, 2002.
[27] M. K. Nicholas, "Self-efficacy and chronic pain," in *Proceedings of Paper Presented at The Annual Conference of The British Psychological Society*, St Andrews, UK, 1989.
[28] A. Asghari and M. K. Nicholas, "Pain self-efficacy beliefs and pain behaviour: a prospective study," *Pain*, vol. 94, pp. 85–100, 2001.
[29] L. Gibson and J. Strong, "The reliability and validity of a measure of perceived functional capacity for work in chronic back pain," *Journal of Occupational Rehabilitation*, vol. 6, no. 1, pp. 59–75, 1996.
[30] M. K. Nicholas, "The pain self-efficacy questionnaire: taking pain into account," *European Journal of Pain*, vol. 11, no. 2, pp. 153–163, 2007.
[31] C. S. Cleeland, "Pain assessment in cancer," in *Effect of Cancer on Quality of Life*, D. Osoba, Ed., pp. 293–305, CRC Press, Boca Raton, FL, USA, 1991.
[32] M. Pelayo-Alvarez, S. Perez-Hoyos, and Y. Agra-Varela, "Reliability and concurrent validity of the palliative outcome scale, the rotterdam symptom checklist, and the brief pain inventory," *Journal of Palliative Medicine*, vol. 16, no. 8, pp. 867–874, 2013.
[33] M. J. Sullivan, S. R. Bishop, and J. Pivik, "The pain catastrophizing scale: development and validation," *Psychological Assessment*, vol. 7, no. 4, pp. 524–532, 1995.
[34] A. Osman, F. X. Barrios, P. M. Gutierrez, B. A. Kopper, T. Merrifield, and L. Grittmann, "The pain catastrophising scale: further psychometric evaluation with adult samples," *Journal of Behavioural Medicine*, vol. 23, no. 4, pp. 351–365, 2000.
[35] R. P. Miller, S. Kori, and D. Todd, "The Tampa Scale: a measure of kinesiophobia," *Journal of Clinical Pain*, vol. 7, no. 1, pp. 51-52, 1991.
[36] E. J. C. M. Swinkels-Meewisse, R. A. H. M. Swinkels, A. L. M. Verbeek, J. W. S. Vlaeyen, and R. A. B. Oostendorp, "Psychometric properties of the Tampa Scale for kinesiophobia and the fear-avoidance beliefs questionnaire in acute low back pain," *Manual Therapy*, vol. 8, no. 1, pp. 29–36, 2003.
[37] R. C. Tait, J. T. Chibnall, and S. Krause, "The pain disability index: psychometric properties," *Pain*, vol. 40, no. 2, pp. 171–182, 1990.
[38] R. C. Tait, C. A. Pollard, R. B. Margolis, P. N. Duckro, and S. J. Krause, "The Pain disability index: psychometric and validity data," *Archives of Physical Medicine and Rehabilitation*, vol. 68, no. 7, pp. 438–441, 1987.
[39] L. M. McCracken, "Learning to live with pain: acceptance of pain predicts adjustment in persons with chronic pain," *Pain*, vol. 74, no. 1, pp. 21–27, 1998.
[40] M .K. Nicholas and A. Asghari, "Investigating acceptance in adjustment to chronic pain: is acceptance broader than we thought?," *Pain*, vol. 124, no. 3, pp. 269–279, 2006.
[41] P. F. Lovibond and S. H. Lovibond, "The structure of negative emotional states: comparison of the Depression Anxiety Stress Scales (DASS) with the beck depression and anxiety inventories," *Behaviour Research and Therapy*, vol. 33, no. 3, pp. 335–343, 1995.
[42] M. M. Antony, P. J. Bieling, B. J. Cox, M. W. Enns, and R. P. Swinson, "Psychometric properties of the 42-item and

21-item versions of the Depression Anxiety Stress Scales (DASS) in clinical groups and a community sample," *Psychological Assessment*, vol. 10, no. 2, pp. 176–181, 1998.
[43] T. Furukawa, R. C. Kessler, T. Slade, and G. Andrews, "The performance of the k6 and k10 screening scales for psychological distress in the australian national survey of mental health and well-being," *Psychological Medicine*, vol. 33, no. 2, pp. 357–362, 2003.
[44] J. M. Newby, A. E. J. Mahoney, E. C. Mason, J. Smith, S. Uppal, and G. Andrews, "Pilot trial of a therapist-supported internet-delivered cognitive behavioural therapy program for health anxiety," *Internet Interventions*, vol. 6, pp. 71–79, 2016.
[45] B. West, K. B. Welch, and A. T. Galecki, *Linear Mixed Models: A Practical Guide Using Statistical Software*, CRC Press, Boca Raton, FL, USA, 2006.
[46] C. Eccleston, E. Fisher, L. Craig, G. B. Duggan, B .A. Rosser, and E. Keogh, "Psychological therapies (Internet-delivered) for the management of chronic pain in adults," *Cochrane Database of Systematic Reviews*, vol. 2, article Cd010152, 2014.
[47] C. May, V. Brcic, and B. Lau, "Characteristics and complexity of chronic pain patients referred to a community-based multidisciplinary chronic pain clinic," *Canadian Journal of Pain*, vol. 2, no. 1, pp. 125–134, 2018.
[48] M. K. Nicholas, A. Asghari, and F. M. Blyth, "What do the numbers mean? Normative data in chronic pain measures," *Pain*, vol. 134, no. 1, pp. 158–173, 2008.
[49] National Pain Summit Initiative, *National Pain Strategy: Pain Management for All Australians*, National Pain Summit Initiative, Sydney, NSW, Australia, 2010.
[50] Agency for Clinical Innovation, *Pain Management Network*, Agency for Clinical Innovation, Chatswood, NSW, Australia, 2017, https://www.aci.health.nsw.gov.au/chronic-pain.

24

Which Seems to Be Worst? Pain Severity and Quality of Life between Patients with Lateral Hip Pain and Low Back Pain

Raúl Ferrer-Peña,[1,2,3] **César Calvo-Lobo**,[4] **Ramón Aiguadé**,[5] **and Josué Fernández-Carnero**[6]

[1]*Physical Therapy Department and Motion in Brains Research Group, Instituto de Neurociencias y Ciencias del Movimiento (INCIMOV), Centro Superior de Estudios Universitarios La Salle, Universidad Autónoma de Madrid, Madrid, Spain*
[2]*Centro de Salud Entrevías, Gerencia de Atención Primaria, Servicio Madrileño de Salud, Madrid, Spain*
[3]*Escuela Internacional de Doctorado, Department of Physical Therapy, Occupational Therapy, Rehabilitation and Physical Medicine, Universidad Rey Juan Carlos, Alcorcón, Spain*
[4]*Nursing and Physical Therapy Department, Faculty of Health Sciences, Universidad de León, Ponferrada, León, Spain*
[5]*Departamento de enfermería y fisioterapia, Universitat de Lleida, Lleida, Spain*
[6]*Department of Physical Therapy, Occupational Therapy, Rehabilitation and Physical Medicine, Universidad Rey Juan Carlos, Alcorcón, Spain*

Correspondence should be addressed to César Calvo-Lobo; cecalvo19@hotmail.com and Ramón Aiguadé; raiguade@dif.udl.cat

Academic Editor: Monika I. Hasenbring

Purpose. The aim of this study was to compare the pain severity, health-related quality of life (HRQoL), and risk of continue having pain with prognostic risk scores (PRS), between patients referring greater trochanteric pain syndrome (GTPS) and chronic low back pain (CLBP). *Methods.* A descriptive, cross-sectional design using nonprobability convenience sampling was performed. A total sample of 102 patients were recruited from two primary health-care centers and divided into GTPS (n = 51) and CLBP (n = 51) groups. The primary outcome was pain severity which was assessed with the Spanish version of the Graded Chronic Pain Scale (GCPS). The secondary outcome was the HRQoL which was measured using the Spanish version of EuroQoL Five Dimensions and Five Levels (EQ-5D-5L) as well as the PRS. *Results.* Significant differences ($P<0.05$) were found within both groups in the pain severity global score with a medium effect size showing greater values for the CLBP group with regards to the GTPS group. The PRS in both groups did not show statistical differences ($P>0.05$). Nevertheless, subjects referring CLBP showed greater levels in the PRS than patients with GTPS. Comparing both groups, the HRQoL showed statistical differences ($P<0.05$) in the "pain/discomfort" domain in the CLBP group with respect to the GTPS group, but not in the other domains. *Conclusions.* Patients who suffered from CLBP showed greater pain severity and HRQoL discomfort with regard to patients with GTPS. Despite greater scores for CLBP, the PRS did not seem to be different between both conditions.

1. Introduction

Worldwide, chronic low back pain (CLBP) may be considered as one of the main musculoskeletal conditions, which causes disability for the life years [1]. CLBP is frequently referred to primary care and physical therapy units [2]. Up to 40% of the population will experience CLBP [3]. The CLBP prevalence increased during the last years with older age distributions and may be associated with the increase of psychological factors such as anxiety or depression [4–6]. Pain severity, disability, and health-related quality of life (HRQoL) did not seem to be associated with degenerative radiological modifications of the lumbar spine [7]. The socioeconomic factors may predict the CLBP disability process more than medical-biological characteristics and generate a strong impact in the Spanish primary care [8].

Recently, the greater trochanteric pain syndrome (GTPS) appeared as a common nonosteoarthritic hip condition reported usually in the primary health-care services [9–11]. This syndrome comprised signs and symptoms such as a lateral hip pain history as well as pain on lateral hip palpation, among other factors [9]. The GTPS prevalence reached 20.2% of the patients referred from primary care to a tertiary care orthopedic spine center. This syndrome was more commonly reported in women than in men, and the magnetic resonance imaging was not frequently associated with neurological findings [12]. In Spain, there is a lack of GTPS prevalence studies, and this may be secondary to the differential diagnosis challenge of lateral hip pain [10]. Among the musculoskeletal conditions, the GTPS may interfere with the HRQoL and the pain severity of patients referred from the primary health-care system [13].

Indeed, GTPS comprised patients' substantial proportion referred from primary health care in order to evaluate CLBP. Primary care physicians should be able to stablish an early diagnosis and prognosis in order to reduce costly patient referrals and avoid unnecessary surgery [12, 14]. GTPS and CLBP may reduce HRQoL and increase the pain severity as well as complicate the prognosis of primary care patients [13]. Indeed, CLBP was shown to be the musculoskeletal condition which generated the greater disability adjusted by life years impairing the healthy life expectancy as well as high chronic pain severity and HRQoL impairment [1, 13]. Nevertheless, up to date prior studies have not specifically compared both common conditions with regard to HRQoL, pain severity, and their prognostic risk scores (PRS) in primary care environments. Although chronic musculoskeletal conditions showed a clearly detrimental effect on the HRQL and the burden of musculoskeletal conditions has been compared with other common chronic diseases [13], the comparison of pain severity levels and quality of life between patients groups with CLBP and GTPS needs to be addressed. We hypothesize that patients with CLBP may show a higher pain severity, a greater impairment of HRQoL, and a higher risk of continue having pain with worse PRS than patients who suffer from GTPS. Therefore, the aim of the present study was to compare the pain severity, HRQoL, and risk of continue having pain with PRS measures, between patients referring GTPS and CLBP.

2. Methods

2.1. Study Design. A descriptive, cross-sectional design using nonprobability convenience sampling was performed. All participants were recruited since September 2016 to February 2017 and diagnosed as GTPS or CLBP by the referenced general practitioner from two primary health-care centers in Madrid, Spain, and were derived to the physical therapy unit. All the subjects gave their written informed consents. This study was accepted by the Southeast Local Research Committee of the Primary Health Care Management (Code 16/15). The reporting of the study followed the "STrengthening the Reporting of OBservational studies in Epidemiology" (STROBE) guidelines [15].

2.2. Subjects. The inclusion criteria for the present study were (1) patients referring low back pain [5, 6] or (2) patients with unilateral lateral hip pain [16], (3) tenderness on palpation at the greater trochanter [9], (4) being diagnosed and derived by a general practitioner, and (5) having pain almost until last 3 months before the assessment time.

The exclusion criteria were (1) presence of other musculoskeletal injury, neurological, or systemic condition that could affect balance/gait [16], (2) cognitive impairment or psychiatric disease, or (3) having surgical or traumatic history or corticoid local injection in previous six months.

2.3. Data Collection. A sociodemographic questionnaire containing gender, age, height, weight, civil state, level of education, and pain intensity was self-reported by the study participants.

2.3.1. Primary Outcome

Pain Severity. The pain severity was assessed by means of the Spanish version of the Graded Chronic Pain Scale (GCPS). This scale is a self-reported instrument consisting of two subscales; the first scale evaluates the pain intensity, and the second scale assesses the perceived disability. The scale is formed by a total of 8 items, 7 of them are 11 points as Likert format, and the other item evaluates the perpetuation of pain, asking the number of pain days in the previous 6 months. The Spanish version of the GCPS has proven to be a valid and reliable instrument for assessing the severity of chronic pain. Concretely, high internal consistency (Cronbach's $\alpha = 0.87$) and intraclass correlation coefficient (ICC = 0.81) have been described [17]. The total score of the scale ranges from 0 to 70 points, the chronic pain perpetuation with the first item, and also have a graduation in five levels with its punctuation [18].

2.3.2. Secondary Outcomes

Health-Related Quality of Life (HRQoL). It was measured by the Spanish version of EuroQoL Five Dimensions and Five Levels (EQ-5D-5L). This self-reported questionnaire has been widely used in the literature to report perceived health quality of life in many conditions and translated into 130 languages [19–21]. The instrument consists of two elements, the first one is a 5-item questionnaire, one for each domain assessed (mobility, self-care, usual activities, pain/discomfort, and anxiety/depression), and five levels on each domain (no problems, slight problems, moderate problems, severe problems, and extreme problems). Patients were asked to fill only one level on each domain (1 to 5). The digits on each domain can be combined on a five digit number ranging from 11111 to 55555. Also, the EQ-5D-5L results can be interpreted by the *Sum Score* that it is a severity index obtained with the summation of the levels in each dimension of the instrument, subtracting 5 points and multiplying the result by 5. It results on a 0-to-100 range new scale where more points mean more severity. Another way to interpret the results on the EQ-5D-5L is by means of the Index (*EQ-Index*); this approach compares the values in the five dimensions with 3125 different hypothetic health states adjusted by country population, being the "0" value assigned to death and "1" to the perfect health status. Values less than 0 are considered in the index, being those statuses interpreted as "worse than being dead."

The second part of the questionnaire is a vertical 20 cm Visual Analogue Scale (*EQ-VAS*) in which subjects are asked to self-rate their health, from 0 "The worst health you can Imagine" to 100 "The best health you can imagine." Finally, the Spanish EQ-5D-5L presented minimal floor and ceiling effects (<3%) and a Cronbach's α of 0.86 [22].

Prognostic Risk Score (PRS). The PRS is an instrument to determine the probability of having pain in the next years. This tool is based on the perspective of a chronic pain continuum health status, nor a unique state of the subjects who referred pain during 3 or 6 months (as the conventional definition of chronic pain). It was calculated for each subject with the rules proposed by Von Korff and Miglioretti [23] and used in other studies [24, 25] with the scoring method described in Table 1. The cut-points were also established in low risk, intermediate risk, possible risk over 50%, and probable risk over 80% for the probability of having pain in the next 5 years in primary health-care samples [23]. In addition, a high level of reliability was demonstrated for the classification of people at high risk (over 80% probability) for suffering from clinically significant back pain at follow-up [24, 25].

2.4. Pain Intensity. The average pain intensity in the last seven days was measured by means of a Visual Analogue Scale (VAS). This scale consists of a horizontal 100 mm line, in which the patients must indicate their pain intensity. At the left side of the line appears the text "no pain" and at the right side appears "worst possible pain." This instrument had demonstrated its validity and reliability measuring the pain intensity, showing ICCs among pain scales from 0.65 to 0.88 with a median r of 0.74 [26, 27].

2.5. Sample Size. Sample size was calculated with the G*Power 3.1.9.2 for Mac OS X (G*Power© from University of Düsseldorf, Germany) to determine a sufficient sample size considering a one-tailed t-test with two groups and a medium effect size to achieve clinically relevant differences (d = 0.50) in the primary variable (pain severity) to obtain a statistical power of 80% using an α error of 0.05. Based on the aforementioned assumptions, we estimated a sample size of at least 102 subjects [28].

2.6. Data Analysis. Data analyses were performed on SPSS for Mac OS X, Version 22.0 (SPSS Inc., Chicago IL) with a 95% confidence interval (CI) and considering statistically significant differences if P value < 0.05. Parametric tests were used because the sample size (greater than 30 subjects per group) was sufficient to be supported by the central limit theorem [29]. The continuous variables are presented as mean and standard deviation (SD), and the categorical variables are presented as absolute numbers and relative frequency (i.e., percentages). A Student's t-test for independent samples was used to compare the quantitative outcomes between subjects with GTPS and CLBP, and the chi-square test was used for the categorical ones. Furthermore, the effect sizes of the primary outcomes were calculated based on the following formula $d = 2t/\sqrt{gdl}$, which is determined by the SD of the groups. Cohen's d size effect may be interpreted as slight (d lower than 0.20), fair (d from 0.20 to 0.49), moderate (d from 0.50 a 0.79), or large (d equal or higher than 0.80) [30].

3. Results

3.1. Sociodemographic Characteristics. A total sample of one hundred and two subjects were analyzed in this study and divided into two groups, one group of patients diagnosed of GTPS (n = 51) and another group of patients with CLBP (n = 51). Sociodemographic variables did not show any statistically significant difference ($P > 0.05$) between both groups. Descriptive variables of both groups are presented in Tables 1 and 2.

3.2. Primary Outcome. Regarding Student's t-test, a statistical significant difference ($P < 0.05$) was found between both groups in the pain severity global score with a medium effect size (mean difference = −7.49; CI 95% from −13.35 to −1.62; d = 0.51) showing greater values of the CLBP group with regard to the GTPS group. The results of the comparison for the other quantitative variables are presented in Table 3.

3.3. Secondary Outcomes. The chi-square test comparing the PRS in both groups did not show statistical differences, as presented in Table 4. Nevertheless, subjects referring CLBP showed greater levels in the PRS than patients with GTPS. Levels of both groups with the cutoff points for primary health-care samples are presented in Table 4 and Figure 1.

Moreover, the chi-square test comparing the HRQoL between groups showed statistical differences ($P < 0.05$) in the "pain/discomfort" domain of the CLBP group with respect to the GTPS group, but not in the other domains, as presented in Table 5.

4. Discussion

To the authors' knowledge, this may be considered as the first study comparing both common conditions, CLBP and GTPS. CLBP seemed to show greater pain severity and HRQoL discomfort with respect to GTPS. The prognostic risk seemed to be similar between both musculoskeletal pathologies. Despite this, there is a tendency towards poorer quality of life, higher pain severity, and prognostic risk in the patients who suffer from CLBP with regard to patients who suffer from GTPS. These findings coincide with prior research about musculoskeletal conditions related to quality of life and pain severity [1, 7–9, 12, 13].

TABLE 1: Description of quantitative sociodemographic variables between GTPS and CLBP groups.

	GTPS group (n = 51) Mean ± SD	CLBP group (n = 51) Mean ± SD	P value (Student's t-test)
Age (years)	48.88 ± 8.52	52.43 ± 12.34	0.095
BMI	26.89 ± 5.53	29.03 ± 5.60	0.054
Pain days, last 6 months	119.31 ± 62.21	136.03 ± 53.80	0.330
Pain intensity (VAS)	35.19 ± 23.56	40.10 ± 23.91	0.150
Chronicity (months)	28.52 ± 47.04	58.22 ± 90.44	0.065

GTPS, greater trochanteric pain syndrome; CBLP, chronic low back pain; SD, standard deviation; BMI, body mass index.

TABLE 2: Description of categorical sociodemographic variables between GTPS and CLBP groups.

	GTPS group (n = 51), n (%)	CLBP group (n = 51), n (%)	P value (chi-square test)
Gender			
Male	9 (17.6%)	18 (35.3%)	0.463
Female	42 (82.4%)	33 (64.7%)	
Civil state			
Single	12 (23.5%)	9 (17.6%)	0.218
Married	33 (64.7%)	28 (54.9%)	
Divorced	4 (7.8%)	7 (13.7%)	
Widower	2 (3.9%)	7 (13.7%)	
Education level			
None	0 (0%)	2 (3.9%)	0.347
Primary	15 (29.4%)	19 (37.3%)	
Secondary	18 (35.3%)	17 (33.3%)	
University	18 (35.3%)	13 (25.5%)	

All data are presented as number and percentage (n(%)). GTPS, greater trochanteric pain syndrome; CLBP, chronic low back pain; $^*P < 0.05$.

TABLE 3: Comparison of quantitative result variables between GTPS and CLBP groups.

	GTPS group (n = 51) Mean ± SD	CLBP group (n = 51) Mean ± SD	Mean differences	95% of CI	Effect size (Cohen's d)
EuroQoL-5D value index	0.683 ± 0.200	0.689 ± 0.201	2.02	−6.34 To 10.38	0.03
EuroQoL-5D VAS	66.73 ± 22.96	64.70 ± 19.45	−0.006	−0.085 To 0.072	0.10
EuroQol-5D sum score	23.03 ± 14.56	24.31 ± 14.52	−1.27	−6.98 To 4.43	0.08
GCPS total score	28.11 ± 14.74	35.60 ± 15.11	−7.49	−13.35 To −1.62	0.51*
Prognostic risk score	14.21 ± 5.78	16.47 ± 5.34	−2.25	−4.44 To −0.06	0.42

SD, standard deviation; CI, confident interval; VAS, Visual Analogue Scale; GCPS, Graded Chronic Pain Scale; GTPS, greater trochanteric pain syndrome; CBLP, chronic low back pain; $^*P < 0.05$.

TABLE 4: Description of the prognostic risk score Categories between GTPS and CLBP groups.

Prognostic risk score	GTPS group (n = 51)	CLBP group (n = 51)	P value (chi-square test)
Low risk	7 (13.7%)	2 (3.9%)	0.233
Intermediate risk	21 (41.2%)	18 (35.3%)	
Possible chronic pain (50% risk)	15 (29.4%)	19 (37.3%)	
Probable chronic pain (80% risk)	8 (15.7%)	12 (23.5%)	

GCPS, Graded Chronic Pain Scale; GTPS, greater trochanteric pain syndrome; CBLP, chronic low back pain.

Here, we show a challenge in the differential diagnosis between both conditions which may commonly be considered as comorbidities in patients referred to primary health-care and physical therapy units [2, 12–14]. Therefore, the palpation skills and the clinical reasoning of physicians and physical therapists should be improved in order to diagnose and classify these primary care patients, avoid unnecessary costs, and provide interventions according to the HRQoL discomfort and pain severity [9–11, 13].

4.1. Implications for Clinical Practice. Although both CLBP and GTPS conditions may be focused as main musculoskeletal disorders for treating in primary health-care environments [12, 14], patients who suffer from CLBP need greater primary care attention to reduce pain severity and increase HRQoL with regard to patients who suffer from GTPS. Interventions such as multidisciplinary rehabilitation approaches should be prioritized in this kind of patients who attend to primary health-care units [31].

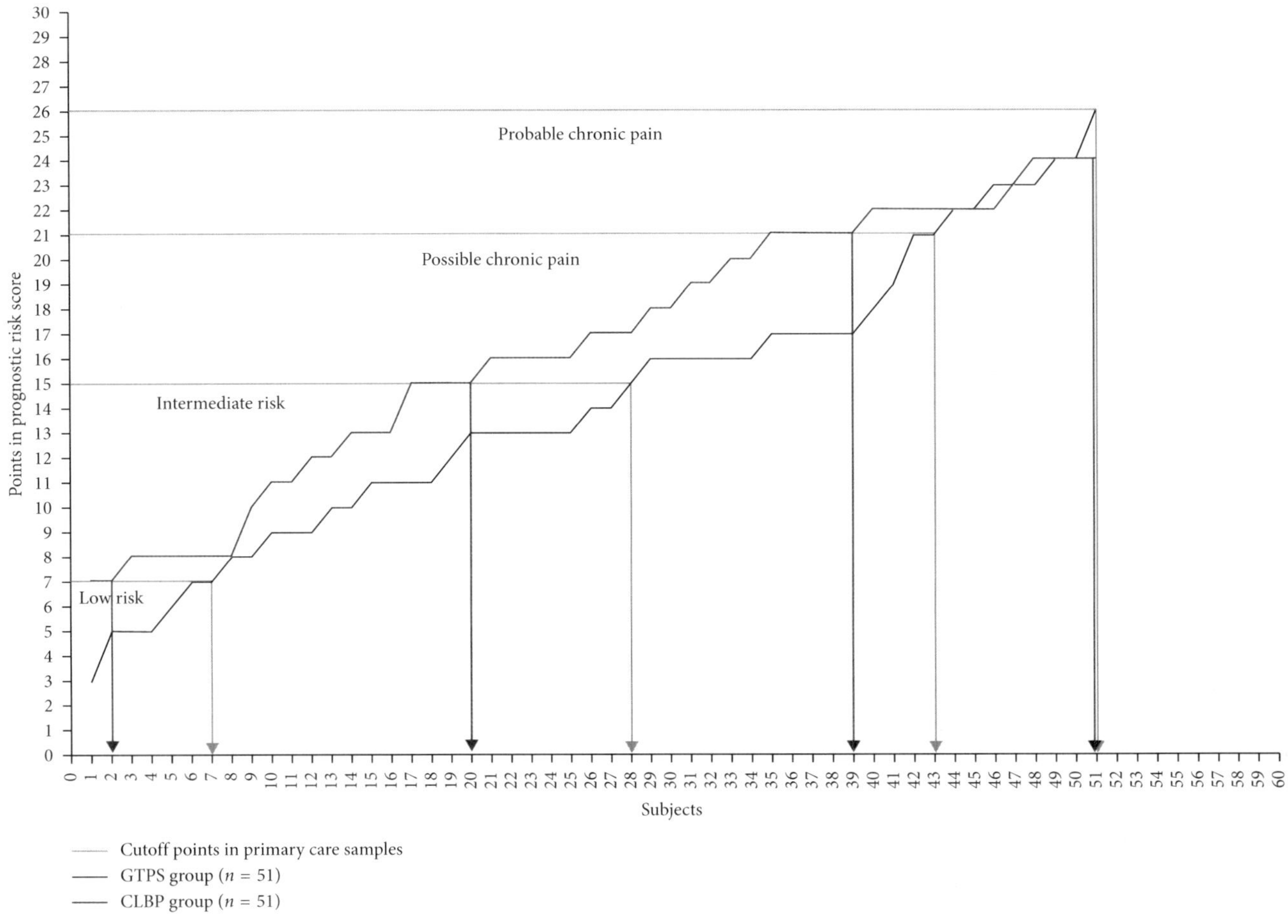

Figure 1: Number of subjects and the relation between GTPS and CLBP patients in PRS. CLBP, chronic low back pain; GTPS, greater trochanteric pain syndrome; PRS, prognostic risk scores.

Table 5: Descriptive data and of five dimensions of EQ-5D and comparison between the GTPS and CLBP groups.

EQ-5D dimension		Groups		*P* value (chi-square test)
		GTPS group (n = 51)	CLBP group (n = 51)	
Mobility	No problem	16 (31.4%)	17 (33.3%)	0.308
	Slight problem	19 (37.3%)	23 (45.1%)	
	Moderate problem	13 (25.5%)	10 (19.6%)	
	Severe problem	3 (5.9%)	0 (0%)	
	Unable to	0 (0%)	1 (2%)	
Self-care	No problem	38 (74.5%)	38 (74.5%)	0.783
	Slight problem	6 (11.8%)	6 (11.8%)	
	Moderate problem	7 (13.7%)	6 (11.8%)	
	Severe problem	0 (0%)	1 (2%)	
	Unable to	0 (0%)	0 (0%)	
Usual activities	No problem	18 (25.3%)	23 (45.1%)	0.436
	Slight problem	23 (45.1%)	15 (29.4%)	
	Moderate problem	9 (17.6%)	12 (23.5%)	
	Severe problem	1 (2%)	1 (2%)	
	Unable to	0 (0%)	0 (0%)	
Pain/discomfort	No problem	4 (7.8%)	1 (2%)	0.024*
	Slight problem	21 (41.2%)	13 (25.5%)	
	Moderate problem	16 (31.4%)	31 (60.8%)	
	Severe problem	10 (19.6%)	6 (11.8%)	
	Unable to	0 (0%)	0 (0%)	

Table 5: Continued.

EQ-5D dimension		Groups		P value (chi-square test)
		GTPS group (n = 51)	CLBP group (n = 51)	
Anxiety/depression	No problem	31 (60.8%)	21 (41.2%)	0.052
	Slight problem	13 (25.5%)	18 (35.3%)	
	Moderate problem	2 (3.9%)	10 (19.6%)	
	Severe problem	3 (5.9%)	1 (2%)	
	Unable to	2 (3.9%)	1 (2%)	

All data are presented as number and percentage (n (%)). EQ-5D, EuroQoL Five Dimensions; GTPS, greater trochanteric pain syndrome; CBLP, chronic low back pain.

4.2. Limitations. Several limitations and methodological aspects should be taken into account regarding the present research. First, physical factors, such as pressure pain thresholds [32], recurrence or physical disability [7], were not assessed. Second, age distributions were not evaluated and may influence psychological aspects [5]. Third, acute and subacute low back pain or GTPS were excluded to include the central sensitization, which commonly occurs in a longer-term process [9, 17, 33]. Although the presence of prior surgeries was an inclusion criterion, former pain experiences of the subjects were not collected and should be considered for future research studies. Finally, individuals from various countries different from Spain and larger sample sizes may be beneficial to reach a study power improvement and find variations among countries [1].

5. Conclusions

Patients who suffered from CLBP showed greater pain severity and HRQoL discomfort with regard to patients with GTPS. Despite greater scores for CLBP, the PRS did not seem to be different between both conditions.

Abbreviations

BMI: Body Mass Index
GCPS: Graded Chronic Pain Scale
EQ-5D: EuroQoL Five Dimensions
GTPS: Greater Trochanteric Pain Syndrome
CBLP: Chronic Low Back Pain
SD: Standard Deviation
CI: Confident Interval
VAS: Visual Analogue Scale.

Ethical Approval

This study was accepted by the Southeast Local Research Committee of the Primary Health Care Management (Code 16/15).

Authors' Contributions

Raúl Ferrer Peña conceived and designed the experiments, performed the experiments, analyzed the data, contributed reagents/materials/analysis tools, wrote the paper, prepared figures and/or tables, and reviewed drafts of the paper. Josué Fernández Carnero, Ramón Aiguadé, and César Calvo Lobo wrote the paper, prepared figures and/or tables, and reviewed drafts of the paper. All authors contributed to the development of concept, design, analyses, interpretation of data, and drafting of the manuscript and revising it critically for important intellectual content. Raúl Ferrer-Peña and César Calvo-Lobo contributed equally to this work.

References

[1] GBD 2013 DALYs and HALE Collaborators CJL, C. J. L. Murray, R. M. Barber et al., "Global, regional, and national disability-adjusted life years (DALYs) for 306 diseases and injuries and healthy life expectancy (HALE) for 188 countries, 1990–2013: quantifying the epidemiological transition," *The Lancet*, vol. 386, no. 10009, pp. 2145–2191, 2015.

[2] J. M. Fritz, J. S. Magel, M. McFadden et al., "Early physical therapy vs usual care in patients with recent-onset low back pain: a randomized clinical trial," *JAMA*, vol. 314, no. 14, pp. 1459–1467, 2015.

[3] P. J. Bennett, C. Patterson, and M. P. Dunne, "Health-related quality of life following podiatric surgery," *Journal of the American Podiatric Medical Association*, vol. 91, no. 4, pp. 164–173, 2001.

[4] D. Palacios-Ceña, C. Alonso-Blanco, V. Hernández-Barrera, P. Carrasco-Garrido, R. Jiménez-García, and C. Fernández-de-las-Peñas, "Prevalence of neck and low back pain in community-dwelling adults in Spain: an updated population-based national study (2009/10–2011/12)," *European Spine Journal*, vol. 24, no. 3, pp. 482–492, 2015.

[5] C. Calvo-Lobo, J. M. Vilar Fernández, R. Becerro-de-Bengoa-Vallejo et al., "Relationship of depression in participants with nonspecific acute or subacute low back pain and no-pain by age distribution," *Journal of Pain Research*, vol. 10, pp. 129–135, 2017.

[6] D. Lopez-Lopez, J. M. Vilar-Fernandez, C. Calvo-Lobo, M. E. Losa-Iglesias, D. Rodriguez-Sanz, and R. Becerro-de-Bengoa-Vallejo, "Evaluation of depression in subacute low back pain: a case control study," *Pain Physician*, vol. 20, no. 4, pp. E499–E505, 2017.

[7] M.-V. Corniola, M. N. Stienen, H. Joswig et al., "Correlation of pain, functional impairment, and health-related quality of life with radiological grading scales of lumbar degenerative

disc disease," *Acta Neurochirurgica*, vol. 158, no. 3, pp. 499–505, 2016.

[8] C. González-Ramírez, J. Montanero-Fernández, and D. Peral-Pacheco, "A multifactorial study on duration of temporary disabilities in Spain," *Archives of Environmental & Occupational Health*, vol. 72, no. 6, pp. 328–335, 2017.

[9] A. M. Fearon, J. M. Scarvell, T. Neeman, J. L. Cook, W. Cormick, and P. N. Smith, "Greater trochanteric pain syndrome: defining the clinical syndrome," *British Journal of Sports Medicine*, vol. 47, no. 10, pp. 649–653, 2013.

[10] J. J. Wilson and M. Furukawa, "Evaluation of the patient with hip pain," *American Family Physician*, vol. 89, no. 1, pp. 27–34, 2014.

[11] A. Brinks, R. M. van Rijn, A. M. Bohnen et al., "Effect of corticosteroid injection for trochanter pain syndrome: design of a randomised clinical trial in general practice," *BMC Musculoskeletal Disorders*, vol. 8, no. 1, p. 95, 2007.

[12] P. J. Tortolani, J. J. Carbone, and L. G. Quartararo, "Greater trochanteric pain syndrome in patients referred to orthopedic spine specialists," *Spine Journal*, vol. 2, no. 4, pp. 251–254, 2002.

[13] F. Salaffi, R. De Angelis, A. Stancati, W. Grassi, MArche Pain, and Prevalence INvestigation Group (MAPPING) study, "Health-related quality of life in multiple musculoskeletal conditions: a cross-sectional population based epidemiological study. II. The MAPPING study," *Clinical and Experimental Rheumatology*, vol. 23, no. 6, pp. 829–839, 2002.

[14] M. Rho, A. Camacho-Soto, A. Cheng et al., "Deconstructing chronic low back pain in the older adult—step by step evidence and expert-based recommendations for evaluation and treatment. Part VIII: lateral hip and thigh pain," *Pain Medicine*, vol. 17, no. 7, pp. 1249–1260, 2016.

[15] E. von Elm, D. G. Altman, M. Egger, S. J. Pocock, P. C. Gøtzsche, and J. P. Vandenbroucke, "The Strengthening the Reporting of Observational Studies in Epidemiology (STROBE) statement: guidelines for reporting observational studies," *Journal of Clinical Epidemiology*, vol. 61, no. 4, pp. 344–349, 2008.

[16] K. Allison, K. L. Bennell, A. Grimaldi, B. Vicenzino, T. V. Wrigley, and P. W. Hodges, "Single leg stance control in individuals with symptomatic gluteal tendinopathy," *Gait and Posture*, vol. 49, pp. 108–113, 2016.

[17] R. Ferrer-Peña, A. Gil-Martínez, J. Pardo-Montero, V. Jiménez-Penick, T. Gallego-Izquierdo, and R. La Touche, "Adaptation and validation of the graded chronic pain scale into Spanish," *Reumatología Clínica*, vol. 12, no. 3, pp. 130–138, 2016.

[18] M. Von Korff, J. Ormel, F. J. Keefe, and S. F. Dworkin, "Grading the severity of chronic pain," *Pain*, vol. 50, no. 2, pp. 133–149, 1992.

[19] M. Herdman, C. Gudex, A. Lloyd et al., "Development and preliminary testing of the new five-level version of EQ-5D (EQ-5D-5L)," *Quality of Life Research*, vol. 20, no. 10, pp. 1727–1736, 2011.

[20] M. Obradovic, A. Lal, and H. Liedgens, "Validity and responsiveness of EuroQol-5 dimension (EQ-5D) versus Short Form-6 dimension (SF-6D) questionnaire in chronic pain," *Health and Quality of Life Outcomes*, vol. 11, no. 1, p. 110, 2013.

[21] M. Oppe, N. J. Devlin, B. van Hout, P. F. M. Krabbe, and F. de Charro, "A program of methodological research to arrive at the new international EQ-5D-5L valuation protocol," *Value Health*, vol. 17, no. 4, pp. 445–453, 2014.

[22] A. Bilbao, L. García-Pérez, J. C. Arenaza et al., "Psychometric properties of the EQ-5D-5L in patients with hip or knee osteoarthritis: reliability, validity and responsiveness," *Quality of Life Research*, pp. 1–12, 2018, In press.

[23] M. Von Korff and D. L. Miglioretti, "A prognostic approach to defining chronic pain," *Pain*, vol. 117, no. 3, pp. 304–313, 2005.

[24] K. M. Dunn, P. R. Croft, C. J. Main, and M. Von Korff, "A prognostic approach to defining chronic pain: replication in a UK primary care low back pain population," *Pain*, vol. 135, no. 1-2, pp. 48–54, 2008.

[25] S. Muller, E. Thomas, K. M. Dunn, and C. D. Mallen, "A prognostic approach to defining chronic pain across a range of musculoskeletal pain sites," *Clinical Journal of Pain*, vol. 29, no. 5, pp. 411–416, 2013.

[26] M. P. Jensen, J. A. Turner, J. M. Romano, and L. D. Fisher, "Comparative reliability and validity of chronic pain intensity measures," *Pain*, vol. 83, no. 2, pp. 157–162, 1999.

[27] M. P. Jensen, P. Karoly, and S. Braver, "The measurement of clinical pain intensity: a comparison of six methods," *Pain*, vol. 27, no. 1, pp. 117–126, 1986.

[28] F. Faul, E. Erdfelder, A.-G. Lang, and A. G. Buchner, "∗Power 3: a flexible statistical power analysis program for the social, behavioral, and biomedical sciences," *Behavior Research Methods*, vol. 39, no. 2, pp. 175–191, 2007.

[29] N. Hazut, S. Medalion, D. A. Kessler, and E. Barkai, "Fractional Edgeworth expansion: corrections to the Gaussian-Lévy central-limit theorem," *Physical Review E*, vol. 91, no. 5, article 052124, 2015.

[30] J. Cohen, "A power primer," *Psychological Bulletin*, vol. 112, no. 1, pp. 155–159, 1992.

[31] K. F. Stein and A. Miclescu, "Effectiveness of multidisciplinary rehabilitation treatment for patients with chronic pain in a primary health care unit," *Scandinavian Journal of Pain*, vol. 4, no. 4, pp. 190–197, 2013.

[32] T. K. Koo, J. Guo, and C. M. Brown, "Test-retest reliability, repeatability, and sensitivity of an automated deformation-controlled indentation on pressure pain threshold measurement," *Journal of Manipulative and Physiological Therapeutics*, vol. 36, no. 2, pp. 84–90, 2013.

[33] J. Nijs, A. Apeldoorn, H. Hallegraeff et al., "Low back pain: guidelines for the clinical classification of predominant neuropathic, nociceptive, or central sensitization pain," *Pain Physician*, vol. 18, no. 3, pp. E333–E346, 2015.

The Effect of Anterior Uterocervical Angle on Primary Dysmenorrhea and Disease Severity

Mefkure Eraslan Sahin,[1] Erdem Sahin,[1] Yusuf Madendag,[2] Ilknur Col Madendag,[3] Ahter Tanay Tayyar,[4] Fatma Özdemir,[2] Gokhan Acmaz,[2] and Iptisam Ipek Muderris[2]

[1]*Department of Obstetrics and Gynecology, Health Sciences University Sivas Sarkışla Government Hospital, Sivas, Turkey*
[2]*Department of Obstetrics and Gynecology, Erciyes University Medicine Faculty, Kayseri, Turkey*
[3]*Department of Obstetrics and Gynecology, Health Sciences University Kayseri Education and Research Hospital, Kayseri, Turkey*
[4]*Department of Obstetrics and Gynecology, Acibadem Maslak Hospital, Istanbul, Turkey*

Correspondence should be addressed to Mefkure Eraslan Sahin; mefkureee@hotmail.com

Academic Editor: Jacob Ablin

Background. Primary dysmenorrhea, defined as painful menstrual cramps originating in the uterus without underlying pathology, is a gynecological disease that affects quality of life and school success. Our goal was to determine the effect of anterior uterocervical angle on primary dysmenorrhea and disease severity. *Methods.* A total of 200 virgin adolescents, 16 to 20 years of age, were included in the study. The Andersch and Milsom scale was used to determine dysmenorrhea severity. Those with pathologies causing secondary dysmenorrhea were excluded from the study. Study subjects were grouped based on severity of pain. Demographic characteristics and uterocervical ultrasonographic measurements were compared among groups. *Results.* Of the 200 participants enrolled in the study, 50 were healthy controls and 150 had primary dysmenorrhea. Those with primary dysmenorrhea had a significant family history of primary dysmenorrhea compared with controls ($P < 0.001$). Age ($P = 0.668$), body mass index ($P = 0.898$), menarche age ($P = 0.915$), and length of menstrual cycles ($P = 0.740$) were similar in all groups. The uterine corpus longitudinal axis, uterine corpus transverse axis, and uterine cervix longitudinal axis were also similar ($P = 0.359$, $P = 0.279$, and $P = 0.369$, resp.). The mean uterocervical angle was 146.8 ± 6.0 in controls and 143.3 ± 7.3 in those with mild pain with no significant difference between the groups. In those with moderate pain, the mean uterocervical angle was 121.2 ± 7.3 compared with 101 ± 9.2 in those with severe pain, which was a significant difference. Additionally, there was also a significant difference in the uterocervical angle among those with mild, moderate, and severe pain ($P < 0.001$). *Conclusion.* Our results indicate that a narrower anterior uterocervical angle is associated with primary dysmenorrhea and disease severity.

1. Introduction

Primary dysmenorrhea (PD), often seen in adolescent girls and women during the reproductive period, is defined as painful menstrual cramps originating from the uterus without underlying pathology. It is a gynecological disease that affects quality of life and school success [1, 2]. PD is characterized by suprapubic pain that starts several hours before menstrual bleeding and lasts a few hours after the culmination of bleeding. Symptoms peak with maximum blood flow and continue for two to three days [3].

The underlying cause of PD is not yet fully understood; however, several factors are known to play a role in the etiopathogenesis. One such factor is increased intrauterine pressure. In women without dysmenorrhea during menstrual bleeding, the basal uterine tonus is below 10 mmHg, and there are three to four rhythmic synchronized contractions every 10 minutes. However, in women with PD, the basal uterine tonus exceeds 10 mmHg, and every 10 minutes, there are four to five contractions without rhythm and coordination. Pressure during contractions can reach 150 to 180 mmHg [4]. When the uterine pressure exceeds the systemic arterial pressure, anaerobic metabolites are released due to ischemia and these metabolites stimulate nerve fibers leading to dysmenorrhea [5].

The uterocervical angle (UCA), which is between the cervical canal and the uterus frontal wall, is a newly investigated ultrasonographic parameter. In the literature, it has been stated that ultrasonographically measured cervical length and UCA can determine the clinical function of the cervix. Recently, Dziadosz et al. reported that in the presence of a large UCA, uterine contents are directly and more easily displaced to the cervix [6]. In another study, Zebitay et al. reported that cervical length and uterine cervical volume were significantly associated with PD in virgin adolescent girls [7].

Menstrual pain which is associated with PD augments during maximum blood flow and uterine pressure increases exceeding the systemic arterial pressure. This process is associated with the length of the cervix, thus it is possible to assume that the pain occurs with the difficult excretion of endometrial tissues. The hypothesis is that if one considers that the excretion of endometrial tissues becomes more difficult, then the UCA is narrow. The presence of a narrow UCA may lead to PD. This study aimed at determining the effect of anterior UCA on PD and disease severity.

2. Materials and Methods

This study was conducted at Sivas Sarkisla Government Hospital in Turkey. The study was approved by the Ethics Committee of Cumhuriyet University (decision number: 2018-01/12) according to the Declaration of Helsinki. Study participants included virgin adolescents aged 16 to 20 years who were referred to the gynecology clinic for complaints of dysmenorrhea.

The Andersch and Milsom scale was used to determine dysmenorrhea severity. Study participants were questioned concerning each of the three categories: work activity, systemic symptoms, and need for analgesics [1, 8, 9]. They were then divided into four groups based upon their level of reported pain as follows: (1) control group, menstruation is not painful and daily activity is unaffected; (2) mild pain group, menstruation is painful but seldom inhibits normal activity, analgesics are seldom required; (3) moderate pain group, daily activity is affected, analgesics are required and give relief so that absence from work or school is unusual; and (4) severe pain group, activity is clearly inhibited, poor effect of analgesics, vegetative symptoms, and severe pain exists.

Patients were excluded from the study if pathologies causing secondary dysmenorrhea existed, including: fibroids, adnexal masses (abscess, ovarian cyst, and hydrosalpinx), gynecological operation history, pelvic inflammatory disease history, presence of urinary or other infections, uterine anomaly, oral contraceptive use, alcohol and cigarette use, or nonsteroidal anti-inflammatory drug use in the last two days.

The longitudinal and transverse axis of the uterine cervix and uterine corpus were measured after ablation by abdominal ultrasonography. Measurements were performed on the midsagittal plane by the same specialized person (MES). The uterine cervical longitudinal axis was measured when at least three of the following five recognition points on the plane were clearly visible: (1) the external cervical os, (2) the internal cervical os, (3) the cervical canal, (4) the cervical/vaginal interface, and (5) the cervical corpus [10]. When the length between the internal and external cervical os could not be measured on a flat plane due to the curvature of the cervical canal, the longitudinal diameter of the uterine cervix was measured as the sum of the possible linear measures taken in part. The longitudinal axis of the uterine corpus was measured on a longitudinal plane extending from the projection point of the endometrium on the uterine corpus to the internal cervical os where the internal cervical os and endometrium were visible the longest. The transverse axis of the uterine corpus was measured on the same plane perpendicular to the uterine corpus longitudinal axis where the uterine corpus was widest. The UCA was defined as the line drawn from the internal os to the external os and the angle formed by the second line passing through the internal cervical os parallel to the lower side of the anterior uterine wall in the internal os [11]. All measurements were performed on the second or third day of the menstrual cycle, and in order to minimalize intra and interobserver variabilities, all measurements were performed by a single sonographer (MES) using the same ultrasonography device (Mindray DC-7 Ultrasound System, China) and a 3.5 MHz abdominal probe (Figure 1).

To determine the number of patients evaluated in our study, we referenced the study conducted by Zebitay et al., entitled "Importance of cervical length in dysmenorrhea etiology" [7]. The Minitab®16 statistical program (Minitab Inc., State College, PA, USA) was used to perform the statistical analysis. The Shapiro–Wilk test was used to assess normality of the data, and Levene's test was used to assess for homogeneity of variances. Values are expressed as mean ± standard deviation. Parametric comparisons were made via a t-test or z-test, and nonparametric comparisons were made via a Mann–Whitney U test. A P value <0.05 was considered statistically significant.

3. Results

Of the 200 virgin adolescents enrolled in the study, 50 were healthy controls and 150 had PD. Demographic characteristics were compared and are shown in Table 1. Age ($P = 0.668$), body mass index ($P = 0.898$), menarche age ($P = 0.915$), and length of menstrual cycles ($P = 0.740$) were similar in all groups. Patients with PD had a significant family history of PD compared with controls ($P < 0.001$).

Table 2 displays a comparison of ultrasonographic measurements among the groups. The uterine corpus longitudinal axis, uterine corpus transverse axis, and uterine cervix longitudinal axis were similar in both control and PD subjects ($P = 0.359$, $P = 0.279$, and $P = 0.369$, resp.). The mean UCA was 146.8 ± 6.0 in control subjects and 143.3 ± 7.3 in those with mild pain, which was not significantly different. The mean UCA was 121.2 ± 7.3 in those with moderate pain and 101.9 ± 9.2 in those with severe pain, which was significantly different. Additionally, UCA was significantly different among those with mild, moderate, and severe pain ($P < 0.001$).

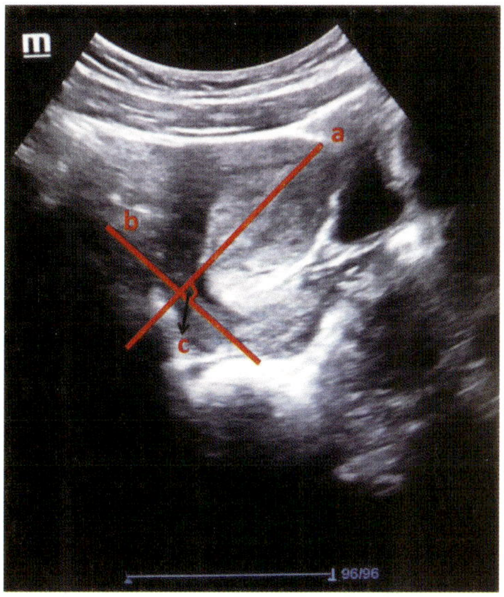

Figure 1: Ultrasonography measurements. (a) Uterine corpus longitudinal axis. (b) Uterine cervix longitudinal axis. (c) Anterior uterocervical angle.

Table 1: Comparison of demographic characteristics among groups.

	Group 1, control $n = 50$	Group 2, mild pain $n = 50$	Group 3, moderate pain $n = 50$	Group 4, severe pain $n = 50$	P value
Age (years)	17.60 ± 1.21^a	17.50 ± 1.28^a	17.68 ± 1.09^a	17.42 ± 0.97^a	0.668
BMI (kg/m^2)	22.68 ± 1.22^a	22.66 ± 1.14^a	22.49 ± 1.07^a	22.52 ± 1.05^a	0.898
Menarche age (years)	12.74 ± 0.80^a	12.82 ± 0.87^a	12.78 ± 0.84^a	12.68 ± 0.99^a	0.915
Length of menstrual cycles (days)	28.22 ± 1.23^a	28.40 ± 1.06^a	28.34 ± 0.79^a	28.42 ± 0.75^a	0.740
Family history of PD n (%)	3 (6%)^a	21 (42%)^b	18 (36%)^b	24 (48%)^b	0 < 001

Note. BMI, body mass index; PD, primary dysmenorrhea. Superscript numbers indicate the absence (a) or presence (b) of statistically significant differences. The Minitab®16 statistical program (Minitab Inc., State College, PA, USA) was used to perform the statistical analysis. The Shapiro–Wilk test was used for normality assumption of the data, and Levene's test was used for the variance homogeneity assumption. Values are expressed as mean ± standard deviation. Parametric comparisons were made via t-test or z-test, and nonparametric comparisons were made via Mann–Whitney U tests. $P < 0.05$ was considered statistically significant.

Table 2: Comparison of ultrasonographic measurements among groups.

	Group 1, control $n = 50$	Group 2, mild pain $n = 50$	Group 3, moderate pain $n = 50$	Group 4, severe pain $n = 50$	P value
Uterine corpus longitudinal axis (mm)	45.60 ± 4.78^a	44.76 ± 2.75^a	46.08 ± 4.77^a	45.94 ± 3.41^a	0.359
Uterine corpus transverse axis (mm)	33.02 ± 2.41^a	33.32 ± 2.18^a	32.46 ± 2.13^a	32.82 ± 2.25^a	0.279
Uterine cervix longitudinal axis (mm)	31.94 ± 2.04^a	32.10 ± 1.60^a	31.66 ± 1.90^a	32.46 ± 1.34^a	0.369
Anterior uterocervical angle	146.8 ± 6.0^a	143.3 ± 7.3^a	121.2 ± 7.3^b	101.9 ± 9.2^c	0 < 001

Note. BMI, body mass index; PD, primary dysmenorrhea. Superscript numbers indicate the absence (a) or presence (b,c) of statistically significant differences. The Minitab®16 statistical program (Minitab Inc., State College, PA, USA) was used to perform the statistical analysis. The Shapiro–Wilk test was used to evaluate the normality assumption of the data and Levene's test was used to assess the variance homogeneity assumption. Values are expressed as mean ± standard deviation. Parametric comparisons were made via t-test or z-test, and nonparametric comparisons were made via Mann–Whitney U test. $P < 0.05$ was considered statistically significant.

4. Discussion

In the present study we aimed at determining the effect of anterior UCA on PD and disease severity. According to our findings, UCA was significantly narrower in patients with PD compared with those without, and lower UCA correlated with severity of disease. UCA seems to be an important anatomical factor in PD etiopathogenesis.

There is evidence in the literature that vasoconstriction-induced hypoxia has a role in the underlying pathogenesis of

PD but the cause is not fully understood [7]. Numerous studies have focused on disease treatment but only one assessed the association of uterine and cervical anatomy with PD. In a study by Zebitay et al., they reported that the length of cervical longitudinal and transverse axis and uterine cervical volume significantly correlated with severity of PD [7]. In the present study, we did not find significant differences in the uterine corpus longitudinal axis, uterine corpus transverse axis, and uterine cervix longitudinal axis among the groups.

In the current study, we did find that narrower UCA is associated with PD and disease severity. Because the material in the uterine cavity will pass through a narrower structure than itself during the ejection of menstrual blood from the uterine cavity, the uterus is in need of a propulsive force due to the resistance that occurs in the form of friction. A narrower UCA will certainly increase this resistance. The relationship between this propulsive force and resistance can be explained by the Navier–Stokes equation, which is the basic motion equation for a viscous fluid, considering the unit volume of fluid, mass conversion, Newton's second law, energy conversion, and the second law of thermodynamics [7, 12]. In cases with a narrower UCA, an increase in uterine contractility may occur to overcome the greater frictional force present during the passage of blood. Parallel to the increased contraction, the UCA will produce a more intense pain sensation. This explains the significant correlation of UCA with pain severity in patients with dysmenorrhea.

In addition, in a prospective observational study over eight years, Juang et al. reported that both gestation length and type of delivery had an effect on PD. The most important improvement occurs after the first delivery. In addition, spontaneous vaginal delivery has the advantage of reducing the severity of dysmenorrhea compared with cesarean birth [13]. Although more prospective studies are needed, it can be assumed that the first birth reduces the severity of dysmenorrhea by changing the UCA and reducing resistance in the cervical canal. Other studies reported that the severity of dysmenorrhea was reduced by cervical dilatation in a recursive manner with artificial methods [4] and hot pad application [14]. The benefits of cervical dilatation in these studies have been explained by the reduction of resistance to cervical excretion due to the formation of a wider cervical canal after dilatation. This helps to reduce the severity of dysmenorrhea due to the reduction of friction and resistance, which decreases prostaglandin release and reduces uterine pressure [4]. These reports clearly show that the anatomy of the cervix is related to the severity of PD and disease. As such, they support the findings of our study.

However, there are some limitations in this study. Measurements were made with empty bladders to maintain normal anatomic position, which increased the difficulty of obtaining measurements.

5. Conclusion

The present study showed that a narrower anterior UCA is associated with PD and disease severity. Further prospective studies with a greater number of patients are required to further substantiate these results.

References

[1] M. I. Tomás-Rodríguez, A. Palazón-Bru, D. R. Martínez-St John, F. Navarro-Cremades, J. V. Toledo-Marhuenda, and V. F. Gil-Guillén, "Factors associated with increased pain in primary dysmenorrhea: analysis using a multivariate ordered logistic regression model," *Journal of Pediatric and Adolescent Gynecology*, vol. 30, no. 2, pp. 199–202, 2017.

[2] M. I. Ortiz, "Primary dysmenorrhea among Mexican university students: prevalence, impact and treatment," *European Journal of Obstetrics and Gynecology and Reproductive Biology*, vol. 152, no. 1, pp. 73–77, 2010.

[3] M. Burnett and M. Lemyre, "No. 345-primary dysmenorrhea consensus guideline," *Journal of Obstetrics and Gynaecology Canada*, vol. 39, no. 7, pp. 585–595, 2017.

[4] M. Y. Dawood, "Primary dysmenorrhea: advances in pathogenesis and management," *Obstetrics and Gynecology*, vol. 108, no. 2, pp. 428–441, 2006.

[5] S. Altunyurt, M. Göl, O. Sezer, and N. Demir, "Primary dysmenorrhea and uterine blood flow: a color Doppler study," *Journal of reproductive medicine*, vol. 50, no. 4, pp. 251–255, 2005.

[6] M. Dziadosz, T. A. Bennett, C. Dolin et al., "Uterocervical angle: a novel ultrasound screening tool to predict spontaneous preterm birth," *American Journal of Obstetrics and Gynecology*, vol. 215, no. 3, pp. 376.e1–376.e7, 2016.

[7] A. G. Zebitay, F. F. Verit, M. N. Sakar, S. Keskin, O. Cetin, and A. I. Ulusoy, "Importance of cervical length in dysmenorrhoea aetiology," *Journal of Obstetrics and Gynaecology*, vol. 36, no. 4, pp. 540–543, 2016.

[8] A. E. Ambresin, R. E. Belanger, C. Chamay, A. Berchtold, and F. Narring, "Body dissatisfaction on top of depressive mood among adolescents with severe dysmenorrhea," *Journal of Pediatric and Adolescent Gynecology*, vol. 25, no. 1, pp. 19–22, 2012.

[9] N. Ozerdogan, D. Sayiner, U. Ayranci, A. Unsal, and S. Giray, "Prevalence and predictors of dysmenorrhea among students at a university in Turkey," *International Journal of Gynecology and Obstetrics*, vol. 107, no. 1, pp. 39–43, 2009.

[10] L. L. Saul, J. T. Kurtzman, C. Hagemann, M. Ghamsary, and D. A. Wing, "Is transabdominal sonography of the cervix after voiding a reliable method of cervical length assessment?," *Journal of Ultrasound in Medicine*, vol. 27, no. 9, pp. 1305–1311, 2008.

[11] J. C. Knight, E. TenBrink, J. Sheng, and A. S. Patil, "Anterior uterocervical angle measurement improves prediction of cerclage failure," *Journal of Perinatology*, vol. 37, no. 4, pp. 375–379, 2017.

[12] M. L. Chavez and C. J. DeKorte, "Valdecoxib: a review," *Clinical Therapeutics*, vol. 25, no. 3, pp. 817–851, 2003.

[13] C. M. Juang, M. S. Yen, N. F. Twu, H. C. Horng, H. C. Yu, and C. Y. Chen, "Impact of pregnancy on primary dysmenorrhea," *International Journal of Gynaecology and Obstetrics*, vol. 92, no. 3, pp. 221–227, 2006.

[14] M. Akin, W. Price, G. Rodriguez Jr., G. Erasala, G. Hurley, and R. P. Smith, "Continuous, low-level, topical heat wrap therapy as compared to acetaminophen for primary dysmenorrhea," *Journal of Reproductive Medicine*, vol. 49, no. 9, pp. 739–745, 2004.

Evaluation of C-Reactive Protein Level in Patients with Pain Form of Temporomandibular Joint Dysfunction

Malgorzata Pihut,[1] Piotr Ceranowicz,[2] and Andrzej Gala[1]

[1]*Prosthodontics Department, Consulting Room of Temporomandibular Joint Dysfunction, Jagiellonian University Medical Collage, 4 Montelupich Str., 31-155 Krakow, Poland*
[2]*Department of Physiology, Faculty of Clinical Physiology, Jagiellonian University Medical College, 16 Grzegorzecka Str., 31-531 Krakow, Poland*

Correspondence should be addressed to Andrzej Gala; galamed@wp.pl

Academic Editor: Klaus Boening

Temporomandibular joint dysfunction is a functional disorder concerned with the abnormal functioning of the muscles of the stomatognathic system and temporomandibular joints involved in the dynamic movements of the jaw and surrounding structures. The aim of the study was to compare the level of C-reactive protein in patients with pain and painless forms of temporomandibular joint dysfunction. *Materials and methods*. The study group consisted of 72 patients who reported to the prosthetic treatment because of temporomandibular joint dysfunction. The study group included 36 patients with pain form of dysfunction, and the control group included 36 patients with painless form of disorder. Each patient underwent specialized examination of functional disorders in order to diagnose the type of dysfunction and was commissioned to carry out a study of the blood test concerned with evaluation of the C-reactive protein (CRP) level in the same analytical laboratory. The results of the investigation were subjected to statistical analysis. The research obtained approval from the Ethics Committee of the Jagiellonian University (KBET/125/L/2013). Level of Evidence for primary research was established as type V. *Results*. The mean values of C-reactive protein levels in both groups were in the normal range and did not differ statistically significantly, which indicates the fact that the pain form of the temporomandibular joint disorders is not associated with inflammation of the soft tissues of the joint. *Conclusion*. Painful form of the temporomandibular joint dysfunctions is not connected with the inflammation of joints.

1. Introduction

Temporomandibular joint dysfunction includes dysfunction of the masticatory muscles of the stomatognathic system and temporomandibular joints and the surrounding structures. They are often associated with abnormal conditions of occlusion. Functional disorders do not include all disorders associated with musculoskeletal organs including inflammatory, degenerative arthritis, and cancer lesions of the muscles (multiple sclerosis, tetany, and dermatomyositis). They are often the result of muscles undergoing prolonged and excessive work and nonphysiological loads occurring in the stomatognathic system [1–4].

The pain form of the disease is manifested by spontaneous pain in the preaural region, accompanied by pain or tenderness of the masseter muscle. Pain that appears during palpation examination of temporomandibular joints is frequently not related to inflammation of the soft tissue around the temporomandibular joints, as it is claimed by several authors [1, 3, 5–9]. The cause of this problem is a long-term overload of the soft tissue causally associated with excessive muscle tension, that sometimes even persists for years [1–4, 6, 9].

C-reactive protein (CPR) was first isolated in the blood serum in 1930 by Tillet and Francis in a bacteriological laboratory in the Rockefeller Institute in New York. Long years of research on the protein allowed for its assessment in a clinical setting. CRP is synthesized primarily by hepatocytes and the Kupffer and Browicz cells and is a cyclic pentamer with a molecular mass of 120 kDa. Its expression was also found in monocytes and lymphocytes. Each of the subunits of the protein is composed of 206 amino acids noncovalently linked together [10–12]. Each amino acid has a single disulfide bridge formed by cysteines at positions 37 and 78. Among the modifying agents of CRP concentration are cytokines and interleukins 1 and 6. The mechanism of stimulation of the biosynthesis of CRP is still not fully understood. CRP is present in healthy individuals in an amount of 0–5 mg/l. There is no evidence of differences of this marker that depends on gender. Currently, it is recognized as an important marker of ongoing inflammation and cancer reaction in the body and one of the major proteins of the acute phase. Its concentration may be increased even thousand-fold within 48 hours of the onset of inflammation. CRP is used as one of the markers of choice in monitoring the acute phase response because the markers increase to a relatively high concentration compared to basal concentration [13–16].

Marking of C-reactive protein concentration is based on the immune reaction of monovalent antibodies against CRP using the methods of radial immunodiffusion, immunoelectrophoresis, immunonephelometry, radioimmunoassay, and enzyme immunoassay. In recent years, the methods are immunoblotting, ELISA assays, and techniques of modern molecular biology [12, 14].

The aim of the study was to evaluate the level of C-reactive protein in patients treated for the pain form of temporomandibular joint dysfunction.

2. Materials and Methods

The study enrolled a group of 72 patients, aged 21 to 48 years, of both sexes, who reported to the prosthodontic treatment in the Consulting Room of Temporomandibular Joint Dysfunction at the Dental Institute at the Jagiellonian University in Cracow, between January 2015 and February 2017, due to the pain and painless forms of the temporomandibular joint dysfunction, and acoustic symptoms, accompanied by excessive tension of the masticatory muscles. Symptoms persisted from 3 to 12 months prior to the beginning of the treatment. All patients were subjected to a specialist functional examination of the masticatory organ using typical procedures: information of spontaneous and provoked ailments, muscles and temporomandibular jaw palpation, functional manipulation, assessment of ranges of mandibular movements, joints' sounds, and dental rating. Patients were consecutively and alternately assigned to the study and control groups, 36 patients in each. The study group consisted of pain form of temporomandibular joint dysfunction and the control group included painless form of this dysfunction.

During the study, we analyzed information concerned with general health and present complaints, and a functional examination of the stomatognathic system was conducted, with particular regard to the nature and intensity of the perceived pain and discomfort of temporomandibular joints and masticatory muscles, which occurred prior to treatment and radiation of pain, the type of sound symptoms (clicks), volume, and the phase of the movement of lowering and lifting the jaw, during which there were tension-type headache and back pain (Table 1). Examination was conducted once.

Functional assessment of the masticatory apparatus and muscles consists of a medical interview and a physical examination. Another important element of a medical interview was to evaluate the patient's posture, facial expression, and the general well-being after the patient enters the surgery. Through a medical interview, detailed information about the current general health condition was revealed (including information about chronic and hereditary diseases); the examining physician obtained information about the patient's surgical treatment and head trauma history within the last 6–8 months and the current medications being taken on daily basis. In this context, particular attention was given to muscle and joint conditions, with a focus on multiple sclerosis, osteoporosis, fibromyalgia, trigeminal neuralgia, hormonal disorders, and autoimmune diseases.

Physical examination started with a facial symmetry test; the oral cavity was examined for the dental and periodontal status and the condition of oral mucosa. If the patient had any missing teeth, the number and location of existing natural teeth in the occlusion support zones were investigated. Dental classification (according to Eichner index or Galasińska–Landsberger classification) was recorded in the patient's medical file. Dental prosthetic restorations, if present, were examined in terms of their clinical value.

A clinical examination of temporomandibular joint consists of palpation and auscultation; palpation was performed simultaneously on both sides of the face by exerting a force of around 400 g per square centimeter. Auscultation was performed with the aid of a double-tube stethoscope. The individual palpation force was measured using an electronic kitchen scale [1, 3, 17, 18].

Factors of inclusion in the study were pain form of temporomandibular joint dysfunction, the required age range, and a good general state of health (particularly with regard to cardiac and metabolic disorders). Good general state of the patients' health means that patients did not suffer from the medical conditions that could have an influence on the level of CRP.

Factors for exclusion from the research included the will (consent) of the patient, the presence of general diseases, traumas, or local inflammations.

All respondents were directed to one external medical analysis laboratory to determine the level of C-reactive protein in the blood serum. For this purpose, the immunoturbidimetric assay was performed for the in vitro quantitative determination of CRP in human serum and plasma using Roche/Hitachi cobas c systems. It was also assumed that the correct level of this marker in patients who show no evidence of inflammation taking account of the above method is 0 to 5 mg/l [12, 14]. All patients underwent ultrasound examination of the temporomandibular joints.

In case of the measure giving the constant results, statistical analysis was based on the traditional methods of calculation: mean values, standard deviation, minimal values, maximal values, standard error of the mean, variance analysis for dependent variables, and post hoc Tukey test for dependent variables being the statistical significance measure.

To compare the dependencies between the results obtained in consecutive clinical tests, the nonparametric

Table 1: A summary of symptoms obtained during functional examination of stomatognathic system conducted in both groups.

Symptoms of temporomandibular joint disorders			Group I		Group II	
			W	M	W	M
Intrinsic pain	Single TMJ	Acute	14	6	0	0
		Dull	6	3	0	0
	Bilaterally	Acute	8	5	0	0
		Dull	1	2	0	0
Mastication pain or/pain presence during lower jaw movements			28	14	0	0
Pain of the TMJs triggered by palpation			20	13	0	0
Pain associated with lower jaw movements			28	17	0	0
Masticatory muscle pain			20	5	0	0
Radiation of pain			8	5	0	0
Sounds, snaps in TMJs	Single TMJ	R	9	1	8	3
		L	2	2	3	1
	Bilaterally	R	4	2	2	3
		L	4	2	2	3
Subjective feeling of increased tension in muscles			22	7	24	6
Constricted opening of the lower jaw			4	1	3	0
Constricted lateral mandibular movements			2	1	3	1
Mandibular deviation during opening			15	5	16	2
Difficulty in chewing			15	14	14	2
Occlusion parafunctions			20	8	21	5
"Closed ear" symptom on the affected TMJ side			2	2	4	2
Sudden hearing impairment			1	0	2	1
Tinnitus			2	0	1	1

Friedman test, Kendall's W, and Wilcoxon signed-rank test (comparing two related samples) were used. For statistical studies, special computer software STATISTICA 2010 was used. A p value less than 0.05 was accepted as statistically significant. The research obtained approval from the Ethics Committee of the Jagiellonian University (KBET/125/L/2013). Clinical Trial Gov. Identifier was registered as well: NCT03065608.

Level of Evidence for primary research was established as type V.

3. Results and Discussion

The study involved 72 patients, ranging from 21 to 48 years, divided into two groups of 36 people. Group I included 24 women and 12 men (mean age 29), and group II control included 27 women and 8 men (mean age 31). Analysis of the results of clinical examinations conducted in both groups show a homogeneous clinical material (sound symptoms in the temporomandibular joint, range of motion of the jaw, abnormal range and symmetry of movement of the jaw, and difficulty in chewing foods) with the exception of pain, which is a factor differentiating patients between group I and II. The results of the clinical examination (symptoms indicating the occurrence of functional disorders) are summarized in Table 1.

In group I, the mean level of CRP was 2.54, the extreme values were 5.9–0.14, median was 2.15, and the standard deviation was 1.54. In group II, the average value of C-reactive protein was 2.69 (peak of 5.2–0.7), median was 2.4, and the standard deviation was 1.87. Average values of amounts of CRP did not significantly differ statistically, since $p > 0.05$. The results of the statistical calculations are graphically depicted in Figures 1 and 2.

None of the examined patients had signs of inflammation in the temporomandibular joints in ultrasound examination (pleural joint).

The authors of many publications [10–16, 19] emphasize the high utility of this marker in the diagnosis and confirmation of the presence of inflammation in the body, which also reflects a severity of current inflammation process. The level of this protein is increased between 6 and 8 hours after the pathogen in the body was found. The normalization of CRP is a valuable indicator of the patient's recovery. One should pay attention to general medical conditions concomitant to dysfunction because, for example, heart problems associated with the occurrence of continuous inflammation of the vascular endothelium will result in increase of CRP level and it will be due to the current associated medical main condition [19].

In the dental treatment specificity, the elevated level of CRP has been found in many diseases, such as periodontal disease, gangrenous pulp, fungal diseases of prosthetic base, or posttraumatic conditions—fractures of the jaws [12, 15]. While the states of inflammation of the temporomandibular joints are rare, and even more, they are not accompanied by temporomandibular joint dysfunction. They take the form of inflammation of the joint capsule (synovitis), the synovial membrane lining the inner surfaces of the bag, capsule ligaments (capsulitis), the retrodiscal tissues, and the area behind the articular disk (retrodiscitis) and inflammation associated with destructive changes in the bone (osteoarthritis). In each of these forms, the main causes of the inflammation for most parts are macrotrauma and mechanical damage. In contrast to functional disorders, when the pain associated with the movements of the mandible is dominant, inflammation is associated with continuous pain [1, 2, 20, 21].

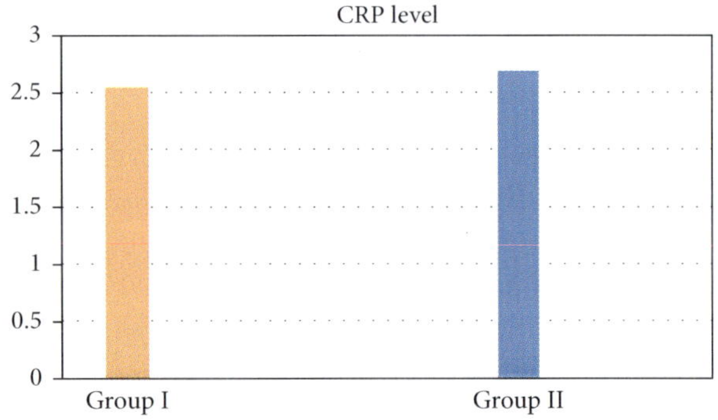

FIGURE 1: Average C-reactive protein values, obtained in both groups, presented graphically.

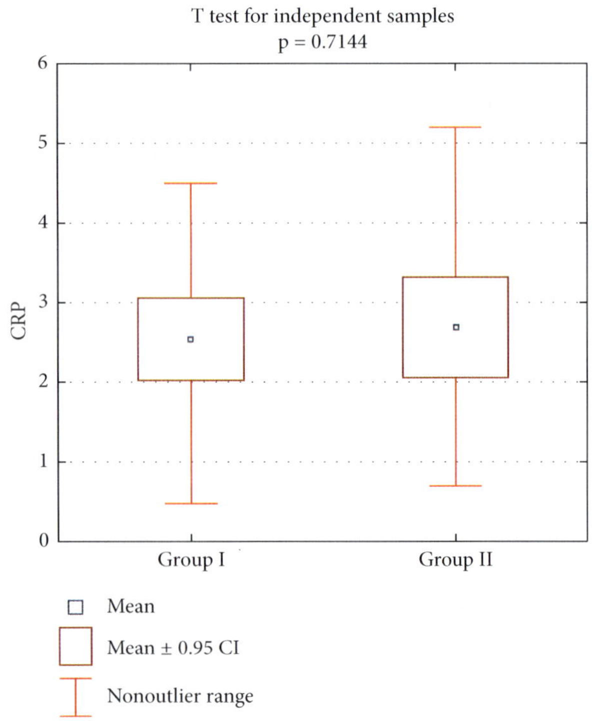

FIGURE 2: Average C-reactive protein values, obtained in both groups, presented in statistical evaluation.

CRP levels in our own study of both groups are in the normal range, and therefore this indicates that the pain form of temporomandibular joint dysfunction of subjects is not associated with the occurrence of the state of the inflammation in the soft tissues and bones of the temporomandibular joints. The presence of pain in the palpable test is often interpreted as an evidence of inflammation of tissues, but it is not confirmed in the clinical and laboratory tests.

Pain in any joint structure is called arthralgia. It would seem that pain is originated from the articular surfaces when the joints are overloaded by the work of muscles. It is impossible because of lack of the innervation of the articular surfaces, so arthralgia can originate only from nociceptors located in the soft tissue of the temporomandibular joints, like disc and capsular ligaments, and retrodiscal tissue [1–3, 16, 21, 22]. The temporomandibular articulation is unique in the body in that the two joints must always move simultaneously. Two distinct movements, rotation and translation, occur in the joint during mandibular opening and closing. Normal movements of the mandible depend on proper function of the temporomandibular joints. If the dysfunction is connected with muscles and joints prolonged overload, it will result as disruption of normal condyle-disc complex spatial relationship. In such a clinical form of dysfunction mainly the retrodiscal ligament is destroyed, and it is responsible for the occurrence of pain. The disc is then dislocated, mostly anteriorly. Meyer [23] describing the rules for the temporomandibular joint examination technique emphasizes that tenderness elicited by the palpation of the joint is invariably associated with joint inflammation.

In general, diseases such as arthritis and temporomandibular joint dysfunction can occur with elevated CRP because of general disease, as indicated by Lin et al. [24]. Nordahl et al. [16] described the progression of radiographic changes of the temporomandibular joint with reference to plasma levels of interleukin-1beta (IL-1beta), C-reactive protein (CRP), and disease duration. They point at the correlation of these factors with the severity of pathological changes. Progression of the overall grade of radiographic changes in the joints occurs in the group of the patients with chronic inflammatory joint disease. Increased levels of CRP are associated with progression of joints' bone loss.

Analyzing the available literature, it can be assumed that the use of studies evaluating CRP levels can be very helpful in diagnosing or excluding the inflammatory component of the temporomandibular joints. Kostrzewa-Janicka et al. indicate that more information could be obtained from synovial fluid of joints, like cytokines and their receptors, which are involved in the pathogenesis of temporomandibular joints. However, it is very difficult to aspirate the proper amount of synovial fluid from such a small joint, although recent advances in arthroscopic surgery allowed the direct examination of these joints [18]. These authors point out that in the case of joint diseases not related to functional disorders, the concentration of neuropeptides, cytokines, leukotrienes, prostaglandins, and catabolic products, identified in the joint's fluid, are correlated with joint pain and presence of surface lesions observed within the joint [18].

The above test results show the importance of information on the general principles of the treatment of pain form of temporomandibular joint dysfunction that the administration of antibiotics in case of pain on the palpation test of the temporomandibular joints may be wrong. Such a clinical situation requires careful verification and use of additional tests to plan an appropriate treatment [1, 2].

This provides valuable information for proper diagnosis and correct treatment in temporomandibular joint dysfunction with the use of occlusal splints and occlusal correction of the teeth contacts and supporting numerous treatments in physiotherapy, such as laser biostimulation, sonophoresis, physiotherapy, and manual therapy. Intraoral splints are commonly used in dental treatment for a variety of conditions. Such splints alter the condyle-disc-fossa relationship, probably by changing the loading status of joints and discs. The antibiotics are not necessary for such a kind of treatment [22].

Despite the etiological factor associated with the psychosocial sphere, this provides valuable information for proper diagnosis, and correct treatment of temporomandibular joint dysfunction is primarily occlusal splint, correction of occlusal contact, and numerous supporting physiotherapy treatments, such as biostimulation laser, sonophoresis, and manual techniques [1, 2, 5, 25–28].

4. Conclusion

Pain form of the temporomandibular joint dysfunctions is not connected with inflammation of the temporomandibular joints.

References

[1] J. Okeson, *Management of Temporomandibular Joint Dysfunction and Occlusion*, Elsevier, St. Louis, MO, USA, 7th edition, 2012.

[2] J. Okeson, "Evolution of occlusion and temporomandibular disorder in orthodontics: past, present, and future," *American Journal of Orthodontics and Dentofacial Orthopedics*, vol. 147, no. 5, pp. S216–S223, 2015.

[3] S. Bender, "Orofacial pain and headache: a review and look at the commonalities," *Current Pain and Headache Reports*, vol. 18, no. 3, p. 400, 2014.

[4] R. L. Gauer and M. J. Semidey, "Diagnosis and treatment of temporomandibular disorders," *American Family Physician Journal*, vol. 91, no. 6, pp. 378–386, 2015.

[5] E.-J. Garcia-Moya, J.-M. Montiel-Company, and J.-M. Almerich-Silla, "Case-control study of craniomandibular disorders in patients with fibromyalgia," *Journal of Clinical and Experimental Dentistry*, vol. 7, no. 2, pp. e293–e298, 2015.

[6] K. Kristensen, P. Stoustrup, A. Küseler, T. Pedersen, M. Twilt, and T. Herlin, "Clinical predictors of temporomandibular joint arthritis in juvenile idiopathic arthritis: a systematic literature review," *Seminars in Arthritis and Rheumatism*, vol. 45, no. 6, pp. 717–732, 2015.

[7] L. Marnall, C. Mold, and T. Du Clos, "C-reactive protein: ligands, receptors and role in inflammation," *Clinical Immunology*, vol. 117, no. 2, pp. 104–111, 2005.

[8] S.-C. Lee, J.-K. Kim, C.-H. Kim, and B.-J. Kim, "Temporomandibular joint disorder from skull-base osteomyelitis: a case report," *Maxillofacial Plastic Reconstructive Surgery*, vol. 37, no. 1, pp. 37–39, 2015.

[9] J. Nickel, L. Iwasaki, M. Beatty, M. Moss, and D. Marx, "Static and dynamic loading effect on temporomandibular joint disc tractional forces," *Journal of Dental Research*, vol. 85, no. 9, pp. 809–813, 2006.

[10] A. Olewicz–Gawlik and P. Hrycaj, "Acute phase protein in rheumatic diseases or just-markers," *Rheumatology*, vol. 45, no. 1, pp. 321–324, 2007.

[11] A. Suosa, R. Okawa, C. Silva, and M. Araujo, "Short-term changes on C-reactive protein (CRP) levels after non-surgical periodontal treatment in systemically healthy individuals," *Clinical Oral Investigations*, vol. 21, no. 1, pp. 477–484, 2017.

[12] U. Orzędała-Koszel, T. Bachanek, and B. Karczemarek-Borowska, "C-reactive protein as a diagnostic agent in inflammation of the mouth and cancer," *Dental and Medical Problems*, vol. 42, no. 1, pp. 131–136, 2005.

[13] T. Bansal, A. Pandey, and K. Asthana, "C-reactive protein (CRP) and its association with periodontal disease-a brief review," *Journal of Clinical and Diagnostic Research*, vol. 8, no. 7, pp. ZE21–ZE24, 2014.

[14] A. Pfutzner and T. Forst, "High-sensitivity C-reactive protein as cardiovascular risk marker in patients with diabetes mellitus," *Diabetes Technology & Therapeutics*, vol. 8, no. 1, pp. 28–36, 2006.

[15] R. Ramamoorthy, V. Nallasamy, R. Reddy, N. Esther, and Y. Maruthappan, "A review of C reactive protein; a diagnostic indicator in periodontal medicine," *Journal of Pharmacy And Bioallied Sciences*, vol. 4, no. 6, pp. 422–426, 2012.

[16] S. Nordahl, P. Alstergren, S. Eliasson, and S. Kopp, "Radiographic signs of bone destruction in the arthritic temporomandibular joint with special reference to markers of disease activity: a longitudinal study," *Rheumatology*, vol. 40, no. 6, pp. 691–694, 2001.

[17] S. Witulski, T. Vogl, S. Rehart, and P. Ottl, "Evaluation of the TMJ by means of clinical TMD examination and MRI diagnostics in patients with rheumatoid arthritis," *BioMed Research International*, vol. 2014, Article ID 328560, 9 pages, 2014.

[18] J. Kostrzewa-Janicka, P. Jurkowski, M. Nędzi-Góra, and E. Mierzwińska-Nastalska, "Inflammatory markers in temporomandibular joint disorders," *Central European Journal of Immunology*, vol. 37, no. 3, pp. 290–293, 2012.

[19] B. Everett, T. Kurth, J. Buring, and P. Ridker, "The relative strength of C-reactive protein and lipid levels as determinants of ischemic stroke compared with coronary heart disease in women," *Journal of the American College of Cardiology*, vol. 48, no. 11, pp. 2235–2242, 2006.

[20] S. Kumar, S. Shah, S. Budhiraja, K. Desai, C. Shah, and D. Mehta, "The effect of periodontal treatment on C-reactive protein: a clinical study," *Journal of Natural Science, Biology and Medicine*, vol. 4, no. 2, pp. 379–382, 2013.

[21] T. Salzberg, B. Overstreet, J. Rogers, J. Califano, A. Best, and H. Schenkein, "C-reactive protein levels in patients with aggressive periodontitis," *Journal of Periodontology*, vol. 77, no. 6, pp. 933–939, 2006.

[22] E. Sindelar, S. Edwards, and S. Herring, "Morphologic changes in the TMJ following splint wear," *The Anatomical Record*, vol. 266, no. 3, pp. 167–176, 2002.

[23] R. Meyer, *Clinical Methods, the History, Physical and Laboratory Examination: The Temporomandibular Joint Examination, Clinical Methods* Chapter 163, Butterworths, Boston, MA, USA, 3rd edition, 1990.

[24] Y.-C. Lin, M.-L. Hsu, J.-S. Yang, T.-H. Liang, S.-L. Chou, and H.-Y. Lin, "Temporomandibular joint disorder in patients with rheumatoid arthritis," *Journal of the Chinese Medical Association*, vol. 70, no. 12, pp. 527–534, 2007.

[25] J. Park and J. Chung, "Inflammatory cytokines and sleep disturbance in patients with temporomandibular disorders," *Journal of Oral & Facial Pain and Headache*, vol. 30, no. 1, pp. 27–33, 2016.

[26] E. Bulet, S. Bulet, I. Etikan, and O. Koseoglu, "The value of routine antibiotic prophylaxis in mandibular third molar surgery; acute phase protein levels as indicator of infection," *Journal of Oral Science*, vol. 43, no. 2, pp. 117–122, 2001.

[27] M. Wieckiewicz, M. Zientek, J. Smardz, D. Zenczak-Wieckiewicz, and N. Grychowska, "Mental status as a common factor for masticatory muscle pain: a systematic review," *Frontiers in Psychology*, vol. 8, 2017.

[28] M. Wieckiewicz, A. Paradowska-Stolarz, and W. Wieckiewicz, "Psychology aspect of bruxism, the most paramount factor influencing teeth grinding," *BioMed Research International*, vol. 2014, Article ID 469187, 7 pages, 2014.

27

Relation between Headache and Mastication Muscle Tone in Adolescents

Ewa Wozniak, Jolanta E. Loster, and Aneta Wieczorek

Department of Dental Prosthetics, Institute of Dentistry at Jagiellonian University, Krakow, Poland

Correspondence should be addressed to Aneta Wieczorek; aneta.wieczorek@uj.edu.pl

Academic Editor: Fabio Antonaci

Headache is a common problem in the population, which decreases the quality of life and makes everyday functioning difficult. It often coexists with typical symptoms of temporomandibular disorders. The objective of the study was to clarify whether there is a relationship between the presence of headache in young volunteers and the mastication muscle tone. *Material and Method.* Volunteers aged 18 years who underwent general dental examination, clinical evaluation, and examination using the dual-axis diagnostic system Research Diagnostic Criteria for Temporomandibular Disorders (RDC/TMD) form in the Polish language version participated in the study. On the basis of the examination results, these individuals were divided into three groups according to RDC results. A group of healthy individuals (axis I value 0), a group of sick individuals (axis I diagnosis Ia, IIa, or IIIa), and a group of individuals suffering from depression (axis II values 1–3) were singled out. Then, volunteers were divided into two groups: group I reporting headache and group II without any pain. In each of these individuals, the contractile activity of the masseter muscles and anterior temporal muscles was recorded bilaterally as the surface electromyographic activity (sEMG) at rest, during swallowing, and maximum clenching. The activity index ranging between +100 (activity of the masseter muscles only) and −100 (activity of the anterior temporal muscles only) was used to indicate the predominance of activity of the study muscles. *Results.* The statistical analysis of data showed that there was a significant relationship between the presence of headache and a change in the mastication muscle tone, expressed as the predominant activity of the temporal muscles, only in the group of sick individuals during maximum clenching. *Summary.* The diversity of sEMG results implies that a change in the mastication muscle tone is not a direct consequence of headache, but it has to be modified by other factors.

1. Introduction

Headache is a common condition which compromises everyday functioning and decreases the quality of life not only in adults. The results of the systematic review covering epidemiological studies on the prevalence of headache among children and adolescents from 32 countries have shown that the problem affects 54.4% of the population on average [1]. The causes of headache vary due to the great number and complexity of anatomical structures, various pathophysiological mechanisms, and effects of psychogenic factors. Temporomandibular disorders (TMD) are among conditions which may manifest with headache. This term covers a broad range of clinical problems that are related to the masticatory muscles, temporomandibular joints, and adjacent tissues [2]. Functional disorders are the most common orofacial pain syndrome due to which patients seek medical help [3]. According to the studies by Solberg et al., 76% of study subjects aged 18–25 years reported signs associated with TMD, and at least one typical sign of TMD was found in 26% [4]. In the past, the diagnosis of temporomandibular disorders was problematic, but today clinicians have diagnostic tools at their disposal that make it much easier to establish the diagnosis and than to apply appropriate treatment strategies. The standardized classification of TMD has become possible owing to the development of research diagnostic criteria for TMD [5]. This diagnostic system takes into account the biopsychological etiology of the analysed problem and comprises two axes: axis I is a set of procedures for clinical evaluation of a patient that lead to a physical diagnosis and axis II uses personal questionnaires with which, through the patient self-evaluation, the psychological dimension of pain, resultant disability, presence of depression, and nonspecific somatic symptoms can be determined. The results of scientific research show that typical symptoms of TMD-pain in the area of the temporomandibular joints and/or muscles of mastication, limited mandibular range of motion, and acoustic symptoms are more common in patients who suffer from primary headache, such as migraine or tension headache, compared to the healthy population [6, 7]. At the same time, the inverse trend has been observed, i.e., an increase in the prevalence of primary headache (in particular migraine) in patients with diagnosed TMD [8]. Moreover, it has been demonstrated that the coexistence of these two conditions exacerbates the typical symptoms of each of them, leading to a higher degree of disability [6]. Therefore, a conclusion can be drawn that procedures appropriate for the treatment of both headache and TMD should be included in the therapeutic management. One of TMD treatment strategies is to apply the therapy using occlusal splints in patients. There are scientific reports which confirm the efficacy of using occlusal splints not only for the elimination of mastication muscle pain and acoustic symptoms in the temporomandibular joints, but also for the treatment of migraine pain [9]. The results of studies involving electromyographic measurements of the mastication muscles indicate that there are effects such as a reduction in the electrical activity of the mastication muscles and equalization of the muscle activity on the left and right sides after the implementation of stabilization splint therapy [10]. Correlations between primary headache and TMD that are noticeable in the symptomatology and effects of similar treatment strategies suggest that there may be a relationship between headache and mastication muscle tone. The objective of the present study was to clarify whether there is a relationship between headache in young volunteers and the mastication muscle tone in the group of healthy individuals, group of individuals suffering from TMD, and group of individuals with diagnosed depression. The initial hypothesis assumed that the predominant activity of anterior temporal muscles would be observed in individuals with headache compared to individuals without any pain.

2. Material and Methods

Individuals aged 18 years were enrolled in the study from among volunteers taking part in the research project. None of these individuals had earlier contact with any of the study doctors or clinical procedures forming an integral part of the research project. Informed consent forms for participation in the project were signed by all subjects, and the study program was approved by the Bioethics Committee of the Jagiellonian University (KBET//89B/2009). The study was conducted in accordance with the Good Clinical Practice guide, Declaration of Helsinki.

The study inclusion criteria included full dental arches. The exclusion criteria included: malocclusions, carious destruction of dental tissues, permanent prosthetic restorations, therapy with botulinum toxin, mental illnesses, and pregnancy. Clinical evaluation was performed in each of the subjects by the same dental practitioner using the RDC/TMD dual-axis diagnostic system. A Polish version of the personal questionnaire forming a part of the RDC/TMD diagnostic algorithm was completed by the project participants themselves [12]. Based on the evaluation results and data from questionnaires, the subjects were assigned to one of 3 groups: group I of healthy individuals (RDC/TMD system axis I value 0), group II of sick individuals (axis I diagnosis Ia, IIa, or IIIa), and group III of individuals with depression or nonspecific somatic symptoms (axis II values 1–3). Each of the subjects was asked to assess the presence and intensity of headache on the day of evaluation using a 4 point scale: 0, no headache; 1, mild headache; 2, moderate headache; and 3, severe headache. All subjects underwent surface electromyography (sEMG) examination using the eight-channel BioEMG III BioPAK Measurement System Electromyograph (BioResearch, Inc., Milwaukee, WI, USA). Measurements of tone of the left and right masseter muscles (LMM, RMM) and the anterior temporal muscle on the left and right sides (LTA, RTA) were performed [13–16]. The first measurement involved the scenario with a position at rest, the second one was performed during maximum clenching, and the third one was taken during swallowing. For each of the scenarios, the activity index (AcI) was calculated, which was to indicate the predominant activity of the masseter muscle or the anterior temporal muscle. The activity index was calculated using the equation introduced by Naeije [17] in accordance with the following formula: $AcI = (RMS_{masseter} - RMS_{temporal})/(RMS_{masseter} + RMS_{temporal}) \times 100$, where RMS is the root mean square. The activity index ranged between +100 (activity of the masseter muscles only) and −100 (activity of the anterior temporal muscles only). The value 0 meant that that there was a balance between the activity of both groups of muscles. The analysis of data consisted of the following steps:

(1) Test for normality of distribution

(2) Evaluation of the impact of presence of headache on the activity index of the mastication muscles in groups I, II, and III at rest

(3) Evaluation of the impact of presence of headache on the activity index of the mastication muscles in groups I, II, and III during maximum clenching

(4) Evaluation of the impact of presence of headache on the activity index of the mastication muscles in groups I, II, and III during swallowing

Statistical calculations were performed using the R 3.1.2 statistical package. The results with the p value < 0.05 were considered to be statistically significant.

3. Results

In total, 106 individuals (27 men and 79 women) aged 18 years were enrolled in the study. There were 74 subjects in the first group, 32 subjects in the second group, and the third group included 47 individuals.

(1) The activity indices of the mastication muscles were normally distributed across all groups under analysis (the p value of the Shapiro–Wilk test above 0.05), therefore the analysis was performed using the parametric Student t-test.

(2) At rest, the differences in the activity index of the mastication muscles between individuals with headache and those without pain were not statistically significant in group I (healthy individuals), group II (sick individuals), and group III (individuals with depression) (group I: $p = 0.589$; group II: $p = 0.641$; group III: $p = 0.404$) (Figures 1–3). Although there was no statistical significance, the activity index in group III indicated the predominance of the anterior temporal muscles in individuals with headache (AcI = −7.78), while in groups I and II, masseter muscles showed greater activity, if headache was present.

(3) During maximum clenching, differences in the activity index of the mastication muscles between individuals with headache and those without headache in the group I were statistically insignificant ($p = 0.088$); however, the activity index value was lower in individuals with headache compared to individuals without pain, which indicated a reduction in predominant activity of the masseter muscles. In the group II, the relationship between the presence of headache and a change in the activity index of the mastication muscles was statistically significant ($p = 0.003$) (Figures 4–6). The mean AcI in sick individuals with headache was nearly 0 (AcI = −0.07), which indicated a balance between the activity of the masseter muscles and anterior temporal muscles, while AcI in sick individuals without pain was definitely positive (AcI = 17.73), which indicated the predominant activity of the masseter muscles. Differences in the activity index of the mastication muscles between individuals with headache and those without headache in the group III were not statistically significant ($p = 0.782$); however, a tendency towards greater activity of the temporal muscles in individuals with pain was noticeable.

(4) During swallowing, differences in the activity index of the mastication muscles between individuals with headache and those without headache were not statistically significant across all study groups (group I: $p = 0.309$; group II: $p = 0.523$; group III: $p = 0.972$) (Figures 7–9). However, the increased activity of the temporal muscles was noticeable in healthy individuals in the case of presence of headache.

4. Discussion

The initial hypothesis of the present study was based on reports by Rodrigues-Bigaton et al. [11] who demonstrated that there was a statistically significant difference in the

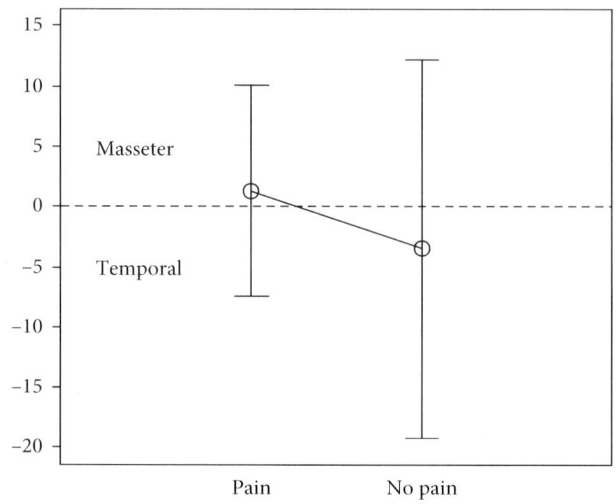

Figure 1: Activity index at rest in group of healthy individuals.

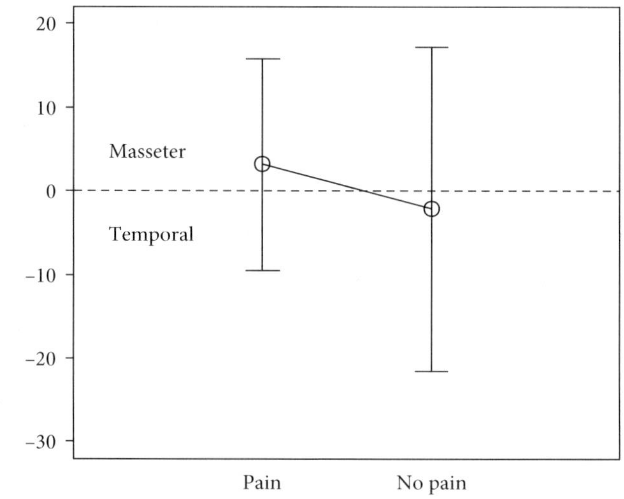

Figure 2: Activity index at rest in group of TMD individuals.

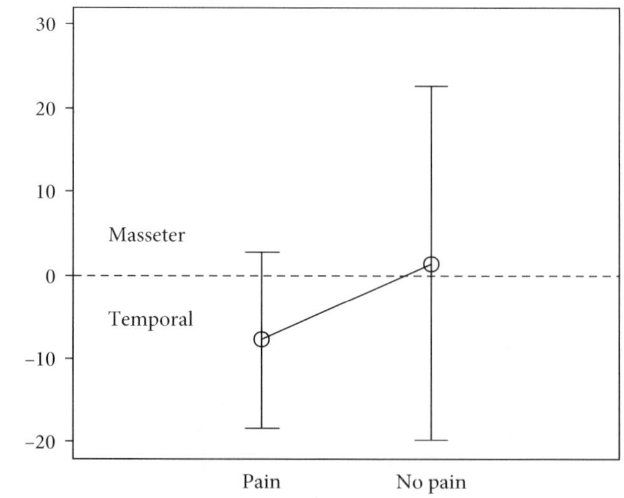

Figure 3: Activity index at rest in group of individuals with depression.

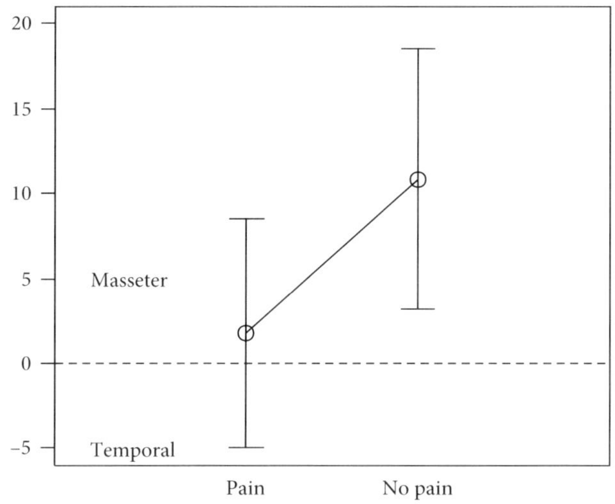

FIGURE 4: Activity index during maximum clenching in group of healthy individuals.

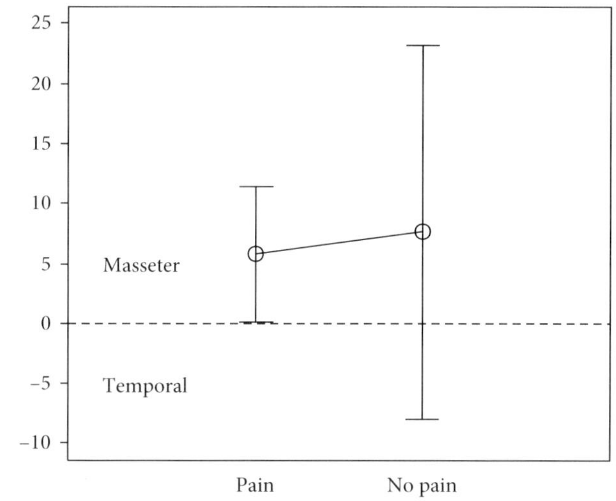

FIGURE 6: Activity index during maximum clenching in group of individuals with depression.

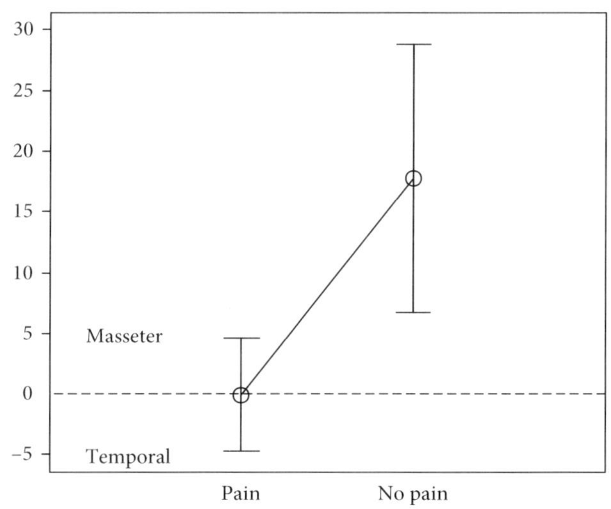

FIGURE 5: Activity index during maximum clenching in group of TMD individuals.

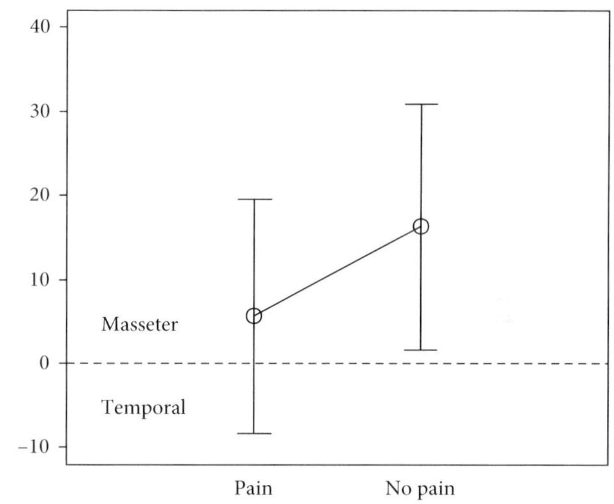

FIGURE 7: Activity index during swallowing in group of healthy individuals.

activity index of the mastication muscles during resting mandibular position in individuals with TMD compared to the healthy control group. In the study conducted by Rodrigues-Bigaton, the difference in the activity index was expressed as the dominance of the temporal muscles in individuals with TMD, so the relationship between the presence of TMD, of which mastication muscle pain is a component, and a change in the mastication muscle tone was demonstrated. The objective of the present study was to clarify whether the analogous relationship between the presence of headache and mastication muscle tone exists. Therefore, the initial hypothesis assumed that there would be a change in the mastication muscle tone expressed as the predominant activity of the temporal muscles in individuals with headache. The initial hypothesis was confirmed only in the group of sick individuals during maximum clenching. The results obtained by Rodrigues-Bigaton are in contrast to this observation. He found no statistically significant differences in the activity index of the mastication muscles between individuals with TMD and the control group in the situation of isometric contraction of the muscles of mastication. Although there was no statistical significance in the present study, tendencies in conformity with the initial assumption were noticeable in groups of individuals with depression in the position at rest and during maximum clenching and healthy individuals during maximum clenching and swallowing. Apart from studies conducted by Rodrigues-Bigaton, the issues related to the impact of mastication muscle pain on changes in the tone of these muscles during different functional activities were addressed by a number of other authors. There are scientific reports which found that there was no significant difference in the sEMG readings from the temporal muscles at rest between individuals with mastication muscle pain and the control

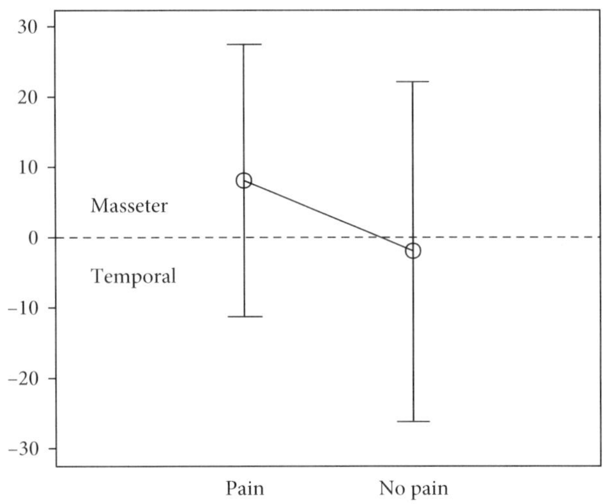

Figure 8: Activity index during swallowing in group of TMD individuals.

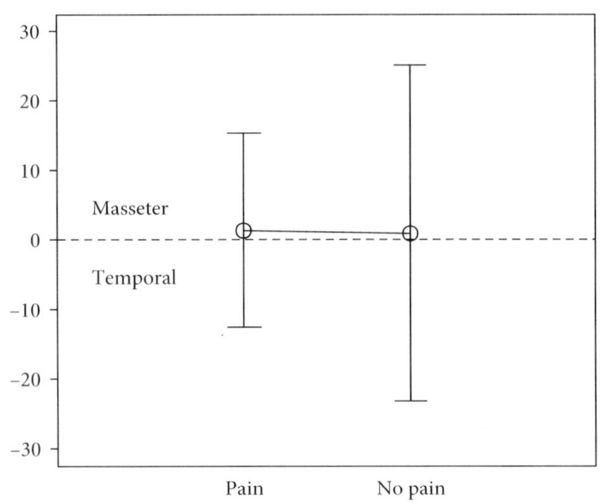

Figure 9: Activity index during swallowing in group of individuals with depression.

group [18]. On the other hand, numerous studies on animals demonstrated that experimentally induced painful stimuli resulted in a short-term increase in the mastication muscle tone recorded in sEMG [19, 20]. The results of studies involving patients with TMD, who reported headache, also confirmed higher sEMG activity of the mandibular elevator muscles at rest in these patients [21]. However, it was observed that there were significant differences in the time of onset and duration of changes recorded in sEMG in individual subjects with pain. Some authors conclude that time parameters, such as onset and duration of changes in sEMG, may be more reliable in the identification of muscle activity patterns that are changed by pain than the amplitude itself of these changes [22]. The diversity of obtained results has provoked the development of contradictory hypotheses to clarify whether an increase in the sEMG reading for the mandible adductor muscles is caused by pain or may be a primary increase in the activity recorded in sEMG is a component of the feedback mechanism which maintains chronic muscle pain. The vicious cycle theory has been developed which assumes that a pain-initiating factor, e.g., abnormality in structure, posture, movement, or stress, leads spontaneously to muscular hyperactivity. It results in increased muscle tone, spasm and fatigue, and finally dysfunction which maintains pain [23]. A weak point of the mentioned theory is that the pathophysiological mechanism linking muscle pain and muscle tone has not been fully explained yet. It has been claimed that pain results in neuroplastic changes in the central nervous system, leading to increased motor neuron activity at supraspinal and segmental levels, of which the effect is slightly increased muscular activity [24]. It was also found that in patients reporting bilateral headache, the EMG readings from the mastication muscles were higher than these recorded in patients with unilateral pain [21]. It suggests that the modulation of muscular activity is not only a direct consequence of peripheral nociceptive mechanism and indicates a response involving the central nervous system as well. However, in the majority of studies, an increase in the EMG activity recorded when pain was present turned out to be so small (of about several μV) that its role in the development of the claimed muscular hyperactivity and maintaining painful impulsation is doubtful; therefore, it seems to have no clinical relevance [23]. In the presented study a slight correlation between headache and a change in tone recorded superficially from the temporal and masseter muscles was confirmed. Some scientific reports assume the possibility that the examined muscles may show normal or slightly changed superficial EMG activity in pain syndromes, but certain specific, small areas within the muscles, so called trigger points, are distinguished by a higher EMG reading. Therefore, it is suspected that continuous activity of several motor units, which persists over a long period of time, may be sufficient for the stimulation of nociceptors [24], while the sEMG reading from the entire muscle remains unchanged. The pain adaptation model is the theory that explains the observed relationships better than the vicious cycle theory. It assumes that pain causes decreased EMG activity in the agonist muscles and results in reduced range of motion and its longer duration [23]. These changes are aimed at preventing further damage to the sensorimotor system. The present study results are in conformity with the mentioned theory: a significant change in the muscle tone was observed in individuals with diagnosed TMD who reported the presence of headache compared to individuals without any pain during maximum clenching of the teeth, i.e., during active contraction. Similar results were obtained by Li et al. [25] who investigated whether unilateral pain from TMD was associated with the occlusion contacts and EMG activity of the mastication muscles. They demonstrated that in individuals with TMD (with pain) the muscle tone measured using sEMG in both masseter muscles and the temporal muscle on the pain side was lower compared to the healthy control group during maximum clenching at maximum intercuspation. The newest model describing the relation between pain and muscle activity, i.e., the integrated pain adaptation model [23], assumes that pain results in a new, optimized recruitment strategy of motor units to minimize pain and maintain homeostasis. This model represents the individual response of the motor system to the multidimensional nature of pain: not only the biological dimension of pain but also psychosocial components of the pain experience are taken into account. Thus, it emphasizes the individual reaction to pain, i.e., factors such as the presence of depression, previous pain experience, social context, and genetic factors that will affect a change in the muscle activity in a unique way. The performed study did not demonstrate that the presence of headache in individuals with depression or psychosomatic symptoms had effect on the mastication muscle tone.

5. Conclusions

Headache has impact on a change in the mastication muscle tone in individuals with diagnosed TMD during maximum clench. The diversity of sEMG results implies that a change in the mastication muscle tone is not a direct consequence of headache, but it has to be modified by other factors.

Acknowledgments

This study was supported by a grant from the Ministry of Education and Research for Jagiellonian University Medical College and completed within MNiSW project no. N N403 589138. The authors would like to express their appreciation to BioResearch (Milwaukee, WI, USA) for their training on the BioEMG and T-scan III systems and help with BIO-FLEX sensors and to Tekscan Inc. (South Boston, MA, USA) for the donation of sensors.

References

[1] C. Wober-Bingol, "Epidemiology of migraine and headache in children and adolescents," *Current Pain and Headache Reports*, vol. 17, no. 6, p. 341, 2013.

[2] R. De Leeuw, *Orofacial Pain: Guidelines for Assessment, Diagnosis and Management*, Quintessence Publishing Co., Chicago, IL, USA, 2008.

[3] S. F. Dworkin, "Temporomandibular disorder (TMD) pain-related disability found related to depression, nonspecific physical symptoms, and pain duration at 3 international sites," *Journal of Evidence Based Dental Practice*, vol. 11, no. 3, pp. 143-144, 2011.

[4] W. K. Solberg, M. W. Woo, and J. B. Houston, "Prevalence of mandibular dysfunction in young adults," *Journal of the American Dental Association*, vol. 98, no. 1, pp. 25–34, 1979.

[5] S. F. Dworkin and L. LeResche, "Research diagnostic criteria for temporomandibular disorders: review, criteria, examinations and specifications, critique," *Journal of Craniomandibular Disorders: Facial & Oral Pain*, vol. 6, no. 4, pp. 301–355, 1992.

[6] S. Mitrirattanakul and R. L. Merrill, "Headache impact in patients with orofacial pain," *Journal of the American Dental Association*, vol. 137, no. 9, pp. 1267–1274, 2006.

[7] D. A. G. Gonçalves, M. E. Bigal, L. C. F. Jales, C. M. Camparis, and J. G. Speciali, "Headache and symptoms of temporomandibular disorder: an epidemiological study," *Headache*, vol. 50, no. 2, pp. 231–241, 2010.

[8] A. L. Franco, D. A. Goncalves, S. M. Castanharo, J. G. Speciali, M. E. Bigal, and C. M. Camparis, "Migraine is the most prevalent primary headache in individuals with temporomandibular disorders," *Journal of Orofacial Pain*, vol. 24, no. 3, pp. 287–292, 2010.

[9] A. A. Quayle, R. J. Gray, R. J. Metcalfe, E. Guthrie, and D. Wastell, "Soft occlusal splint therapy in the treatment of migraine and other headaches," *Journal of Dentistry*, vol. 18, no. 3, pp. 123–129, 1990.

[10] V. Scopel, G. S. Alves da Costa, and D. Urias, "An electromyographic study of masseter and anterior temporal muscles in extra-articular myogenous TMJ pain patients compared to an asymptomatic and normal population," *Cranio*, vol. 23, no. 3, pp. 194–203, 2005.

[11] D. Rodrigues-Bigaton, K. C. Berni, A. F. Almeida, and M. T. Silva, "Activity and asymmetry index of masticatory muscles in women with and without dysfunction temporomandibular," *Electromyography and Clinical Neurophysiology*, vol. 50, no. 7-8, pp. 333–338, 2010.

[12] M. A. Osiewicz, F. Lobbezoo, B. W. Loster, M. Wilkosz, M. Naeije, and R. Ohrbach, "Research diagnostic criteria for temporomandibular disorders (RDC/TMD): the Polish version of a dual-axis system for the diagnostic of TMD," *Journal of Stomatology*, vol. 66, no. 5, pp. 576–649, 2013.

[13] T. Sierpinska, P. Jacunski, J. Kuc, M. Golebiewska, A. Wieczorek, and S. Majewski, "Effect of the dental arches morphology on the masticatory muscles activities in normal occlusion young adults," *Cranio*, vol. 33, no. 2, pp. 134–141, 2015.

[14] A. Wieczorek, J. Loster, and B. W. Loster, "Relationship between occlusal force distribution and the activity of masseter and anterior temporalis muscles in asymptomatic young adults," *BioMed Research International*, vol. 2013, Article ID 354017, 7 pages, 2013.

[15] A. Wieczorek and J. E. Loster, "Activity of the masticatory muscles and occlusal contacts in young adults with and without orthodontic treatment," *BMC Oral Health*, vol. 15, no. 1, 2015.

[16] J. E. Loster, M. A. Osiewicz, M. Groch, W. Ryniewicz, and A. Wieczorek, "The prevalence of TMD in Polish young adults," *Journal of Prosthodontics*, vol. 26, no. 4, pp. 284–288, 2017.

[17] M. Naeije, R. S. McCarroll, and W. A. Weijs, "Electromyographic activity of the human masticatory muscles during submaximal clenching in the inter-cuspal position," *Journal of Oral Rehabilitation*, vol. 16, no. 1, pp. 63–70, 1989.

[18] R. F. Majewski and E. N. Gale, "Electromyographic activity of anterior temporal area pain patients and non-pain subjects," *Journal of Dental Research*, vol. 63, no. 10, pp. 1228–1231, 1984.

[19] X.-M. Yu, B. J. Sessle, H. Vernon, and J. W. Hu, "Effects of inflammatory irritant application to the rat temporomandibular joint on jaw and neck muscle activity," *Pain*, vol. 60, no. 2, pp. 143–149, 1995.

[20] J. Y. Ro, P. Svensson, and N. F. Capra, "Effects of experimental muscle pain on electromyographic activity of masticatory muscles in the rat," *Muscle Nerve*, vol. 25, no. 4, pp. 576–584, 2002.
[21] C. Bodere and S. H. Tea, "Activity of masticatory muscles in subjects with different orofacial pain conditions," *Pain*, vol. 116, no. 1, pp. 33–41, 2005.
[22] B. Hatef, S. Talebian, F. Hashemirad, and M. Ghaffarpour, "Effect of pain on the timing pattern of masseter muscle activity during the open-close-clench cycle in the migraine without aura and tension type headaches," *Iranian Journal of Neurology*, vol. 11, no. 4, pp. 146–150, 2012.
[23] C. Peck, G. Murray, and T. Gerzina, "How does pain affect jaw muscle activity? The integrated pain adaptation model," *Australian Dental Journal*, vol. 53, no. 3, pp. 201–207, 2008.
[24] L. Bendtsen and C. Fernández-de-la-Peñas, "The role of muscles in tension-type headache," *Current Pain and Headache Reports*, vol. 15, no. 6, pp. 451–458, 2011.
[25] B.-Y. Li, L.-J. Zhou, S.-X. Guo, Y. Zhang, L. Lu, and M.-Q. Wang, "An investigation on the simultaneously recorded occlusion contact and surface electromyographic activity for patients with unilateral temporomandibular disorders pain," *Journal of Electromyography and Kinesiology*, vol. 28, pp. 199–207, 2016.

Effects of Gabapentinoids Premedication on Shoulder Pain and Rehabilitation Quality after Laparoscopic Cholecystectomy: Pregabalin versus Gabapentin

Mohamed Said Nakhli,[1,2] **Mohamed Kahloul**,[1,2] **Chawki Jebali**,[2,3] **Walid Frigui**,[1] **and Walid Naija**[1,2]

[1]*Department of Anesthesia and Intensive Care, Sahloul Academic Hospital, Sousse, Tunisia*
[2]*University of Medicine "Ibn Al Jazzar", Sousse, Tunisia*
[3]*Emergency Medical Service, Sahloul Academic Hospital, Sousse, Tunisia*

Correspondence should be addressed to Mohamed Said Nakhli; mohamedsaid.nakhli@rns.tn

Academic Editor: Massimiliano Valeriani

Introduction. Gabapentinoids are increasingly used in preoperative premedication despite controversial results. The aim of our study was to evaluate the effects of preemptive use of gabapentin or pregabalin on postoperative shoulder pain and rehabilitation quality after laparoscopic cholecystectomy. *Methods.* This is a clinical trial comparing the effects of a preoperative premedication with 600 mg of gabapentin or 150 mg of pregabalin versus placebo on postoperative pain and recovery quality after laparoscopic cholecystectomy. Premedication was taken 2 hours before the surgery beginning. Ninety patients were included and randomized into 3 groups (gabapentin, pregabalin, and placebo). The anesthetic protocol was the same for all patients. Primary endpoint was the shoulder pain intensity at the 48th postoperative hour. Secondary endpoints were postoperative nausea and vomiting (PONV), sleep quality during the first night, and the onset time for the first standing position. *Results.* During the first 48 postoperative hours, the gabapentin and pregabalin groups had significantly lower shoulder pain than the placebo group ($p < 0.05$). In gabapentinoids groups, the incidence of PONV was lower and the sleep quality during the first postoperative night was better with significant results. Mean Spiegel scores were 22.43 ± 1.45, 22.30 ± 1.44, and 17.17 ± 1.66, respectively, in pregabalin, gabapentin, and placebo groups ($p < 0.05$). The delay for the first standing position was 14.9 ± 4.9 hours in the pregabalin group, 9.7 ± 3.6 hours in the gabapentin group, and 21.6 ± 2.1 hours in the placebo group. No superiority was found between gabapentin and pregabalin. *Conclusion.* Preemptive premedication with gabapentinoids can enhance postoperative rehabilitation quality after laparoscopic cholecystectomy by reducing postoperative shoulder pain, decreasing PONV incidence, and improving sleep quality during the first postoperative night. This trial is registered with ClinicalTrial.gov (NCT03241875).

1. Introduction

Laparoscopic cholecystectomy is one of the most widely performed surgeries in the world [1]. Its postoperative follow-up is usually simple allowing ambulatory practices [1, 2]. However, postoperative pain, especially scapular ones, seems to be a hindrance to a quick postoperative recovery [3]. In fact, postoperative shoulder pain is a common side effect after laparoscopic procedures. It seems to have a multifactorial mechanism, but the most reported theory is carbon dioxide gas persistence between the right diaphragm and the hepatic dome. It appears mainly after patient verticalization and it may remain even after standard analgesic medications. In addition, the high emetic potential of laparoscopic procedures with an incidence exceeding 75% when no specific prophylaxis is prescribed can extend the length of hospital stay [4].

Gabapentin and pregabalin are two drugs belonging to the gabapentinoids family. They are classically known as antiepileptic treatments. However, they have been used in other conditions such as neuropathic, diabetic, and post-herpetic pain [5]. They have few drug interactions and side effects with close pharmacokinetic profiles justifying their interest in the perioperative context [5, 6].

Preemptive administration of gabapentinoids can reduce postoperative pain intensity even after laparoscopic surgery [7]. It can also alleviate preoperative anxiety and stress response to surgical stimuli and decreases anesthetic consumption and postoperative nausea and vomiting (PONV) [6, 8–10].

The aim of this study was to evaluate the effects of preemptive use of gabapentin or pregabalin on postoperative shoulder pain and recovery parameters after laparoscopic cholecystectomy.

2. Methods

After obtaining institutional ethic committee approval and patients' informed consent, this randomized, double-blind clinical trial was conducted jointly between the anesthesia and the visceral surgery departments of Sahloul Teaching Hospital (Sousse, Tunisia). This study was conducted between December 2016 and August 2017. This trial was registered with ClinicalTrial.gov (NCT03241875).

Patients aged 18–65 years, with American Society of Anesthesiologists (ASA) physical status 1 and 2, and scheduled for laparoscopic cholecystectomy under general anesthesia were enrolled in this study. Exclusion criteria were as follows: allergy to gabapentin or pregabalin, history of psychiatric disorders, chronic neuroleptic treatment, history of renal and/or hepatic disorders, pregnant and/or breastfeeding women, complicated lithiasis pathology, conversion to laparotomy, and perioperative complications (surgical difficulties, difficult intubation, bronchospasm, anaphylaxis, etc).

Fixing the α risk at 0.05 and the study power at 80% and hoping a 30% decrease in shoulder pain intensity at the 48th hour postoperatively, the minimum sample size was estimated at 29 patients per group. Sample calculation was made by the software Epi Info 6.0.

Patients were randomized into 3 groups of 30 each. Patients of group 1 received 150 mg of pregabalin (2 capsules of 75 mg), those of group 2 received 600 mg of gabapentin (2 capsules of 300 mg), and those of group 3 received 2 capsules of placebo. Capsules were arranged in nontransparent and numbered envelopes. They were given to patients during preoperative visit to be taken 2 hours before arrival in the operating room. No other premedication was prescribed.

In the operating room, all patients had standard monitoring (electrocardiogram, noninvasive blood pressure, pulse oximetry, capnography, anesthetic gas analyzer, and neuromuscular monitoring). Anesthesia induction was carried out by propofol at the dose of 3 mg/kg, remifentanil at the dose of 1 μg/kg over one minute, and cisatracurium at the dose of 0.15 mg/kg. Anesthesia was maintained by isoflurane in a mixture of 50% oxygen and 50% air. Remifentanil doses and expired isoflurane concentrations were adjusted intraoperatively to maintain a hemodynamic profile (arterial pressure and heart rate) not exceeding ±20% from baseline. Cisatracurium was reinjected at the dose of 0.03 mg/kg depending on neuromuscular blockade monitoring. PONV risk was assessed by the Apfel score (a four-criteria score used to estimate the probability of experiencing PONV) and prevented by dexamethasone 8 mg and ondansetron 4 mg. Normal saline was used for intraoperative vascular loading at the dose of 4 ml/kg/h. Tidal volume was fixed at 6 ml/kg of ideal weight, and respiratory rate was adjusted to maintain EtCO2 between 30 and 35 mmHg.

Postoperative analgesia was anticipated 30 minutes before the end of surgery by 1 g of paracetamol and 20 mg of nefopam. All patients were extubated in the operating room after complete decurarization. They were monitored in the post-anesthesia care unit for one hour and then transferred to the visceral surgery ward. Postoperative analgesia was performed with 1 g of paracetamol and 20 mg of nefopam given four times a day. Postoperative vomiting was managed by 4 mg of ondansetron.

Primary endpoint was shoulder pain intensity at the 48th postoperative hour assessed by the Visual Analog Scale (VAS) ranging from 0 to 10. Secondary endpoints were PONV incidence, sleeping quality assessed by Spiegel Scale (a very simple and widely used scale with six questions about sleep; total score below 15 signifies a pathological sleep and a score above 20 signifies a good sleep), and time for the first standing position.

Statistical analysis was performed using SPSS software version 20.0 for windows (IBM Corp., USA). Categorical variables were expressed in percentages. Normal distribution of continuous variables was tested using the Kolmogorov–Smirnov test. They were expressed as means or medians according to their distribution.

Categorical variables were analyzed using chi-squared test. Student's t-test was used to compare means of normally distributed variables, whereas the Mann–Whitney test was used for non-normally distributed ones. A value of $p < 0.05$ was considered to be statistically significant.

3. Results

This study enrolled 90 patients undergoing scheduled laparoscopic cholecystectomy. All of them were followed up until the end of the study. Demographic characteristics were comparable between all groups. Insufflation pressure and duration of surgery, anesthesia, and pneumoperitoneum were also comparable between the 3 groups (Table 1).

At the 48th hour after surgery, the overall incidence of postoperative shoulder pain was 51.1%. It was 13.3% in the pregabalin group, 12.2% in the gabapentin group, and 25.6% in the control group ($p = 0.003$). Postoperative shoulder pain occurred after the 6th postoperative hour in all cases. Its intensity at rest and at exertion was significantly lower in the gabapentinoids groups than in the control one. When comparing the pregabalin group to the gabapentin one according to postoperative shoulder pain intensity, no significant difference was found (Figure 1).

PONV incidence was significantly higher in the control group than in the gabapentinoids ones; however, they were

TABLE 1: Sociodemographic and intraoperative characteristics.

	Group 1 $n = 30$	Group 2 $n = 30$	Group 3 $n = 30$	p
Age (years)	42.7 ± 13.7	47.1 ± 13.1	43.5 ± 13.6	0.433
BMI (kg/m^2)	26.3 ± 2.4	28.1 ± 4.5	25.6 ± 3.3	0.081
Gender n (%)				
Male	7 (23.3)	6 (20)	6 (20)	0.93
Female	23 (76.7)	24 (80)	24 (80)	
Apfel score: n (%)				
1	4 (13.3)	6 (20)	4 (13.3)	
2	26 (86.7)	24 (80)	25 (83.3)	0.61
3	0 (0)	0 (0)	1 (3.3)	
ASA status n (%)				
1	26 (86.6)	23 (76.6)	25 (83.3)	0.58
2	4 (13.4)	7 (23.4)	5 (16.7)	
Surgery duration (min)	51 ± 14.4	56.2 ± 17.7	50.7 ± 15.9	0.398
Pneumoperitoneum duration (min)	37.6 ± 15.2	37.3 ± 16.3	37.1 ± 13.6	0.983
Insufflation pressure (mmHg)	11.6 ± 0.6	11.6 ± 0.7	11.5 ± 0.7	0.72
Anesthesia duration (min)	63.1 ± 16	68 ± 18.4	63.9 ± 15.5	0.47

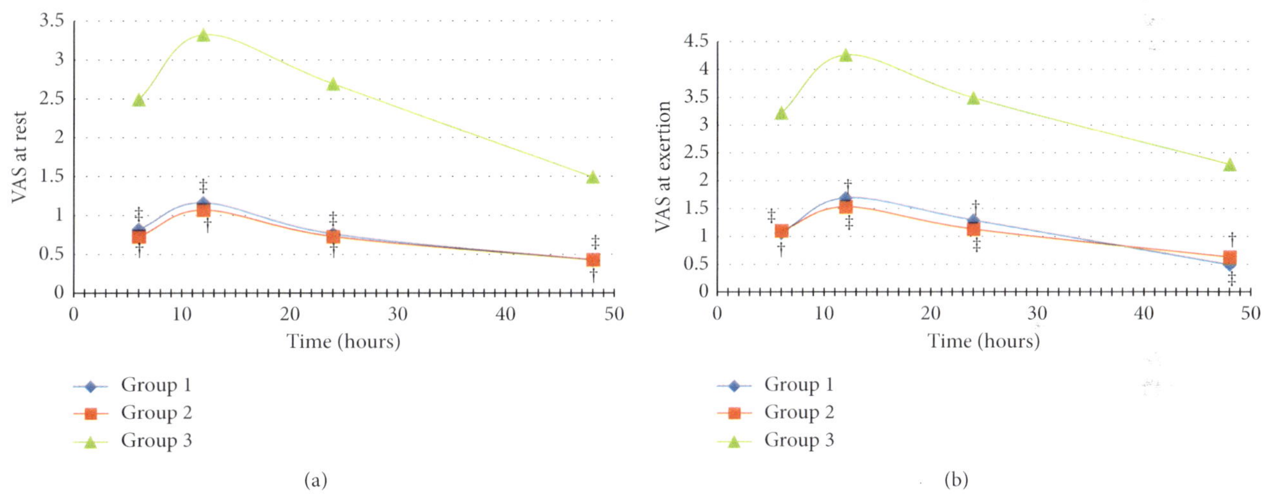

FIGURE 1: Postoperative shoulder pain intensity ((a) at rest and (b) at exertion). $^\dagger p < 0.05$ between groups 1 and 3. $^\ddagger p < 0.05$ between groups 2 and 3.

TABLE 2: Effects of gabapentinoids on PONV, sleep quality, and first standing position.

	Group 1 $n = 30$	Group 2 $n = 30$	Group 3 $n = 30$
Postoperative nausea n (%)			
2nd hour	4 (13.3)†	8 (26.7)‡	25 (83.3)
6th hour	5 (16.7)†	2 (6.7)‡	22 (73.3)
12th hour	0 (0)†	3 (10)‡	12 (40)
Postoperative vomiting n (%)			
2nd hour	5 (16.7)†	4 (13.3)‡	21 (70)
6th hour	1 (3.3)†	4 (13.3)‡	12 (40)
12th hour	0 (0)†	0 (0)‡	4 (13.3)
Spiegel score (mean)	$22.43 \pm 1.45^\dagger$	$22.30 \pm 1.44^\ddagger$	17.17 ± 1.66
Time for the first standing position (hr)	$14.9 \pm 4.9^\dagger$	$9.7 \pm 3.6^\ddagger$	21.6 ± 2.1

$^\dagger p < 0.05$ between groups 1 and 3. $^\ddagger p < 0.05$ between groups 2 and 3.

at the same risk of PONV as assessed by the Apfel score. No difference was found when comparing the pregabalin group to the gabapentin group (Table 2).

During the first postoperative night, sleeping quality was significantly better in gabapentinoids groups ($p < 0.05$). Average Spiegel scales were 22.43 ± 1.45 in the pregabalin group, 22.30 ± 1.44 in the gabapentin group, and 17.17 ± 1.66 in the control group. Sleeping quality was comparable between the pregabalin group and gabapentin group (Table 2).

Postoperative deambulation was significantly earlier in the gabapentinoids groups. No significant difference was found between the pregabalin and gabapentin groups (14.9 ± 4.9 hours in the pregabalin group, 9.7 ± 3.6 hours in the gabapentin group, and 21.6 ± 2.1 hours in the control group; $p < 0.05$) (Table 2).

Dizziness was the unique type of side effects documented in the gabapentinoids groups (9 patients in the gabapentin group versus 11 patients in the pregabalin group). This adverse effect was reported only before anesthesia induction.

4. Discussion

Our results suggest that a premedication with a gabapentinoid (150 mg of pregabalin or 600 mg of gabapentin) can reduce the intensity of postoperative shoulder pain after laparoscopic cholecystectomy. It can also reduce the incidence of PONV, shorten the time to the first standing position, and improve sleep quality during the first postoperative night. However, no superiority was found when comparing the two gabapentinoids.

Gabapentin and pregabalin are known as antiepileptic drugs. However, they have other reported uses due to their analgesic and anxiolytic effects [5, 10, 11]. They have comparable pharmacokinetic characteristics. The half-life of elimination is around 6 to 8 hours. The bioavailability is about 35 to 60% for gabapentin and 90% for pregabalin. Peak plasma concentration is reached in less than 2 hours for gabapentin versus 30 to 120 min for pregabalin [9, 12].

Several studies have shown the effect of gabapentinoids use as anesthetic adjuvant in the reduction of postoperative pain and analgesic requirements [7, 9, 10, 13–17]. Main studied surgeries were laparoscopic cholecystectomy, hysterectomy, mastectomy, and tonsillectomy. A low dose ranging from 600 to 1200 mg of gabapentin and from 150 to 300 mg of pregabalin was used in these trials without any reported significant adverse effect [18–20].

Although a single preemptive administration was the most prescribed modality, other studies kept the treatment for 2 to 5 days postoperatively. The meta-analysis of Lam et al. including 74 protocols of pregabalin use in different surgeries did not found any significant difference in postoperative pain reduction when comparing a single preemptive administration to an extended postoperative administration. When comparing different gabapentinoids drugs especially for laparoscopic cholecystectomy, findings are in favour of pregabalin [21].

Mishra et al. compared 150 mg of pregabalin to 900 mg of gabapentin in postoperative pain after laparoscopic cholecystectomy. Pain intensity and analgesic requirements were significantly lower in the pregabalin group at the expense of an increase in postoperative sedation [15]. Similar results were found by Eidy et al. by their clinical trial showing a significant decrease in postoperative pain and pethidine requirements in the pregabalin group compared to the gabapentin group [13].

Although analgesic effects of gabapentinoids are well described in postoperative pain, few data are available about the postoperative shoulder pain which is particularly frequent in post-laparoscopic surgery. It has a mechanical mechanism, as it is related to residual gas in the peritoneal cavity and it occurs mainly after patients' mobilization. Valadan et al. conducted a clinical trial enrolling 40 patients scheduled for laparoscopic ovarian surgery. After premedication with 600 mg of gabapentin, a significant decrease in the intensity of postoperative shoulder pain at rest and at exertion was noted up to the 12th hour postoperatively [8]. This analgesic effect was found with smaller dose of gabapentin (150 mg) in the study of Nutthachote et al. enrolling patients scheduled for laparoscopic gynecologic surgeries [22]. However, other studies showed different results [23]. For instance, the postoperative shoulder pain reduction due to preemptive premedication by gabapentinoids started at the 6th postoperative hour and reached more than 70% at the 12th postoperative hour. The same results were found for pain intensity following trocar insertion. In a systematic review analyzing 52 trials and enrolling 1774 patients, Tiippana et al. had evaluated the effect of preemptive gabapentin and pregabalin administration in postoperative pain after various surgical procedures. The postoperative pain intensity reduction started at the second postoperative hour [6].

Analgesic effects of gabapentinoids are due to their anxiolytic, antinociceptive, and opioid-like characteristics which are mainly explained by a central neural sensitization. Gabapentinoids have also an antihyperalgesic effect by their interaction with voltage-gated calcium channels of the spinal cord and the dorsal root ganglia [24]. Finally, a probable modulation of glutamate receptors by gabapentinoids has been reported [25].

By reducing postoperative pain, gabapentinoids seems to be interesting in inducing a quick postoperative rehabilitation allowing ambulatory practices after laparoscopic cholecystectomy.

However, the high incidence of nausea and vomiting after laparoscopic procedures must be considered before patient discharge as it compromises the oral intake. Various pharmacological treatments are usually used in the operating room for antiemetic purpose. Dexamethasone–ondansetron association is the most prescribed medication. Recently, several studies have evaluated the antiemetic effects of gabapentinoids with controversial results.

In a quantitative analysis of evidence from randomized controlled clinical trials, Achuthan et al. evaluated gabapentin prophylaxis for PONV in abdominal surgeries. Seventeen studies enrolling 1605 patients were analyzed. The incidence of nausea was reduced by 24% and the incidence of vomiting was reduced by 38% in the gabapentin group [26]. Ho et al. found similar results in a systematic review concluding to a lower incidence of PONV due to a preemptive gabapentin administration (RR 0.58; CI 95% 0.39–0.86) [19]. Gabapentinoids antiemetic properties are not well described. Several hypotheses have been reported such as a reduction of opioid requirements during and after anesthesia, a reduction of anesthetic gas consumption, and a reduction of tachykinin activity [27].

Finally, given analgesic and antiemetic properties of gabapentinoids, together with their sedative characteristics, an improvement in patients sleep quality especially during the first postoperative night was expected and evaluated in our study.

Lunn et al. evaluated analgesic and sedative effects of perioperative gabapentin in a double-blind trial enrolling patients scheduled for total knee replacement. Assessed by the Nonrestorative Sleep Scale (NRSS), the quality of sleep was better in the gabapentin group during the first two postoperative nights [28].

However, Eloy et al. found different results when they studied the effect of gabapentin on postoperative pain and sleep quality in patients undergoing total knee arthroplasty, total hip arthroplasty, or a hip fracture repair. Their findings indicate that gabapentin does not improve sleep quality assessed by the Pittsburg Sleep Quality Index. The small dose of gabapentin and the small study sample must be considered in results interpretation [29]. Assessed by Spiegel score, sleep quality in our study was better in gabapentinoids groups without significant difference between gabapentin and pregabalin.

Preemptive premedication with 600 mg of gabapentin or 150 mg of pregabalin improves several parameters of postoperative rehabilitation after laparoscopic cholecystectomy. It reduces significantly the intensity of postoperative shoulder pain, decreases the incidence of PONV, improves the quality of sleep during the first night, and shortens the time to first standing position. However, some limitations should be considered such as the nonevaluation of analgesic requirements during the postoperative period and the absence of the pharmacoeconomic component in our study.

5. Conclusion

Preemptive premedication with gabapentin or pregabalin before laparoscopic cholecystectomy can be interesting in postoperative rehabilitation allowing ambulatory practices. In fact, it can reduce postoperative shoulder pain and PONV incidence. It can also improve the sleep quality during the first postoperative night. However, the optimal doses of gabapentinoids and the duration of treatment are not yet well established.

References

[1] U. F. Teixeira, M. B. Goldoni, M. C. Machry, P. N. Ceccon, P. R. Fontes, and F. L. Waechter, "Ambulatory laparoscopic cholecystectomy is safe and cost-effective: a Brazilian single center experience," *Arquivos de Gastroenterologia*, vol. 53, no. 2, pp. 103–107, 2016.

[2] J. Bueno Lledó, P. Granero Castro, I. Gomez et al., "Twenty-five years of ambulatory laparoscopic cholecystectomy," *Cirugía Española*, vol. 94, no. 8, pp. 429–441, 2016.

[3] M. Jiménez Fuertes and D. Costa Navarro, "Outpatient laparoscopic cholecystectomy and pain control: a series of 100 cases," *Cirugía Española*, vol. 93, no. 3, pp. 181–186, 2015.

[4] C. Zhou, Y. Zhu, Z. Liu, and L. Ruan, "5HT3 antagonists versus dexamethasone in the prevention of PONV in patients undergoing laparoscopic cholecystectomy: a meta-analysis of RCTs," *Biomed Research International*, vol. 2016, Article ID 8603409, 7 pages, 2016.

[5] D. Moulin, A. Boulanger, A. J. Clark et al., "Pharmacological management of chronic neuropathic pain: revised consensus statement from the Canadian Pain Society," *Pain Research and Management*, vol. 19, no. 6, pp. 328–335, 2014.

[6] E. M. Tiippana, K. Hamunen, V. K. Kontinen, and E. Kalso, "Do surgical patients benefit from perioperative gabapentin/pregabalin? A systematic review of efficacy and safety," *Anesthesia and Analgesia*, vol. 104, no. 6, pp. 1545–1556, 2007.

[7] A. Agarwal, S. Gautam, D. Gupta, S. Agarwal, P. K. Singh, and U. Singh, "Evaluation of a single preoperative dose of pregabalin for attenuation of postoperative pain after laparoscopic cholecystectomy," *British Journal of Anaesthesia*, vol. 101, no. 5, pp. 700–704, 2008.

[8] M. Valadan, S. Banifatemi, and F. Yousefshahi, "Preoperative gabapentin to prevent postoperative shoulder pain after laparoscopic ovarian cystectomy: a randomized clinical trial," *Anesthesiology and Pain Medicine*, vol. 5, no. 6, article e31524, 2015.

[9] C. Y. Chang, C. K. Challa, J. Shah, and J. D. Eloy, "Gabapentin in acute postoperative pain management," *BioMed Research International*, vol. 2014, Article ID 631756, 7 pages, 2014.

[10] H. Clarke, S. Pereira, D. Kennedy et al., "Gabapentin decreases morphine consumption and improves functional recovery following total knee arthroplasty," *Pain Research and Management*, vol. 14, no. 3, pp. 217–222, 2009.

[11] F. Imani and P. Rahimzadeh, "Gabapentinoids: gabapentin and pregabalin for postoperative pain management," *Anesthesiology and Pain Medicine*, vol. 2, no. 2, pp. 52-53, 2012.

[12] A. Ghai, M. Gupta, S. Hooda, D. Singla, and R. Wadhera, "A randomized controlled trial to compare pregabalin with gabapentin for postoperative pain in abdominal hysterectomy," *Saudi Journal of Anaesthesia*, vol. 5, no. 3, pp. 252–257, 2011.

[13] M. Eidy, M. R. Fazel, H. Abdolrahimzadeh, A. R. Moravveji, E. Kochaki, and M. Mohammadzadeh, "Effects of pregabalin and gabapentin on postoperative pain and opioid consumption after laparoscopic cholecystectomy," *Korean Journal of Anesthesiology*, vol. 70, no. 4, pp. 434–438, 2017.

[14] P. Gupta, A. Saxena, and L. Chaudhary, "Effect of pregabalin premedication on the requirement of anesthetic and analgesic drugs in laparoscopic cholecystectomy: randomized comparison of two doses," *Anesthesia: Essays and Researches*, vol. 11, no. 1, pp. 330–333, 2017.

[15] R. Mishra, M. Tripathi, and H. C. Chandola, "Comparative clinical study of gabapentin and pregabalin for postoperative analgesia in laparoscopic cholecystectomy," *Anesthesia: Essays and Researches*, vol. 10, no. 2, pp. 201–206, 2016.

[16] F. Frouzanfard, M. R. Fazel, A. Abolhasani, E. Fakharian, G. Mousavi, and A. Moravveji, "Effects of gabapentin on pain and opioid consumption after abdominal hysterectomy," *Pain Research and Management*, vol. 18, no. 2, pp. 94–96, 2013.

[17] A. Yeganeh Mogadam, M. R. Fazel, and S. Parviz, "Comparison of analgesic effect between gabapentin and diclofenac

on post-operative pain in patients undergoing tonsillectomy," *Archives of Trauma Research*, vol. 1, no. 3, pp. 108–111, 2012.
[18] R. W. Hurley, S. P. Cohen, K. A. Williams, A. J. Rowlingson, and C. L. Wu, "The analgesic effects of perioperative gabapentin on postoperative pain: a meta-analysis," *Regional Anesthesia and Pain Medicine*, vol. 31, no. 3, pp. 237–247, 2006.
[19] K. Y. Ho, T. J. Gan, and A. S. Habib, "Gabapentin and postoperative pain-a systematic review of randomized controlled trials," *Pain*, vol. 126, no. 1, pp. 91–101, 2006.
[20] R. K. Seib and J. E. Paul, "Preoperative gabapentin for postoperative analgesia: a meta-analysis," *Canadian Journal of Anesthesia*, vol. 53, no. 5, pp. 461–469, 2006.
[21] D. M. Lam, S. W. Choi, S. S. Wong, M. G. Irwin, and C. W. Cheung, "Efficacy of pregabalin in acute postoperative pain under different surgical categories: a meta-analysis," *Medicine*, vol. 94, no. 46, article e1944, 2015.
[22] P. Nutthachote, P. Sirayapiwat, W. Wisawasukmongchol, and S. Charuluxananan, "A randomized, double-blind, placebo-controlled trial of oral pregabalin for relief of shoulder pain after laparoscopic gynecologic surgery," *Journal of Minimally Invasive Gynecology*, vol. 21, no. 4, pp. 669–673, 2014.
[23] S. H. Chang, H. W. Lee, H. K. Kim, S. H. Kim, and D. K. Kim, "An evaluation of perioperative pregabalin for prevention and attenuation of postoperative shoulder pain after laparoscopic cholecystectomy," *Anesthesia and Analgesia*, vol. 109, no. 4, pp. 1284–1286, 2009.
[24] D. McClelland, R. M. Evans, L. Barkworth, D. J. Martin, and R. H. Scott, "A study comparing the actions of gabapentin and pregabalin on the electrophysiological properties of cultured DRG neurones from neonatal rats," *BMC Pharmacology*, vol. 4, no. 1, p. 14, 2004.
[25] N. M. Doha, A. Rady, and S. R. El Azab, "Preoperative use of gabapentin decreases the anesthetic and analgesic requirements in patients undergoing radical mastectomy," *Egyptian Journal of Anaesthesia*, vol. 26, no. 4, pp. 287–291, 2010.
[26] S. Achuthan, I. Singh, S. B. Varthya, A. Srinivasan, A. Chakrabarti, and D. Hota, "Gabapentin prophylaxis for postoperative nausea and vomiting in abdominal surgeries: a quantitative analysis of evidence from randomized controlled clinical trials," *British Journal of Anaesthesia*, vol. 114, no. 4, pp. 588–597, 2015.
[27] V. K. F. Kong and M. G. Irwin, "Gabapentin: a multimodal perioperative drug?," *British Journal of Anaesthesia*, vol. 99, no. 6, pp. 775–786, 2007.
[28] T. H. Lunn, H. Husted, M. B. Laursen, L. T. Hansen, and H. Kehlet, "Analgesic and sedative effects of perioperative gabapentin in total knee arthroplasty: a randomized, double-blind, placebo-controlled dose-finding study," *Pain*, vol. 156, no. 12, pp. 2438–2448, 2015.
[29] J. D. Eloy, C. Anthony, S. Amin, M. Caparó, M. C. Reilly, and S. Shulman, "Gabapentin does not appear to improve postoperative pain and sleep patterns in patients who concomitantly receive regional anesthesia for lower extremity orthopedic surgery: a randomized control trial," *Pain Research and Management*, vol. 2017, Article ID 2310382, 5 pages, 2017.

Changes in Pain Perception following Psychotherapy: The Mediating Role of Psychological Components

Susanna Zanini,[1] Alessandra Voltolini,[1] Gaia Gragnano,[2] Emilia Fumagalli,[1] and Francesco Pagnini[2,3]

[1]Clinical Psychology Service, ASST Grande Ospedale Metropolitano Niguarda, Piazza Dell'Ospedale Maggiore 3, 20162 Milan, Italy
[2]Department of Psychology, Università Cattolica del Sacro Cuore, Largo Agostino Gemelli 1, 20123 Milan, Italy
[3]Department of Psychology, Harvard University, 33 Kirkland Street, Cambridge, MA 02138, USA

Correspondence should be addressed to Francesco Pagnini; francesco.pagnini@unicatt.it

Academic Editor: Michihiro Osumi

Chronic pain is frequently associated with significant psychological issues, such as depression or anxiety. Psychological treatments, such as psychotherapy, can often alleviate both psychological and pain symptoms. However, there is limited research about the association between psychological symptoms and perceived pain in the context of psychotherapeutic interventions. We conducted a retrospective study that analyzed, in a hospital context, how changes in psychological functioning and well-being were associated with pain reduction. Thirty-seven records of patients with chronic pain attending psychotherapy in a public hospital were included. All patients were assessed before psychotherapy, as well as after 6 and 10 months, with self-reported questionnaires about pain, anxiety, depression, and psychological functioning. Results indicate that reductions in anxiety, depression, psychological problems, risk factors, and well-being are strongly related with a reduction in pain, further confirming the hypothesis that psychological morbidity is associated with pain severity.

1. Introduction

Pain is an unpleasant and distressing feeling that is often caused by an intense or damaging stimulus [1]. While pain is influenced by the stimulus intensity, it is also connected to cognitive and emotional factors, which can modulate the painful experience [2]. Therefore, similar painful stimuli may lead to different experiences among the individuals, on the base of contexts and psychological characteristics [3]. Considering the importance of the cognitive and emotional components in the experience of pain, psychological interventions, such as psychotherapy, could play an important role in pain rehabilitation and management [4].

Reactive psychological symptoms, such as depression and anxiety, may have an important role in the exacerbation of pain perception [5]. For example, de Heer and colleagues [6] have found, over a large sample of people with chronic pain, that depressive and anxiety disorders were associated with increased pain-related disability. This association with depression and anxiety remains stable over time [7, 8]. It has also been suggested that depression and pain may share similar neuroplastic changes in the central nervous system [9], which would explain the positive impact of antidepressants on the pain symptomatology [10]. Similarly, in the framework of a randomized controlled trial, the reduction of depression following an online cognitive-behavioral intervention was associated with pain decrease [11].

Psychosocial pain treatments, including psychotherapy, proved to be effective in reducing pain and promoting increased quality of life [12]. Most research, as it is often the case in clinical psychology, has been conducted in *true-experiment settings*, providing high internal validity for the results, but not necessarily generalizing to the actual clinical contexts. For this reason, we planned a study that analyses

Table 1: Sample characteristics.

N	37
Sex (N, %)	Male: 13 (35.13%) Female: 24 (64.87%)
Age (mean, SD)	58.32 (13.26)
Disease (N, %)	Rheumatological conditions: 11 (29.72%) Nephrological conditions: 11 (29.72%) Nononcological chronic pain: 15 (40.54%)
Marital status (N, %)	Never married: 5 (13.51%) Married: 23 (62.16%) Divorced: 3 (8.1%) Widowed: 6 (16.21%)
Education (N, %)	Elementary school: 8 (21.62%) Middle school: 5 (13.51%) High school: 17 (45.94%) Degree: 7 (19.91%)
Job (N, %)	Office worker: 8 (21.62%) Factory worker: 4 (10.81%) Professional: 6 (16.21%) Educator/teacher: 5 (13.51%) Health professionals: 2 (5.4%) Retired: 8 (24.32%) Unemployed: 3 (8.1%)
Treatment (N, %)	Individual sessions: 29 (78.37%) Group sessions: 8 (21.62%)

data from a hospital setting. We aimed at verifying whether the hypothesis of an association between psychological symptoms and perceived pain would be confirmed in the mainframe of psychotherapeutic interventions.

2. Materials and Methods

We conducted a retrospective cohort study based on medical records collected by the Service of Psychology at ASST Grande Ospedale Metropolitano Niguarda. Specifically, we selected the requests for pain management that involved a psychotherapeutic intervention. Medical records included psychological questionnaires about pain, anxiety, depression, and psychological morbidity.

We selected all the records that met the following criteria: outpatients with chronic, nononcological pain treated at Rheumatology, Pain Service, or Nephrology units at Niguarda Ca' Granda Hospital in Milan; who successfully attended a psychotherapeutic intervention with either Susanna Zanini or Alessandra Voltolini; with a defined chronic pain diagnosis for more than 3 months; and who were 18 or older. To access the service, patients provided informed consent about the fact that their data could be used for scientific analysis, resulting in publication only in aggregated forms.

All patients ($n = 37$) were assessed before beginning psychotherapy (first ambulatory session) and after 6 and 10 months.

The records included the following scales:

(i) *QUID*: Italian pain questionnaire [13], which is a self-report instrument assessing pain characteristics. It includes a semantic interval scale consisting of 42 pain descriptors and is divided into four main classes: sensory, affective, evaluative, and mixed. The items can be combined together to provide a total pain score.

(ii) *HADS*: Hospital Anxiety and Depression Scale [14] for the assessment of anxiety and depression in hospitalized patients. The scale does not include items that refer to physical aspects of anxiety and depression, and it is widely used in the hospital setting.

(iii) *CORE-OM*: Clinical Outcomes in Routine Evaluation-Outcome Measure [15] for the assessment of psychological distress. It is a widely used scale with adequate reliability (α 0.75–0.95) developed to evaluate the outcome of psychological therapy. The questionnaire is composed of four subscales: functioning, problems, well-being, and risks. Item scores range from 0 to 4 (higher scores indicate more distress).

2.1. Interventions. The psychotherapeutic interventions were conducted by two experienced psychotherapists (Susanna Zanini; Alessandra Voltolini), either in individual or group settings, on the base of patients' needs. The average duration of the treatments was 10 months. The two psychotherapists were trained in cognitive-behavioral therapy (CBT; Alessandra Voltolini) [16] and short-term integrated therapy (Susanna Zanini) [17, 18].

CBT is generally based on the "A-B-C" (Antecedent-Belief-Consequence) model and aims at changing dysfunctional thoughts, emotions, and behaviors [19]. Some of the strategies promoted by CBT are problem solving, decision-making, scheduling, relaxation techniques, mindfulness training, role-playing, and others. The short-term, focus-based, integrated psychotherapy includes different therapeutic theories and techniques: a short psychoanalytic model, the cognitive-behavioral model, and the developmental model, which include life-cycle theories and findings from resilience researches [17]. The integration among different models allows the selection of the therapeutic strategy that best fit to every specific patient, according to his/her needs. Moreover, it allows to combine together techniques from different approaches or to use them sequentially [20].

2.2. Analysis. The mediation effect that resilience could exert on pain over the course of psychotherapy was explored with linear mixed models [21]. Time points were formatted as time variant to consider changes over time, and the random effect was used to account for intrasubject variability. We referred to an autoregressive (AR1) covariance matrix with heterogeneous variances across different assessments (this matrix provided better fit indexes than the "unstructured" covariance matrix) [22]. We followed the same procedure to analyze the effects of resilience on anxiety and depression. Linear mixed models were also used to explore repeated measures trends. Bonferroni correction was used

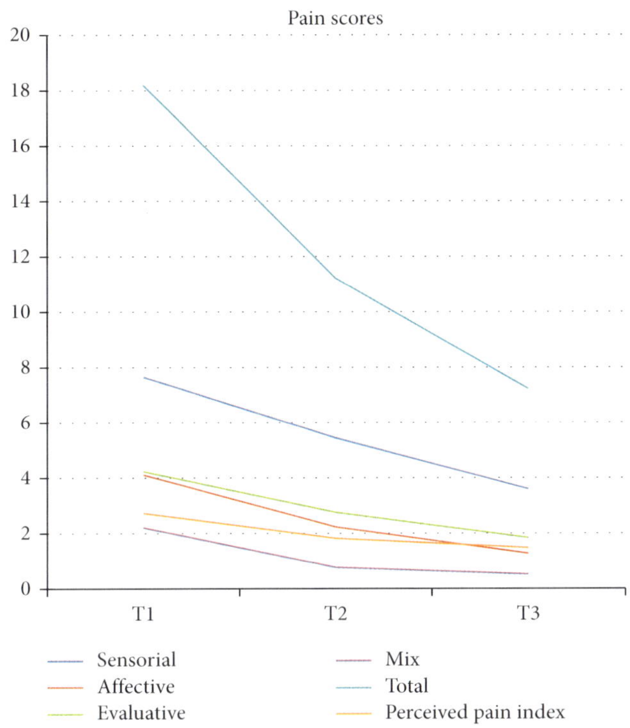

Figure 1: Time changes in pain scores.

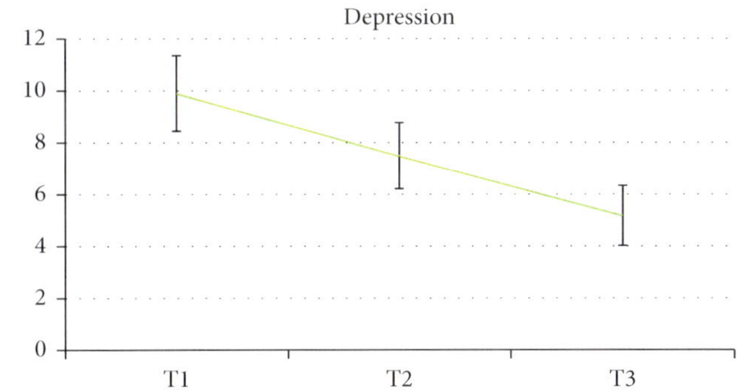

Figure 2: Time changes in depression scores.

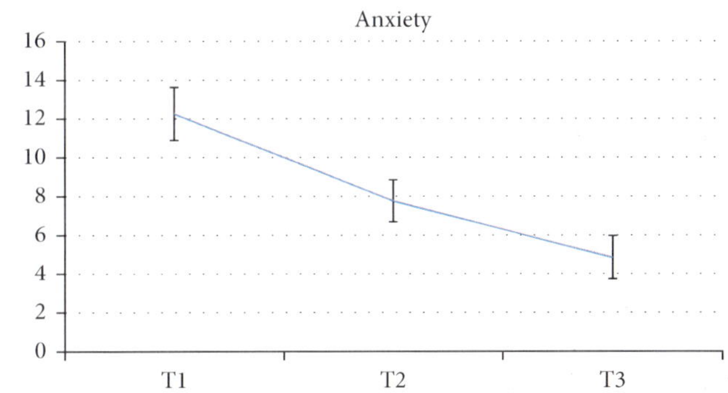

Figure 3: Time changes in anxiety scores.

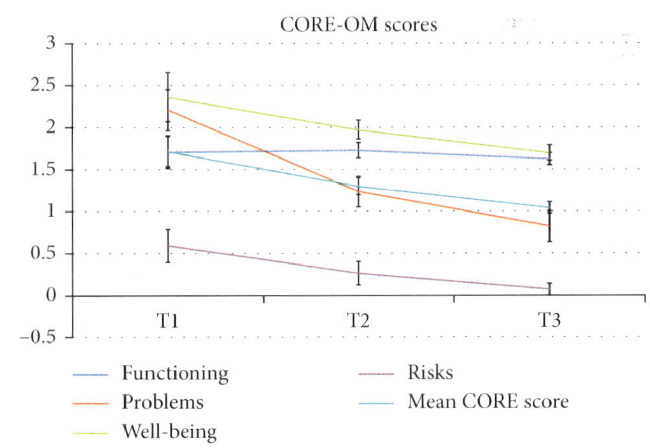

Figure 4: Time changes in the CORE-OM scores.

to account for multiple analyses. Data were analyzed with SPSS software.

3. Results and Discussion

Table 1 reports the descriptive statistics of the sample, including demographic and clinical data.

In time, there was a significant reducing trend among the three assessment times for pain and pain subscales ($p < 0.001$), anxiety ($p < 0.001$), and depression ($p < 0.001$). All CORE-OM scales showed significant reductions ($p < 0.001$ for all), with the only exception of functioning, which remained stable over time ($F(2, 42.580) = 1.880$, $p = 0.165$). Time trends are reported in Figures 1–4.

Results from linear mixed models indicate that changes in both anxiety and depression strongly predicted total pain scores and specific pain components. All the subscales from the CORE-OM, with the exclusion of functioning, successfully predicted QUID scores, including both the total and the subscales. Beta scores, significance, and confidence intervals are detailed in Table 2.

As expected, we found strong correlations between psychological aspects and pain perceptions. Both pain and psychological morbidity significantly decreased over time. That is not surprising, as participants were all in psychotherapy and also treated for pain management in the hospital setting. The reduction of psychological symptoms, including anxiety and depression, resulted in association with pain reduction in all the assessed components. Interestingly, the scale functioning of the CORE-OM, which refer to general, interpersonal, and social functioning, did not result in association with pain. Accounting for this exception, our data draw a clear picture of strong associations between the psychological domains and the chronic pain experience. Results are in line with the previous research [23], and extend the association, sometimes found in controlled studies, in a natural setting (i.e., hospital).

The retrospective and observational nature of the study does not allow making a causal inference. In particular, the lack of a control group does not allow us to state that psychotherapy is what has brought to a reduction of the "negative" outcomes. From the perspective that we can honestly have with this study, we can observe and document

Table 2: Linear mixed modeling.

	Total QUID			Sensorial			Affective			Evaluative			Mix		
	β	p	95% CI	β	p	95% CI	β	p	95% CI	β	p	95% CI	β	p	95% CI
Anxiety	1.092	0.000	0.789 to 1.396	0.400	0.000	0.264 to 0.536	0.257	0.000	0.184 to 0.331	0.231	0.000	0.137 to 0.324	0.178	0.000	0.126 to 0.229
Depression	1.051	0.000	0.621 to 1.481	0.350	0.003	0.135 to 0.566	0.228	0.004	0.116 to 0.339	0.276	0.000	0.153 to 0.400	0.181	0.000	0.115 to 0.245
Functioning	1.191	0.630	−3.714 to 6.096	0.582	0.506	−1.541 to 2.706	0.177	0.804	−1.366 to 1.720	0.814	0.223	−0.5102 to 2.139	−0.144	0.769	−1.193 to 0.904
Problems	6.158	0.000	4.661 to 6.656	2.168	0.000	1.500 to 2.837	1.537	0.001	0.951 to 2.123	1.485	0.000	0.974 to 1.996	1.027	0.000	0.714 to 1.340
Well-being	6.287	0.000	3.552 to 9.022	2.469	0.000	1.261 to 3.676	1.162	0.005	0.382 to 1.941	1.615	0.000	0.857 to 2.373	0.882	0.000	0.423 to 1.340
Risks	12.961	0.002	8.525 to 17.398	4.769	0.000	3.214 to 6.324	3.115	0.000	2.109 to 4.121	2.480	0.001	1.407 to 3.553	1.840	0.000	1.187 to 2.493

Note. QUID: Italian questionnaire of pain.

the neat associations that anxiety, depression, psychological problems, risk factors, and well-being have with pain in all the assessed facets.

4. Conclusions

In a hospital setting, archives from outpatients with chronic pain attending psychotherapy and regular pain management were analyzed for associations between psychological factors and pain reduction. Results from this naturalistic setting indicate an association between psychological morbidity and pain severity.

References

[1] H. Merskey, "Pain terms: a list with definitions and notes on usage. Recommended by the IASP subcommittee on taxonomy," *Pain*, vol. 6, pp. 249–252, 1979.

[2] C. Villemure and C. M. Bushnell, "Cognitive modulation of pain: how do attention and emotion influence pain processing?," *Pain*, vol. 95, no. 3, pp. 195–199, 2002.

[3] A. L. Burke, J. L. Mathias, and L. A. Denson, "Psychological functioning of people living with chronic pain: a meta-analytic review," *British Journal of Clinical Psychology*, vol. 54, no. 3, pp. 345–360, 2015.

[4] R. R. Edwards, R. H. Dworkin, M. D. Sullivan, D. C. Turk, and A. D. Wasan, "The role of psychosocial processes in the development and maintenance of chronic pain," *Journal of Pain*, vol. 17, no. 9, pp. T70–T92, 2016.

[5] A. K. Woo, "Depression and anxiety in pain," *Reviews in Pain*, vol. 4, no. 1, pp. 8–12, 2010.

[6] E. W. de Heer, M. M. J. G. Gerrits, A. T. F. Beekman et al., "The association of depression and anxiety with pain: a study from NESDA," *PloS One*, vol. 9, no. 10, article e106907, 2014.

[7] M. M. Gerrits, H. W. J. van Marwijk, P. van Oppen, H. van der Horst, and B. W. J. H. Penninx, "Longitudinal association between pain, and depression and anxiety over four years," *Journal of Psychosomatic Research*, vol. 78, no. 1, pp. 64–70, 2015.

[8] M. M. Gerrits, P. van Oppen, S. S. Leone, H. W. J. van Marwijk, H. E. van der Horst, and B. W. Penninx, "Pain, not chronic disease, is associated with the recurrence of depressive and anxiety disorders," *BMC Psychiatry*, vol. 14, no. 1, p. 187, 2014.

[9] T. Nekovarova, A. Yamamotova, K. Vales, A. Stuchlik, J. Fricova, and R. Rokyta, "Common mechanisms of pain and depression: are antidepressants also analgesics?," *Frontiers in Behavioral Neuroscience*, vol. 8, p. 99, 2014.

[10] N. B. Finnerup, N. Attal, S. Haroutounian et al., "Pharmacotherapy for neuropathic pain in adults: a systematic review and meta-analysis," *Lancet Neurology*, vol. 14, no. 2, pp. 162–173, 2015.

[11] M. Buhrman, M. Syk, O. Burvall, T. Hartig, T. Gordh, and G. Andersson, "Individualized guided Internet-delivered cognitive-behavior therapy for chronic pain patients with comorbid depression and anxiety: a randomized controlled trial," *Clinical Journal of Pain*, vol. 31, no. 6, pp. 504–516, 2015.

[12] M. A. Day, D. M. Ehde, and M. P. Jensen, "Psychosocial pain management moderation: the limit, activate, and enhance model," *Journal of Pain*, vol. 16, no. 10, pp. 947–960, 2015.

[13] G. De Benedittis, R. Massel, R. Nobili, and A. Pieri, "The Italian pain questionnaire," *Pain*, vol. 33, no. 1, pp. 53–62, 1988.

[14] A. S. Zigmond and R. P. Snaith, "The hospital anxiety and depression scale," *Acta Psychiatrica Scandinavica*, vol. 67, no. 6, pp. 361–370, 1983.

[15] J. M. C. Evans, F. Margison, M. Barkham, K. Audin, J. Connell, and G. McGrath, "CORE: clinical outcomes in routine evaluation," *Journal of Mental Health*, vol. 9, no. 3, pp. 247–255, 2000.

[16] J. S. Beck, "Cognitive-behavioral therapy," in *Clinical Textbook of Addictive Disorders*, pp. 474–501, Guilford Press, New York, NY, USA, 2011.

[17] F. Pagnini, S. Zanini, and M. C. Gislon, "Patient's needs and psychotherapy integration," *International Journal of Psychotherapy*, vol. 17, no. 3, pp. 20–23, 2013.

[18] G. C. Zapparoli, "An integrative approach to severe emotional disorders," *Psychoanalytic Psychotherapy*, vol. 13, no. 1, pp. 19–30, 1999.

[19] R. Dudley and W. Kuyken, "Formulation in cognitive-behavioural therapy," in *Formulation in Psychology and*

Psychotherapy; Making Sense of People's Problems, Routledge, Abingdon, UK, 2006.

[20] G. C. Zapparoli, "Resistance to change in the psychotic patient," *Psychoanalytic Psychotherapy*, vol. 13, no. 1, pp. 31–40, 1999.

[21] A. Field, *Discovering Statistics using IBM SPSS Statistics*, Sage, London, UK, 2013.

[22] R. H. Heck, S. L. Thomas, and L. N. Tabata, *Multilevel and Longitudinal Modeling with IBM SPSS*, Routledge, Abingdon, UK, 2013.

[23] G. Castelnuovo, E. M. Giusti, G. M. Manzoni et al., "Psychological considerations in the assessment and treatment of pain in neurorehabilitation and psychological factors predictive of therapeutic response: evidence and recommendations from the Italian consensus conference on pain in neurorehabilitation," *Frontiers in Psychology*, vol. 7, 2016.

30

Medicinal Plants of the Family Lamiaceae in Pain Therapy

Cristina M. Uritu,[1] Cosmin T. Mihai,[1] Gabriela-Dumitrita Stanciu,[1] Gianina Dodi,[1] Teodora Alexa-Stratulat,[1] Andrei Luca,[1] Maria-Magdalena Leon-Constantin,[1] Raluca Stefanescu,[1] Veronica Bild,[1] Silvia Melnic,[2] and Bogdan I. Tamba[1]

[1]*"Grigore T. Popa" University of Medicine and Pharmacy, 700115 Iasi, Romania*
[2]*Institute of Chemistry, Academy of Sciences of Moldova, MD-2028 Chisinau, Moldova*

Correspondence should be addressed to Silvia Melnic; silmel_sm@yahoo.com

Academic Editor: Gokhan Zengin

Recently, numerous side effects of synthetic drugs have lead to using medicinal plants as a reliable source of new therapy. Pain is a global public health problem with a high impact on life quality and a huge economic implication, becoming one of the most important enemies in modern medicine. The medicinal use of plants as analgesic or antinociceptive drugs in traditional therapy is estimated to be about 80% of the world population. The Lamiaceae family, one of the most important herbal families, incorporates a wide variety of plants with biological and medical applications. In this study, the analgesic activity, possible active compounds of Lamiaceae genus, and also the possible mechanism of actions of these plants are presented. The data highlighted in this review paper provide valuable scientific information for the specific implications of Lamiaceae plants in pain modulation that might be used for isolation of potentially active compounds from some of these medicinal plants in future and formulation of commercial therapeutic agents.

1. Introduction

Pain comes in many forms: acute, chronic, visceral, inflammatory, or neuropathic [1, 2]. It is not simply a result of tissue damage but also reflects the influence of many psychological variables such as attention, anxiety, stress [3], suggestion, or previous experiences and may have a significant genetic contribution [4]. Pain accompanies most pathologies present in current medical practice, and 25% percent of Americans, for example, experience pain on a daily basis. Having the numbers on its side, pain became a global public health problem and a leading cause of disability all over the world [5].

As life expectancy is rising and chronical pathologies along with it, the prevalence of accompanying pain is expected to increase yearly, with higher prevalence in elderly patients, where the treatment is also more sensitive [6, 7]. Considering the above, new therapeutic agents with increased efficacy, less side effects, and lower costs and leading to an improved quality of life [8–11] should become one of the primary objectives in modern medical research, together with constant monitoring [12] of the previous mentioned aspects.

The medicinal use of plants as analgesic drugs in folk medicine is an ancient tradition, far older than the current sciences of medicine in developing countries [13, 14]. According to estimations, up to 70,000 plant species are used ethnomedicinally worldwide. Effects of herbal extracts have been studied by different pain tests including writhing test, light tail flick test, tail immersion test, hot-plate test, and formalin test [15].

The exploration for new analgesic combinations from the enormous arrays of medicinal plant resources is growing. This is because such information holds guarantees for the finding of new therapeutic agents capable of inhibiting, decreasing, or relieving pain [16–28]. Plants characterize a vast natural supply of appreciated compounds that might achieve primary importance for the expansion of novel drugs [29]. The survey of the effectiveness of plant-based remedies used in the folk medicine has given great reflections because they are cheap and have reduced side effects.

According to the World Health Organization (WHO), about 80% of the world population still relies mainly on plant-based drugs [30], thus lowering at the same time the impact of self-medication side effects [6]. The data in biomedical literature presenting plants with medicinal capabilities are very similar to the array of publications depicting the modulatory effects certain ones have over pain perception.

The Lamiaceae family, one of the most important herbal families, incorporates a wide variety of plants with biological and medical applications. The most known members of this family are a variety of aromatic spices like thyme, mint, oregano, basil, sage, savory, rosemary, self-heal, hyssop, lemon balm, and some others with more limited use [31].

Our main objective was to perform a review of this literature for the specific implications of Lamiaceae family plants in pain modulation and thus aid the constant search for new potential agents of natural origin with analgesic effects.

2. Materials and Methods

The search strategy employed in this review includes internationally accepted databases, namely, ScienceDirect, Scopus, Web of Science, and PubMed, using specific keywords of both whole plant products and plant extracts, pain, and analgesic and antinociceptive effects. For investigation, a combination of keywords was used [pain; analgesic; antinociceptive; plant extract] + [*Betonica officinalis*; *Glechoma hederacea*; *Hyptis pectinata*; *Lavandula*; *Leonurus cardiaca*; *Lamium*; *Melissa officinalis*; *Mentha*; *Marrubium vulgare*; *Origanum*; *Ocimum*; *Rosmarinus officinalis*; *Salvia*;*Satureja hortensis*; *Stachys lavandulifolia*; *Scutellaria lateriflora*; *Sideritis*; *Teucrium*; *Thymus*; *Ziziphora tenuior*] + [Lamiaceae; botanical genus]. Case reports, case studies, *in vivo* and *in vitro* relevant studies, and comparative studies were included in this search strategy. Additionally, text books and potentially relevant reviews were explored and included in the reference list. The literature search was confined to the period between 2003 and December 2017. Several articles before 2000 were also included in order to point out the universal interest in natural products with potential applicability in therapy. The dynamic character of the field is reflected in the number of recent publications. For example, a search with the keywords "Lamiaceae family and pain" in ScienceDirect yields 152 titles in 2015, 111 in 2016, and 129 in 2017, and 23 papers will be published in the first months of the next year (Figure 1).

3. Species of the Lamiaceae Family with Potential Analgesic/Antinociceptive Effects

3.1. Rosmarinus Genus. *Rosmarinus* in the Lamiaceae family is a genus of woody, perennial herbs with fragrant evergreen needle-like leaves that is native to the Mediterranean Basin.

3.1.1. Rosmarinus officinalis. *Rosmarinus officinalis* L., commonly called rosemary, is a Mediterranean shrubby herb and widely spread in European, American, and Asian countries. It is a common spice used worldwide for culinary, medicinal, and commercial uses, including the fragrance and food industries [32]. The leaves of rosemary (fresh or dries) are used for their characteristic aroma in cooking or consumed in small amounts as herbal tea, while rosemary extracts are regularly used for their natural antioxidant active proprieties to improve the shelf life of perishable foods. Recently, rosemary extracts (E392) have been approved as a safe and effective natural antioxidant for food preservation by the European Union [33].

Phytochemical studies have revealed that leaves contain 0.5% to 2.5% volatile oil. The major components of rosemary oil include monoterpene hydrocarbons (alpha and beta-pinene), camphene, limonene, camphor (10% to 20%), borneol, cineole, linalool, and verbinol. Rosemary contains a widespread variety of volatile and aromatic components. Flavonoids in the plant consist of diosmetin, diosmin, genkwanin, luteolin, hispidulin, and apigenin [34–41]. Additionally, terpenoid components from rosemary consist of the triterpenes oleanolic and ursolic acid and the diterpene carnosol. Phenols in rosemary comprise caffeic, chlorogenic, labiatic, neochlorogenic, and rosmarinic acids. Rosemary covers high amounts of salicylates [42–48].

Modern pharmacological studies have indicated that rosemary and its constituents, especially caffeic acid derivatives such as rosmarinic acid, have various traditional uses in ethnomedicine including analgesic, anti-inflammatory, anticarcinogenic, antirheumatic, spasmolytic, antihepatotoxic, atheroscl erotic, carminative, and choleretic applications [44–54], protection against UV and gamma radiation, and amelioration of stress [43].

The powdered leaves are used as an effective natural flea and tick repellent. Activity against certain bacteria including *Staphylcoccus aureus*, *Staphylococcus albus*, *Vibrio cholerae*, *Escherichia coli*, and *Corynebacterium* has been observed. One study found that rosemary oil is most active against "meat spoiling" Gram-negative (*Pseudomonas*) and Gram-positive (*Lactobacillus*) bacteria [49].

Even though rosemary oil is used safely as a food flavoring spice and whole leaves are used as a potherb for seasoning, ingestion of great quantities can be associated with toxicity characterized by stomach and intestinal irritation and kidney damage. While rosemary oil is irritating to rabbit skin, it is not usually considered to be a sensitizer for human skin [55].

Bioactive compounds such as flavonoids, diterpenes, phenols, and triterpenes from plant sources have been traditionally extracted by a conventional solid-liquid extraction. Nevertheless, this extraction technique presents several disadvantages, mainly because it is an arduous, time-consuming process that requires a high consumption of solvents, and in some cases provides low recovery. For that reason, in last years, new promising extraction methods are arising, which introduce some form of additional energy in order to facilitate the transfer of solutes from the sample to solvent in a faster process [54]. Thus, microwave-assisted

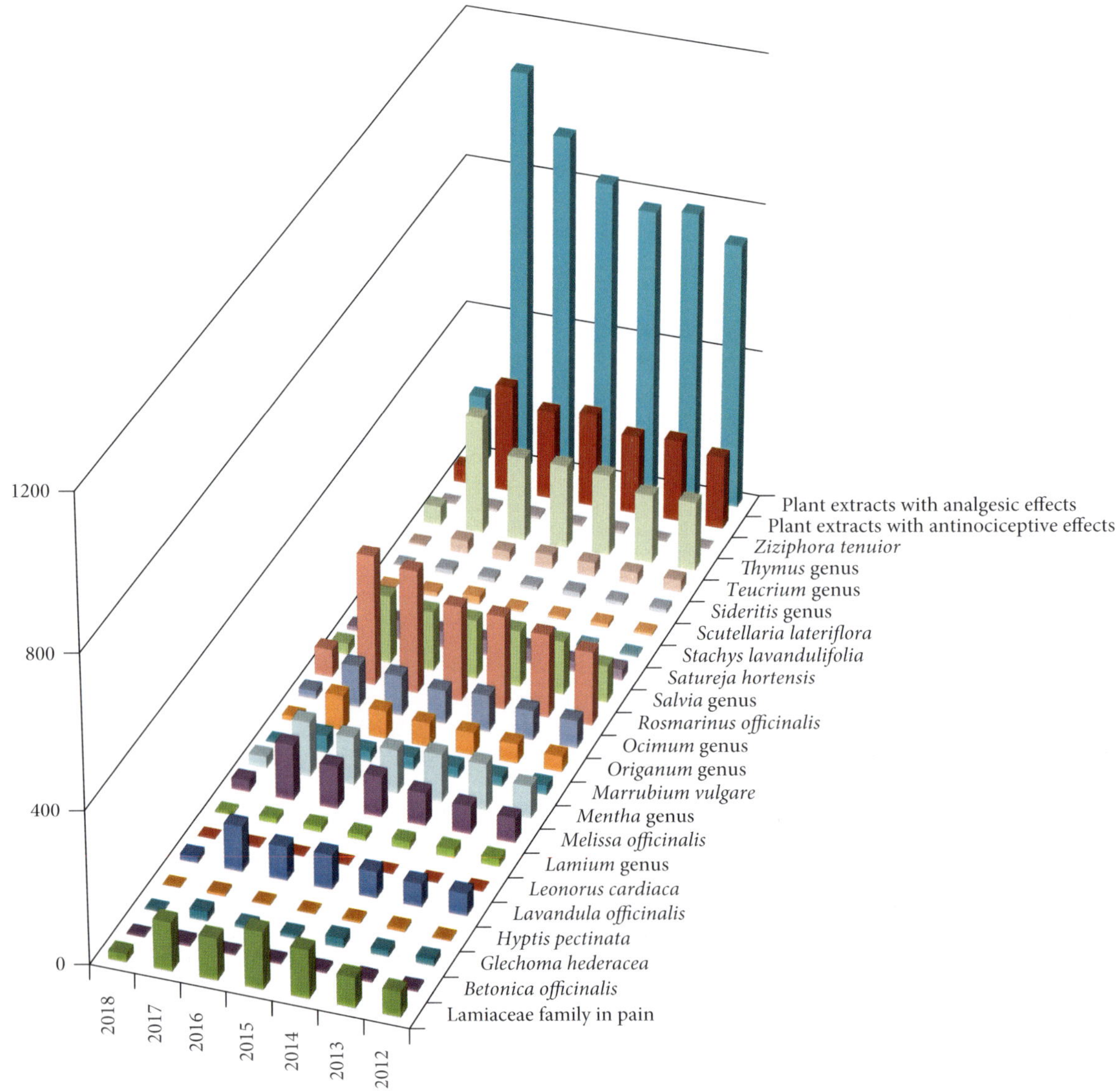

Figure 1: Number of publications according to ScienceDirect.

extraction [56] and/or ultrasound-assisted ethanol, acetone, or *n*-hexane extraction represent alternatives to the conventional method, improving the speed and efficiency of the extraction process and reducing the consumption of solvents [57].

Previous studies have revealed that the rosemary extract may have analgesic and anti-inflammatory effects [58–62]. Therefore, data have shown that the ethanolic extract of rosemary inhibited acetic acid-induced pain in mice with an ED50 of 108.84 mg/kg^{-1} [23]. Furthermore, the extract inhibited the time mice spent licking and shaking induced by formalin injections. Nevertheless, the extract did not display any anti-inflammatory activity as evaluated by uric acid induced-hind limb edema in rats [23]. In an experiment conducted by Emami et al. [34], the effects of *R. officinalis* extract and its major constituent, carnosol, on plasma corticosterone levels and activity of the enzymes cyclooxygenase types 1 and 2 (COX1 and COX2) reduced pain in phase 2 of the formalin test, which was not inhibited by naloxone and/or memantine. In addition, pretreatment of the animals with *R. officinalis* extract and/or carnosol reduced the formalin-induced inflammation. Moreover, the extract and carnosol did not affect plasma corticosterone levels compared with the control group. Interestingly, both the extract and carnosol inhibited COX1 and COX2 activities. Going one step further, one can conclude that *R. officinalis* extract and carnosol suppress pain and inflammation induced by formalin injection, which may be due to inhibition of the activity of COX1 and COX2 enzymes.

3.2. Marrubium Genus. *Marrubium* is a genus of flowering plants that are included in the Lamiaceae family and are found in the temperate regions of Europe, North Africa, and Asia as far east as the Xinjiang region, and some species are also naturalized as far as North and South America. *Marrubium*, known as horehound or hoarhound, counts approximately 40 species of flowering plants native to the temperate countries of Europe, northern Africa, and Asia.

3.2.1. Marrubium vulgare. *Marrubium vulgare* L., commonly named as "marimba" or "marroio" in Brazil and white horehound in Europe, is regularly used in traditional medicine to cure a diversity of maladies [63, 64].

Phytochemical investigations on different parts of *M. vulgare* have reported the presence of alkaloids, lactones, steroids, tannins, a series of phenylpropanoid esters, diterpenoids [65], and flavonoids [64], together with their derivatives. Marrubiin, a furano labdane diterpenoid, was found to be the major chemotaxonomic marker isolated from leaves of the plant and exhibits potent antinociceptive properties and vasorelaxant activity [66–68].

Marrubiin, the main active ingredient of *M. vulgare*, seems to be generated as an artifact from premarrubiin during the extraction procedure when high temperatures are involved in extraction or concentration [69].

The leaves and stems are known to have antiseptic, antispasmodic, antidiabetic, diuretic, strongly expectorant, and tonic roles [70, 71]. The intensive modern research and clinical trials have confirmed several capabilities traditionally described to *M. vulgare*, such as antimicrobial against Gram-positive bacteria, antioxidant, analgesic [66, 67], anti-inflammatory [71], and anti-oedematogenic [72]. Furthermore, extracts of this plant have shown some effects on type II diabetes [73] and, recently, on neurological disorders [74, 75]. One study found that marrubiin has dose-related antinociceptive effects. The antinociceptive properties were observed using different routes of administration (systemic and oral), and the effect was sustained over a long period of time.

The great potencies observed in the writhing test and formalin-influenced pain test propose that marrubiin acts by some peripheral mechanism. In the hot-plate test, marrubiin did not increase the latency period of pain induced by the thermal stimuli. Reducing the lactone ring of marrubiin with the formation of marrubiinic acid and two esterified derivatives has conditioned the successful analgesic effect influencing the number of writhes in mice. Marrubiinic acid exhibited a high analgesic effect that has been long established in other experimental models of pain, suggesting the possibility to use it as a new and useful analgesic agent [67]. Marrubiin does not prove any cytotoxicity against 66 cancer cell lines according to the NIH PubMed website [Marrubiin-Compound Summary (CID 73401)]. *In vivo* experimental studies have documented an LD50 of 370 mg/kg body weight [68], and recent data have highlighted a safety limit up to 100 mg/kg body weight when injected into mice [71].

3.3. Sideritis Genus. *Sideritis* genus counts more than 150 species of plants that are situated primarily in the Mediterranean area and also in Atlantic regions, North Africa, and even Norway, with apparent differences in composition between the same species corresponding to the geographical place of provenience [76]. The species have been used as flavoring agents, widely as ingredients for tea preparation or with medicinal purposes [77] in some areas being listed as an endangered plant. Although the use in traditional medicine has been extensive in the abovementioned places, *Sideritis* species have reduced usage in western medicine [78], because medical literature are offering data mostly on the *scardica*, *lotsy*, and *stricta* species.

3.3.1. Sideritis scardica. *S. scardica* Gris. is also known as "Greek tea" or "mountain tea." The components of *scardica* have been studied through various methods for their presence as well as medical role in both animal and human studies.

By using chromatographic separations (HPLC) and mass spectrometry, one study found six different flavonoid aglycones: luteolin, apigenin, hypolaetin, 4′-*O*-methylhypolaetin, isoscutellarein, and 4′-*O*-methylisoscutellarein [79], and also other components like sterols, coumarins, flavonoids, essential oil, iridoids, terpenoids, and glycosides [76]. The presence of phenolic antioxidants (catechins) correlating to the antioxidant activity of Greek mountain tea was also established [80].

Gas chromatography with mass spectrometry (GC-MS) analysis demonstrated that the composition of *S. scardica* oil samples, however, varies from region to region. In the oil from Macedonia, for example, α-cadinol is predominant as compared to the Bulgarian version of the same plant oil which contains mostly diterpenic compounds and octadecenol. Interestingly, none contained menthol, nerol, or geraniol, which are the major components in the *S. scardica* oil from Yugoslavia [81].

For an overview of the *Sideritis* species in the Balkan area, mountain tea was analyzed by mass spectrometry coupled to high-performance liquid chromatography with diode-array detection. The analysis found that it contains 90% phenylethanoid glycosides and flavonoid acetylglycosides [82]. Turkish *S. scardica* oil has β-pinene in abundance as compared to the Greek version which contains α-pinene primarily. Both these varieties are mainly rich in monoterpene hydrocarbons unlike the ones from Macedonia and Bulgaria, which are poor in these compounds [83]. Significant differences in components have also been proven between the fresh and dried versions of the plant material [84].

An analysis of urine samples from humans who received oral administration of *S. scardica* showed that the flavonoid metabolites were dominant in urine samples and that hypolaetin and isoscutellarein had the largest number of metabolites (methylhypolaetin and methylisoscutellarein glucuronides) together with apigenin [85].

The pharmacological activity of *S. scardica* is attributed to the high content of flavonoid and phenolic compounds. Studies have demonstrated that plants from the *Sideritis* genus have antioxidant, anti-inflammatory, diuretic, antibacterial, analgesic, and antifungal effects [86]. In experimental ex vivo models, *S. scardica* showed a capacity to inhibit human serotonin transporter (hSERT) greater than in rat models [77]. Accordingly, the *in vivo* test in rats showed that *S. scardica* extract administered orally has been associated with psychostimulant and antidepressive effects, being classified as perhaps a substitute for adaptogens and thus useful for other pathologies correlated with depressive or altered mental status like sleep apnea or increased cardiovascular risks [87–89].

The antibacterial activity seems to be influenced by the method of obtaining the extract: carbon dioxide extraction being superior to hydrodistillation and is attributed partially to diterpenes and fatty acids and their derivates and also to other momentarily unknown elements that might be involved [90] but with a certain degree of effect on different types of pathogens.

The antioxidant activity was widely demonstrated, probably due to the content of catechins but not limited to this and has multiple health benefits and implications in pain treatment proving a possible valuable agent in limiting the use of analgesics, anti-inflammatory, and antipyretic forms of self-medication [6, 91].

In vivo models demonstrated the anti-inflammatory effects of *S. scardica* over a model of carrageenan-induced rat paw edema and proved gastroprotective activity over ethanol-induced acute stress ulcer in rats and also a promising cytotoxic activity [92], attributing in part to flavonoid constituents (apigenin and luteolin) that can induce cell-cycle arrest and cellular apoptosis *in vitro* [93]. *In vivo* models demonstrated a preventive capacity of *S. scardica* over Aβ-induced memory impairments in transgenic and nontransgenic mice and proved a possible positive effect in Alzheimer's disease, fully rescuing neuronal loss in transgenic mice, thus being flagged as a possible treatment forimproving memory in healthy adults and in dementia patients [78].

The usage of *S. scardica* in traditional and modern medicine has demonstrated various degrees of effectiveness with promising beneficial health results in a long series of pathologies from prevention of anemia, anxiety disorders, major depression, cardiovascular disease, attention-deficit hyperactivity disorder, mental impairment, or neurodegenerative diseases [77] to rheumatic problems [94], inflammatory pain, gastric ulcer [93], pulmonary pathologies (common cold, lung emphysema, bronchitis, and asthma) [85], and also an effective cytotoxic activity [92, 95]. The anti-inflammatory and edema-reducing capabilities should be considered as the basis for further studies of *S. scardica* implication in pain modulation.

3.3.2. Sideritis lotsyi. *Sideritis lotsyi* Pit. contains tetracyclic diterpenes (ent-kaur-16-ene and epicandicandiol 7β-mono acetate-18-palmitate), rhoiptelenol, hydrocarbon ent-trachy lobane, amyrin, trachinodiol, a rare diterpene 16β,18-dihy droxy-ent-atisane, and 5-hydroxy-3,7,4′-trimethoxyflavone, but the content is different between *S. lotsyi* and *S. lotsyi* var. *mascaensis* [96]. *S. lotsyi* var. *mascaensis* extracts were studied in a comprehensive analysis for the antimicrobial activity, toxicity, and anti-inflammatory and analgesic proprieties.

A dose of 2 g/kg body weight *S. lotsyi* extracts administered orally in mice did not show any toxic effects; however, a dose of only 250 mg/kg ethanol extract administered orally has shown analgesic proprieties on the visceral pain produced during the writhing test, and the chloroform fraction demonstrated antinociceptive effect. The same extracts manifested anti-inflammatory effect on the early, histamin-mediated, phase of paw inflammation, but much more significant effects were observed in ear inflammation with topical administration. Contrary to *S. scardica*, no antimicrobial effect was noted [97].

3.3.3. Sideritis stricta. *Sideritis stricta* Benth. is listed as an endangered plant and is being used as an aromatic and medicinal plant containing essential oils with antimicrobial, cytotoxic, antiviral, and antioxidant properties [98]. The diterpenes composition was identified as sideroxol, 7-acetyl sideroxol, 7-epicandicandiol, linearol (5), ent-7α,15β,18-trihydroxy-kaur-16-ene, ent-7α-acetyl,15,18-dihydroxy-kaur-16-ene, foliol, sideridiol, siderol, and the recently identified ent-1β-hydroxy-7α-acetyl-15β,16β-epoxykaurane [99] together with two flavonoid glycosides and a phenolic fraction by means of spectroscopic evidence [100]. Although phenolic compounds did not manifest anti-inflammatory proprieties, the flavonoid glycosides show both anti-inflammatory and antinociceptive capabilities when combined [100]. Similarly to *S. lotsyi*, the acetone extract of *S. stricta* showed lower antimicrobial activity as compared to gentamicin [99], and no extensive data with the implications of *S. stricta* over pain are published.

3.4. Thymus Genus. *Thymus* genus, part of the Lamiaceae family, consists of over 350 species of aromatic plants with evergreen leaves. Geographically, these plants extend to Asia, North Africa, and Europe. Although more than one species is cultivated for culinary (cheese and liqueur flavor agent) or ornamental use, the most extensively studied in literature is *Thymus vulgaris*. Used for thousands of years in traditional medicine, the effects of *Thymus* species in medicine is wide, from antimicrobial and anti-inflammatory to possible treatment for dementia or oncological pathologies through apigenin [101].

3.4.1. Thymus vulgaris. GC-MS and GC-FID analyses revealed that the main active components in one type of *Thymus vulgaris* L. essential oil are thymol (41.0%), geraniol (26.4%), thujanol (42.2% *cis*-sabinene hydrate and 7.3% *trans*-sabinene hydrate), and linalool (72.5%) [102], and others also contain borneol and carvacrol. The chemotypes of thyme are determined based on oil compositions. Geographical provenience and weather influence the chemotype and composition [103], which was demonstrated by a study comparing essential oils from two regions of France (linalool chemotype with 76.2% linalool and thymol chemotype with 47.1% thymol) and two regions of Serbia (geraniol chemotype with 59.8% geraniol and sabinene hydrate chemotype with 30.8% *cis*-sabinene hydrate) [104].

The terpenoids associated with *T. vulgaris* anesthethic capabilities are thymol (2-isopropyl-5-methylphenol) and eugenol (4-allyl-2-methoxyphenol) [105]; moreover, thymol inhibits synthetisation of vitamin K and is implicated in the inhibition of platelet aggregation [106], resulting in potential anticoagulant activity [107].

In animals, hydroalcoholic extracts of propolis *T. vulgaris* showed promising results in the treatment of dermal leishmaniasis or *Tetranychus urticae* [108, 109]. *T. vulgaris* also has a spasmolytic, antimicrobial, anti-inflammatory, immunomodulatory, and antioxidant capabilities, these effects being attributed to the thymol contained in the volatile thyme oil [110]. Confirming the effect of *T. vulgaris* on respiratory pathologies and the spasmolytic effects underlined in *ex vivo* studies [111], a study also has indicated its promising potential for the treatment of gastrointestinal pathologies in animal models without any toxic potential.

By inhibiting, *in vivo*, TNF-α, lipopolysaccharide inflammatory induced cell influx, IL-6, protein concentration in bronchoalveolar lavage fluid, and NF-κB activation in the lung, thymol could be a promising therapeutical agent for acute lung injury [112].

The inhibitory role over the nitric oxide (NO) by limiting iNOS mRNA expression plays a major role in the anti-inflammatory proprieties of *T. vulgaris* extracts [113]. Also, because of the antioxidant capabilities and being an inhibitor of acetylcholinesterase, *T. vulgaris* could be a promising therapeutic agent for neurodegenerative disorders like dementia or Alzheimer's disease [114].

In vitro activity of *T. vulgaris* oil confirmed a high antibacterial activity over Gram-positive and also Gram-negative bacteria, though the effect was smaller on the latter [102].

In traditional medicine and in clinical practice, *T. vulgaris* is used, and *T. vulgaris* shows promising results on inflammatory skin disorders [115], scabies, herpes, wounds, alopecia, dental plaque [116], ringworm, and headaches [106]. Moreover, *T. vulgaris* showed a promising insecticidal effect on *Culex pipiens*, the vector for lymphatic filariasis [117], demonstrating an increased importance in many fields.

Probably in part due to the anti-inflammatory and antioxidant capabilities, *Thymus* extracts demonstrated analgesic, anti-inflammatory, and antipyretic activity in mouse models of pain. Therefore, the authors concluded that the extracts of *Thymus* may be used against pain, pyrexia, and inflammation [118], correlating with other similar findings that position *T. vulgaris* as a modulator agent over acute and chronic pain [119]. In clinical practice, comparative effects of *T. vulgaris* and ibuprofen on pain severity associated with primary dysmenorrhea were found [120].

3.4.2. Thymus pulegioides. *Thymus pulegioides* L. belongs to the genus *Thymus*, and together with three other species, it has a different phenolic content than *T. vulgaris* [121]. It grows on the European continent, and it is used as an antiseptic in local regions of Portugal [122].

In phytochemical analysis, *Thymus pulegioides* was found to have a high flavonoid content, tannins, and hydroxycinnamic acids. The *T. pulegioides* oil, in one analysiss, was characterized by the presence of high amounts of thymol and carvacrol [122]. The dose-dependent scavenging effect and the chelating activity of *T. pulegioides* are moderate to high, with an increased acetylcholinesterase inhibition [114]. A study in Italy places *T. pulegioides* among the first medicinal plants in traditional medicine and the second most relevant in respiratory pathologies usage [123].

It has an important antioxidant role [124], but as an anti-inflammatory agent, it elicits cell-type-dependent response [125]. Another consideration that increases the medicinal importance of *T. pulegioides* is that it has demonstrated considerable antifungal capacities [122]; however, more data are required to quantify its effect in pain modulation.

3.5. Satureja Genus. *Satureja* genus consists of aromatic plants of the Lamiaceae family that are related to rosemary and thyme. It is native to the North African region, southern and southeastern European regions, and the Middle East and Central Asian parts of the globe. A few species found on the American continent were formerly included in *Satureja* genus but were thereafter moved to other genera.

3.5.1. Satureja hortensis. *Satureja hortensis* L., also known as summer savory (culinary herbs), is an annual aromatic plant with origin in the Mediterranean region and wide distribution in the Mediterranean Sea region, Black Sea, Central and Southern Europe, Asia Minor, and Siberia, but nowadays cultivated worldwide [126]. The floral parts and leaves from the plant are used as aromatic spice. It is also used in medicinal purposes as decoctions, plasters, and compresses.

The main constituents of the plant were carvacrol, γ-terpinene, p-cymene, α-terpinene, and myrcene. The only notable sesquiterpene is β-bisabolene [126].

Regarding the biological activity, extracts from *S. hortensis* are covering a large spectrum of pathological conditions [127–132]: antimicrobial activity, antioxidant activity, cytotoxic activity, insecticidal activity, fumigant toxicity, insect repellant activity, antinociceptive and analgesic activity, antileishmanial activity, genotoxic activity, anti-inflammatory activity, effects on immune system, effects on productive performance, acaricidal activity, antidiarrheal activity, relaxant effect (antispasmoidal activity), antigenotoxic activity, antihepatoma activity, contact toxicity and persistence, effect on vitality and healthiness of cereals, molluscicidal activity, larvicidal activity, anti-helmintic activity, inhibition on blood platelet adhesion, aggregation and secretion, effect on rhinosinusitis, amyloid beta protein aggregation inhibitory activity, and matrix metalloproteinase inhibitory activity.

Concerning the analgesic activity, *S. hortensis* extracts (hydroalcoholic extract, polyphenolic fraction, and essential oil of the aerial parts of the herb) were evaluated by use of tail flick, formalin, and acetic acid-induced writhing tests in mice. Results showed that, in the light tail flick test, neither the essential oil nor the extracts could exert any significant effect. The hydroalcoholic extract (2000 mg/kg, p.o.) and the essential oil (200 mg/kg, p.o.) inhibited the mice writhing responses caused by acetic acid. In the formalin test, hydroalcoholic extract (500–2000 mg/kg, p.o.), polyphenolic fraction (250–1000 mg/kg, p.o.), and the essential oil (50–200 mg/kg, p.o.) showed analgesic activity, and pretreatment with naloxone (1 mg/kg, i.p.) or caffeine (20 mg/kg, i.p.) failed to reverse this antinociceptive activity. Authors suggested that antinociceptive effect could be due to the involvement of opioid and adenosine receptors in the antinociception mediation [133].

3.6. Stachys Genus. *Stachys* genus is one of the largest genera in the flowering plant family of Lamiaceae. Estimates of the number of species in the genus are ranging between 300 and about 450.

3.6.1. Stachys lavandulifolia. *Stachys lavandulifolia* Vahl., a type of *Stachys*, also known as mountain tea (Chay-e-Kouhi) has been distributed in a variety of climatic conditions including diverse areas of Europe, Asia, Africa, and Australia. The plant is known as Chay-e-kouhi in Persian, whereas in English it is called Betony. Also, its common names include heal-all, self-heal, woundwort, betony, lamb's ears, and hedge nettle [134].

Based on recent studies on this herb, 79 compounds were identified, representing 98.2% of the essential oil, in which the major components were germacrene-D (13.2%), β-phellandrene (12.7%), β-pinene (10.2%), myrcene (9.4%), α-pinene (8.4%), and Z-β-ocimene (5.8%). In another study, spathulenol (35.0%) and caryophyllene oxide (25.6%) were the main components of the oil [135]. Another study revealed the existence of α-thujone (0.3%–32.3%), Δ-cadinene (11.6%) and 1,4-methano-1H-indene (10.1%) [136].

The aqueous extract obtained from the aerial parts of *S. lavandulifolia* is used in antipyretic, anti-inflammatory, spasmolytic, sedative, and hypnotic treatment [137]. Also, this plant has antibacterial, antioxidant, anxiolytic, analgesic, and wound-healing effects. Decoctions or infusions of *Stachys* are applied as tonics to treat skin or taken internally for stomach disorders [138].

Some other biological activities of *S. lavandulifolia* were signaled, and the main of those being possibility of abortion depending on the dosage in animals, useful in controlling premenstrual syndrome (PMS) and primary dysmenorrhea symptoms, helps in strengthening stomach and preventing gastric ulcers caused by alcohol consumption, and useful in treating *Leishmania major*. Being useful to treat fatigue, nausea, and vomiting associated with primary dysmenorrhea, it could be a potentially effective treatment for dysmenorrhea, particularly because of its antipyretic and spasmolytic effects. As an undesired effect, it gives rise to failure in fetus survival and, consequently, abortion. Its action on insomnia is approved. It is also known for its antidepressive and appetite-stimulating effects [139, 140].

For the evaluation of the analgesic effect, hydroalcoholic, polyphenolic, and boiled extracts of the aerial parts from *S. lavandulifolia* were prepared, and their analgesic effects were studied in mice using formalin, acetic acid-induced writhing, and light tail flick tests. Results showed that all the tested extracts were able to reduce the abdominal constrictions in acetic acid-induced writhing test. These extracts also significantly ($P < 0.001$) suppressed both phases of the formalin test. In the light tail flick test, none of the extracts showed analgesic activity [141].

In another study regarding antinociceptive effects of *S. lavandulifolia* extracts, the implication of essential oil (EOSl) and (−)-α-bisabolol (BIS), its main compound, was studied in algogen-induced orofacial nociceptive behavior in mice. Authors have shown that the treatment with EOS1 and BIS has significantly reduced pain in different orofacial pain tests on mice, but BIS proved to be more effective, significantly reducing nociceptive behavior in all tests including both phases of the formalin test [142].

3.6.2. Stachys officinalis (Synonym Betonica officinalis). It is commonly known as wood betony, purple betony, woundwort, or Bishop's wort; it is a perennial herb found in dry grassland, meadows, and open woods in most of Europe, western Asia, North and South America, Africa, and tropical regions. For centuries, *Betonica officinalis* herbs (roots and aerial parts) were used in traditional folk medicine for numerous purposes, either internally as tea or externally as compresses or baths. The beneficial properties include anti-inflammatory [143], antibacterial [144], antifungal, antioxidant [145, 146], and hypotensive activity [147]. Important analgesic effects and implications in the treatment of respiratory tract, gastrointestinal tract, nervous and cardiac systems, and skin and gynecological disorders were also observed. Also, a variety of *Betonica* species are used in food industry to improve the taste in preparation of jelly or yogurt, or as seasonings and flavorings [148].

The chemical composition of *Betonica officinalis* includes polyphenols such as tannins, phenolic acids, flavonoids, alkaloids trigonelline, and stachydrine (a pyrrolidine alkaloid), iridoids, diterpenes, phenylethanoid glycosides, fatty acids, betaine, volatile oils, and choline [149, 150]. According to the literature data, phenylethanoid glycosides, triterpenoids, and flavonoids are considered to be the active components responsible for the biological actions of the genus *Stachys*, but the anti-inflammatory or analgesic effects, or components of it, have not been elucidated completely so far.

3.6.3. Stachys inflata. A hydroalcoholic extract of *Stachys inflata* Benth., one of the *Stachys* species from Iran, induced antinociception and anti-inflammatory effects in two well-characterized inflammatory models in rats: carrageenan-induced paw edema and formalin-induced paw licking [151]. Intraperitoneal injection of the hydroalcoholic extract of the aerial parts from nonflowering stems of *S. inflata*, 60 min before induction of inflammation, was capable of attenuating both early and delayed phases of carrageenan-induced inflammation with a dose-related inhibition over the dose range of 50–200 mg/kg. Compared to a standard nonsteroidal anti-inflammatory drug, indomethacin, the hydroalcoholic extract of *S. inflata* inhibited the inflammation more effectively than indomethacin. Moreover, all three doses of the extract significantly inhibited the pain associated with the second phase (inflammatory component) of the formalin test, but with no effect against the first phase (0–5 min).

The obtained data suggest that the anti-inflammatory activity of hydroalcoholic extract of *S. inflata* may be related to the inhibition of the release or synthesis of cyclooxygenase products and polymorphonuclear leukocytes accumulation determined by myeloperoxidase activity. The effects of *S. inflata* extracts (200 mg/kg) on inflammation and myeloperoxidase activity were confirmed by histological examination where the extract considerably reduced the morphological injury and neutrophil infiltration in a carrageenan-induced model of local inflammation.

The results presented in this study are taken as the basis for further investigation on the exact mode of action of individual constituents of the extract. Several components quantified in *Stachys* extracts demonstrated *in vivo* anti-inflammatory and antinociceptive activity in carrageenan-induced hind paw edema and *p*-benzoquinone-induced abdominal constriction tests [100].

3.6.4. Stachys byzantina. Khanavi et al. [152] proved that acetone and methanol extracts of *S. byzantina* K. Koch, a species of *Stachys*, native to Turkey, Armenia, and Iran, play a significant role in the inhibition of pain and inflammatory processes by using two inflammatory models, namely, formalin test and carrageenan-induced paw edema.

Dried and finely powdered aerial parts were extracted with acetone at room temperature for 2 weeks in order to isolate and identify an acyclic diterpene ester (phytyl nonadecanoate), two normal alkanes (tritriacontane and hentriacontane), one fatty acid (oleic acid), and two sterols (stigmasterol and lawsaritol). Structures were established by conventional methods of analysis and confirmed by ^{1}H, ^{13}C NMR, and mass spectral analysis. All three doses of acetone/methanol extracts of *Stachys byzantina* (50, 100, and 200 mg/kg), administered by intraperitoneal injections, significantly inhibited the pain associated with the second phase (inflammatory component) of the formalin test, and the effect of the low dose was predominant. Compared to indomethacin (high dose of 5 mg/kg) as a nonsteroidal anti-inflammatory drug, the extracts decreased licking response in the late phase significantly, with the maximum inhibitory response obtained with 50 mg/kg of the extract.

The authors assumed that the analgesic effects of the extracts are probably mediated by interactions with inflammatory mediators (arachidonic acid metabolites), since the antinociceptive activities were observed in late phase (20 min after formalin injection). In the carrageenan-induced paw edema, both extracts revealed dose-related inhibitory effects, in both early and delayed phases, over the dose range 50–200 mg/kg, similar to a high dose of indomethacin (5 mg/kg). The present data demonstrated that the anti-inflammatory activity of acetone and methanol extracts of *S. byzantina* is probably related to the inhibition of the synthesis or release of COX2 products.

3.7. Glechoma Genus. Glechoma genus is composed of flowering plants in the mint family first described in 1753. This genus is distributed in both northern Asia and Europe. In Asia, however, it is most predominantly seen in China, and it is closely related to *Marmoritis*.

3.7.1. Glechoma hederacea. Glechoma hederacea L., more commonly known as ground ivy, is a perennial herb with creeping stem that can be found throughout Northern Europe and the neighboring regions of Asia. The aerial parts of the plant (consumed as salad or tea) have been used in both Asian and European traditional medicine as a remedy for several digestive, pulmonary, skeletal, and inflammatory conditions [153]. Active components include several polyphenols such as chlorogenic acid, caffeic acid, ferulic acid, rutin, genistin, rosmarinic acid, quercetin, or genistein [153] and triterpenoids such as ursolic acid and oleanoic acid [154, 155]. Additionally, studies report that *G. hederacea* leaves contain polyunsaturated fatty acids [156] and a type of insecticidal lectin called Gleheda [157].

Current preclinical data indicate that *G. hederacea* has several pharmacological effects. As such, hot water extracts of ground ivy have been shown to exhibit antibacterial, anticancer, insecticidal, and platelet-stimulating activity [157, 158]. Currently, there are no studies specifically addressing ground ivy's effect on pain. However, existing data point out that the plant has potent anti-inflammatory effects. An *in vitro* study revealed that incubating activated macrophages with a ground ivy decoction (3 h in boiling distilled water) led to a significant decrease in nitric oxide production. Furthermore, the authors noted that the expression of some inflammatory cytokines such as IL-12p70 and TNFα was significantly decreased [159]. Similarly, Kim et al. demonstrated that several compounds found in *G. hederacea* inhibit NF-κB production [154]. *In vivo*, hot water *G. hederacea* extract was shown to have an anti-inflammatory effect in a rat model of hepatic inflammation: rats that received 0.5 g/kg *G. hederacea* extract daily for four weeks were shown to have significantly lower levels of inflammatory cell infiltration/activation in the liver [153]. Additionally, several inflammatory markers, such as NF-κB, TNF-α, IL-1β, and IL-6, were decreased in these animals when compared with the control group.

Other possible mechanisms that make ground ivy a potential candidate as coanalgesic include its effects on extracellular calcium (Ca) levels [160] and on oxidation. Purified ethyl acetate extracts of ground ivy showed a strong antioxidant activity when used as a food additive in two different types of food (pork lard and sunflower oil) [161].

There are no reported side effects following *G. hederacea* administration. However, one *in vitro* study showed that *G. hederacea* ethanol extract concentrations exceeding 100 μg/dl are cytotoxic [160], and several studies now focus on the plant's ability to kill different types of cancer cells [162]. Due to its ability to target and kill cancerous cells, those extracts should also be included in preclinical screenings addressing pediatric cancerous cells (e.g., insulinomas being one of the most frequently encountered types of neuroendocrine pancreatic tumors [163]).

3.8. Scutellaria Genus. Scutellaria genus includes over 350 species, many of which have been used in traditional medicine and are documented to have medical proprieties.

3.8.1. Scutellaria lateriflora. Scutellaria lateriflora L., also known as American skullcap, is a member of *Scutellaria* genus and is native to North America and is best known for its sedative and anxiolytic effects. The plant is still widely used by herbal medicine practitioners for insomnia, nervous anorexia, headaches, depression, panic attacks, and fibromyalgia [164, 165]. Most often, it is prescribed as a tincture, although teas and tablets are also commercially available, with wide variability depending on the manufacturer and species of *Scutellaria* used [166]. Although rare, possible side effects of chronic treatment include drowsiness, mild digestive upset, and vivid dreaming [165].

The first clinical study assessing skullcap's effect on mood was performed on nineteen patients and had positive results [167]. In 2014, Brock et al. published the results of a larger randomized controlled clinical trial designed to assess the effect of a *S. lateriflora* extract on mood in healthy volunteers. Results indicated that global mood was significantly enhanced in individuals who received 350 mg of plant extract for two weeks without negative effects on energy and cognition [164]. Taking into account the fact that anxiety is a well-known enhancer of pain perception [168], *S. lateriflora* extracts could have clinical value as co-analgesics. Additionally, ethanolic and aqueous *S. lateriflora* extracts have been shown to have potent antioxidant effects, reducing ROS and lipid peroxides in tissue homogenates [169], most likely due to the flavonoids it contains.

S. lateriflora contains several active compounds such as baicalin (40 mg/g in a 50% EtOH extract), baicalein (33 mg/g in a 95% EtOH), GABA (1.6 mg/g in EtOH and H_2O extracts), and glutamine (31 mg/g in H_2O extract) [170]. Other flavonoids found in *S. lateriflora* include wogonin, oroxylin A, genkwanin, hesperetin, quercetin, rutin, naringenin, chrysin, and daidzein [167]. While its anxiolytic effects are probably related to some of the flavonoids that bind to one of the serotonin receptors [171], *S. lateriflora*'s antioxidant activity is most likely due to its content of baicalein and its glucuronide, baicalin.

Baicalein can be extracted from *S. lateriflora* through alkali solution and acid isolation methods; for a high-purity extract (99.35%), hydrolysis of baicalin and column chromatography purification can be used [172]. As an isolated compound, baicalein has shown not only antioxidant activity but also significant anti-inflammatory activity in several *in vitro* and *in vivo* models, which has made it an interesting drug to be screened as an analgesic.

One study used several extracts from a plant of the *Scutellaria* genus and found that baicalein has a significant analgesic effect in the carrageenan-induced rat paw inflammatory model [173]. Similarly, baicalein was found to significantly decrease pain-related behavior and c-fos expression (a surrogate marker for pain intensity) in the spinal dorsal horn of animals exposed to painful stimuli [174]. A combination of baicalin and catechins was assessed in three widely used animal pain models and was found to have analgesic effects in visceral, nociceptive, and inflammatory pain [175].

Baicalin has also shown some efficacy in neuropathic pain: an *in vivo* study on spinal nerve ligation rats showed that tactile allodynia and thermal hyperalgesia were reversed by intrathecal baicalin administration. Additionally, baicalin significantly enhanced the effect of morphine in neuropathic animals, most likely by suppressing histone deacetylase 1 expression in the spinal dorsal horn [176]. The compound was also shown to be effective in cancer-induced bone pain: both intrathecal and oral baicalin administration reduced cytokine expression and inhibited pain-related signals as assessed by behavioral and biochemical tests [177, 178] in an animal model.

This compound most likely exerts its analgesic effects through modulating the inflammatory process. Baicalein's anti-inflammatory activity can partly be explained by its inhibitory effects on lipoxygenases—enzymes that play a key role in leukotriene and lipoxin synthesis, thus initiating the inflammatory response. Deschamps et al. found that baicalein inhibits both human platelet 12-lipoxygenase and human reticulocyte 15-lipoxygenase-1 [179]. Additionally, Hsieh et al. showed that baicalein inhibits IL-1β and TNF-α through modulation of the NK-κB pathway [180] while other authors found that it inhibits protein expression of inducible nitric oxide synthase [181] and COX2 gene expression [182]. Pretreatment with baicalein increased the concentration of antioxidant enzymes such as SOD, catalase, and GSH in an *in vivo* model of myocardial ischemic injury [183] and protected cells against lipid membrane peroxidation [184]. However, it is very likely that, taking into account the fact that baicalein is effective also in non-inflammatory types of pain, it has other analgesic mechanisms as well. One hypothesis states that baicalein binds to the $GABA_A$ receptor, which has a modulatory effect on pain because GABA is the main inhibitory neurotransmitter. When directly injected into the central nervous system, baicalein has strong sedative and anxiolytic effects due to GABA binding [185]. Also, a recently published article indicated that through GABA modulation, baicalin could be used in orofacial pain modulation [186]. Another study also suggested that baicalein modulates both intracellular and extracellular calcium levels [187], which may play a role in cell signaling and pain transmission.

3.9. Ocimum Genus. Ocimum genus species are amongst the best-known medicinal plants, with historical reports of their antimicrobial, immunomodulatory, antistress, anti-inflammatory, antiulcer, antidiabetic, hepatoprotective, chemoprotective, antihyperlipidemic, cardioprotective, antioxidant, antitussive, radioprotective, memory enhancing, antiarthritic, antifertility, antihypertensive, anticoagulant, anticataract, anthelmintic, and antinociceptive activity [188]. As such, several members of the genus such as

Ocimum sanctum, *Ocimum gratissimum*, or *Ocimum micranthum* have played a significant part in different traditional medicines and are currently considered as potential sources for innovative drugs.

3.9.1. Ocimum sanctum. *Ocimum sanctum* Linn., also known as tulsi, is an indigenous plant commonly found in India [189]. In Ayurvedic medicine, it is used in the form of a fresh leaf extract or a decoction with hot water to alleviate muscular pain, joint pain, and severe headache [190]. It contains (−)-linalool (30–40%), eugenol (8–30%), and methyl chavicol (15–27%). Minor constituents are (+)-delta-cadinene, 3-carene, α-humulene, citral, and (−)-*trans*-caryophyllene [191]. In recent years, the interest for evaluating the potential benefits of *O. sanctum* extracts in several conditions has significantly increased, especially in the anticancer, antimicrobial, and neurobiology fields. A double-blind clinical trial assessed the effects of oral ethanolic extract of *O. sanctum* on healthy volunteers and concluded that the drug has immunomodulatory effects and can be given for a period of four weeks without any significant side effects [192]. Although less numerous, there are some studies that have assessed the effect of *O. sanctum* extracts on different types of pain, most often inflammatory or neuropathic.

In vitro, *O. sanctum* leaf extracts exhibited significant anti-inflammatory effects in LPS-stimulated monocytic cells, reducing cytokine production and decreasing TNF-α secretion [193]. Different types of dried leaf extracts were also shown to be effective in reducing carrageenan-induced and leukotriene-induced paw edema [194]. More recently, a triple-blind randomized clinical study compared an ethanolic extract of *O. sanctum* with chlorhexidine mouthwash in regards to their effect on dental plaque and gingival inflammation and found that the two are equivalent. Additionally, the *O. sanctum* extract was better tolerated and had no side effects [195].

Regarding its effect on other pain models, there are several studies that have demonstrated that *O. sanctum* extracts alleviate neuropathic pain. The method of preparation was similar in most study designs: dried tulsi leaves were reduced to coarse powder and then extracted with a mixture of methanol and water (3 : 1) [189, 190] in order to obtain an oral preparation. 50 mg/kg b.w. of *O. sanctum* extract attenuated sciatic nerve transection-induced axonal degeneration, reduction of nociceptive threshold, and motor in-coordination [190]. Kaur et al. orally administered 100 mg/kg b.w. or 200 mg/kg b.w. of *O. sanctum* to rats that underwent chronic constriction injury in the sciatic nerve and found that the extract alleviated cold-induced hyperalgesia, mechanical allodynia, and paw-heat hyperalgesia [196]. In another study, a 200 mg/kg b.w. dose of the extract was used, and the authors concluded that it is effective in preventing vincristine-induced neuropathic pain in rats [189]. The same dose of *O. sanctum* extract was administered in rats with surgically induced focal cerebral ischemia/reperfusion injury and was shown to reduce both neurological deficit and oxidative damage [197].

3.9.2. Ocimum gratissimum. *Ocimum gratissimum* L. is widely found in several geographical regions in South America and Africa [198, 199] and still used as a medicinal plant with analgesic activity [198]. It contains several proanthocyanidins, which have been shown to exhibit significant antioxidant activity, and tannins, saponins, steroids, alkaloids, terpenoids, flavonoids, phenols, and cardiac glycosides [200]. *O. gratissimum* essential oil was orally administered to mice with chronic constriction injury and effectively alleviated neuropathic pain most likely due to eugenol's antihyperalgesic activity [199]. The same group demonstrated the efficacy of the aforementioned essential oil for increasing paw withdrawal latency in the hot-plate test and for decreasing formalin-induced hind paw inflammation and pain-evoked behaviors [201]. Another team used the essential oil of *O. gratissimum* in a model of visceral pain (the writhing test) and in the formalin test with equally favorable results [202]. Similar analgesic activity was demonstrated by *O. gratissimum* aqueous and hydroalcoholic extracts in two animal pain models: the acetic acid writhing test and the hot-plate test [198], indicating that it is efficient in nociceptive, neuropathic and inflammatory pain.

trans-Caryophyllene, a sesquiterpene from *O. gratissimum*, was shown to have dose-dependent analgesic effects in several experimental models of acute and chronic pain such as the formalin test, chronic constriction injury, and the hot-plate test. The authors evaluated the potential mechanisms responsible for the substance's properties and found that the analgesic effect was reversed by several types of antagonists [203], thus indicating the involvement of both the opioid and endocannabinoid system [204].

3.9.3. Ocimum micranthum. *Ocimum micranthum* Willd. or *Ocimum campechianum* Mill., more commonly known as Amazonian or Peruvian basil, has similar anti-inflammatory and antianalgesic effects in several animal models of pain, although it has been reported as less effective on the hot-plate test [205]. The difference in efficacy between plants is most likely due to their different compositions that additionally vary according to the geographical area. While some authors believe that the saponins these plants contain are responsible for their effect on pain [189], others have suggested that the volatile oil eugenol is in fact the most potent antioxidant and anti-inflammatory compound [197].

3.10. Lamium Genus. *Lamium* genus contains almost 40 herbaceous plants, some of which have been used as remedies for various conditions such as trauma, putrescence, paralysis, leucorrhoea, hypertension, or inflammation [206]. The *Lamium* species contain different concentrations of iridoids, flavonoids, phenylpropanoids, benzoxazinoids, and essential oil [207], which vary according to species and geographical area of cultivation. Although widely used in traditional medicine, there are only few studies that investigate the potential analgesic effects of this genus. One study screened several plants of the *Lamium* genus and concluded that *Lamium purpureum* has potent antioxidant effects, being able to rapidly scavenge free radicals in several *in vitro* assays [150].

Another screening study assessed potential anti-inflammatory and antinociceptive effects of different *Lamium* species and concluded that *Lamium garganicum* L. and *L. purpureum* L. extracts are as effective as indomethacin, a reference anti-inflammatory drug. In this study, all extracts were prepared by methanolic extraction of air-dried and powdered aerial plant parts (25 g plant in 250 mL methanol), which was then concentrated to dryness, suspended in water, partitioned, and lyophilized. The study showed that 200 mg/kg body weight of *L. garganicum* or *L. purpureum* methanolic extracts alleviate inflammatory pain in a model of ear edema and in carrageenan-induced and prostaglandin E2-induced hind paw edema [206].

3.11. Teucrium Genus. *Teucrium* genus contains several mostly perennial plants commonly referred to as germanders.

3.11.1. Teucrium polium. *Teucrium polium* L. is a perennial wild-growing plant, widely spread in several regions such as South-Western Asia, Europe, and North Africa [208], and has been used in traditional medicine for the treatment of inflammations, rheumatism, diabetes, and ulcers. Two major components of the dried leaf plant extract are flavons and flavonoids [209]; the essential oil contains α-pinene (25.769%) and myrcene (12.507), and the methanolic extract contains sinapic acid (15.553 mg/g) and eugenol (6.805 mg/g) [210]. A preclinical study showed that intraperitoneal administration of 100 or 200 mg/kg b.w. per day for two weeks reduced pain-related behavior in the diabetic rat formalin test [211]. A larger dose of 500 mg/kg body weight of ethanolic extract of *T. polium* inhibited carrageenan-induced inflammation and reduced granuloma formation [212]. Another study compared the effect of morphine and *T. polium* extract on the tail flick latency and found the two to be comparable in efficacy [213]. Both the total extract and the essential oil of the plant exhibited analgesic effects on the acetic acid-induced writhing test, thus suggesting it might be effective in visceral pain [214]. Subsequently, a triple-blind, randomized, clinical trial was designed in order to assess the plant's effects on dysmenorrhea. Seventy female students were randomly assigned to receive either *T. polium* powder every six hours for the first three days of their menstrual cycle or 250 mg mefenamic acid. Study results indicated that the two are equally effective, thus concluding that *T. polium* is effective in this type of pain [209].

3.11.2. Teucrium hyrcanicum. *Teucrium hyrcanicum* L., also known as "Purple Tails" is a plant native to Iran, which has been also shown to exhibit analgesic and anti-inflammatory activities in carrageenan-induced paw edema, acetic acid-induced writhing, tail flick, and formalin pain tests [215]. A recent study used a methanolic extract of dried aerial parts of *T. hycranicum* and observed that the high flavonoid content of the plant has significant antioxidant effects [216].

3.11.3. Teucrium chamaedrys. *Teucrium chamaedrys* L., also known as "The wall germander," is an evergreen subshrub native to the Mediterranean region of Europe and North Africa, and to the Middle East. It has been used in traditional English medicine as part of the Portland Powder for treating rheumatism and gout [217]. A preclinical study identified teucrioside as the main active ingredient of the plant and concluded that it is effective in inhibiting calcineurin, thus potentially playing a role in reducing inflammatory states [218].

3.12. Hyptis Genus. *Hyptis* genus, also known in Brazil as "sambacaitá" or "canudinho," is a genus of aromatic plants in the Lamiaceae family [219]. The genus *Hyptis* consists of approximately 400 species distributed from the southern United States to Argentina [220] and exhibits a major morphological diversity in the Brazilian Cerrado [221].

3.12.1. Hyptis pectinata. *Hyptis pectinata* L. Poit. is present very common in gardens, and it is frequently used as tea (decoctions or infusions) and mouthwash to treat inflammation due to being considered a natural antiphlogistic. In Brazilian folk medicine, the infusion of the fresh leaves is used to treat inflammations, bacterial infections, pain, gastrointestinal disorders, skin infections, nasal congestion, fever, cramps, inflammation, orofacial painful conditions and wound healing [222], fungal infections, and HIV.

Also, the plant has cytotoxicity and insecticide properties [223]. *H. pectinata* has an important neurogenic and inflammatory orofacial antinociceptive effects, without interference in the motor performance. The mechanism is currently unknown but seems to be related to vanilloid and glutamate receptors. The opioid system seems unlikely to participate in the antinociception caused by the extract [224]. The local application of dental gel based on *H. pectinata* has anti-inflammatory effect and also prevents alveolar bone resorption and weight loss in animals with periodontitis [223]. The healing effect of *H. pectinata* suggests that this plant may have antileishmanial action [219].

The aqueous extract of *H. pectinata* possesses anti-edematogenic properties in the carrageenan-induced paw edema model. The association of the aqueous extract of *H. pectinata* leaves at 200 mg/kg with intraoperative laser therapy can stimulate liver regeneration and cause a reduction in liver mitochondrial respiratory function without altering its phosphorylative activity [225].

The antinociceptive effects of *H. pectinata* can be seen in the volatile oil [226]. The major constituents of oil are 1,8-cineole (12.46%), α-pinene (20.51%), and β-pinene (13.54%). β-Pinene may be considered a partial agonist of μ-opioid receptors [227]. Franco et al. [228] suggested that the essential oils have both peripheral and central analgesic actions without opioid system influence, although the central activity was more discrete. GC-MS analysis showed that β-caryophyllene (40.90%) and caryophyllene oxides (30.05%) were the main compounds present in the oil.

In 2011, Raymundo published the results that *H. pectinata* essential oil shows peripheral and central antinociceptive effects, likely mediated by opioid and cholinergic receptors, and anti-inflammatory activity through the inhibition of nitric oxide and PGE2 production [229]. The involvement of the opioid system in the antinociceptive activity of *H. pectinata* essential oil was evaluated in the hot-plate model by pretreating mice with an opioid antagonist, naloxone. The results suggest that naloxone reversed the antinociceptive activity of the essential oil. The antinociceptive effects were observed in other tests like acetic acid or hot-plate [230].

3.13. Melissa Genus. *Melissa* genus contains the perennial herbs from the Lamiaceae family, native from Europe and Asia but cultivated and naturalized in many other places.

3.13.1. Melissa officinalis. *Melissa officinalis* L., also known as lemon balm, English balm, garden balm, balm mint, common balm, melissa, sweet balm, and heart"s delight, is an aromatic herb from the mint family (Lamiaceae) that includes two subspecies: *Melissa officinalis* L. subsp. *officinalis,* the common cultivated lemon balm, and *Melissa officinalis* L. subsp. *altissima*, naturalized in New Zealand and known as bush balm. The first information about the usage of the plant was found in Greece, 2000 years ago. In 2007, Khare [231] published the results that the plant has antidepressant, antispasmodic, antihistaminic, and antiviral properties and can be used in cases of anxiety, neurosis and nervous excitability, palpitation and headache, and also in hyperthyroidism.

The known major components of lemon balm are hydroxycinnamic acid derivatives, particularly rosmarinic acid, caffeic acids, chlorogenic acid, and metrilic acid [232, 233], tannins [234], flavonoids, including luteolin, luteolin 7-*O*-beta-D-glucopyranoside, apigenin 7-*O*-beta-D-glucopyranoside, and luteolin 3′-*O*-beta-D-glucuronopyranoside [235, 236], monoterpene glycosides [237], sesquiterpenes, including β-caryophyllene and germacrene [237], triterpenes [238], and volatile oils, including citronellal, citral a (geranial), citral b (neral), methyl citronellate, ocimene, citronellol, geraniol, nerol, β-caryophyllene, β-caryophyllene oxide, linalool, and etheric oil [239].

M. officinalis exhibit antiviral effects against Newcastle disease virus, Semliki forest virus, influenza virus, myxoviruses, vaccinia [240], and herpes simplex virus types 1 and 2 [241], HIV-1 [242]. The antiviral effects are mediated by tannin and polyphenol constituents, rosmarinic, caffeic, and ferulic acids [240].

M. officinalis has antibacterial effects and can be used to treat oropharyngeal diseases produced by anaerobic and facultative aerobic periodontal bacteria like *Porphyromonas gingivalis*, *Prevotella* spp., *Fusobacterium nucleatum*, *Capnocytophaga gingivalis*, *Veillonella parvula*, *Eikenella corrodens*, *Peptostreptococcus micros*, and *Actinomyces odontolyticus* [243].

Englberger suggests that rosmarinic acid has anti-inflammatory effects because it reduces paw edema induced by cobra venom factor in rats and inhibit passive cutaneous anaphylaxis in rats at doses of 1–100 mg/kg by mouth. The same author says that rosmarinic acid has antithrombotic effects because it inhibits the classical pathway convertase and the alternative pathway convertase [244].

M. officinalis has antithyroid effects (inhibit the binding of bovine TSH to human thyroid plasma membranes and adenylate cyclase, inhibit the extrathyroidal enzymatic T4-5′-deiodination to both T3-and T4-5′-deiodination) [245], spasmolytic effects (observed only in *in vitro* studies on isolated duodenum of rat) [246], sedative effects (dose-dependent sedation, inducing sleep and potentiating sub-hypnotic and hypnotic doses of pentobarbital) [246], and cardiovascular effects (significant reduction in the cardiac rate by the stimulation of cardiac muscarinic receptors) [247, 248].

3.14. Origanum Genus. *Origanum* is a genus of herbaceous perennials and subshrubs in the Lamiaceae family, native to Europe, North Africa, and much of temperate Asia and can be found in open or mountainous environments. A few species also naturalized in North America and other regions. The plants have strongly aromatic leaves and abundant tubular flowers with long-lasting coloured bracts. The genus includes *Origanum vulgare* L. or common marjoram and *Origanum majorana* L. or sweet marjoram, the two species of *Origanum* that can be used with medicinal purposes.

3.14.1. Origanum vulgare. *O. vulgare* is an aromatic, woody-based perennial, native to the stony slopes and rocky mountain areas at a wide range of altitudes in the Mediterranean area (Portugal and Andalusia), Europe (including the British Isles), and south and central Asia [249].

The difference between these two plants is almost indistinguishable (taste aside) to the amateur gardener. In technical terms, the difference between marjoram and oregano is based on the shape of the calyx and not the leaves, how hairy they are, or the growth habit.

There are a lot of information about *Origanum*. So, Hippocrates used *O. majorana* as an antiseptic agent. The ancient Greeks consider *Origanum* as a symbol of love, honour, and happiness. Aristotle declares that *Origanum* is an antipoison. The people from old Egypt used *Origanum* to disinfect and preserve food [250].

The major compound of *Origanum* oil is terpinen-4-ol (26%), *cis*-sabinene (13.3%), *o*-cymene (9.3%), g-terpinen (5.8%), *trans*-sabinene (5.7%), *p*-menth-1-en-8-ol (5.1%), b-thujene (4.9%), and α-terpinen (3.5%). The extracts obtained by supercritical CO_2 presented higher concentrations of oxygenated monoterpenes, without significant differences between fractions 1 and 2. A study from Iran shows that the composition of essential oils in *O. vulgare* was dominant in β-caryophyllene, germacrene D, and *cis*-sabinene hydrate [251]. Another study from Italy shows that the main components of essential oil in the *O. vulgare* ssp. *vulgare* were β-caryophyllene, thymol, terpinen-4-ol, and *p*-cymene [252]. Biochemical compounds of *O. majorana* are the essential oil and tannins. The difference between the essential oil obtained from *O. vulgare* and *O. majorana* is in quantity (0.67% and 1.5%) [253]. The maximum quantity was obtained in the full flowering stage. The major component is germacrene D for *O. vulgare* and terpinen-4-ol for *O. majorana* [254].

In the folk medicine, *Origanum* was used to treat several illnesses such as spasmodic, antimicrobial, digestive, expectorant, and aromatic for the whooping and convulsive coughs [255, 256]. *O. vulgare* (oregano) and *O. majorana* (marjoram) inhibit the growth of the bacteria and fungus (inhibited the growth of *Candida albicans*) [257] and the synthesis of the microbial metabolites [258, 259]. The leaves of *Origanum* were used to cure diabetes, insomnia, catarrh, and asthma [260]. *O. majorana* has stimulatory properties and vasodilatatory activity [261]. By acting also on cardiovascular system and being used as an adjuvant for diabetes control, *Origanum* subsp. could both prevent and treat more complex diseases associative developed as: atrial fibrillation development [262–265].

3.15. Ziziphora Genus. *Ziziphora* genus is an aromatic herb of the Lamiaceae family, native to Ukraine, Russia, Siberia, Central Asia, Xinjiang, Afghanistan, Irancaner, Turkey, and Middle East. *Ziziphora* species were used as culinary herb in Iran [266].

In traditional medicine, *Ziziphora* is used as infusion, decoction, and maceration for various purposes such as sedative, stomach tonic, heart disorders, common cold, inflammation, carminative, diarrhea, expectorant, coughing, antiseptic, migraine, fever, and depression. Moreover, essential oils are used for treating some diseases such as edema, insomnia, lung abscess, tracheitis, hemorrhoids, and hypertension [267]. The antimicrobial activity of the essential oil of *Salmonella typhi* Vi-positive makes it useful in the treatment of typhoid fever, too. The plant extract can modulate immune response by induction of CD40 expression on DCs and cytokine production and inhibition of T-cell stimulating activity of dendritic cells in high concentration [268].

3.15.1. Ziziphora tenuior. *Ziziphora tenuior* L. may possess an antidepressant-like effect, and its effect is similar to fluoxetine [269]. The composition of the ethanolic extract of *Ziziphora tenuior* contains two new flavonoids named as "ziziphorin A and ziziphorin B," 1-hentetracontanol [270], ursolic acid [271], oleanolic acid (5) [272], β-sitosterol-3-O-β-glucoside [273], and apigenin [274].

The composition of *Z. tenuior* essential oil may therefore vary with plant genetics, environmental conditions, extraction methods, and geographic origin, including climate, soil, elevation, and topography. The main components of *Z. tenuior*, which are identified by GC/MS analysis of the extracts, are 53.977% of *p*-menth-3-en-8-ol, 38.481% of pulegone, and 1.651% of *p*-menth-3,8-diene. The essential oil also contained smaller percentages of β-pinene; 4aα-, 7α-, and 7aα-nepetalactone; α-thujene; caryophyllene oxide; limonene; E-caryophyllene; and terpinolene. *p*-Menth-3-en-8-ol and pulegone are the main components of *Z. tenuior*, and they are responsible for the antimicrobial activities of the essential oil [275]. Essential oils of *Z. tenuior* aerial parts were characterized by high levels of oxygenated monoterpenes, especially pulegone [276].

3.16. Salvia Genus. *Salvia* genus belongs to the subfamily Nepetoideae in the Lamiaceae family. In traditional medicine, salvia is one of the oldest medicinal plants used by humans, and it is considered as a universal panacea, used for its antibacterial, antiviral, antioxidative, antimalarial, anti-inflammatory, antidiabetic, cardiovascular, and antitumor effects.

Salvia can be used as infusion, tincture with diuretic, hemostatic, and spasmolytic activities, volatile oils with antiseptic role, and essential oil with antimicrobial effect.

The pharmacological effects of *Salvia* essential oils are based on the presence of more than 100 active compounds, which can be categorized into monoterpene hydrocarbons, oxygenated monoterpenes, sesquiterpene hydrocarbons, diterpenes, nonisoprenoid compounds and oxygenated sesquiterpenes [277, 278]. The most abundant components are 1,8-cineole, camphor, and a wide variety of thujenes [279].

Analysis made by spectrophotometry and HPLC shows that *Salvia officinalis* L. has the highest total content (1.785 g %) expressed in gram equivalent caffeic acid, and the highest value for rosmarinic acid (728.68 mg %). Rosmarinic acid is the major component, and it has adstringent, anti-iflammatory, antibacterial, and antiviral activity [280]. *S. officinalis* is the most valuable species in terms of biologically active principal contents compared to other species studied, followed by *Salvia verticillata* L. and *Salvia glutinosa* L. [281].

3.17. Leonurus Genus. *Leonurus* genus natively grows in the temperate zone of Asia and Europe and was lately adapted in America and Africa. About 24 species of *Leonurus* have been identified, of which 13 species are spread in China. Plants belonging to *Leonurus* genus are traditionally used for antigynecological disorder in East Asia, and as sedative in Europe. Chemical investigations of the genus enriched the natural products library and also enlarged the pharmacological applications of this traditional herb [282].

3.17.1. Leonurus cardiaca. *Leonurus cardiaca* L. is a perennial herb widespread in Europe, throughout the plains and hills, as well as in East Asia to the Himalayas and eastern Siberia, Northern Africa, and North America [283]. The common name of *L. cardiaca* is motherwort, but it is also known as throw-wort, lion's ear, or lion's tail. For centuries, motherwort extract has been used as a medicinal plant to treat cardiac and vascular diseases, especially tachycardia associated with anxiety, tension, and stress, and also for hypertension to reduce the risk of thrombosis to inhibit artery calcification formation [284].

The ethanolic extract has been prepared by adding 96% ethanol over aerial parts of the plants for 24–36 hours. The supernatant was collected and concentrated by vacuum distillation at a temperature of 50°C. The extract was completely dried under sterile conditions using an autoclave at temperatures lower than 50°C.

In the aerial parts of *L. cardiaca*, many compounds were identified: terpene compounds: monoterpenes (iridoids: leonuride, ajugoside, galiridoside, and reptoside) [285], diterpenes (of clerodane, furanolabdane, and labdane types) [286], triterpenes (ursolic acid, oleanolic acids, corosolic acid, euscaphic acid, and ilelatifol D) [287], nitrogen-containing compounds (leonurine, stachydrine, and amine choline), and phenylpropanoids (lavandulifolioside), as well as flavonoids, phenolic acids, volatile oils, sterols (β-sitosterol and stigmasterol), and tannins. The phenolic compounds comprise phenylpropanoid glycosides such as lavandulifolioside (arabinoside) [288], phenolic acids such as chlorogenic, rosmarinic, caffeic, *p*-coumaric, *p*-hydroxybenzoic, vanillic, and ferulic acids, and phenolic glycoside [289]. The volatile oils mainly contain sesquiterpenes such as germacrene D, epicedrol, β-caryophyllene, α-humulene, and spathulenol and monoterpenes such as α-pinene and dehydro-1,8 cineole [290, 291]. Of these, ursolic acid proved a stronger anti-inflammatory activity than indomethacin and acetylsalicylic acid, and furanolabdane-type diterpenes inhibited abdominal cramps more effectively than the parallel-given aspirin or acetaminophen.

Pharmacological studies have established that *L. cardiaca* possesses additional antimicrobial [286, 292], antioxidant [289, 293], anti-inflammatory [294, 295], antinociceptive [296], neuroprotective [297], sedative [298], and even anticancer effects [299]. The findings obtained by Rezaee-Asl and coworkers, using the *formalin*, *tail flick*, and *hot-plate* tests, assess that central and peripheral mechanisms are involved in the antinociceptive activity of the motherwort extract. According to the tail flick test of this study, *L. cardiaca* extract only at the maximum dose (500 mg/kg) could alleviate the pain in all times of tail flick test, whereas the lower doses (125 and 250 mg/kg) reduced only late pain. The formalin test showed that the *L. cardiaca* extract at a dose of 500 mg/kg and 250 mg/kg was more effective in the first and second phases, suggesting peripheral and central antinociceptive mechanism. The second phase of the formalin test is related to a peripheral inflammatory process [296].

As a conclusion, the studies concerning the analgesic activity of *L. cardiaca* extract afford a justification for the use of this plant in pain and inflammatory disorders. Further research should be accomplished for the isolation of new phytochemicals and to fully understand the antinociceptive mechanism exhibited by the plant extract.

As undesirable effects, one can mention the potential to increase the risk of bleeding due to its antithrombotic and antiplatelet effects, and the synergistic sedative effect when associated with benzodiazepines, which may result in coma [300].

3.18. Mentha Genus. *Mentha* is a genus of plants in the Lamiaceae family, with an estimated number of 13 to 18 species, lacking the exact distinction between them [301]. Hybridization between some of the species occurs naturally. The genus has a wide distribution across Europe, Africa, Asia, Australia, and North America. While the *Mentha* species can be found in many environments, most grow best in wet surroundings and moist soils. The mint stems grow 10–120 cm tall and tend to spread uncontrollably over an indeterminate area; hence, they are sometimes considered invasive. The most common and popular mints for commercial cultivation are *Mentha piperita*, *Mentha spicata*, *Mentha gracilis*, *Mentha arvensis*, and *Mentha suaveolens*. Mint was originally used as a medicinal herb to relieve stomachache and chest pains [302].

3.18.1. Mentha piperita. *Mentha piperita* L. (peppermint) is a hybrid of *M. spicata* and *M. aquatica*. This plant was cultivated since the time of ancient Egyptians and established in the Icelandic Pharmacopoeia of the thirteenth century. The list of benefits and uses of peppermint as a folk remedy or alternative medical therapy include biliary maladies, dyspepsia, enteritis, flatulence, gastritis, intestinal colic, and spasms of the bile duct, gallbladder, or gastrointestinal (GI) tract [303].

The phytochemical occurrence in peppermint leaves and oil depends on plant maturity, variety, geographical origin, and processing methods' conditions [304–307]. As fatty acids, there have been found palmitic, linoleic, and linolenic acids [308]. The main components identified in the volatile oil of peppermint are menthol (33–60%), menthone (15–32%), isomenthone (2–8%), 1,8-cineole (eucalyptol) (5–13%), menthyl acetate (2–11%), menthofuran (1–10%), limonene (1–7%), β-myrcene (0.1–1.7%), β-caryophyllene (2–4%), pulegone (0.5–1.6%), and carvone (1%) [304, 309]. The fresh leaves contain 1.2–3.9% (v/w) of essential oil, while the dried leaves is reported to contain only 21% of the original oil [310].

Carotenoids, chlorophylls, α- and γ-tocopherols, and ascorbic acid have also been reported in the plant extract [311]. The major minerals in dried peppermint leaves include K, Ca, Mg, and Na, along with smaller amounts of Fe, Mn, Zn, and Cu and trace amounts of Cr, I, and Se [312]. The polyphenols isolated from peppermint leaves include mainly eriocitrin and rosmarinic acid, luteolin 7-*O*-rutinoside, and hesperidin [313, 314].

The extraction of essential oils has been approached through different techniques, of which hydrodistillation is still the most common to achieve volatile oils from medicinal plants, including *Mentha* [315]. In order to diminish the extraction time and for higher extraction yields along with an increased quality extracts, a number of extraction procedures have also been implemented, such as microwave-assisted extraction, pressurized solvent extraction, supercritical fluid extraction, and ultrasound-assisted extraction [316–319].

In vitro and *in vivo* pharmacological studies have proved multiple therapeutic effects, which are mentioned as follows: antioxidant capacity (radical scavenging capacity being higher than that of *M. aquatica* or *M. longifolia*) [46, 320], antitumor activity on different cell lines [321, 322], antiallergenic activity [323, 324], antiviral activity with significant results on herpes simplex viruses (HSV-1 and HSV-2) and against human immunodeficiency virus-1 (HIV-1) [242, 325–327], antibacterial activity against different bacterial strains, including Gram-positive cocci and rods and Gram-negative rods (e.g., *S. aureus*, *Salmonella enteritidis*, *Shigella sonnei*, some strains of *E. coli*, *Heli cobacter pylori*, *Haemophilus influenzae*, *Streptococcus pneumoniae*, *Streptococcus pyogenes*, and many other pathogens) [328–331], modulatory effects on hepatic and renal functions [332–334], nervous system actions as analgesic and local anesthetic, and anti-inflammatory actions [335, 336].

The antinociceptive activity of *M. piperita* aqueous extract has been investigated by Yousef A. Taher using *in vivo* tests on mice [336]. According to these studies, the plant extract showed inhibition of acetic acid-induced abdominal constrictions in mice at both 200 and 400 mg/kg doses. The hot-plate test has shown that administration of *M. piperita* aqueous extract (using the same abovementioned doses) caused a significant latency of the response to thermal stimulation. The carrageenan-induced paw edema test disclosed an increase in paw thickness; hence, it is assumed that the aqueous extract has a noninflammatory pain reliever activity, in contrast with previous research when the phytochemical compounds were obtained by the ethanolic extraction [335]. On the other hand, the methanolic extract of different *Mentha* species displayed different analgesic effects, indicating that these effects are species- and extract-form dependent [337, 338]. These findings indicate that the phytochemicals present in the *M. piperita* extract exhibit analgesic effect arising from both CNS and peripheral actions since the response appears to both thermal and chemical pain stimuli. A similar efficacy is characteristic of central analgesics, such as morphine, which inhibits equally inflammatory and noninflammatory pains. The results concerning analgesic effects produced by *M. piperita* strongly recommend this plant as pain reducing and encourage further studies for a better understanding of the nociception mechanism in order to find new options in pain therapy, with less side effects.

Toxicology studies of peppermint oil and its components completed in animals have shown no adverse effects or histopathological modifications. There are no chronic toxicity studies of peppermint in humans, although the use of peppermint oil has been reported as contraindicated in patients with bile duct, gallbladder, and liver disorders. The use of peppermint oil capsules in patients with GI reflux, hiatal hernia, or kidney stones needs also caution [339].

3.18.2. Mentha spicata. *Mentha spicata* L., also known as spearmint, originated in Bangladesh and is traditionally used as herbal remedy for various disorders. Hajjaj Yousuf et al. have performed a study which aimed at evaluating the analgesic, anti-inflammatory, and antipyretic effects of *M. spicata* on animal models, using hot-plate, acetic acid-induced writhing test, carrageenan-induced rat paw edema, and yeast-induced pyrexia methods [340]. The hot-plate results suggest a centrally antinociceptive action with a higher pain inhibition at 180 minutes after administration, being comparable to a standard drug. The acetic acid-induced writhing method evaluates the peripherally analgesic action, which took place through inhibition of local peritoneal receptors, most probably by inhibition of cyclooxygenase activity. The anti-inflammatory effect was maintained at a significant level for a 6-hour period, showing efficiency in the late phase of inflammation due to the presence of certain components that interfere with the release of prostaglandins.

Many other research studies on *Mentha* species such *as M. longifolia* [341], *M. arvensis* [342], or *M. villosa* [343] were also carried out regarding the analgesic activity. Although the phytochemical occurrence is not identical, different mechanisms have been consequently involved in achieving the antinociception, with competitive results.

3.19. Lavandula Genus. *Lavandula* genus includes more than 39 known species, mostly distributed in Arabia, Mediterranean Coasts, Asia, Middle East, and Northern Africa. *Lavandula officinalis, Lavandula angustifolia*, *Lavandula hybrida*, and *Lavandula vera* have been considered as antidepressive, antispasmodic, antiflatulent, antiemetic, diuretic, anticonvulsant, antibacterial, antiepileptogenic, antioxidant, antibacterial, antifungal, sedative, antinociceptive, and gastroprotective effects [344–348]. Lavender comprised over 100 constituents, among which the primary components are polyphenols, anthocyanins, carotenoids, linalool and linalyl acetate, α-pinene, limonene, 1,8-cineole, *cis*- and *trans*-ocimene, 3-octanone, camphor, caryophyllene, terpinen-4-ol, and flavonoids [349, 350].

3.19.1. Lavandula angustifolia. *Lavandula angustifolia* Mill. is one of the most famous aromatic and medicinal plants [351] used in fresh state or dry condition, containing 1–6% volatile oils (monoterpenic compounds, alcohols, and esters), triterpenic acids, coumarins, flavones, resins, and polyphenols [352]. As medicinal activity, *L. angustifolia* extracts or essential oils possess antispastic, carminative, analgesic, sedative, hypotensive, antiseptic, antimicrobial, antifungic, diuretic, and general tonic action, but little information on lavender analgesic properties is available in the literature.

3.19.2. Lavandula officinalis. *Lavandula officinalis* Chaix is used in traditional and herbal medicine for the treatment of pain and in the reduction of the inflammatory pain. In pharmacological and biological tests, extracts, fractions, and essential oils of *L. officinalis* are reported to have analgesic effects. The literature data show that *L. officinalis* extract contains linalool, acetate linalool, monotril, sesquiterpene, luteolin, ursolic acid, coumarin, and umbelliferone.

Hajhashemi and Ghannadi [349] showed that the aquatic, alcoholic, and phenolic extracts have antinociception effects in the second phase of the formalin test, but only the phenolic and alcoholic extracts had been able to prevent the first phase of the formalin test. Barocelli et al. (2004) [353] proved that *L. officinalis* leaves inhalation attenuates pain evoked by hot-plate test, and stomach graze induced by high-dose administration of ethanol and ascetic acid. Husseini et al. (2015) [354] demonstrated that *L. officinalis* hydroalcoholic extracts inhibit inflammation and pain induced by formalin and cyclooxygenase (COX) type 1 and 2 activity in mice, using the formalin and hot-plate tests. The administration of the extract (100, 200, 250, 300, 400, and 800 mg/kg, i.p.) has inhibitory effects on inflammation induced by formalin injection into the animals hind paw, effects equal to morphine, dexamethasone, and indomethacin. The extract in 100, 200, and 300 mg/kg significantly reduced heat-induced pain and COX activity in dose-dependent manner.

3.19.3. Lavandula hybrida. In 2004, Barocelli et al. [353] demonstrated the antinociceptive and the gastroprotective effects of orally administered (100 mg/kg) or inhaled *Lavandula hybrida* Reverchon "Grosso" essential oil, and its principal constituents linalool and linalyl acetate in rodents. In the hot-plate test, the analgesic activity was observed after oil inhalation was inhibited by naloxone, atropine, and mecamylamine pretreatment, suggesting the involvement of opioidergic as well as cholinergic pathways. Therefore, the lavender oil reveals an interesting analgesic activity mainly relevant after inhalation, at doses devoid of sedative side effect, suggesting the interest for potential application of this oil in aromatherapy.

4. Identification of Secondary Metabolites

The identification of secondary metabolites from essential oils was achieved by gas chromatography coupled with mass spectrometry and from aqueous or alcoholic extracts by liquid chromatography coupled with mass spectrometry. Due to the high selectivity and sensitivity, mass spectrometry coupled to separation techniques such as gas chromatography and liquid chromatography represents a valuable technique for the qualitative and quantitative analysis of chemical substances present in essential oils and plant extracts.

The determination of the chemical composition belonging to essential oils for the following 14 species of the Lamiaceae family of plants: *Hyptis pectinata* [357], *Lavandula angustifolia* [349], *Lavandula officinalis* [356], *Leonurus cardiaca* [290], *Lamium purpureum* [357], *Melissa officinalis* [358], *Mentha spicata* [359], *Marrubium vulgare* [360], *Origanum vulgare* [361], *Ocimum basilicum* [362], *Rosmarinus officinalis* [363], *Salvia officinalis* [364], *Satureja hortensis*, and *Thymus vulgaris* [365], included in most of the scientific articles follow the same steps: (i) collection of flowering aerial parts and drying of the plant material, (ii) hydrodistillation of the dried plant material using a Clevenger apparatus for 1 to 5 hours, (iii) drying the essential oil using anhydrous sodium sulfate (Na_2SO_4), storing the essential oil in the dark at 4°C, i.v. injection of 0.1–1 μl of the essential oil in the capillary column of a gas chromatograph, and separation of the chemical compounds, (v) ionization and detection of each volatile substance in a mass spectrometer, and (vi) identification of the components performed based on their retention indices established in relation with a series of *n*-alkanes (C_8–C_{32}) and based on the mass spectra stored in NIST 21, NIST 107, Wiley spectral libraries, or reported in scientific articles.

The volatile substances isolated from the 14 species of plants and analyzed by gas chromatography coupled with mass spectrometry are presented for each of the essential oils in Table 1.

The chemical compounds identified by LC-ESI-MS in extracts prepared for the 9 species of plants that are included in the Lamiaceae family are also presented in Table 2.

Yalçin and the collaborators showed, using HPLC-ESI-MS, that the *n*-butanol extract of *Lamium garganicum* subsp. *Laevigatum*, which was previously shown to possess anti-inflammatory and antinociceptive activity, contains nine iridoid glycosides [366].

The decoction prepared from *Melissa officinalis* dry leaves was filtered through a Whatman no. 4 filter paper, frozen and lyophilized. The phenolic compounds were separated and analyzed by HPLC coupled with an ESI-triple quadrupole-ion trap mass spectrometer using the negative-ion mode. The identification of the phenolic compounds was carried out based on the comparison of their retention time, UV-Vis, and mass spectra with those obtained from solutions prepared with standard substances. For the compounds for which no standard substance was available, the identification was performed based on the scientific literature [367].

Based on the UHPLC-ESI-MS data reported by Martina Cirlini et al. [368], the methanolic extract of *Mentha spicata* contains 88% of rosmarinic acid derivatives when calculating the amount of rosmarinic acid derivatives as percentage of the total amount of detected phenols. For the salvianolic acids, a percentage of 5.6% of the total amount of detected phenols was calculated.

Taamalli and collaborators reported the analyses of the methanolic extract of *Mentha pulegium* performed using an UPLC-ESI-QTOF mass spectrometer coupled with a liquid chromatograph and detected metabolites from the following groups: hydroxybenzoic acids, hydroxycinnamic acids, flavanols, flavones, flavanones, flavonols, organic acids, nucleosides, amino acids, and fatty acids [56]. In the methanolic extract of *Mentha pulegium*, the authors identified a very high amount of gallocatechin.

In the case of the plant *Marrubium vulgare*, Amessis-Ouchemoukh Nadia and collaborators prepared the methanolic extract and analyzed it using an UHPLC-ESI-QTOF instrument. The mass spectra were acquired in the negative-ion mode and showed the presence of the metabolites presented in Table 2 [369].

Anna Vallverdú-Queralt et al. identified the phenolic compounds present in the ethanolic acidified extract of

Table 1: Compounds identified by GC-MS in essential oil.

Number	Compound	Plant name: *Hyptis pectinata*	*Lavandula angustifolia*	*Lavandula officinalis*	*Leonurus cardiaca*	*Lamium purpureum*	*Melissa officinalis*	*Mentha spicata*	*Marrubium vulgare*	*Origanum vulgare*	*Ocimum basilicum*	*Rosmarinus officinalis*	*Salvia officinalis*	*Satureja hortensis*	*Thymus vulgaris*	References
1	Sabinene	+				+	+	+		+			+			[355, 357–359, 361, 364]
2	β-Pinene	+	+	+	+	+	+	+				+	+	+		[355, 357, 359–361, 363–365]
3	1-Octen-3-ol	+					+			+						[355, 358, 361]
4	Limonene	+			+	+	+	+					+	+	+	[290, 355, 357, 358, 364, 365]
5	β-(E)-Ocimene	+	+			+	+			+						[349, 355, 357, 358, 361]
6	Linalool	+	+	+					+	+	+	+	+		+	[349, 355, 356, 360–363]
7	α-Copaene	+		+		+	+				+					[355, 356, 357, 358, 362]
8	β-Elemene	+				+					+					[355, 357, 362]
9	β-Caryophyllene	+	+	+	+	+	+	+	+	+		+	+	+	+	[349, 355–359, 361, 363–365]
10	Aromadendrene	+											+			[355, 364]
11	cis-Muurola-3,5-diene	+														[355]
12	α-Humulene	+		+	+		+		+	+	+		+			[290, 355, 356, 358, 360–362, 364]
13	Germacrene D	+	+		+	+	+		+	+	+					[290, 349, 355, 358, 360–362]
14	cis-β-Guaiene	+														[355]
15	γ-Patchoulene	+														[355]
16	Germacrene A	+														[355]
17	γ-Cadinene	+			+	+	+			+	+					[290, 355, 357, 358, 361, 362]
18	trans-Calamenene	+														[355]
19	Germacrene B	+		+												[355, 356]
20	Caryophyllene oxide	+			+		+						+			[290, 355, 358, 364]
21	1,10-Di-epi-cubenol	+														[355]
22	Calamusenone	+														[355]
23	Cyperotundone	+														[355]
24	α-Thujene		+			+				+		+	+	+		[349, 357, 361, 363–365]
25	α-Pinene		+	+	+	+	+	+	+	+		+	+	+	+	[290, 349, 356–361, 363–365]
26	α-Fenchene		+										+			[349, 364]
27	Camphene		+	+					+	+		+	+	+	+	[349, 356, 360, 361, 363–365]
28	Delta-3-carene		+													[349]
29	1,8-Cineole		+	+			+	+	+		+	+	+			[349, 356, 358–360, 362–364]
30	γ-Terpinene		+	+			+	+		+			+	+	+	[349, 356, 358, 359, 361, 364, 365]
31	Terpinolene		+		+		+					+		+	+	[290, 349, 358, 363–365]
32	Camphor		+	+					+			+	+			[349, 356, 360, 363, 364]
33	Borneol		+						+			+	+	+	+	[349, 360, 363–365]

TABLE 1: Continued.

Number	Compound	Plant name														References
		Hyptis pectinata	*Lavandula angustifolia*	*Lavandula officinalis*	*Leonurus cardiaca*	*Lamium purpureum*	*Melissa officinalis*	*Mentha spicata*	*Marrubium vulgare*	*Origanum vulgare*	*Ocimum basilicum*	*Rosmarinus officinalis*	*Salvia officinalis*	*Satureja hortensis*	*Thymus vulgaris*	
34	Lavandulol		+													[349]
35	4-Terpineol		+	+			+	+					+	+		[349, 356, 358, 359, 364, 365]
36	**α**-Terpineol		+	+			+	+		+			+	+	+	[349, 356, 358, 359, 361, 364, 365]
37	Linalyl acetate		+							+			+			[349, 361, 364]
38	Bornyl acetate		+	+			+				+	+	+			[349, 356, 358, 362–364]
39	cis-**β**-Farnesene		+													[349]
40	Verbenene			+												[356]
41	1,3,5-cycloheptatriene			+												[356]
42	3-Octanone			+		+										[356, 357]
43	**β**-myrcene			+		+	+	+		+		+	+	+	+	[356, 357–359, 361, 364–365]
44	3-Octanol			+		+										[356, 357]
45	**α**-Phellandrene			+						+		+		+		[356, 361, 363, 365]
46	*o*-Isopropenyl toluene			+												[356]
47	**α**-Terpinene			+			+			+				+	+	[356, 358, 361, 364, 365]
48	*p*-Cymene			+	+		+	+		+			+	+	+	[290, 356, 358, 359, 361, 364, 365]
49	Linalool oxide			+												[356]
50	Methyl benzoate			+												[356]
51	Thujancis			+												[356]
52	D-fenchyl alcohol			+												[356]
53	Pinocarveol			+												[356]
54	Isopinocamphone			+									+			[356, 364]
55	Pinocarvone			+												[356]
56	Pinocamphone			+									+			[356, 364]
57	Naphthalene			+												[356]
58	*p*-Cymen-8-ol			+									+			[356, 364]
59	Myrtenol			+												[356]
60	Verbenone			+												[356]
61	*trans*-Carveol			+				+								[356, 359]
62	**β**-Citronellol			+					+							[356, 360]
63	Pulegone			+			+	+								[356, 358, 359]
64	Piperitone			+				+								[356, 359]
65	Cinnamaldehyde			+												[356]
66	Thymol			+			+			+				+	+	[356, 358, 361, 364, 365]
67	2-Hydroxy-4-isopropyl-1-methylbenzene			+												[356]
68	Carvacrol			+						+			+	+	+	[356, 361, 364, 365]
69	Piperitenone			+			+									[356, 358]
70	**α**-Cubebene			+												[356]
71	Thymyl acetate			+												[356]
72	Farnesene			+		+					+					[356, 357, 362]
73	**β**-Acoradiene			+												[356]
74	**α**-Cedrene			+												[356]
75	Spathulenol			+	+		+				+			+		[290, 356, 358, 362, 365]

Table 1: Continued.

Number	Compound	Plant name														References
		Hyptis pectinata	*Lavandula angustifolia*	*Lavandula officinalis*	*Leonurus cardiaca*	*Lamium purpureum*	*Melissa officinalis*	*Mentha spicata*	*Marrubium vulgare*	*Origanum vulgare*	*Ocimum basilicum*	*Rosmarinus officinalis*	*Salvia officinalis*	*Satureja hortensis*	*Thymus vulgaris*	
76	Butylidenephthalide			+												[356]
77	3N Butylphthalide			+												[356]
78	Butylidene dihydrophthalide			+												[356]
79	3-Methyl butanal				+											[290]
80	(E,E)-2,4-Hexadienal				+											[290]
81	Benzaldehyde				+											[290]
82	Dehydro-1,8-cineole				+											[290]
83	Phenylacetaldehyde				+											[290]
84	*p*-Menth-1,5-dien-8-ol				+											[290]
85	Dodecane				+											[290]
86	Dihydroedulan I				+											[290]
87	(E)-**α**-ionone				+											[290]
88	**β**-Humulene				+											[290]
89	Geranyl acetone				+											[290]
90	(E)-**β**-ionone				+											[290]
91	**β**-Selinene				+											[290]
92	Eugenyl acetate				+											[290]
93	(E)-nerolidol				+											[290]
94	*trans*-Sesquisabinene hydrate				+											[290]
95	Presilphiperfolan-8-ol				+											[290]
96	**β**-Atlantol				+											[290]
97	Epi-cedrol				+											[290]
98	**α**-Bisabolol				+											[290]
99	(2E, 6E)-farnesol				+											[290]
100	8-Cedren-13-ol acetate				+											[290]
101	6,10,14-Trimethyl-2-pentadecanone				+											[290]
102	(2Z, 6E)-farnesyl acetate				+											[290]
103	Methyl-linolenate				+											[290]
104	Allo-aromadendrene epoxide				+											[290]
105	Eicosane				+											[290]
106	Heneicosane				+											[290]
107	(E)-3-hexen-1-ol					+										[349]
108	Heptanal					+										[357]
109	1-Octen-3-one					+										[357]
110	(E,E)-2,4-Heptadienal					+										[357]
111	Z-**β**-ocimene					+	+			+						[356, 357, 361]
112	Undecane					+										[357]
113	Nonanal					+										[357]
114	Decanal					+										[357]
115	**β**-Cyclocitral					+										[357]
116	N-tridecane					+										[357]
117	Delta-elemene					+				+						[357, 361]
118	(E)-**β**-damascenone					+										[357]
119	**β**-bourbonene					+		+	+	+						[290, 357, 359, 361]
120	(E)-**β**-farnesene					+										[357]
121	Farnesane					+										[357]
122	Bicyclogermacrene					+	+							+		[357, 358, 365]
123	*n*-Pentadecane					+										[357]

Table 1: Continued.

Number	Compound	Plant name														References
		Hyptis pectinata	*Lavandula angustifolia*	*Lavandula officinalis*	*Leonurus cardiaca*	*Lamium purpureum*	*Melissa officinalis*	*Mentha spicata*	*Marrubium vulgare*	*Origanum vulgare*	*Ocimum basilicum*	*Rosmarinus officinalis*	*Salvia officinalis*	*Satureja hortensis*	*Thymus vulgaris*	
124	(E)-hydrate de sabinene						+									[358]
125	*p*-Menth-3,8-diene						+									[358]
126	Z-hydrate de sabinene						+						+			[358, 365]
127	1-Octen-3-ol acetate						+									[358]
128	3-Octenyl acetate						+									[358]
129	*p*-Menth-3-en-8-ol						+									[358]
130	Menthone						+	+								[358, 359]
131	Isomenthone						+	+	+						+	[358–360, 364]
132	Neomenthol						+									[358]
133	Z-Piperitone oxide						+									[358]
134	Pseudodisphenol						+									[358]
135	Isopulegyl acetate 1						+									[358]
136	Neomenthylacetate						+	+								[358, 359]
137	Diosphenol						+									[358]
138	Menthylacetate						+	+								[358, 359]
139	Piperitenone oxide						+									[358]
140	(E)-jasmone						+									[358]
141	Nepetalactone						+									[358]
142	*p*-Menth-1,2,3-triol						+									[358]
143	**α**-Gurjunene						+									[358]
144	Cadina-3,5-diene						+									[358]
145	Delta-cadinene						+		+							[358, 360]
146	Viridiflorol						+									[358]
147	1,10-Di-epi-cubenol						+									[358]
148	**α**-cadinol						+				+					[358, 362]
149	2-Octanol							+								[359]
150	Menthol							+								[359]
151	Isomenthol							+								[359]
152	Dihydrocarveol							+					+		+	[359, 364]
153	Carvone							+		+						[357, 359]
154	*cis*-Carveol							+								[359]
155	*trans*-Anethole							+								[359]
156	Menthyl camphor							+								[359]
157	Eugenol							+			+					[359, 362]
158	*N*-trimethylsilyl trifluoroacetamide								+							[360]
159	*N,N'*-bis(trimethylsilyl) trifluoroacetamide								+							[360]
160	**α**-Thujone								+							[360]
161	1-Vinyl cyclohexane								+							[360]
162	Geraniol								+				+			[360, 364]
163	Citronellyl formate								+							[360]
164	**α**-Muurolene								+							[360]
165	**α**-Amorphene								+		+					[360, 362]
166	Neoalloocimene								+							[360]
167	Neryl acetate								+							[360]
168	Ledene								+							[360]

TABLE 1: Continued.

Number	Compound	Plant name														References
		Hyptis pectinata	*Lavandula angustifolia*	*Lavandula officinalis*	*Leonurus cardiaca*	*Lamium purpureum*	*Melissa officinalis*	*Mentha spicata*	*Marrubium vulgare*	*Origanum vulgare*	*Ocimum basilicum*	*Rosmarinus officinalis*	*Salvia officinalis*	*Satureja hortensis*	*Thymus vulgaris*	
169	β-Bisabolene								+	+				+		[360, 361, 365]
170	α-Agarofuran								+							[360]
171	γ-Eudesmol								+							[360]
172	Furan-2-one, 4-phenyltetrahydro								+							[360]
173	β-Cubebene								+							[360]
174	Citronellyl butanoate								+							[360]
175	Geranyl tiglate								+							[360]
176	Cyclononasiloxane, octadecamethyl								+							[360]
177	Eicosamethylcyclodecasiloxane								+							[360]
178	β-Phellandrene									+			+		+	[361, 365]
179	Carvacrol methyl ether									+				+		[361, 365]
180	Allo-aromadendrene									+	+		+			[361, 362, 364]
181	*cis*-Epoxy-ocimen										+					[362]
182	*cis*-Caryophyllene										+					[362]
183	α-Guaiene										+					[362]
184	Delta-guaiene										+					[362]
185	*cis*-Calamenene										+					[362]
186	Epi-bicyclosesquiphellandrene										+					[365]
187	β-Eudesmol										+					[362]
188	α-Selinene										+					[362]
189	Zingiberene										+					[362]
190	Tricyclene											+				[360]
191	*o*-Cymene											+	+		+	[358, 363, 364]
192	Trifluoroacetyl-α-															
Terpineol											+					[363]
193	Carene											+				[363]
194	*cis*-α-Terpineol											+				[363]
195	2-Bornanone											+				[363]
196	Isoborneol											+			+	[363, 364]
197	*trans*-Pinocarveol												+			[364]
198	(-)-Citronellal												+		+	[363]
199	Myrtenal												+		+	[363]
200	Myrtenol												+		+	[363]
201	Isobornyl acetate												+			[363]
202	β-Cedrene												+			[363]
203	γ-Gurjunene												+			[363]
204	α-7-Epi-selinene												+			[363]
205	Carvacrol acetate													+		[361]

Table 2: Compounds identified by HPLC-ESI-MS in aqueous and alcoholic extracts.

Number	Compound	Plant name									References
		Lamium garganicum subsp. *Laevigatum*	*Melissa officinalis*	*Mentha spicata*	*Mentha pulegium*	*Marrubium vulgare*	*Origanum vulgare*	*Ocimum basilicum*	*Rosmarinus officinalis*	*Salvia officinalis*	
1	Lamalbidee	+									[366]
2	Sesamoside	+									[366]
3	Lamiide	+									[366]
4	6-β-OH ipolamiide	+									[366]
5	Shanzhiside methyl ester	+									[366]
6	Dehydropenstemoside	+									[366]
7	8-*O*-acetyl shanzhiside methyl ester	+									[366]
8	6-Syringyl-8-*O*-acetyl shanzhiside methyl ester	+									[366]
9	3-(3,4-Dihydroxyphenyl)-lactic acid		+								[367]
10	Caftaric acid		+	+							[367, 372]
11	Caffeic acid hexoside		+				+				[367, 370]
12	Fertaric acid		+								[367]
13	Caffeic acid		+	+		+	+	+	+	+	[367, 369, 370, 372, 373]
14	Sulfated rosmarinic acid		+								[367]
15	Yunnaneic acid E		+								[367]
16	Prolithospermic acid		+								[367]
17	Lithospermic acid A isomer		+								[367]
18	Chicoric acid		+								[367]
19	Salvianolic acid C derivative		+								[367]
20	Sagerinic acid		+	+							[367, 372]
21	*cis*-Rosmarinic acid		+								[367]
22	*trans*-Rosmarinic acid		+								[367]
23	Salvianolic acid A isomer		+								[367]
24	Protocatechuic acid			+			+	+		+	[370–373]
25	Hydroxybenzoic acid			+						+	[372, 373]
26	Hydroxyphenyllactic acid			+							[372]
27	Luteolin-8-C-glucoside (orientin)			+							[372]
28	3′-Caffeoylquinic (neochlorogenic acid)			+			+				[370, 372]
29	Coumaric acid			+			+				[370, 372]
30	Salvianolic acid F			+							[372]
31	Dicaffeic acid			+							[372]
32	5′-Caffeoylquinic (chlorogenic acid)			+	+		+	+		+	[56, 370–373]
33	Feruloylquinic acid			+							[372]
34	Rosmarinic acid-*O*-caffeic acid			+							[372]

Table 2: Continued.

Number	Compound	Plant name									References
		Lamium garganicum subsp. *Laevigatum*	*Melissa officinalis*	*Mentha spicata*	*Mentha pulegium*	*Marrubium vulgare*	*Origanum vulgare*	*Ocimum basilicum*	*Rosmarinus officinalis*	*Salvia officinalis*	
35	Rosmarinic acid-rutinoside			+							[372]
36	Salvianolic acid J isomer			+							[372]
37	Luteolin-rutinoside			+	+				+		[56, 372]
38	Rosmarinic acid-*O*-hexoside			+			+				[370, 372]
39	Luteolin-hexoside			+					+	+	[372, 373]
40	Luteolin-7-glucuronide			+				+	+	+	[371–373]
41	Salvianolic acid B/E isomer			+							[372]
42	Narirutin (naringenin-7-*O*-rutinoside)			+							[372]
43	Salvianolic acid D			+							[372]
44	Salvianolic acid E			+	+						[56, 372]
45	Rosmarinic acid			+	+		+	+	+	+	[56, 370–373]
46	Sagerinic acid isomer			+							[372]
47	Salvianolic acid A derivative			+							[372]
48	Lithospermic acid			+	+						[56, 372]
49	Salvianolic acid B			+	+						[56, 372]
50	Dehydrorosmarinic acid			+							[372]
51	Rosmarinic acid dihexoside			+							[372]
52	Salvianolic acid A			+							[372]
53	Apigenin				+	+	+	+	+		[56, 369–372]
54	Hydroxybenzoic acid hexose isomer 1				+					+	[56, 373]
55	Vanillyl alcohol				+						[8]
56	Dihydroxybenzoic acid hexose				+						[8]
57	Vanillic acid hexose				+		+				[4, 8]
58	Syringic acid				+		+	+			[56, 370, 371]
59	Hydroxybenzoic acid hexose isomer 2				+						[8]
60	Dihydroxybenzoic acid				+						[8]
61	Syringic acid hexose				+						[8]
62	Caffeic acid glucuronide isomer 1				+						[8]
63	Caffeic acid glucuronide isomer 2				+						[56]
64	*p*-Coumaric acid				+			+	+		[56, 371, 372]
65	Salvianolic acid I				+						[56]
66	Salvianolic acid H				+						[56]
67	Isosalvianolic acid B				+						[56]
68	Eukovoside				+						[56]

TABLE 2: Continued.

Number	Compound	Plant name									References
		Lamium garganicum subsp. *Laevigatum*	*Melissa officinalis*	*Mentha spicata*	*Mentha pulegium*	*Marrubium vulgare*	*Origanum vulgare*	*Ocimum basilicum*	*Rosmarinus officinalis*	*Salvia officinalis*	
69	Salvianolic acid C				+						[56]
70	Catechin-4-ol-*O*-glycopyranoside				+						[56]
71	Gallocatechin isomer 1				+						[56]
72	(+)-Catechin hydrated				+						[56]
73	Diosmin				+						[56]
74	Acacetin rutinoside				+						[56]
75	Hesperidin				+						[56]
76	Isosakuranetin-*O*-rutinoside				+						[56]
77	Syringetin				+						[56]
78	Jaceidin isomer 1				+						[56]
79	Geshoidin					+					[369]
80	Decaffeoylverbascoside					+					[369]
81	Sacranoside A					+					[369]
82	Marruboside					+					[369]
83	Forsythoside B (isomer 1)					+					[369]
84	Forsythoside B (isomer 2)					+					[369]
85	Verbascosin					+					[369]
86	Luteolin-*O*-glucoside					+				+	[369, 373]
87	Alyssonoside					+					[369]
88	Leukoceptoside A					+					[369]
89	Apigenin-*O*-glucoside					+					[369]
90	Deacetylforskolin (isomer 1)					+					[369]
91	Preleosibirin					+					[369]
92	Deacetylforskolin (isomer 2)					+					[369]
93	Garcinone E (isomer 1)					+					[369]
94	Terniflorin (isomer 1)					+					[369]
95	Garcinone E (isomer 2)					+					[369]
96	Luteolin					+		+	+		[369, 371, 372]
97	Premarrubiin (isomer 1)					+					[369]
98	Terniflorin (isomer 2)					+					[369]
99	Premarrubiin (isomer 2)					+					[369]
100	Deacetylforskolin (isomer 3)					+					[369]
101	Terniflorin (isomer 3)					+					[369]
102	Deacetylforskolin (isomer 4)					+					[369]
103	Deacetylforskolin (isomer 5)					+					[369]
104	Marrulibacetal A (isomer 1)					+					[369]
105	Marrulibacetal A (isomer 2)					+					[369]
106	Premarrubiin (isomer 3)					+					[369]
107	Premarrubiin (isomer 4)					+					[369]

TABLE 2: Continued.

Number	Compound	Plant name									References
		Lamium garganicum subsp. *Laevigatum*	*Melissa officinalis*	*Mentha spicata*	*Mentha pulegium*	*Marrubium vulgare*	*Origanum vulgare*	*Ocimum basilicum*	*Rosmarinus officinalis*	*Salvia officinalis*	
108	Anisofolin A (isomer 1)					+					[369]
109	Anisofolin A (isomer 2)					+					[369]
110	Marrubenol					+					[369]
111	Gallic acid						+	+			[372, 373]
112	*p*-Hydroxybenzoic acid						+	+	+		[371, 372]
113	*m*-Hydroxybenzoic acid						+				[370]
114	Coumaric acid-*O*-hexoside						+				[370]
115	Cryptochlorogenic acid (4-*O*-caffeoylquinic acid)						+				[370]
116	Homovanilic acid						+				[370]
117	Apigenin-C-hexoside-C-hexoside						+				[370]
118	4-*O*-*p*-coumaroylqunic acid						+				[370]
119	Kaempferol-*O*-dihexoside						+				[370]
120	Ferulic acid						+	+			[370, 371]
121	Kaempferol-3-*O*-rutinoside						+	+			[370, 371]
122	Quercetin-3-*O*-glucoside						+	+			[370, 371]
123	Kaempferol-3-*O*-glucoside						+				[370]
124	Dicaffeoylquinic acid						+				[370]
125	Hesperidin						+				[370]
126	Apigenin-7-*O*-glucoside						+	+	+		[370–372]
127	Kaempferol						+	+			[370, 371]
128	Quercetin						+	+			[370, 371]
129	Hesperidin (hesperetin-7-*O*-rutinoside)						+		+		[370, 371]
130	Rosmanol						+		+		[370, 372]
131	Carnosic acid						+		+	+	[370, 372, 373]
132	Quercetin-3-*O*-rutinoside (rutin)							+			[371]
133	Quercetin-3-*O*-malonylglucoside							+			[371]
134	Apigenin-7-*O*-glucuronide							+		+	[371, 373]
135	Eugenol							+			[371]
136	Coniferaldehyde							+			[371]
137	Isothymusin							+			[371]
138	Kaempferide							+			[371]
139	Cirsiliol							+			[371]
140	Cirsimaritin							+			[371]
141	Cirsilineol							+			[371]
142	Nevadensin							+			[371]
143	Acacetin							+			[371]

Table 2: Continued.

Number	Compound	Plant name									References
		Lamium garganicum subsp. *Laevigatum*	*Melissa officinalis*	*Mentha spicata*	*Mentha pulegium*	*Marrubium vulgare*	*Origanum vulgare*	*Ocimum basilicum*	*Rosmarinus officinalis*	*Salvia officinalis*	
144	5-Desmethylsinensetin							+			[371]
145	Methyleugenol							+			[371]
146	Salvigenin							+			[371]
147	Methoxyeugenol							+			[371]
148	Gardenin B							+			[371]
149	Apigenin-7,4-dimethylether							+			[371]
150	Oleanolic acid							+			[371]
151	Ursolic acid							+			[371]
152	Galloylglucose							+			[371]
153	Etylprotocatechuate							+			[371]
154	Methylgallate							+			[371]
155	Sinapinic acid							+			[371]
156	Methylprotocatechuate							+			[371]
157	Vanillic acid							+			[371]
158	Ethyl caffeate							+			[371]
159	Medioresinol								+		[372]
160	Isorhamnetin-3-*O*-hexoside								+		[372]
161	Homoplantaginin (hispidulin 7-glucoside)								+		[372]
162	Dihydroxy-dimethoxyflavone derivative								+		[372]
163	Dihydroxy-dimethoxyflavone								+		[372]
164	Medioresinol derivative								+		[372]
165	Luteolin-3′-acetyl-*O*-glucuronide								+		[372]
166	Medioresinol-glucuronide								+		[372]
167	Eriodictyol								+		[372]
168	Isorhamnetin-rutinoside								+		[372]
169	Isorhamnetin								+		[372]
170	Trihydroxy-methoxyflavone								+		[372]
171	Methylrosmarinate								+		[372]
172	Apigenin-7-*O*-rutinoside								+		[372]
173	Hispidulin-rutinoside								+		[372]
174	Hesperetin								+		[372]
175	5,6,7,10-Tetrahydro-7-hydroxyrosmariquinone derivative								+		[372]
176	Cirsimaritin								+		[372]
177	Carnosol methyl ether isomer								+		[372]

Table 2: Continued.

Number	Compound	Plant name									References
		Lamium garganicum subsp. *Laevigatum*	*Melissa officinalis*	*Mentha spicata*	*Mentha pulegium*	*Marrubium vulgare*	*Origanum vulgare*	*Ocimum basilicum*	*Rosmarinus officinalis*	*Salvia officinalis*	
178	Rosmanol quinone								+		[372]
179	Epirosmanol								+		[372]
180	Carnosol quinone								+		[372]
181	Isosakuranetin								+		[372]
182	Genkwanin								+		[372]
183	Carnosic acid hexoside								+		[372]
184	Rosmanol isomer								+		[372]
185	Carnosol								+		[372]
186	Carnosic acid quinone								+		[372]
187	4′-Methoxytectochrysin								+		[372]
188	Rosmadial								+		[372]
189	Rosmaridiphenol								+		[372]
190	5,6,7,10-Tetrahydro-7-hydroxyrosmariquinone								+		[372]
191	12-*O*-methylcarnosic acid								+		[372]
192	Betulinic acid								+		[372]
193	Salvianic acid A									+	[373]
194	Protocatechuoyl-hexose									+	[373]
195	Dimethoxybenzoic acid									+	[373]
196	Coumaroyl hexose									+	[373]
197	Caffeoyl-fructosyl-glucose									+	[373]
198	Coumaroyl-apiosyl-glucose-isomer									+	[373]
199	Chlorogenic acid isomer									+	[373]
200	Methyldihydrojasmonic acid isomer									+	[373]
201	Feruloyl-glucose isomer									+	[373]
202	Salvianolic acid I isomer									+	[373]
203	Saponarin (apigenin-6-C-glucoside-7-*O*-glucoside)									+	[373]
204	Salvianolic F isomer									+	[373]
205	Luteolin diglucuronide									+	[373]
206	Eriocitrin									+	[373]
207	Hydroxy-luteolin-glucuronide									+	[373]
208	Methylmelitric acid A									+	[373]
209	Apigenin-diglucuronide									+	[373]
210	Sagecoumarin									+	[373]
211	Luteolin-rutinoside isomer									+	[373]
212	Apigenin rutinoside isomer									+	[373]
213	Apigenin hexoside									+	[373]

Table 2: Continued.

Number	Compound	Plant name									References
		Lamium garganicum subsp. *Laevigatum*	*Melissa officinalis*	*Mentha spicata*	*Mentha pulegium*	*Marrubium vulgare*	*Origanum vulgare*	*Ocimum basilicum*	*Rosmarinus officinalis*	*Salvia officinalis*	
214	Hispiludin-glucuronide									+	[373]
215	Salvianolic acid B									+	[373]
216	Salvianolic acid K isomer									+	[373]
217	Carnosol isomer									+	[373]
218	Epirosmanol									+	[373]
219	Carnosic acid isomer									+	[373]

Origanum vulgare (Table 2) [370]. After the first extraction with a hydroalcoholic solvent, the extracted plant material was centrifuged, dried, ground, and stored. An aliquot of 1 g of extracted and dried plant material was subjected to extraction, 3 times, with 5 mL of 50% aqueous ethanol containing 0.1% formic acid. All the supernatants were combined, and the organic solvent was evaporated under nitrogen flow. The dried residue was dissolved in 0.1% formic acid and subjected to solid-phase extraction using mixed-mode anion-exchange cartridges in order to reduce potential interferences from plant extracts. For accurate mass measurement, the separation and mass spectrometric analyses were performed using a LC-ESI-LTQ-Orbitrap mass spectrometer operated in negative-ion mode. The quantification of the compounds identified was performed using a triple-quadrupole mass spectrometer.

Pandey and Kumar performed extraction of dried leaves of *Ocimum basilicum* using 80% aqueous methanol [371]. A liquid chromatograph coupled to an ESI-Q-TOF mass spectrometer was used for the identification of the compounds, and the results are summarized in Table 2.

5. *In Vivo* Evaluation of Phytochemicals Analgesic Activity

Over the decades, just a few studies tried to find alternatives to the classical treatment of pain, such as the application of the Lamiaceae phytochemicals.

Marrubiin, the broadly known diterpenoid lactone, has been associated with the bitter principle of the horehound (*Marrubium vulgare*, *M. deserti* de Noe, *M. alysson*, and *M. thessalum*) and other traditionally important Lamiaceae species (*Leonotis leonurus*, *L. nepetifolia*, and *Phlomis bracteosa*) [67, 374–379]. According to recent literature, extensive pharmacological studies have revealed that *marrubiin* shows a suite of activities such as antinociceptive, antispasmodic, antihypertensive, antidiabetic, gastroprotective, anti-inflammatory, antimicrobial, anticancerous, antioxidant, and antihepatotoxic [65, 67, 71–73, 75, 374, 376–378].

Over time, the antinociceptive profile of marrubiin was analyzed in some animal models of pain. De Jesus et al.'s [64] results showed that marrubiin reveals potent and dose-related antinociceptive effects in mice, whose calculated ID50 values (μmol/kg, i.p.) were as follows: 2.2 in the writhing test, 6.6 (first phase) and 6.3 (second phase) in the formalin-induced pain test, and 28.8 when evaluated over the capsaicin test. These findings show that it is more potent than some other well-known analgesic drugs. The antinociception produced by the marrubiin is not reversed by naloxone when analyzed against the writhing test. Its exact mechanism of action remains however still to be determined, but the results suggest that marrubiin, like the hydroalcoholic extract of *M. vulgare*, does not interact with opioid systems.

Analgesic activity success was obtained by reducing lactonic function of the *marrubiin*, in the formation of marrubiinic acid and two esterified derivatives, which have shown significant analgesic effect on the writhing test in mice [68, 374]. The pharmacological studies specified that marrubiinic acid presents an important ($p < 0.05$) and dose-dependent antinociceptive effect, against the writhing test, in intraperitoneal administration, with ID50 value of 12 μmol/kg, being about 11-fold more active than the standard drugs used as reference, but less active than marrubiin [64].

Marrubiinic acid, given orally, at a dose of 50 mg/kg, produced a marked analgesic effect, reducing $76 \pm 0.9\%$ of the number of abdominal constrictions induced by acetic acid, which may recommend that it can be well absorbed by the gastrointestinal tract. However, it was not effective in abolishing pain in a nonopioid way, showing the lack of antinociceptive effects in the hot-plate test [64]. When verified against the capsaicin test, it provided more direct evidence of the analgesic potential on neurogenic pain, causing an inhibition of $37.3 \pm 3.8\%$ at 10 mg/kg of capsaicin-induced licking, signifying its involvement with the antagonism of vanilloid receptor [74].

The specific mechanism underlying the antinociceptive action of marrubiinic acid has yet to be determined, but it is unlikely that it is associated with the interaction of opioid peptides. Although marrubiinic acid displayed lesser analgesic properties than marrubiin, it is more potent than some clinically used drugs. In summary, these results show that it could be used as a model to obtain new and more potent analgesic drugs [67].

In 2013, the analgesic activity of the aqueous extracts obtained from leaves (AEL) and stems (AES) of *Rosmarinus officinalis*, as well as its isolated compound—rosmarinic acid (RA)—were analyzed by Lucarini et al. [379]. The analysis is based upon abdominal constriction and formalin tests in mice. The extracts were used at doses of 100, 200, and 400 mg·kg^{-1}, and the compounds were tested at 10, 20, and 40 mg·kg^{-1}. Orally administered AEL, AES, and RA were not significantly active at any of the doses tested during the abdominal constriction test; the acetyl ester derivative of RA presented significant analgesic activity. These data recommend that the analgesic effects of the acetyl derivative of RA function through a peripheral-mediated mechanism. The acetyl ester derivative of RA is theoretically applicable as a new lead compound for the management of pain.

Takaki et al. [23] investigated the antinociceptive effects of rosemary essential oil (REO) using the acetic acid-induced writhing and hot-plate tests in mice. REO is very common in folk medicine because of its antispasmodic, analgesic, antirheumatic, and carminative effects. In the hot-plate test, the administration of REO in doses of 125, 250, and 500 mg/kg revealed unremarkable effects on response latency, whereas control injection of meperidine induced significant antinociceptive effects.

Moreover, the REO inhibited licking and shaking induced by formalin injections. Instead, at doses of 70, 125, and 250 mg/kg, REO displayed a substantial antinociceptive effect in the acetic acid-induced abdominal writhing test compared with control animals. The results suggest that REO possesses peripheral antinociceptive activity. Similarly, Martinez et al. [363] described the antinociceptive effect of this essential oil using a rat model of arthritic pain. The essential oil with intraperitoneal administration in doses of 100, 300, and 600 mg/kg determined a dose-dependent antinociceptive effect, manifested as a remarkable reduction of the dysfunction in the pain-induced functional impairment model in the rat, mostly at high doses. Emami et al. [34] indicate that rosemary essential oil can inhibit carrageenan-induced paw edema tests in rats and acetic acid-induced writhing model of visceral pain and hot-plate tests in mice, suggesting that rosemary essential oil possesses anti-inflammatory and peripheral antinociceptive activity [23, 380, 381].

Investigations of the effects of carnosol as one of the constituents of rosemary essential oil extract have also shown that carnosol inhibited LPS-stimulated nitric oxide production (LPS (lipopolysaccharide)) in Raw 264.7 cells and reduced inflammation [382]. Moreover, carnosol inhibited proinflammatory leukotrienes in intact polymorph nuclear leukocytes [383], inhibited 5-lipoxygenase, antagonized mobilization of intracellular calcium ions, and inhibited cyclooxygenase type 2 (COX2) in inflamed skin in male Balb/C mice [384].

A recent work demonstrated that extracts from *R. officinalis* can control pain by inhibiting its progression during a persistent noxious condition. As an essential characteristic, rosemary extract prevents damage to the nervous system. Thus, rosemary applies effects on the origins of neuropathic pain and offers a mean to directly modulate nervous signaling. The antineuropathic effects are mainly due to the terpenoid fraction in a mecamylamine-reversed manner, suggesting a pharmacodynamic role of nicotinic acetylcholine receptors [385, 386].

Husseini et al. [355] analyzed the effects of *L. officinalis* hydroalcoholic extract on pain induced by formalin and also cyclooxygenase (COX) type 1 and 2 activity in mice. The administration of the extract intraperitoneally in doses of 100, 200, 250, 300, 400, and 800 mg/kg, respectively, produces significant analgesic and anti-inflammatory activity in the chronic phase of the formalin test and also in hot-plate test in mice with no noted effect on the acute phase of the formalin test.

Moreover, this inhibitory effect is equal to the effects of morphine (10 mg/kg, s.c.), dexamethasone (10 mg/kg, i.p.), and indomethacin (10 mg/kg, i.p.). The extract in doses of 100, 200, and 300 mg/kg significantly reduced heat-induced pain and also reduced COX activity in a dose-dependent manner, where the inhibitory effect on COX1 activity was 33% and on COX2 activity was 45%. Therefore, these results indicate that the possible mechanism of analgesic and anti-inflammatory effects of the extract may be through modulation of COX2 activity.

Other studies [349] have also revealed that the extract of *L. officinalis* leaves might inhibit the formalin-induced chronic pain, abdomen writhing, and carrageenan-evoked edema. High doses of the essential oils and polyphenolic fraction of *L. officinalis* have similar effects by blocking acetic acid evoked pain [353]. This pharmacological activity could be derived from the contribution of various active principles composing the whole oil such as linalool, myrcene, and 1–8 cineole, previously proved to possess antinociceptive proprieties [387–389]. However, administration of the essential oil with naloxone, atropine, and mecamylamine could eliminate the analgesic effect of the extract, which indicates that the analgesic activity of the extract is dependent on cholinergic and opioid systems [349].

The antinociceptive and analgesic effects of the essential oil of *Mentha* spp. (EOM) leaves and its major constituent, piperitenone oxide (PO), were investigated in mice [390]. After an oral administration of 200 mg/kg of EOM and PO, the antinociceptive activity was demonstrated by an important reduction in the acetic acid-induced number of writhings and the second phase of the formalin test, while in the similar range of doses, they did not interfere with the nociception associated with the hot-plate and tail immersion tests. The hot-plate and tail immersion tests are reported to be useful tests in discriminating analgesic agents acting primarily at the spinal medulla level and at higher central nervous system levels (positive results) from those acting through peripheral mechanisms (negative results) [391].

These findings suggest that EOM and PO are acting by peripheral mechanisms. In addition, EOM caused a reduction in the paw licking time for the second phase of the formalin test, when administered at higher doses (100 and 200 mg/kg). At 100 and 200 mg/kg, PO reduced this second phase to 8.3 ± 2.7 s ($N = 12$) and 3.0 ± 1.2 s ($N = 10$), respectively. The antinociceptive activity induced by EOM and PO in the writhing and formalin tests was not altered by naloxone, demonstrating that their actions do not depend on opioid receptors [392], supporting the anti-inflammatory hypothesis for their mechanism of action. Thus, it is reasonable to suggest that EOM and PO have an analgesic activity, which is probably indirect and attributed to the anti-inflammatory activity, which does not involve the central nervous system [393].

6. Future Perspectives and Conclusions

The Lamiaceae family includes numerous known species that are used as traditional medicine. The present review summarizes the general aspects, traditional uses, pharmacology, and *in vitro* and *in vivo* studies of *Betonica officinalis, Glechoma hederacea, Hyptis pectinata, Lavandula* genus, *Leonurus cardiaca, Lamium* genus, *Melissa officinalis, Mentha* genus, *Marrubium vulgare, Origanum* genus, *Ocimum* genus, *Rosmarinus officinalis, Salvia* genus, *Satureja hortensis, Stachys lavandulifolia, Scutellaria lateriflora, Sideritis* genus, *Teucrium* genus, *Thymus* genus, and *Ziziphora tenuior*, belonging to Lamiaceae botanical genus. The above-referred studies reported that the abovementioned medicinal plants have potent analgesic and antinociceptive activity. The findings of this review are promising, regarding new potential therapeutic agents with possible modulation in pain therapy. Most of the extracts identified did not present any toxic capabilities or known side effects and were at least as efficient as currently used synthetic drugs. Overall, although promising information evidence the efficacy of Lamiaceae genus in the treatment of pain associated disorders, the data are too preliminary and mostly fail to explain the exact cellular and molecular mechanisms of action and the respective active compounds. Therefore, future studies should be focused on investigating mechanisms of actions, realistic dosages, clinical efficacy, and safety of the extracts and active compounds in pain treatment. This review covers a useful approach for further identification of new compounds from various medicinal plants, which may be effective in pain management.

Authors' Contributions

All authors contributed equally to this work.

References

[1] R. Masuda, J. Ajimi, and T. Murata, "Pharmacotherapy for neuropathic pain in Japan," *Journal of Nippon Medical School*, vol. 84, no. 6, pp. 258–267, 2017.

[2] B. I. Tamba, M.-M. Leon, and T. Petreus, "Common trace elements alleviate pain in an experimental mouse model," *Journal of Neuroscience Research*, vol. 91, no. 4, pp. 554–561, 2013.

[3] A. Iuliana Alexa, A. Cantemir, A. Ciobica et al., "Preliminary data regarding decreased catalase specific activity in the tears as a result of environmental stress," *Revista de Chimie-Bucharest*, vol. 68, no. 1, 2017.

[4] K. Zorina-Lichtenwalter, M. Parisien, and L. Diatchenko, "Genetic studies of human neuropathic pain conditions," *Pain*, p. 1, 2017.

[5] F. Gedin, M. Skeppholm, K. Burström, V. Sparring, M. Tessma, and N. Zethraeus, "Effectiveness, costs and cost-effectiveness of chiropractic care and physiotherapy compared with information and advice in the treatment of non-specific chronic low back pain: study protocol for a randomised controlled trial," *Trials*, vol. 18, no. 1, p. 613, 2017.

[6] I. D. Alexa, A. G. Pancu, A. I. Moroşanu et al., "The impact of self-medication with NSAIDS/analgesics in a north-eastern region of Romania," *Farmacia*, vol. 62, 2014.

[7] A. Scurrah, C. T. Shiner, J. A. Stevens, and S. G. Faux, "Regional nerve blockade for early analgesic management of elderly patients with hip fracture-a narrative review," *Anaesthesia*, 2017, In press.

[8] I. Gardikiotis, D. Azoicai, M. Popa, A. M. Manole, and M. Iorga, "The impact of body image and self-perceived physical ability on the well-being after mastectomy without reconstruction," *Jurnalul de Chirurgie*, vol. 11, no. 4, pp. 143–149, 2015.

[9] A. Luca, T. Alexa, A. Dondaş, I.-M. Crăcană, M. Bădescu, and C. Bohotin, "The effects of riboflavin and methylene blue on nociception and visceral pain," *Revista Medico-Chirurgicala a Societatii De Medici Si Naturalisti Din Iasi*, vol. 119, no. 2, pp. 466–472, 2015.

[10] R. Cobzaru, A.-M. Dumitrescu, A. Glodeanu, M. Leon, S. Constantin, and M. Luca, "Pain and physical deformity elephantiasis," *Revista Medico-Chirurgicala a Societatii De Medici Si Naturalisti Din Iasi*, vol. 117, pp. 29–32, 2013.

[11] D. M. Iurea (Rata), M. Popa, J.-F. Chailan, B. I. Tamba, I. Tudorancea, and C. A. Peptu, "Ibuprofen-loaded chitosan/poly(maleic anhydride-alt-vinyl acetate) submicronic capsules for pain treatment," *Journal of Bioactive and Compatible Polymers*, vol. 28, no. 4, pp. 368–384, 2013.

[12] M. Iorga, L.-Z. Sztankovszky, C. Soponaru, and I. Gardikiotis, "Pharmacists' attitude and practices about drug dispensing in Romania," *Farmacia*, vol. 63, no. 4, pp. 601–606, 2015.

[13] R. Ullah, S. Ahmad, A. Atiq et al., "Quantification and antibacterial activity of flavonoids in coffee samples," *African Journal of Traditional, Complementary and Alternative Medicines*, vol. 12, no. 4, p. 84, 2015.

[14] M. Ayaz, M. Junaid, F. Ullah et al., "Molecularly characterized solvent extracts and saponins from *Polygonum hydropiper* L. show high anti-angiogenic, anti-tumor, brine shrimp, and fibroblast NIH/3T3 cell line cytotoxicity," *Frontiers in Pharmacology*, vol. 7, p. 74, 2016.

[15] F. Haq, H. Ahmad, R. Ullah, and Z. Iqbal, "Species diversity and ethno botanical classes of the flora of Allai valley District Battagram, Pakistan," *International Journal of Plant Research*, vol. 2, no. 4, pp. 111–123, 2012.

[16] M. Anilkumar, "Ethnomedicinal plants as anti-inflammatory and analgesic agents," *Research Signpost*, vol. 37661, pp. 267–293, 2010.

[17] T. Alexa-Stratulat, A. Luca, M. Bădescu, C.-R. Bohotin, and I. D. Alexa, "Nutritional modulators in chemotherapy-induced neuropathic pain," in *Nutritional Modulators of Pain in the Aging Population*, Elsevier, pp. 9–33, New York, NY, USA, 2017.

[18] B. I. Tamba and T. Alexa-Stratulat, "Trace elements alleviate pain in mice and humans," in *Nutritional Modulators of Pain in the Aging Population*, Elsevier, pp. 199–216, New York, NY, USA, 2017.

[19] C. Peptu, R. Rotaru, L. Ignat et al., "Nanotechnology approaches for pain therapy through transdermal drug delivery," *Current Pharmaceutical Design*, vol. 21, no. 42, pp. 6125–6139, 2015.

[20] T. Alexa, A. Marza, T. Voloseniuc, and B. Tamba, "Enhanced analgesic effects of tramadol and common trace element coadministration in mice," *Journal of Neuroscience Research*, vol. 93, no. 10, pp. 1534–1541, 2015.

[21] B. I. Tamba, A. Dondas, M. Leon et al., "Silica nanoparticles: preparation, characterization and in vitro/in vivo biodistribution studies," *European Journal of Pharmaceutical Sciences*, vol. 71, pp. 46–55, 2015.

[22] M. Silion, D. Hritcu, I. M. Jaba et al., "In vitro and in vivo behavior of ketoprofen intercalated into layered double hydroxides," *Journal of Materials Science: Materials in Medicine*, vol. 21, no. 11, pp. 3009–3018, 2010.

[23] I. Takaki, L. E. Bersani-Amado, A. Vendruscolo et al., "Anti-inflammatory and antinociceptive effects of *Rosmarinus officinalis* L. essential oil in experimental animal models," *Journal of Medicinal Food*, vol. 11, no. 4, pp. 741–746, 2008.

[24] I. M. Jaba, D. Vasincu, G. Manolidis, I. Haulică, and O. C. Mungiu, "Experimental data regarding the implications of certain minimum structure enkephalin-like peptides in nociceptive processing," *Romanian Journal of Physiology*, vol. 41, no. 1-2, pp. 119–126, 2004.

[25] T. Alexa, A. Luca, A. Dondas, and C. R. Bohotin, "Preconditioning with cobalt chloride modifies pain perception in mice," *Experimental and Therapeutic Medicine*, vol. 9, no. 10, pp. 1465–1469, 2015.

[26] A. Luca, T. Alexa, A. Dondaş et al., "Pain modulation by curcumin and ascorbic acid in mice," *Revista Medico-Chirurgicala a Societatii De Medici Si Naturalisti Din Iasi*, vol. 118, no. 2, pp. 346–351, 2015.

[27] D. C. Ababei, S. Besche Chiriac, W. Bild et al., "Synergistic effects of the doxepin-candesartan combination on the

thermoalgesic sensibility in mice," *Farmacia*, vol. 65, pp. 726–730, 2017.

[28] B. I. Tamba, T. Petreus, M.-M. L. Constaintian, C. Rezus, M. Floria, and E. Rezus, "Heavy metal trace elements induced antinociception in an experimental mouse model," *Revista de Chimie*, vol. 66, no. 7, pp. 976–982, 2015.

[29] B. B. Kakoti, P. Pradhan, S. Borah, K. Mahato, and M. Kumar, "Analgesic and anti-inflammatory activities of the methanolic stem bark extract of *Nyctanthes arbor-tristis* Linn," *BioMed Research International*, vol. 2013, Article ID 826295, 6 pages, 2013.

[30] M. Bahmani, H. Shirzad, M. Majlesi, N. Shahinfard, and M. Rafieian-Kopaei, "A review study on analgesic applications of Iranian medicinal plants," *Asian Pacific Journal of Tropical Medicine*, vol. 7, pp. S43–S53, 2014.

[31] M. Bekut, S. Brkić, N. Kladar, G. Dragović, N. Gavarić, and B. Božin, "Potential of selected Lamiaceae plants in anti(retro) viral therapy," *Pharmacological Research*, 2017, In press.

[32] M. R. al-Sereiti, K. M. Abu-Amer, and P. Sen, "Pharmacology of rosemary (*Rosmarinus officinalis* Linn.) and its therapeutic potentials," *Indian Journal of Experimental Biology*, vol. 37, no. 2, pp. 124–130, 1999.

[33] G. Altinier, S. Sosa, R. P. Aquino, T. Mencherini, R. Della Loggia, and A. Tubaro, "Characterization of topical antiinflammatory compounds in *Rosmarinus officinalis* L.," *Journal of Agricultural and Food Chemistry*, vol. 55, no. 5, pp. 1718–1723, 2007.

[34] F. Emami, H. Ali-Beig, S. Farahbakhs et al., "Hydroalcoholic extract of rosemary (*Rosmarinus officinalis* L.) and its constituent carnosol inhibit formalin-induced pain and inflammation in mice," *Pakistan Journal of Biological Sciences*, vol. 16, no. 7, pp. 309–316, 2013.

[35] J. I. Sotelo-Félix, D. Martinez-Fong, P. Muriel, R. L. Santillán, D. Castillo, and P. Yahuaca, "Evaluation of the effectiveness of *Rosmarinus officinalis* (Lamiaceae) in the alleviation of carbon tetrachloride-induced acute hepatotoxicity in the rat," *Journal of Ethnopharmacology*, vol. 81, no. 2, pp. 145–154, 2002.

[36] J. M. Visanji, D. G. Thompson, and P. J. Padfield, "Induction of G2/M phase cell cycle arrest by carnosol and carnosic acid is associated with alteration of cyclin A and cyclin B1 levels," *Cancer Lett*, vol. 237, pp. 130–136, 2006.

[37] N. Okamura, H. Haraguchi, K. Hashimoto, and A. Yagi, "Flavonoids in *Rosmarinus officinalis* leaves," *Phytochemistry*, vol. 37, no. 5, pp. 1463–1466, 1994.

[38] F. J. Señoráns, E. Ibañez, S. Cavero, J. Tabera, and G. Reglero, "Liquid chromatographic-mass spectrometric analysis of supercritical-fluid extracts of rosemary plants," *Journal of Chromatography A*, vol. 870, no. 1-2, pp. 491–499, 2000.

[39] M. A. Thorsen and K. S. Hildebrandt, "Quantitative determination of phenolic diterpenes in rosemary extracts. Aspects of accurate quantification," *Journal of Chromatography A*, vol. 995, pp. 119–125, 2003.

[40] L. Almela, B. Sánchez-Muñoz, J. A. Fernández-López, M. J. Roca, and V. Rabe, "Liquid chromatograpic–mass spectrometric analysis of phenolics and free radical scavenging activity of rosemary extract from different raw material," *Journal of Chromatography A*, vol. 1120, no. 1-2, pp. 221–229, 2006.

[41] P. Ramírez, M. R. García-Risco, S. Santoyo, F. J. Señoráns, E. Ibáñez, and G. Reglero, "Isolation of functional ingredients from rosemary by preparative-supercritical fluid chromatography (Prep-SFC)," *Journal of Pharmaceutical and Biomedical Analysis*, vol. 41, no. 5, pp. 1606–1613, 2006.

[42] J. Dörrie, K. Sapala, and S. J. Zunino, "Carnosol-induced apoptosis and downregulation of Bcl-2 in B-lineage leukemia cells," *Cancer Letters*, vol. 170, no. 1, pp. 33–39, 2001.

[43] A.-H. Lo, Y.-C. Liang, S.-Y. Lin-Shiau, C.-T. Ho, and J.-K. Lin, "Carnosol, an antioxidant in rosemary, suppresses inducible nitric oxide synthase through down-regulating nuclear factor-κB in mouse macrophages," *Carcinogenesis*, vol. 23, no. 6, pp. 983–991, 2002.

[44] S.-C. Huang, C.-T. Ho, S.-Y. Lin-Shiau, and J.-K. Lin, "Carnosol inhibits the invasion of B16/F10 mouse melanoma cells by suppressing metalloproteinase-9 through down-regulating nuclear factor-κB and c-Jun," *Biochemical Pharmacology*, vol. 69, no. 2, pp. 221–232, 2005.

[45] J. Del Campo, M. J. Amiot, and C. Nguyen-The, "Antimicrobial effect of rosemary extracts," *Journal of Food Protection*, vol. 63, no. 10, pp. 1359–1368, 2000.

[46] B. Bozin, N. Mimica-Dukic, I. Samojlik, and E. Jovin, "Antimicrobial and antioxidant properties of rosemary and sage (*Rosmarinus officinalis* L. and *Salvia officinalis* L., Lamiaceae) essential oils," *Journal of Agricultural and Food Chemistry*, vol. 55, no. 19, pp. 7879–7885, 2007.

[47] I. Rasooli, M. H. Fakoor, D. Yadegarinia, L. Gachkar, A. Allameh, and M. B. Rezaei, "Antimycotoxigenic characteristics of *Rosmarinus officinalis* and *Trachyspermum copticum* L. essential oils," *International Journal of Food Microbiology*, vol. 122, no. 1-2, pp. 135–139, 2008.

[48] W. A. Bernardes, R. Lucarini, M. G. Tozatti et al., "Antimicrobial activity of *Rosmarinus officinalis* against oral pathogens: relevance of carnosic acid and carnosol," *Chemistry & Biodiversity*, vol. 7, no. 7, pp. 1835–1840, 2010.

[49] B. Ouattara, R. E. Simard, R. A. Holley, G. J. Piette, and A. Bégin, "Antibacterial activity of selected fatty acids and essential oils against six meat spoilage organisms," *International Journal of Food Microbiology*, vol. 37, no. 2-3, pp. 155–162, 1997.

[50] J. Yamamoto, K. Yamada, A. Naemura, T. Yamashita, and R. Arai, "Testing various herbs for antithrombotic effect," *Nutrition*, vol. 21, no. 5, pp. 580–587, 2005.

[51] M. Haloui, L. Louedec, J. B. Michel, and B. Lyoussi, "Experimental diuretic effects of *Rosmarinus officinalis* and *Centaurium erythraea*," *Journal of Ethnopharmacology*, vol. 71, no. 3, pp. 465–472, 2000.

[52] T. Bakırel, U. Bakırel, O. Ü. Keleş, S. G. Ülgen, and H. Yardibi, "In vivo assessment of antidiabetic and antioxidant activities of rosemary (*Rosmarinus officinalis*) in alloxan-diabetic rabbits," *Journal of Ethnopharmacology*, vol. 116, no. 1, pp. 64–73, 2008.

[53] F. A. Fahim, A. Y. Esmat, H. M. Fadel, and K. F. Hassan, "Allied studies on the effect of *Rosmarinus officinalis* L. on experimental hepatotoxicity and mutagenesis," *International Journal of Food Sciences and Nutrition*, vol. 50, no. 6, pp. 413–427, 1999.

[54] L. Pérez-Fons, M. T. GarzÓn, and V. Micol, "Relationship between the antioxidant capacity and effect of rosemary (*Rosmarinus officinalis* L.) polyphenols on membrane phospholipid order," *Journal of Agricultural and Food Chemistry*, vol. 58, no. 1, pp. 161–171, 2010.

[55] L. Fernandez, S. Duque, I. Sanchez, D. Quiñones, F. Rodriguez, and J. L. Garcia-Abujeta, "Allergic contact dermatitis from rosemary (*Rosmarinus officinalis* L.)," *Contact Dermatitis*, vol. 37, no. 5, pp. 248-249, 1997.

[56] A. Taamalli, D. Arráez-Román, E. Ibañez, M. Zarrouk, A. Segura-Carretero, and A. Fernández-Gutiérrez, "Optimization of microwave-assisted extraction for the characterization

of olive leaf phenolic compounds by using HPLC-ESI-TOF-MS/IT-MS 2," *Journal of Agricultural and Food Chemistry*, vol. 60, no. 3, pp. 791–798, 2012.

[57] C. Proestos and M. Komaitis, "Application of microwave-assisted extraction to the fast extraction of plant phenolic compounds," *LWT-Food Science and Technology*, vol. 41, no. 4, pp. 652–659, 2008.

[58] C.-H. Peng, J.-D. Su, C.-C. Chyau et al., "Supercritical fluid extracts of rosemary leaves exhibit potent anti-inflammation and anti-tumor effects," *Bioscience, Biotechnology, and Biochemistry*, vol. 71, no. 9, pp. 2223–2232, 2007.

[59] M. M. Chan, C. T. Ho, and H. I. Huang, "Effects of three dietary phytochemicals from tea, rosemary and turmeric on inflammation-induced nitrite production," *Cancer Letters*, vol. 96, no. 1, pp. 23–9, 1995.

[60] K.-I. Inoue, H. Takano, A. Shiga et al., "Effects of volatile constituents of a rosemary extract on allergic airway inflammation related to house dust mite allergen in mice," *International Journal of Molecular Medicine*, vol. 16, pp. 315–319, 2005.

[61] K. Inoue, H. Takano, A. Shiga et al., "Effects of volatile constituents of rosemary extract on lung inflammation induced by diesel exhaust particles," *Basic Clinical Pharmacology Toxicology*, vol. 99, no. 1, pp. 52–57, 2006.

[62] M. E. González-Trujano, E. I. Peña, A. L. Martínez et al., "Evaluation of the antinociceptive effect of *Rosmarinus officinalis* L. using three different experimental models in rodents," *Journal of Ethnopharmacology*, vol. 111, no. 3, pp. 476–482, 2007.

[63] C. Meyre-Silva and V. Cechinel-Filho, "A review of the chemical and pharmacological aspects of the genus *marrubium*," *Current Pharmaceutical Design*, vol. 16, no. 31, pp. 3503–3518, 2010.

[64] R. A. De Jesus, V. Cechinel-Filho, A. E. Oliveira, and V. Schlemper, "Analysis of the antinociceptive properties of marrubiin isolated from *Marrubium vulgare*," *Phytomedicine*, vol. 7, no. 2, pp. 111–115, 2000.

[65] C. A. Rodrigues, A. O. S. Savi, V. Schlemper, F. Reynaud, and V. Cechinel-Filho, "An improved extraction of marrubiim from *Marrubium vulgare*," *Chromatographia*, vol. 47, no. 7-8, pp. 449-450, 1998.

[66] M. M. de Souza, R. A. P. de Jesus, V. Cechinel-Filho, and V. Schlemper, "Analgesic profile of hydroalcoholic extract obtained from *Marrubium vulgare*," *Phytomedicine*, vol. 5, no. 2, pp. 103–107, 1998.

[67] C. Meyre-Silva, R. A. Yunes, V. Schlemper, F. Campos-Buzzi, and V. Cechinel-Filho, "Analgesic potential of marrubiin derivatives, a bioactive diterpene present in *Marrubium vulgare* (Lamiaceae)," *Il Farmaco*, vol. 60, no. 4, pp. 321–326, 2005.

[68] O. Popoola, A. Elbagory, F. Ameer, and A. Hussein, "Marrubiin," *Molecules*, vol. 18, no. 8, pp. 9049–9060, 2013.

[69] K. Yousefi, S. Hamedeyazdan, M. Torbati, and F. Fathiazad, *Chromatographic fingerprint analysis of marrubiin in Marrubium vulgare L. via HPTLC Technique*, vol. 6, pp. 131–136, 2016.

[70] A. P. Novaes, C. Rossi, C. Poffo et al., "Preliminary evaluation of the hypoglycemic effect of some Brazilian medicinal plants," *Therapie*, vol. 56, no. 4, pp. 427–430.

[71] H. K. Stulzer, M. P. Tagliari, J. A. Zampirolo, V. Cechinel-Filho, and V. Schlemper, "Antioedematogenic effect of marrubiin obtained from *Marrubium vulgare*," *Journal of Ethnopharmacology*, vol. 108, no. 3, pp. 379–84, 2006.

[72] A. Herrera-Arellano, L. Aguilar-Santamaría, B. García-Hernández, P. Nicasio-Torres, and J. Tortoriello, "Clinical trial of *Cecropia obtusifolia* and *Marrubium vulgare* leaf extracts on blood glucose and serum lipids in type 2 diabetics," *Phytomedicine*, vol. 11, no. 7-8, pp. 561–566, 2004.

[73] I. E. Orhan, R. Belhattab, F. S. Şenol, A. R. Gülpinar, S. Hoşbaş, and M. Kartal, "Profiling of cholinesterase inhibitory and antioxidant activities of *Artemisia absinthium*, *A. herba-alba*, *A. fragrans*, *Marrubium vulgare*, *M. astranicum*, *Origanum vulgare* subsp. *glandulossum* and essential oil analysis of two Artemisia species," *Industrial Crops and Products*, vol. 32, no. 3, pp. 566–571, 2010.

[74] D. Julius, M. J. Caterina, M. A. Schumacher, M. Tominaga, T. A. Rosen, and J. D. Levine, "The capsaicin receptor: a heat-activated ion channel in the pain pathway," *Nature*, vol. 389, no. 6653, pp. 816–824, 1997.

[75] G. Çitoğlu and F. Aksit, "Occurence of marrubiin and ladanein in *Marrubium trachyticum* Boiss. from Turkey," *Biochemical Systematics and Ecology*, vol. 30, no. 9, pp. 885-886, 2002.

[76] B. Janeska, M. Stefova, and K. Alipieva, "Assay of flavonoid aglycones from the species of genus *Sideritis* (Lamiaceae) from Macedonia with HPLC-UV DAD," *Acta Pharmaceutica*, vol. 57, no. 3, 2007.

[77] R. Knörle, "Extracts of *Sideritis scardica* as triple monoamine reuptake inhibitors," *Journal of Neural Transmission*, vol. 119, no. 12, pp. 1477–1482, 2012.

[78] J. Hofrichter, M. Krohn, T. Schumacher et al., "Alzheimer's β-amyloidosis mouse models and aged C57Bl/6 mice," *Journal of Alzheimer's Disease*, vol. 53, no. 3, pp. 967–80, 2016.

[79] J. P. Stanoeva and M. Stefova, "Evaluation of the ion trap MS performance for quantification of flavonoids and comparison to UV detection," *Journal of Mass Spectrometry*, vol. 47, no. 11, pp. 1395–1406, 2012.

[80] V. Samanidou, A. Tsagiannidis, and I. Sarakatsianos, "Simultaneous determination of polyphenols and major purine alkaloids in Greek *Sideritis* species, herbal extracts, green tea, black tea, and coffee by high-performance liquid chromatography-diode array detection," *Journal of Separation Science*, vol. 35, no. 4, pp. 608–615, 2012.

[81] E. Kostadinova, D. Nikolova, K. Alipieva et al., "Chemical constituents of the essential oils of *Sideritis scardica* Griseb. and *Sideritis raeseri* Boiss and Heldr. from Bulgaria and Macedonia," *Natural Product Research*, vol. 21, no. 9, pp. 819–823, 2007.

[82] J. Petreska, G. Stefkov, S. Kulevanova, K. Alipieva, V. Bankova, and M. Stefova, "Phenolic compounds of mountain tea from the Balkans: LC/DAD/ESI/MSn profile and content," *Natural Product Communications*, vol. 6, no. 1, pp. 21–30, 2011.

[83] A. B. Trendafilova, M. N. Todorova, L. N. Evstatieva, and D. V. Antonova, "Variability in the essential-oil composition of *Sideritis scardica* Griseb. from native Bulgarian Populations," *Chemistry & Biodiversity*, vol. 10, no. 3, pp. 484–492, 2013.

[84] B. Qazimi, G. Stefkov, M. Karapandzova, I. Cvetkovikj, and S. Kulevanova, "Aroma compounds of mountain tea (*Sideritis scardica* and *S. raeseri*) from western Balkan," *Natural Product Communications*, vol. 9, pp. 1369–72, 2014.

[85] J. Petreska Stanoeva and M. Stefova, "Assay of urinary excretion of polyphenols after ingestion of a cup of mountain tea (*Sideritis scardica*) measured by HPLC-DAD-ESI-MS/MS," *Journal of Agricultural and Food Chemistry*, vol. 61, no. 44, pp. 10488–10497, 2013.

[86] E. González-Burgos, M. E. Carretero, and M. P. Gómez-Serranillos, "*Sideritis spp.*: uses, chemical composition and

pharmacological activities—a review," *Journal of Ethnopharmacology*, vol. 135, no. 2, pp. 209–225, 2011.
[87] C. M. Ghiciuc, L. C. Dima-Cozma, R. M. Bercea et al., "Imbalance in the diurnal salivary testosterone/cortisol ratio in men with severe obstructive sleep apnea: an observational study," *Brazilian Journal of Otorhinolaryngology*, vol. 82, no. 5, pp. 529–535, 2016.
[88] W. Dimpfel, "Pharmacological classification of herbal extracts by means of comparison to spectral EEG signatures induced by synthetic drugs in the freely moving rat," *Journal of Ethnopharmacology*, vol. 149, no. 2, pp. 583–589, 2013.
[89] O. Mitu, M. Roca, M.-M. Leon, A. Gherasim, M. Graur, and F. Mitu, "Association of health-related quality of life with cardiovascular risk factors and subclinical atherosclerosis in non-diabetic asymptomatic adults," *Biomedical Research*, vol. 27, 2016.
[90] V. Tadić, D. Bojović, I. Arsić et al., "Chemical and antimicrobial evaluation of supercritical and conventional *Sideritis scardica* Griseb., Lamiaceae extracts," *Molecules*, vol. 17, no. 3, pp. 2683–2703, 2012.
[91] F. Danesi, S. Saha, P. A. Kroon et al., "Bioactive-rich *Sideritis scardica* tea (mountain tea) is as potent as *Camellia sinensis* tea at inducing cellular antioxidant defences and preventing oxidative stress," *Journal of the Science of Food and Agriculture*, vol. 93, no. 14, pp. 3558–3564, 2013.
[92] V. Tadić, I. Jeremic, S. Dobric et al., "Anti-inflammatory, gastroprotective, and cytotoxic effects of *Sideritis scardica* extracts," *Planta Medica*, vol. 78, no. 5, pp. 415–427, 2012.
[93] I. Jeremic, V. Tadic, A. Isakovic et al., "The mechanisms of in vitro cytotoxicity of mountain tea, *Sideritis scardica*, against the C6 glioma cell line," *Planta Medica*, vol. 79, pp. 1516–1524, 2013.
[94] E. Rezuş, A. Grigoriu, and C. Rezuş, "Aggressive nature of rheumatic arthritis with citrullinated cyclic peptide antibodies," *Revista Medico-Chirurgicala a Societatii De Medici Si Naturalisti Din Iasi*, vol. 113, no. 1, pp. 73–78, 2009.
[95] M. Todorova and A. Trendafilova, "*Sideritis scardica* Griseb., an endemic species of Balkan peninsula: traditional uses, cultivation, chemical composition, biological activity," *Journal of Ethnopharmacology*, vol. 152, no. 2, pp. 256–265, 2014.
[96] B. M. Fraga, M. G. Hernández, C. Fernández, and J. M. H. Santana, "A chemotaxonomic study of nine Canarian *Sideritis* species," *Phytochemistry*, vol. 70, no. 8, pp. 1038–1048, 2009.
[97] M. Hernández-Pérez and R. M. Rabanal Gallego, "Analgesic and antiinflammatory properties of *Sideritis lotsyi* var. Mascaensis," *Phytotherapy Research*, vol. 16, no. 3, pp. 264–266, 2002.
[98] D. Ö. Yavuz, "Optimization of regeneration conditions and in vitro propagation of *Sideritis Stricta* Boiss & Heldr," *International Journal of Biological Macromolecules*, vol. 90, pp. 59–62, 2016.
[99] T. Kilic, "Isolation and biological activity of new and known isolation and biological activity of new and known diterpenoids from *Sideritis stricta* Boiss. & Heldr.," *Molecules*, vol. 11, no. 4, pp. 257–262, 2006.
[100] E. Küpeli, F. P. Sahin, E. Yeşilada, I. Caliş, and N. Ezer, "In vivo anti-inflammatory and antinociceptive activity evaluation of phenolic compounds from *Sideritis stricta*," *Zeitschrift für Naturforschung C*, vol. 62, no. 7-8, pp. 519–525, 2007.
[101] C.-H. Kang, I. M. N. Molagoda, Y. H. Choi, C. Park, D.-O. Moon, and G.-Y. Kim, "Apigenin promotes TRAIL-mediated apoptosis regardless of ROS generation," *Food and Chemical Toxicology*, vol. 111, pp. 623–630, 2018.
[102] E. Schmidt, J. Wanner, M. Hiiferl et al., "Chemical composition, olfactory analysis and antibacterial activity of *Thymus vulgaris* chemotypes geraniol, 4-thujanol/terpinen-4-ol, thymol and linalool cultivated in southern France," *Natural Product Communications*, vol. 7, pp. 1095–1098, 2012.
[103] V. Vaičiulytė, R. Butkienė, and K. Ložienė, "Effects of meteorological conditions and plant growth stage on the accumulation of carvacrol and its precursors in *Thymus pulegioides*," *Phytochemistry*, vol. 128, pp. 20–26, 2016.
[104] P. Satyal, B. L. Murray, R. L. McFeeters, and W. N. Setzer, "Essential oil characterization of *Thymus vulgaris* from various geographical locations," *Foods*, vol. 5, no. 4, p. 78, 2016.
[105] H. Tsuchiya, "Hironori, anesthetic agents of plant origin: a review of phytochemicals with anesthetic Activity," *Molecules*, vol. 22, no. 8, p. 1369, 2017.
[106] M. Akram and A. Rashid, "Anti-coagulant activity of plants: mini review," *Journal of Thrombosis and Thrombolysis*, vol. 44, no. 3, pp. 406–411, 2017.
[107] K. Okazaki, K. Kawazoe, and Y. Takaishi, "Human platelet aggregation inhibitors from thyme (*Thymus vulgaris* L.)," *Phytotherapy Research*, vol. 16, no. 4, pp. 398-399, 2002.
[108] M. Soosaraei, M. Fakhar, S. Hosseini Teshnizi, H. Ziaei Hezarjaribi, and E. S. Banimostafavi, "Medicinal plants with promising antileishmanial activity in Iran: a systematic review and meta-analysis," *Annals of Medicine and Surgery*, vol. 21, pp. 63–80, 2017.
[109] A. Ebadollahi, J. J. Sendi, and A. Aliakbar, "Efficacy of nanoencapsulated *Thymus eriocalyx* and *Thymus kotschyanus* essential oils by a mesoporous material MCM-41 against *Tetranychus urticae* (Acari: Tetranychidae)," *Journal of Economic Entomology*, vol. 110, no. 6, pp. 2413–2420, 2017.
[110] K. Schönknecht, H. Krauss, J. Jambor, and A. M. Fal, "Treatment of cough in respiratory tract infections-the effect of combining the natural active compounds with thymol," *Wiadomosci Lekarskie*, vol. 69, no. 6, pp. 791–798, 2016.
[111] H. Ayrle, M. Mevissen, M. Kaske et al., "Medicinal plants–prophylactic and therapeutic options for gastrointestinal and respiratory diseases in calves and piglets? A systematic review," *BMC Veterinary Research*, vol. 12, no. 1, p. 89, 2016.
[112] L. Wan, D. Meng, H. Wang et al., "Preventive and therapeutic effects of thymol in a lipopolysaccharide-induced acute lung injury mice model," *Inflammation*, vol. 41, no. 1, 2017.
[113] E. Vigo, A. Cepeda, R. Perez-Fernandez, and O. Gualillo, "In-vitro anti-inflammatory effect of *Eucalyptus globulus* and *Thymus vulgaris*: nitric oxide inhibition in J774A.1 murine macrophages," *Journal of Pharmacy and Pharmacology*, vol. 56, no. 2, pp. 257–263, 2004.
[114] M. Kindl, B. Blažeković, F. Bucar, and S. Vladimir-Knežević, "Antioxidant and anticholinesterase potential of six *Thymus* species," *Evidence-Based Complementary and Alternative Medicine*, vol. 2015, Article ID 403950, 10 pages, 2015.
[115] M. Alabdullatif, I. Boujezza, M. Mekni et al., "Enhancing blood donor skin disinfection using natural oils," *Transfusion*, vol. 57, no. 12, pp. 2920–2927, 2017.
[116] E. Basch, C. Ulbricht, P. Hammerness, A. Bevins, and D. Sollars, "Thyme (*Thymus vulgaris* L.), thymol.," *Journal of Herbal Pharmacotherapy*, vol. 4, no. 1, pp. 49–67, 2004.
[117] E. A. El Zayyat, M. I. Soliman, N. A. Elleboudy, and S. E. Ofaa, "Bioefficacy of some Egyptian aromatic plants on

Culex pipiens (Diptera: Culicidae) adults and larvae," *Journal of Arthropod-Borne Diseases*, vol. 11, no. 1, pp. 147–155, 2017.

[118] M. I. Qadir, A. Parveen, K. Abbas, and M. Ali, "Analgesic, anti-inflammatory and anti-pyretic activities of *Thymus linearis*," *Pakistan Journal of Pharmaceutical Sciences*, vol. 29, no. 2, pp. 591–594, 2016.

[119] A. A. Taherian, M. Babaei, A. A. Vafaei, M. Jarrahi, M. Jadidi, and H. Sadeghi, "Antinociceptive effects of hydroalcoholic extract of *Thymus vulgaris*," *Pakistan Journal of Pharmaceutical Sciences*, vol. 22, pp. 83–89, 2009.

[120] H. Salmalian, R. Saghebi, A. A. Moghadamnia et al., "Comparative effect of *Thymus vulgaris* and ibuprofen on primary dysmenorrhea: a triple-blind clinical study," *Caspian Journal of Internal Medicine*, vol. 5, no. 2, pp. 82–88, 2014.

[121] M. Orłowska, I. Stanimirova, D. Staszek, M. Sajewicz, T. Kowalska, and M. Waksmundzka-Hajnos, "Optimization of extraction based on the thin-layer chromatographic fingerprints of common thyme," *Journal of AOAC International*, vol. 97, no. 5, pp. 1274–1281, 2014.

[122] E. Pinto, C. Pina-Vaz, L. Salgueiro et al., "Antifungal activity of the essential oil of *Thymus pulegioides* on *Candida*, *Aspergillus* and *Dermatophyte* species," *Journal of Medical Microbiology*, vol. 55, no. 10, pp. 1367–1373, 2006.

[123] S. Vitalini, M. Iriti, C. Puricelli, D. Ciuchi, A. Segale, and G. Fico, "Traditional knowledge on medicinal and food plants used in Val San Giacomo (Sondrio, Italy)—an alpine ethnobotanical study," *Journal of Ethnopharmacology*, vol. 145, no. 2, pp. 517–529, 2013.

[124] S. Schaffer, G. P. Eckert, W. E. Müller et al., "Hypochlorous acid scavenging properties of local Mediterranean plant foods," *Lipids*, vol. 39, no. 12, pp. 1239–1247, 2004.

[125] K. Stalińska, A. Guzdek, M. Rokicki, and A. Koj, "Transcription factors as targets of the anti-inflammatory treatment. A cell culture study with extracts from some Mediterranean diet plants," *Journal of Physiology and Pharmacology*, vol. 56, no. 1, pp. 157–169, 2005.

[126] J. Novak, L. Bahoo, U. Mitteregger, and C. Franz, "Composition of individual essential oil glands of savory (*Satureja hortensis* L., Lamiaceae) from Syria," *Flavour and Fragrance Journal*, vol. 21, no. 4, pp. 731–734, 2006.

[127] S. Momtaz and M. Abdollahi, "An update on pharmacology of *Satureja* species; from antioxidant, antimicrobial, antidiabetes and anti-hyperlipidemic to reproductive stimulation," *International Journal of Pharmacology*, vol. 6, pp. 454–461, 2010.

[128] B. Tepe and M. Cilkiz, "A pharmacological and phytochemical overview on *Satureja*," *Pharmaceutical Biology*, vol. 54, no. 3, pp. 375–412, 2016.

[129] F. Nikaein, S. Babajafari, S. Mazloomi et al., "The effects of *Satureja hortensis* L. Dried leaves on serum sugar, lipid profiles, hs-CRP, and blood pressure in metabolic syndrome patients: a double-blind randomized clinical trial," *Iranian Red Crescent Medical Journal*, vol. 19, no. 1, 2017, p. e34931.

[130] F. Jafari, F. Ghavidel, and M. M. Zarshenas, "A critical overview on the pharmacological and clinical aspects of popular *Satureja* species," *Journal of Acupuncture & Meridian Studies*, vol. 9, no. 3, pp. 118–127, 2016.

[131] P. Mašković, V. Veličković, M. Mitić et al., "Summer savory extracts prepared by novel extraction methods resulted in enhanced biological activity," *Industrial Crops and Products*, vol. 109, pp. 875–881, 2017.

[132] S. Ceker, G. Agar, L. Alpsoy, G. Nardemir, and H. E. Kizil, "Antagonistic effects of *Satureja hortensis* essential oil against AFB, on human lymphocytes in vitro," *Cytology and Genetics*, vol. 48, no. 5, pp. 327–332, 2014.

[133] V. Hajhashem, B. Zolfaghari, and A. Yousefi, "Antinociceptive and anti-inflammatory activities of *Satureja hortensis* seed essential oil, hydroalcoholic and polyphenolic extracts in animal models," *Medical Principles and Practice*, vol. 21, no. 2, pp. 178–182, 2012.

[134] M. Mohammadhosseini, A. Akbarzadeh, and H. Hashemi-Moghaddam, "Gas chromatographic-mass spectrometric analysis of volatiles obtained by HS-SPME-GC-MS technique from *Stachys lavandulifolia* and evaluation for biological activity: a review," *Journal of Essential Oil Bearing Plants*, vol. 19, no. 6, pp. 1300–1327, 2016.

[135] K. Javidnia, F. Mojab, and S. A. Mojahedi, "Chemical constituents of the essential oil of *Stachys lavandulifolia* Vahl from Iran," *Journal of Essential Oil Bearing Plants*, vol. 19, no. 6, pp. 174–178, 2003.

[136] A. G. Pirbalouti and M. Mohammadi, "Phytochemical composition of the essential oil of different populations of *Stachys lavandulifolia* Vahl," *Asian Pacific Journal of Tropical Biomedicine*, vol. 3, no. 2, pp. 123–128, 2013.

[137] L. Rouzbeh, "Antimicrobial activity and chemical composition of essential oils of *Stachys lavandulifolia* Vahl. from Mazandaran, Iran," *Journal of Medicinal Plants Research*, vol. 6, no. 24, pp. 4149–4158, 2012.

[138] M. Oztürk, M. E. Duru, F. Aydoğmuş-Oztürk et al., "GC-MS analysis and antimicrobial activity of essential oil of *Stachys cretica* subsp. *smyrnaea*," *Natural Product Communications*, vol. 4, no. 1, pp. 109–114, 2009.

[139] B. Minae, M. Sardari, H. Sharifi, M. Sedigh Rahim Abadi, and O. Sadeghpour, "*Stachys lavandulifolia* Vahl. and its relation with marmazad activities in traditional manuscripts," *Iranian Red Crescent Medical Journal*, vol. 17, no. 11, p. e19932, 2015.

[140] M. Modarresi, L. Hosseinzadeh, N. Nematy, Z. M. Siavash-Haghighi, and K. Ghanbari, "Acute and subchronic toxicological evaluation of *Stachys lavandulifolia* aqueous extract in Wistar rats," *Research in Pharmaceutical Sciences*, vol. 9, no. 3, pp. 165–72, 2014.

[141] V. Hajhashemi, A. Ghannadi, and S. Sedighifar, "Analgesic and anti-inflammatory properties of the hydroalcoholic, polyphenolic and boiled extracts of *Stachys lavandulifolia*," *Research in Pharmaceutical Sciences*, vol. 1, pp. 92–98, 2007.

[142] R. S. S. Barreto, J. S. S. Quintans, R. K. L. R. S. Amarante et al., "Evidence for the involvement of TNF-α and IL-1β in the antinociceptive and anti-inflammatory activity of *Stachys lavandulifolia* Vahl. (Lamiaceae) essential oil and (-)-α-bisabolol, its main compound, in mice," *Journal of Ethnopharmacology*, vol. 191, pp. 9–18, 2016.

[143] E. Háznagy-Radnai, Á. Balogh, S. Czigle, I. Máthé, J. Hohmann, and G. Blazsó, "Antiinflammatory activities of Hungarian *Stachys* species and their iridoids," *Phytotherapy Research*, vol. 26, no. 4, pp. 505–509, 2012.

[144] H. D. Skaltsa, C. Demetzos, D. Lazari, and M. Sokovic, "Essential oil analysis and antimicrobial activity of eight *Stachys* species from Greece," *Phytochemistry*, vol. 64, no. 3, pp. 743–752, 2003.

[145] G. Paun, E. Neagu, C. Albu, V. Moroeanu, and G.-L. Radu, "Antioxidant activity and inhibitory effect of polyphenolic-rich extract from *Betonica officinalis* and *Impatiens noli-tangere* herbs on key enzyme linked to type 2 diabetes," *Journal of the Taiwan Institute of Chemical Engineers*, vol. 60, pp. 1–7, 2016.

[146] I. Šliumpaitė, P. R. Venskutonis, M. Murkovic, and O. Ragažinskienė, "Antioxidant properties and phenolic composition of wood betony (*Betonica officinalis* L., syn. *Stachys officinalis* L.)," *Industrial Crops and Products*, vol. 50, pp. 715–722, 2013.
[147] E. Russo, *Handbook of Psychotropic Herbs: A Scientific Analysis of Herbal Remedies for Psychiatric Conditions*, Haworth Herbal Press, Binghamton, NY, USA, 2001.
[148] F. Conforti, F. Menichini, C. Formisano et al., "Comparative chemical composition, free radical-scavenging and cytotoxic properties of essential oils of six *Stachys* species from different regions of the Mediterranean area," *Food Chemistry*, vol. 116, no. 4, pp. 898–905, 2009.
[149] G. Paun, E. Neagu, V. Moroeanu et al., "Phytochemical analysis and in vitro biological activity of *Betonica officinalis* and *Salvia officinalis* extracts," *Romanian Biotechnological Letters*, vol. 22, no. 4, 2017.
[150] A. Matkowski and M. Piotrowska, "Antioxidant and free radical scavenging activities of some medicinal plants from the Lamiaceae," *Fitoterapia*, vol. 77, no. 5, pp. 346–353, 2006.
[151] N. Maleki, A. Garjani, H. Nazemiyeh et al., "Potent anti-inflammatory activities of hydroalcoholic extract from aerial parts of *Stachys inflata* on rats," *Journal of Ethnopharmacology*, vol. 75, no. 2-3, pp. 213–218, 2001.
[152] M. Khanavi, M. Sharifzadeh, A. Hadjiakhoondi, and A. Shafiee, "Phytochemical investigation and anti-inflammatory activity of aerial parts of *Stachys byzanthina* C. Koch," *Journal of Ethnopharmacology*, vol. 97, no. 3, pp. 463–468, 2005.
[153] Y.-Y. Wang, S.-Y. Lin, W.-Y. Chen et al., "*Glechoma hederacea* extracts attenuate cholestatic liver injury in a bile duct-ligated rat model," *Journal of Ethnopharmacology*, vol. 204, pp. 58–66, 2017.
[154] J. Kim, S. Song, I. Lee et al., "Anti-inflammatory activity of constituents from *Glechoma hederacea* var. longituba," *Bioorganic & Medicinal Chemistry Letters*, vol. 21, no. 11, pp. 3483–3487, 2011.
[155] H. Ohigashi, H. Takamura, K. Koshimizu, H. Tokuda, and Y. Ito, "Search for possible antitumor promoters by inhibition of 12-O-tetradecanoylphorbol-13-acetate-induced Epstein-Barr virus activation; ursolic acid and oleanolic acid from an anti-inflammatory Chinese medicinal plant, *Glechoma hederacea* L.," *Cancer Letters*, vol. 30, no. 2, pp. 143–151, 1986.
[156] H. Kühn, R. Wiesner, L. Alder, and T. Schewe, "Occurrence of free and esterified lipoxygenase products in leaves of *Glechoma hederacea* L. and other Labiatae.," *European Journal of Biochemistry*, vol. 186, no. 1-2, pp. 155–62, 1989.
[157] T. Singh, J. H. Wu, W. J. Peumans et al., "Carbohydrate specificity of an insecticidal lectin isolated from the leaves of *Glechoma hederacea* (ground ivy) towards mammalian glycoconjugates," *Biochemical Journal*, vol. 393, no. 1, pp. 331–41, 2006.
[158] Y. Kumarasamy, P. J. Cox, M. Jaspars, L. Nahar, and S. D. Sarker, "Biological activity of *Glechoma hederacea*," *Fitoterapia*, vol. 73, no. 7-8, pp. 721–723, 2002.
[159] H.-J. An, H.-J. Jeong, J.-Y. Um, H.-M. Kim, and S.-H. Hong, "*Glechoma hederacea* inhibits inflammatory mediator release in IFN-γ and LPS-stimulated mouse peritoneal macrophages," *Journal of Ethnopharmacology*, vol. 106, no. 3, pp. 418–424, 2006.
[160] J. K. Hwang, M. Erkhembaatar, D. R. Gu et al., "*Glechoma hederacea* suppresses RANKL-mediated osteoclastogenesis," *Journal of Dental Research*, vol. 93, no. 7, pp. 685–690, 2014.
[161] M. Milovanovic, D. Zivkovic, and B. Vucelic-Radovic, "Antioxidant effects of *Glechoma hederacea* as a food additive," *Natural Product Communications*, vol. 5, no. 1, pp. 61–63, 2010.
[162] A. Belščak-Cvitanović, K. Durgo, A. Bušić, J. Franekić, and D. Komes, "Phytochemical attributes of four conventionally extracted medicinal plants and cytotoxic evaluation of their extracts on human laryngeal carcinoma (HEp2) cells," *Journal of Medicinal Food*, vol. 17, no. 2, pp. 206–217, 2014.
[163] I. Miron, S. Diaconescu, G. Aprodu, I. Ioniuc, M. R. Diaconescu, and L. Miron, "Diagnostic difficulties in a pediatric insulinoma," *Medicine*, vol. 95, no. 11, 2016, p. e3045.
[164] C. Brock, J. Whitehouse, I. Tewfik, and T. Towell, "American skullcap (*Scutellaria lateriflora*): a randomised, double-blind placebo-controlled crossover study of its effects on mood in healthy volunteers," *Phytotherapy Research*, vol. 28, no. 5, pp. 692–698, 2014.
[165] C. Brock, J. Whitehouse, I. Tewfik, and T. Towell, "American skullcap (*Scutellaria lateriflora*): an ancient remedy for today's anxiety?," *British Journal of Wellbeing*, vol. 1, no. 4, pp. 25–30, 2010.
[166] J. Gao, A. Sanchez-Medina, B. A. Pendry, M. J. Hughes, G. P. Webb, and O. Corcoran, "Validation of a HPLC method for flavonoid biomarkers in skullcap (*Scutellaria*) and its use to illustrate wide variability in the quality of commercial tinctures," *Journal of Pharmacy & Pharmaceutical Sciences*, vol. 11, no. 1, pp. 77–87, 2008.
[167] J. Li, Y.-H. Wang, T. J. Smillie, and I. A. Khan, "Identification of phenolic compounds from *Scutellaria lateriflora* by liquid chromatography with ultraviolet photodiode array and electrospray ionization tandem mass spectrometry," *Journal of Pharmaceutical and Biomedical Analysis*, vol. 63, pp. 120–127, 2012.
[168] J. L. Rhudy and M. W. Meagher, "Fear and anxiety: divergent effects on human pain thresholds," *Pain*, vol. 84, no. 1, pp. 65–75, 2000.
[169] M. Lohani, M. Ahuja, M. A. Buabeid et al., "Anti-oxidative and DNA protecting effects of flavonoids-rich *Scutellaria lateriflora*," *Natural Product Communications*, vol. 8, pp. 1415–1418, 2013.
[170] R. Awad, J. T. Arnason, V. Trudeau et al., "Phytochemical and biological analysis of skullcap (*Scutellaria lateriflora* L.): a medicinal plant with anxiolytic properties," *Phytomedicine*, vol. 10, no. 8, pp. 640–649, 2003.
[171] S. Gafner, C. Bergeron, L. L. Batcha et al., "Inhibition of [3H]-LSD binding to 5-HT7 receptors by flavonoids from *Scutellaria lateriflora*," *Journal of Natural Products*, vol. 66, no. 4, pp. 535–537, 2003.
[172] J. Jianjun and D. Huiru, "Preparation of high-purity baicalein from *Scutellaria baicalensis* Georgi," *Natural Product Research*, vol. 22, no. 16, pp. 1410–1412, 2008.
[173] C.-C. Lin and D.-E. Shieh, "The anti-inflammatory activity of *Scutellaria rivularis* extracts and its active components, baicalin, baicalein and wogonin," *American Journal of Chinese Medicine*, vol. 24, no. 1, pp. 31–36, 1996.
[174] S. Yoo, S. Han, Y. S. Park, J.-H. Lee, U. Oh, and S. W. Hwang, "Lipoxygenase inhibitors suppressed carrageenan-induced Fos-expression and inflammatory pain responses in the rat," *Molecules and Cells*, vol. 27, no. 4, pp. 417–422, 2009.
[175] M. Yimam, L. Brownell, M. Hodges, and Q. Jia, "Analgesic effects of a standardized bioflavonoid composition from *Scutellaria baicalensis* and *Acacia catechu*," *Journal of Dietary Supplements*, vol. 9, no. 3, pp. 155–65, 2012.

[176] C.-H. Cherng, K.-C. Lee, C.-C. Chien et al., "Baicalin ameliorates neuropathic pain by suppressing HDAC1 expression in the spinal cord of spinal nerve ligation rats," *Journal of the Formosan Medical Association*, vol. 113, no. 8, pp. 513–520, 2014.

[177] S. Hu, Y. Chen, Z.-F. Wang et al., "The analgesic and antineuroinflammatory effect of baicalein in cancer-induced bone pain, evidence-based complement," *Alternative Medicine*, vol. 2015, Article ID 973524, 8 pages, 2015.

[178] A. C. Pinzariu, S. A. Pasca, A. Sindilar et al., "Adipose tissue remodeling by prolonged administration of high dose of vitamin D3 in rats treated to prevent sarcopenia," *Revista de Chimie-Bucharest*, vol. 68, pp. 2139–2143, 2017.

[179] J. D. Deschamps, V. A. Kenyon, and T. R. Holman, "Baicalein is a potent in vitro inhibitor against both reticulocyte 15-human and platelet 12-human lipoxygenases," *Bioorganic & Medicinal Chemistry*, vol. 14, pp. 4295–4301, 2006.

[180] C.-J. Hsieh, K. Hall, T. Ha, C. Li, G. Krishnaswamy, and D. S. Chi, "Baicalein inhibits IL-1β- and TNF-α-induced inflammatory cytokine production from human mast cells via regulation of the NF-κB pathway," *Clinical and Molecular Allergy*, vol. 5, no. 1, p. 5, 2007.

[181] I. Wakabayashi, "Inhibitory effects of baicalein and wogonin on lipopolysaccharide-induced nitric oxide production in macrophages," *Pharmacology & Toxicology*, vol. 84, no. 6, pp. 288–91, 1999.

[182] K. J. Woo, J. H. Lim, S.-I. Suh et al., "Differential inhibitory effects of baicalein and baicalin on LPS-induced cyclooxygenase-2 expression through inhibition of C/EBPβ DNA-binding activity," *Immunobiology*, vol. 211, no. 5, pp. 359–368, 2006.

[183] M. Kumar, E. R. Kasala, L. N. Bodduluru, V. Dahiya, and M. Lahkar, "Baicalein protects isoproterenol induced myocardial ischemic injury in male Wistar rats by mitigating oxidative stress and inflammation," *Inflammation Research*, vol. 65, no. 8, pp. 613–622, 2016.

[184] Y. Xie, X. Song, X. Sun et al., "Identification of baicalein as a ferroptosis inhibitor by natural product library screening," *Biochemical and Biophysical Research Communications*, vol. 473, no. 4, pp. 775–780, 2016.

[185] R. S. M. de Carvalho, F. S. Duarte, and T. C. M. de Lima, "Involvement of GABAergic non-benzodiazepine sites in the anxiolytic-like and sedative effects of the flavonoid baicalein in mice," *Behavioural Brain Research*, vol. 221, no. 1, pp. 75–82, 2011.

[186] H. Yin, J. P. Bhattarai, S. M. Oh, S. J. Park, D. K. Ahn, and S. K. Han, "Baicalin activates glycine and γ-aminobutyric acid receptors on substantia gelatinosa neurons of the trigeminal subsnucleus caudalis in juvenile mice," *American Journal of Chinese Medicine*, vol. 44, no. 2, pp. 389–400, 2016.

[187] A. Woo, C. Cheng, and M. Waye, "Baicalein protects rat cardiomyocytes from hypoxia/reoxygenation damage via a prooxidant mechanism," *Cardiovascular Research*, vol. 65, no. 1, pp. 244–253, 2005.

[188] N. Mahajan, S. Rawal, M. Verma, M. Poddar, and S. Alok, "A phytopharmacological overview on *Ocimum* species with special emphasis on *Ocimum sanctum*," *Biomedicine & Preventive Nutrition*, vol. 3, no. 2, pp. 185–192, 2013.

[189] G. Kaur, A. S. Jaggi, and N. Singh, "Exploring the potential effect of *Ocimum sanctum* in vincristine-induced neuropathic pain in rats," *Journal of Brachial Plexus and Peripheral Nerve Injury*, vol. 5, p. 3, 2010.

[190] A. Muthuraman, V. Diwan, A. S. Jaggi, N. Singh, and D. Singh, "Ameliorative effects of *Ocimum sanctum* in sciatic nerve transection-induced neuropathy in rats," *Journal of Ethnopharmacology*, vol. 120, no. 1, pp. 56–62, 2008.

[191] P. Bhattacharyya and A. Bishayee, "*Ocimum sanctum* Linn. (Tulsi): an ethnomedicinal plant for the prevention and treatment of cancer," *Anti-Cancer Drugs*, vol. 24, no. 7, pp. 659–66, 2013.

[192] S. Mondal, S. Varma, V. D. Bamola et al., "Double-blinded randomized controlled trial for immunomodulatory effects of Tulsi (*Ocimum sanctum* Linn.) leaf extract on healthy volunteers," *Journal of Ethnopharmacology*, vol. 136, pp. 452–456, 2011.

[193] S. S. Choudhury, L. Bashyam, N. Manthapuram, P. Bitla, P. Kollipara, and S. D. Tetali, "*Ocimum sanctum* leaf extracts attenuate human monocytic (THP-1) cell activation," *Journal of Ethnopharmacology*, vol. 154, no. 1, pp. 148–155, 2014.

[194] S. Singh, D. K. Majumdar, and H. M. Rehan, "Evaluation of anti-inflammatory potential of fixed oil of *Ocimum sanctum* (holybasil) and its possible mechanism of action," *Journal of Ethnopharmacology*, vol. 54, no. 1, pp. 19–26, 1996.

[195] D. Gupta, D. Bhaskar, R. Gupta et al., "A randomized controlled clinical trial of *Ocimum sanctum* and chlorhexidine mouthwash on dental plaque and gingival inflammation," *Journal of Ayurveda and Integrative Medicine*, vol. 5, p. 109, 2014.

[196] G. Kaur, A. Bali, N. Singh, and A. S. Jaggi, "Ameliorative potential of *Ocimum sanctum* in chronic constriction injury-induced neuropathic pain in rats," *Anais da Academia Brasileira de Ciências*, vol. 87, no. 1, pp. 417–429, 2015.

[197] A. Ahmad, M. M. Khan, S. S. Raza et al., "*Ocimum sanctum* attenuates oxidative damage and neurological deficits following focal cerebral ischemia/reperfusion injury in rats," *Neurological Sciences*, vol. 33, no. 6, pp. 1239–1247, 2012.

[198] N. Okiemy-Andissa, M. Miguel, A. Etou, J. Ouamba, M. Gbeassor, and A. Abena, "Analgesic effect of aqueous and hydroalcoholic extracts of three congolese medicinal plants: *Hyptis suavolens*, *Nauclea latifolia* and *Ocimum gratissimum*," *Pakistan Journal of Biological Sciences*, vol. 7, no. 9, pp. 1613–1615, 2004.

[199] L. Paula-Freire, G. Molska, M. Andersen, and E. Carlini, "*Ocimum gratissimum* essential oil and its isolated compounds (eugenol and myrcene) reduce neuropathic pain in mice," *Planta Medica*, vol. 82, no. 3, pp. 211–216, 2015.

[200] E. O. Igbinosa, E. O. Uzunuigbe, I. H. Igbinosa, E. E. Odjadjare, N. O. Igiehon, and O. A. Emuedo, "In vitro assessment of antioxidant, phytochemical and nutritional properties of extracts from the leaves of *Ocimum gratissimum* (Linn)," *African Journal of Traditional, Complementary and Alternative Medicines*, vol. 10, no. 5, pp. 292–298, 2013.

[201] L. I. G. Paula-Freire, M. L. Andersen, G. R. Molska, D. O. Köhn, and E. L. A. Carlini, "Evaluation of the antinociceptive activity of *Ocimum gratissimum* l. (Lamiaceae) essential oil and its isolated active principles in mice," *Phytotherapy Research*, vol. 27, no. 8, pp. 1220–1224, 2013.

[202] M. Rabelo, E. P. Souza, P. M. G. Soares, A. V. Miranda, F. J. A. Matos, and D. N. Criddle, "Antinociceptive properties of the essential oil of *Ocimum gratissimum* L. (Labiatae) in mice," *Brazilian Journal of Medical and Biological Research*, vol. 36, no. 4, pp. 521–524, 2003.

[203] L. I. G. Paula-Freire, M. L. Andersen, V. S. Gama, G. R. Molska, and E. L. A. Carlini, "The oral administration of *trans*-caryophyllene attenuates acute and chronic pain in mice," *Phytomedicine*, vol. 21, no. 3, pp. 356–362, 2014.

[204] S. Katsuyama, H. Mizoguchi, H. Kuwahata et al., "Involvement of peripheral cannabinoid and opioid receptors in β-caryophyllene-induced antinociception," *European Journal of Pain*, vol. 17, no. 5, pp. 664–675, 2013.
[205] J. de Pinho, A. Silva, B. Pinheiro et al., "Antinociceptive and antispasmodic effects of the essential oil of *Ocimum micranthum*: potential anti-inflammatory properties," *Planta Medica*, vol. 78, no. 7, pp. 681–685, 2012.
[206] E. K. Akkol, F. N. Yalçın, D. Kaya, İ. Çalış, E. Yesilada, and T. Ersöz, "In vivo anti-inflammatory and antinociceptive actions of some *Lamium* species," *Journal of Ethnopharmacology*, vol. 118, no. 1, pp. 166–172, 2008.
[207] K. Alipieva, L. Evstatieva, N. Handjieva, and S. Popov, "Comparative analysis of the composition of flower volatiles from *Lamium* L. species and *Lamiastrum galeobdolon* Heist. ex Fabr.," *Z. Naturforsch. C.*, vol. 58, no. 11-12, pp. 779–782, 2003.
[208] S. Bahramikia and R. Yazdanparast, "Phytochemistry and medicinal properties of *Teucrium polium* L. (Lamiaceae)," *Phytotherapy Research*, vol. 26, no. 11, pp. 1581–1593, 2012.
[209] K. Abadian, Z. Keshavarz, F. Mojab, H. Alavi Majd, and N. M. Abbasi, "Comparison the effect of mefenamic acid and *Teucrium polium* on the severity and systemic symptoms of dysmenorrhea," *Complementary Therapies in Clinical Practice*, vol. 22, pp. 12–15, 2016.
[210] S. Purnavab, S. Ketabchi, and V. Rowshan, "Chemical composition and antibacterial activity of methanolic extract and essential oil of Iranian *Teucrium polium* against some of phytobacteria," *Natural Product Research*, vol. 29, no. 14, pp. 1376–1379, 2015.
[211] T. Baluchnejadmojarad, M. Roghani, and F. Roghani-Dehkordi, "Antinociceptive effect of *Teucrium polium* leaf extract in the diabetic rat formalin test," *Journal of Ethnopharmacology*, vol. 97, no. 2, pp. 207–210, 2005.
[212] M. Tariq, A. M. Ageel, M. A. al-Yahya, J. S. Mossa, and M. S. al-Said, "Anti-inflammatory activity of *Teucrium polium*," *International Journal of Tissue Reactions*, vol. 11, no. 4, pp. 185–188, 1989.
[213] M. Shahraki, H. MirShekari, and M. J. Palan, "The comparison of nociceptive effect of *Teucrium polium* and morphine in female rats," *Horizons Medical Science*, vol. 12, no. 1, pp. 10–14, 2006.
[214] M. Abdollahi, H. Karimpour, and H. R. Monsef-Esfehani, "Antinociceptive effects of *Teucrium polium* L total extract and essential oil in mouse writhing test," *Pharmacological Research*, vol. 48, pp. 31–35, 2003.
[215] A. Farshchi, G. Ghiasi, and A. A. Asl, "Antinociceptive and antiinflammatory effects of *Teucrium hyrcanicum* aqueous extract in male mice and rats," *Physiol Pharmacol*, vol. 14, no. 1, pp. 78–84, 2010.
[216] F. Golfakhrabadi, F. Yousefbeyk, T. Mirnezami, P. Laghaei, M. Hajimahmoodi, and M. Khanavi, "Antioxidant and antiacetylcholinesterase activity of *Teucrium hyrcanicum*," *Pharmacognosy Research*, vol. 7, no. 5, pp. S15–S19, 2015.
[217] C. Nencini, P. Galluzzi, F. Pippi, A. Menchiari, and L. Micheli, "Hepatotoxicity of *Teucrium chamaedrys* L. decoction: role of difference in the harvesting area and preparation method," *Indian J. Pharmacol*, vol. 46, no. 2, pp. 181–184, 2014.
[218] T. A. K. Prescott, N. C. Veitch, and M. S. J. Simmonds, "Direct inhibition of calcineurin by caffeoyl phenylethanoid glycosides from *Teucrium chamaedrys* and *Nepeta cataria*," *Journal of Ethnopharmacology*, vol. 137, no. 3, pp. 1306–1310, 2011.
[219] R. A. Falcao, P. L. A. do Nascimento, S. A. de Souza et al., "Antileishmanial phenylpropanoids from the leaves of *Hyptis pectinata* (L.) Poit," *Evidence-Based Complementary and Alternative Medicine*, vol. 2013, p. 460613, 2013.
[220] S. A. de L. Bordignon, "*Hyptis tetracephala* (Labiatae), nova espécie do sul do Brasil," *Napaea*, vol. 8, pp. 1–3, 1992.
[221] R. Harley, Evolution and distribution of Eriope (Labiatae) and its relation in Brazil, in P. Vanzolini and W. Heyer, Eds., Proc. a Work. Neotrop. Distrib. Patterns, Academia Brasileira de Ciências, Rio de Janeiro, Brazil, pp. 71–121, 1988.
[222] M. D. Bispo, R. H. Mourão, E. M. Franzotti et al., "Antinociceptive and antiedematogenic effects of the aqueous extract of *Hyptis pectinata* leaves in experimental animals," *Journal of Ethnopharmacology*, vol. 76, no. 1, pp. 81–86, 2001.
[223] M. S. Paixão, M. S. Melo, N. P. Damascena et al., "*Hyptis pectinata* gel prevents alveolar bone resorption in experimental periodontitis in rats," *Revista Brasileira de Farmacognosia*, vol. 25, no. 1, pp. 35–41, 2015.
[224] M. S. Paixão, M. S. Melo, M. G. B. Oliveira et al., "*Hyptis pectinata*: redox protection and orofacial antinociception," *Phytotherapy Research*, vol. 27, no. 9, pp. 1328–1333, 2013.
[225] G. B. Melo, R. L. Silva, V. A. Melo et al., "Enhancement of liver regeneration by the association of *Hyptis pectinata* with laser therapy," *Digestive Diseases and Sciences*, vol. 50, no. 5, pp. 949–954, 2005.
[226] M. F. Arrigoni-Blank, R. Silva-Mann, D. A. Campos et al., "Morphological, agronomical and pharmacological characterization of *Hyptis pectinata* (L.) Poit germplasm," *Revista Brasileira de Farmacognosia*, vol. 15, no. 4, pp. 298–303, 2005.
[227] C. Liapi, G. Anifandis, G. Anifantis et al., "Antinociceptive properties of 1,8-cineole and beta-pinene, from the essential oil of *Eucalyptus camaldulensis* leaves, in rodents," *Planta Medica*, vol. 73, no. 12, pp. 1247–54, 2007.
[228] C. R. P. Franco, Â. R. Antoniolli, A. G. Guimarães et al., "Bioassay-guided evaluation of antinociceptive properties and chemical variability of the essential oil of *Hyptis fruticosa*," *Phytotherapy Research*, vol. 25, no. 11, pp. 1693–1699, 2011.
[229] L. J. R. P. Raymundo, C. C. Guilhon, D. S. Alviano et al., "Characterisation of the anti-inflammatory and antinociceptive activities of the *Hyptis pectinata* (L.) Poit essential oil," *Journal of Ethnopharmacology*, vol. 134, no. 3, pp. 725–732, 2011.
[230] J. F. Sarmento-Neto, L. G. Do Nascimento, C. F. B. Felipe, and D. P. De Sousa, "Analgesic potential of essential oils," *Molecules*, vol. 21, pp. 1–29, 2016.
[231] C. P. Khare, *Indian Medicinal Plants*, Springer New York, New York, NY, USA, 2007.
[232] I. Agata, H. Kusakabe, T. Hatano, S. Nishibe, and T. Okuda, "Melitric acids A and B, new trimeric caffeic acid derivatives from *Melissa officinalis*," *Chemical & Pharmaceutical Bulletin*, vol. 41, no. 9, pp. 1608–1611, 1993.
[233] K. Triantaphyllou, G. Blekas, and D. Boskou, "Antioxidative properties of water extracts obtained from herbs of the species Lamiaceae," *International Journal of Food Sciences and Nutrition*, vol. 52, no. 4, pp. 313–317, 2001.
[234] M. Felklová, L. Nátherová, and K. Dusková, "Tannin compounds in leaves of *Melissa officinalis* L., invaded by *Septoria melissae* Desm," *Ceskoslovenska Farmacie*, vol. 18, no. 9, pp. 457–460, 1969.
[235] M. Mrlianová, D. Tekel'ová, M. Felklová, V. Reinöhl, and J. Tóth, "The influence of the harvest cut height on the quality

of the herbal drugs *Melissae folium* and *Melissae herba*," *Planta Medica*, vol. 68, no. 2, pp. 178–80, 2002.
[236] J. Patora, T. Majda, J. Góra, and B. Klimek, "Variability in the content and composition of essential oil from lemon balm (*Melissa officinalis* L.) cultivated in Poland," *Acta Poloniae Pharmaceutica*, vol. 60, no. 5, pp. 395–400, 2003.
[237] J. Mikus, M. Harkenthal, D. Steverding, and J. Reichling, "In vitro effect of essential oils and isolated mono- and sesquiterpenes on *Leishmania major* and *Trypanosoma brucei*," *Planta Medica*, vol. 66, no. 4, pp. 366–368, 2000.
[238] C. H. Brieskorn and W. Krause, "Further triterpenes from *Melissa officinalis* L (author's transl)," *Archiv der Pharmazie*, vol. 307, no. 8, pp. 603–12, 1974.
[239] E. Sarer and G. Kökdil, "Constituents of the essential oil from *Melissa officinalis*," *Planta Medica*, vol. 57, no. 1, pp. 89-90, 1991.
[240] E. C. Herrmann and L. S. Kucera, "Antiviral substances in plants of the mint family (Labiatae). II. Nontannin polyphenol of *Melissa officinalis*," *Proceedings of the Society for Experimental Biology and Medicine*, vol. 124, pp. 869–874, 1967.
[241] M. S. Lawrence, P. Stojanov, P. Polak et al., "Mutational heterogeneity in cancer and the search for new cancer-associated genes," *Nature*, vol. 499, no. 7457, pp. 214–218, 2013.
[242] K. Yamasaki, M. Nakano, T. Kawahata et al., "Anti-HIV-1 activity of herbs in Labiatae," *Biological & Pharmaceutical Bulletin*, vol. 21, no. 8, pp. 829–833, 1998.
[243] L. Iauk, A. M. Lo Bue, I. Milazzo, A. Rapisarda, and G. Blandino, "Antibacterial activity of medicinal plant extracts against periodontopathic bacteria," *Phytotherapy Research*, vol. 17, no. 6, pp. 599–604, 2003.
[244] W. Englberger, U. Hadding, E. Etschenberg et al., "Rosmarinic acid: a new inhibitor of complement C3-convertase with anti-inflammatory activity," *International Journal of Immunopharmacology*, vol. 10, no. 6, pp. 729–737, 1988.
[245] M. Auf'mkolk, J. C. Ingbar, S. M. Amir et al., "Inhibition by certain plant extracts of the binding and adenylate cyclase stimulatory effect of bovine thyrotropin in human thyroid membranes," *Endocrinology*, vol. 115, no. 2, pp. 527–534, 1984.
[246] R. Soulimani, J. Fleurentin, F. Mortier, R. Misslin, G. Derrieu, and J. M. Pelt, "Neurotropic action of the hydroalcoholic extract of *Melissa officinalis* in the mouse," *Planta Medica*, vol. 57, no. 2, pp. 105–109, 1991.
[247] R. Gazola, D. Machado, C. Ruggiero, G. Singi, and M. Macedo Alexandre, "*Lippia alba, Melissa officinalis* and *Cymbopogon citratus*: effects of the aqueous extracts on the isolated hearts of rats," *Pharmacological Research*, vol. 50, no. 5, pp. 477–480, 2004.
[248] T. Anca, P. Alin Constantin, C. Roxana Gabriela et al., "Toxic effects of magnesium nitrate on cardiac muscle tissue of *Gallus domesticus* embryos and chicks," *Revista de Chimie-Bucharest*, vol. 68, pp. 1343–1349, 2017.
[249] F. Sahin, M. C. Güllüce, D. Daferera et al., "Biological activities of the essential oils and methanol extract of *Origanum vulgare* in the Eastern Anatolia region of Turkey," *Food Control*, vol. 15, no. 7, pp. 549–557, 2004.
[250] P. Prerna and N. Vasudeva, "*Origanum majorana* L.phytopharmacological review," *Indian Journal of Natural Products and Resources*, vol. 6, pp. 261–267, 2015.
[251] M. Barazandeh, "Identification of the essential oil composition from *Origanum majorana* L.," *Journal of Pajohesh & Sazandegi*, vol. 14, pp. 38–40, 2000.
[252] M. Melegari, F. Severi, M. Bertoldi et al., "Chemical characterization of essential oils of some *Origanum vulgare* L. subspecies of various origin," *Revista Brasileira de Plantas Medicinais*, vol. 16, no. 4, pp. 21–28, 1995.
[253] R. Baranauskienė, P. R. Venskutonis, E. Dambrauskienė, and P. Viškelis, "Harvesting time influences the yield and oil composition of *Origanum vulgare* L. ssp. vulgare and ssp. hirtum," *Industrial Crops and Products*, vol. 49, pp. 43–51, 2013.
[254] S. Tahmasebi, A. Majd, A. Mehrafarin, and P. Jonoubi, "Comparative ontogenetic survey of the essential oil composition in *Origanum vulgare* L., and *Origanum majorana* L.," *Acta Biologica Szegediensis*, vol. 60, pp. 105–111, 2016.
[255] H. J. Dorman and S. G. Deans, "Antimicrobial agents from plants: antibacterial activity of plant volatile oils," *Journal of Applied Microbiology*, vol. 88, no. 2, pp. 308–316, 2000.
[256] I. Novák, É. Zámbori-Németh, H. Horváth, Z. Seregély, and K. Kaffka, "Study of essential oil components in different *Origanum* species by GC and sensory analysis," *Acta Alimentaria*, vol. 32, no. 2, pp. 141–150, 2003.
[257] B. Lakhrissi, A. Boukhraz, M. Barrahi, H. El, and M. Ouhssine, "Antifungal activity of essential oil of oregano (*Origanum vulgare*)," *International Journal of Research Studies in Science, Engineering and Technology*, vol. 3, pp. 14–17, 2016.
[258] M. Marino, C. Bersani, and G. Comi, "Impedance measurements to study the antimicrobial activity of essential oils from Lamiaceae and Compositae," *International Journal of Food Microbiology*, vol. 67, no. 3, pp. 187–95, 2001.
[259] H. Baydar, O. Sagdic, G. Ozkan, and T. Karadogan, "Antibacterial activity and composition of essential oils from *Origanum*, *Thymbra* and *Sartureja* species with commercial importance in Turkey," *Food Control*, vol. 15, no. 3, pp. 169–172, 2004.
[260] J. H. Cano and G. Volpato, "Herbal mixtures in the traditional medicine of eastern Cuba," *Journal of Ethnopharmacology*, vol. 90, no. 2-3, pp. 293–316, 2004.
[261] E. Vági, B. Simándi, Á. Suhajda, and É. Héthelyi, "Essential oil composition and antimicrobial activity of *Origanum majorana* L. extracts obtained with ethyl alcohol and supercritical carbon dioxide," *Food Res. Int*, vol. 38, no. 1, pp. 51–57, 2005.
[262] M. Floria and V. L. Drug, "Atrial fibrillation and gastroesophageal reflux disease: from the cardiologist perspective," *World Journal of Gastroenterology*, vol. 21, no. 10, pp. 3154–3156, 2015.
[263] M. Floria, D. Blommaert, M. Lacrosse et al., "Assessment of left atrial shape and volume in structural remodeling secondary to atrial fibrillation," *Journal of Interventional Cardiac Electrophysiology*, vol. 25, no. 3, pp. 167–170, 2009.
[264] M. Floria, O. Barboi, C. Rezus et al., "Atrial fibrillation and gastro-oesophageal reflux disease-controversies and challenges," *Current Pharmaceutical Design*, vol. 21, no. 26, pp. 3829–3834, 2015.
[265] E. Rezus, M. Floria, A. Grigoriu, B. I. Tamba, and C. Rezus, "Cardiovascular risk factors in chronic inflammatory rheumatic diseases: modern assessment and diagnosis," *Current Vascular Pharmacology*, vol. 13, no. 6, pp. 716–724, 2015.
[266] S. Talebi, A. Rezakhanlou, and G. S. Isfahani, "Trichome plasticity in *Ziziphora tenuior* L. (Labiatae) in Iran: an ecological review," *Annals of Biological Research*, vol. 3, pp. 668–672, 2012.
[267] F. Senejoux, C. Girard, P. Kerram et al., "Mechanisms of vasorelaxation induced by *Ziziphora clinopodioides* Lam.

(Lamiaceae) extract in rat thoracic aorta," *Journal of Ethnopharmacology*, vol. 132, no. 1, pp. 268–273, 2010.

[268] A. Azadmehr, R. Latifi, S. Mosalla, R. Hajiaghaee, and M. Shahnazi, "Immunomodulatory effects of *Ziziphora tenuior* L. extract on the dendritic cells," *DARU Journal of Pharmaceutical Sciences*, vol. 22, no. 1, p. 63, 2014.

[269] H. H. Gharetapeh, S. A. Maleki, and J. Asgharpanah, "Antidepressant effects of *Ziziphora tenuior* L. hydroalcoholic extract in animal models of depression," *International Journal of Farming and Allied Sciences*, vol. 3, no. 6, pp. 664–668, 2014.

[270] E. M. Z. Michielin, A. A. Salvador, C. A. S. Riehl, A. Smânia, E. F. A. Smânia, and S. R. S. Ferreira, "Chemical composition and antibacterial activity of *Cordia verbenacea* extracts obtained by different methods," *Bioresource Technology*, vol. 100, no. 24, pp. 6615–6623, 2009.

[271] U. Ahmed and A. U. Rahman, *Handbook of Natural Product Data*, Elsevier, Amsterdam, Netherlands, 1994.

[272] S. Shiow-Yunn, H. Feng-Lin, and L. Yu-Chan, "Two gallates from *Quercus glauca*," *Phytochemistry*, vol. 31, no. 7, pp. 2465–2468, 1992.

[273] B. Voirin, "UV spectral differentiation of 5-hydroxy- and 5-hydroxy-3-methoxyflavones with mono-(4′), di-(3′,4′) or tri-(3′,4′,5′)-substituted B rings," *Phytochemistry*, vol. 22, pp. 2107–2145, 1983.

[274] R. Mehmood, M. Imran, A. Malik, and R. B. Tareen, "Ziziphorins A and B. new flavonoids from *Ziziphora tenuior*," *Zeitschrift für Naturforschung B*, vol. 65, no. 11, pp. 1397–1400, 2010.

[275] T. Darbandi, B. Honarvar, M. Sinaei, and A. Rezaei, "Extraction of *Ziziphora tenuior* essential oil using supercritical CO_2," *European Journal of Experimental Biology*, vol. 2, no. 3, pp. 687–695, 2013.

[276] A. G. Pirbalouti, A. Amirkhosravi, F. Bordbar, and B. Hamedi, "Diversity in the chemical composition of essential oils of *Ziziphora tenuior* as a potential source of pulegone," *Chemija*, vol. 24, no. 3, pp. 234–239, 2013.

[277] Z. H. Fu, H. Wang, X. Hu, Z. Sun, and C. Han, "The pharmacological properties of *Salvia* essential oils," *Journal of Applied Pharmaceutical Science*, vol. 3, no. 7, pp. 122–127, 2013.

[278] K. Szentmihályi, C. Csedo, and M. Then, "Comparative study on tannins, flavonoids, terpenes and mineral elements of some *Salvia* species," *Acta Horticulturae*, vol. 629, pp. 463–470, 2004.

[279] A. Russo, C. Formisano, D. Rigano et al., "Chemical composition and anticancer activity of essential oils of Mediterranean sage (Salvia officinalis L.) grown in different environmental conditions," *Food and Chemical Toxicology*, vol. 55, pp. 42–47, 2013.

[280] M. Coisin, R. Necula, V. Grigoras, E. Gille, E. Rosenhech, and M. Zamfirache, "Phytochemical evaluation of some *Salvia* species from Romanian flora," *Biologie vegetală*, vol. 58, no. 1, pp. 35–44, 2012.

[281] A.-V. Pop (Cuceu), T. Maria, S. A. Sonia et al., "Comparative study regarding the chemical composition of essential oils of some salvia species," *Hop and Medicinal Plants*, 2014.

[282] R.-H. Zhang, Z.-K. Liu, D.-S. Yang, X.-J. Zhang, H.-D. Sun, and W.-L. Xiao, "Phytochemistry and pharmacology of the genus *Leonurus*: the herb to benefit the mothers and more," *Phytochemistry*, vol. 147, pp. 167–183, 2018.

[283] K. Wojtyniak, M. Szymański, and I. Matławska, "*Leonurus cardiaca* L. (Motherwort): a review of its phytochemistry and pharmacology," *Phytotherapy Research*, vol. 27, no. 8, pp. 1115–1120, 2013.

[284] Motherwort Benefits, Uses and Side Effects, Assessment report on Leonurus cardiaca L., herba EMA/HMPC/127430/2010.

[285] M. Wichtl, *Herbal Drugs and Phytopharmaceuticals: A Handbook for Practice on a Scientific Basis*, Medpharm, Guildford, UK, 2004.

[286] V. Agnihotri, H. ElSohly, T. Smillie, I. Khan, and L. Walker, "New Labdane diterpenes from *Leonurus cardiaca*," *Planta Medica*, vol. 74, no. 3, pp. 1288–1290, 2008.

[287] G. Janicsák, K. Veres, A. Zoltán Kakasy, and I. Máthé, "Study of the oleanolic and ursolic acid contents of some species of the Lamiaceae," *Biochemical Systematics and Ecology*, vol. 34, no. 5, pp. 392–396, 2006.

[288] K. Miłkowska-Leyck, B. Filipek, and H. Strzelecka, "Pharmacological effects of lavandulifolioside from *Leonurus cardiaca*," *Journal of Ethnopharmacology*, vol. 80, no. 1, pp. 85–90, 2002.

[289] J. Bernatoniene, A. Kucinskaite, R. Masteikova, Z. Kalveniene, G. Kasparaviciene, and A. Savickas, "The comparison of antioxidative kinetics in vitro of the fluid extract from maidenhair tree, motherwort and hawthorn," *Acta Poloniae Pharmaceutica*, vol. 66, no. 4, pp. 415–421, 2009.

[290] K. Morteza-Semnani, M. Saeedi, and M. Akbarzadeh, "The essential oil composition of *Leonurus cardiaca* L.," *Journal of Essential Oil Research*, vol. 20, pp. 107–109, 2008.

[291] D. Mockutë, G. Bernotienë, and A. Judþentienë, "Storage-induced changes in essential oil composition of *Leonurus cardiaca* L. plants growing wild in Vilnius and of commercial herbs," *Chemija*, vol. 16, no. 2, pp. 29–32, 2005.

[292] A. A. Sattar, V. Bankova, A. Kujumgiev et al., "Chemical composition and biological activity of leaf exudates from some Lamiaceae plants," *Pharmazie*, vol. 50, pp. 62–65, 1995.

[293] S. Jafari, A. Moradi, A. Salaritabar, A. Hadjiakhoondi, and M. Khanavi, "Determination of total phenolic and flavonoid contents of *Leonurus cardiaca* L. in compare with antioxidant activity," *Research Journal of Biological Sciences*, vol. 5, pp. 484–487, 2010.

[294] M. S. Ali, S. A. Ibrahim, S. Jalil, and M. I. Choudhary, "Ursolic acid: a potent inhibitor of superoxides produced in the cellular system," *Phytotherapy Research*, vol. 21, no. 6, pp. 558–561, 2007.

[295] X. Song, T. Wang, Z. Zhang et al., "Leonurine exerts anti-inflammatory effect by regulating inflammatory signaling pathways and cytokines in LPS-induced mouse mastitis," *Inflammation*, vol. 38, pp. 79–88, 2015.

[296] M. Rezaee-Asl, M. Sabour, V. Nikoui et al., "The study of analgesic effects of *Leonurus cardiaca* L. in mice by formalin, tail flick and hot plate tests," *International Scholarly Research Notices*, vol. 2014, pp. 1–5, 2014.

[297] J. Qi, Z. Y. Hong, H. Xin, and Y. Z. Zhu, "Neuroprotective effects of leonurine on ischemia/reperfusion-induced mitochondrial dysfunctions in rat cerebral cortex," *Biological & Pharmaceutical Bulletin*, vol. 33, no. 12, pp. 1958–1964, 2010.

[298] K. B. Ovanesov, I. M. Ovanesova, and E. B. Arushanian, "Effects of melatonin and motherwort tincture on the emotional state and visual functions in anxious subjects," *Eksperimental'naia i klinicheskaia farmakologiia*, vol. 69, no. 6, pp. 17–9, 2006.

[299] J. Tao, P. Zhang, G. Liu et al., "Cytotoxicity of Chinese motherwort (YiMuCao) aqueous ethanol extract is non-apoptotic and estrogen receptor independent on human breast cancer cells," *Journal of Ethnopharmacology*, vol. 122, pp. 234–239, 2009.

[300] A. Tachjian and V. Maria, "Use of herbal products and potential interactions in patients with cardiovascular diseases," *Journal of the American College of Cardiology*, vol. 55, no. 6, pp. 515–525, 2011.

[301] J. Bunsawat, N. E. Elliott, K. L. Hertweck, E. Sproles, and L. A. Alice, "Phylogenetics of *Mentha* (Lamiaceae): evidence from chloroplast DNA sequences," *Systematic Botany*, vol. 29, no. 4, pp. 959–964, 2004.

[302] D. L. McKay and J. B. Blumberg, "A review of the bioactivity and potential health benefits of peppermint tea (*Mentha piperita* L.)," *Phytotherapy Research*, vol. 20, no. 8, pp. 619–633, 2006.

[303] D. L. McKay and J. B. Blumberg, "A review of the bioactivity and potential health benefits of peppermint tea (*Mentha piperita* L.)," *Phytotherapy Research*, vol. 20, no. 8, pp. 619–633, 2006.

[304] C. Gherman, M. Culea, and O. Cozar, "Comparative analysis of some active principles of herb plants by GC/MS," *Talanta*, vol. 53, no. 1, pp. 253–262, 2000.

[305] J. A. Pino, P. Borges, M. A. Martinez et al., "Essential oil of *Mentha piperita* L. grown in Jalisco," *Journal of Essential Oil Research*, vol. 14, no. 3, pp. 189-190, 2002.

[306] M. L. Ruiz del Castillo, G. Santa-María, M. Herraiz, and G. P. Blanch, "A comparative study of the ability of different techniques to extract menthol from *Mentha piperita*," *Journal of Chromatographic Science*, vol. 41, no. 7, pp. 385–389, 2003.

[307] M. C. S. G. Blanco, L. C. Ming, M. O. M. Marques, and O. A. Bovi, "Drying temperature effects in peppermint essential oil content and composition," *Acta Horticulturae*, no. 569, pp. 95–98, 2002.

[308] M. Maffei and S. Scannerini, "Seasonal variations in fatty acids from non-polar lipids of developing *peppermint* leaves," *Phytochemistry*, vol. 31, no. 2, pp. 479–484, 1992.

[309] R. J. Clark and R. C. Menary, "Variations in composition of peppermint oil in relation to production areas," *Economic Botany*, vol. 35, no. 1, pp. 59–69, 1981.

[310] B. Fatih, K. Madani, M. Chibane, and P. Duez, "Chemical composition and biological activities of *Mentha* species," in *Aromatic and Medicinal Plants–Back to Nature*, InTech, Bronx, NY, USA, 2017.

[311] E. Capecka, A. Mareczek, and M. Leja, "Antioxidant activity of fresh and dry herbs of some *Lamiaceae* species," *Food Chemistry*, vol. 93, no. 2, pp. 223–226, 2005.

[312] A. Lozak, K. Sołtyk, P. Ostapczuk, and Z. Fijałek, "Determination of selected trace elements in herbs and their infusions," *Science of the Total Environment*, vol. 289, no. 1–3, pp. 33–40, 2002.

[313] F. M. ScienceDirect, P. Valentão, P. B. Andrade, F. Ferreres, and R. M. Seabra, *Food Chemistry*, Applied Science Publishers, London, UK, 2001.

[314] W. Zheng and S. Y. Wang, "Antioxidant activity and phenolic compounds in selected herbs," *Journal of Agricultural and Food Chemistry*, vol. 49, no. 11, pp. 5165–5170, 2001.

[315] M. Gavahian, A. Farahnaky, R. Farhoosh, K. Javidnia, and F. Shahidi, "Extraction of essential oils from *Mentha piperita* using advanced techniques: microwave versus ohmic assisted hydrodistillation," *Food and Bioproducts Processing*, vol. 94, pp. 50–58, 2015.

[316] B. Kaufmann and P. Christen, "Recent extraction techniques for natural products: microwave-assisted extraction and pressurised solvent extraction," *Phytochemical Analysis*, vol. 13, no. 2, pp. 105–113, 2002.

[317] L. Wang and C. L. Weller, "Recent advances in extraction of nutraceuticals from plants," *Trends in Food Science and Technology*, vol. 17, no. 6, pp. 300–312, 2006.

[318] T. J. Mason, F. Chemat, and M. Vinatoru, "The extraction of natural products using ultrasound or microwaves," *Current Organic Chemistry*, vol. 15, no. 2, pp. 237–247, 2011.

[319] L. Petigny, S. Périno, M. Minuti, F. Visinoni, J. Wajsman, and F. Chemat, "Simultaneous microwave extraction and separation of volatile and non-volatile organic compounds of boldo leaves. From lab to industrial scale," *International Journal of Molecular Sciences*, vol. 15, no. 5, pp. 7183–7198, 2014.

[320] S. Dragland, H. Senoo, K. Wake, K. Holte, and R. Blomhoff, "Several culinary and medicinal herbs are important sources of dietary antioxidants," *Journal of Nutrition*, vol. 133, no. 5, pp. 1286–1290, 2003.

[321] S. K. G. Abirami and P. Nirmala, "A comparative–invitro study of anticancer effect of *Mentha piperita*, *Ocimum basilicum* and *Coleus aromaticus* against human laryngeal epidermoid carcinoma (HEP-2) cell lines," *Journal of Medicinal Plants Studies*, vol. 2, no. 1, 2014.

[322] P. Ferreira, T. Cardoso, F. Ferreira, M. Fernandes-Ferreira, P. Piper, and M. J. Sousa, "*Mentha piperita* essential oil induces apoptosis in yeast associated with both cytosolic and mitochondrial ROS-mediated damage," *FEMS Yeast Research*, vol. 14, 2014.

[323] T. Inoue, Y. Sugimoto, H. Masuda, and C. Kamei, "Antiallergic effect of flavonoid glycosides obtained from *Mentha piperita* L.," *Biological and Pharmaceutical Bulletin*, vol. 25, no. 2, pp. 256–259, 2002.

[324] A. Sato and H. Tamura, "High antiallergic activity of 5,6,4′-trihydroxy-7,8,3′-trimethoxyflavone and 5,6-dihydroxy-7,8,3′,4′-tetramethoxyflavone from eau de cologne mint (*Mentha* × *piperita* citrata)," *Fitoterapia*, vol. 102, pp. 74–83, 2015.

[325] A. Schuhmacher, J. Reichling, and P. Schnitzler, "Virucidal effect of peppermint oil on the enveloped viruses herpes simplex virus type 1 and type 2 in vitro," *Phytomedicine*, vol. 10, no. 6-7, pp. 504–510, 2003.

[326] J. Omidian, F. Sheikhi-Shooshtari, and M. Fazeli, "Inhibitory effect of *Mentha Piperita* extracts against herpes simplex virus isolated from eye infection," *Iranian Journal of Virology*, vol. 8, no. 1, pp. 35–41, 2014.

[327] R. Singh, M. A. M. Shushni, and A. Belkheir, "Antibacterial and antioxidant activities of *Mentha piperita* L.," *Arabian Journal of Chemistry*, vol. 8, no. 3, pp. 322–328, 2015.

[328] P. Horváth and J. Koščová, "In vitro antibacterial activity of *Mentha* essential oils against *Staphylococcus aureus*," *Folia Veterinaria*, vol. 61, no. 3, pp. 71–77, 2017.

[329] S. Inouye, H. Yamaguchi, and T. Takizawa, "Screening of the antibacterial effects of a variety of essential oils on respiratory tract pathogens, using a modified dilution assay method," *Journal of Infection and Chemotherapy*, vol. 7, no. 4, pp. 251–254, 2001.

[330] Y. Shahbazi, "Chemical composition and in vitro antibacterial activity of *Mentha spicata* essential oil against common food-borne pathogenic bacteria," *Journal of Pathogens*, vol. 2015, Article ID 916305, 5 pages, 2015.

[331] I. Rasooli, P. Owlia, M. Taghizadeh, S. D. A. Astaneh, and S. M. Sharafi, "Protective effects of bioactive phytochemicals from *Mentha piperita* with multiple health potentials.," *Pharmacognosy Magazine*, vol. 6, no. 23, pp. 147–153, 2010.

[332] P. P. Maliakal and S. Wanwimolruk, "Effect of herbal teas on hepatic drug metabolizing enzymes in rats," *Journal of Pharmacy and Pharmacology*, vol. 53, no. 10, pp. 1323–1329, 2001.

[333] A. F. Khalil, H. O. Elkatry, and H. F. El Mehairy, "Protective effect of peppermint and parsley leaves oils against hepatotoxicity on experimental rats," *nnals of Agricultural Sciences*, vol. 60, no. 2, pp. 353–359, 2015.

[334] N. Ullah, M. A. Khan, T. Khan, A. H. Asif, and W. Ahmad, "Mentha piperita in nephrotoxicity–a possible intervention to ameliorate renal derangements associated with gentamicin," *Indian Journal of Pharmacology*, vol. 46, no. 2, pp. 166–170, 2014.

[335] A. H. Atta and A. Alkofahi, "Anti-nociceptive and anti-inflammatory effects of some Jordanian medicinal plant extracts," *Journal of Ethnopharmacology*, vol. 60, no. 2, pp. 117–124, 1998.

[336] Y. A. Taher, "Antinociceptive activity of *Mentha piperita* leaf aqueous extract in mice," *Libyan Journal of Medicine*, vol. 7, no. 1, p. 16205, 2012.

[337] A. H. Atta and K. A. EL-Sooud, "The antinociceptive effect of some Egyptian medicinal plant extracts," *Journal of Ethnopharmacology*, vol. 95, no. 2-3, pp. 235–238, 2004.

[338] L. Moreno, R. Bello, E. Primo-Yúfera, and J. Esplugues, "Pharmacological properties of the methanol extract from *Mentha suaveolens* Ehrh.," *Phytotherapy Research*, vol. 16, no. 1, pp. S10–S13, 2002.

[339] B. Nair, "Final report on the safety assessment of *Mentha piperita* (peppermint) oil, *Mentha piperita* (peppermint) leaf extract, *Mentha piperita* (peppermint) leaf, and *Mentha piperita* (peppermint) leaf water," *International Journal of Toxicology*, vol. 20, no. 3, pp. 61–73, 2001.

[340] P. M. H. Yousuf, N. Y. Noba, M. Shohel, R. Bhattacherjee, and B. K. Das, "Analgesic, anti-inflammatory and antipyretic effect of *Mentha spicata* (Spearmint)," *British Journal of Pharmaceutical Research*, vol. 3, no. 4, pp. 854–864, 2013.

[341] G. J. Amabeoku, S. J. Erasmus, J. A. O. Ojewole, and J. T. Mukinda, "Antipyretic and antinociceptive properties of *Mentha longifolia* Huds. (Lamiaceae) leaf aqueous extract in rats and mice," *Methods and Findings in Experimental and Clinical Pharmacology*, vol. 31, no. 10, p. 645, 2009.

[342] N. N. Biswas, S. Saha, and M. K. Ali, "Antioxidant, antimicrobial, cytotoxic and analgesic activities of ethanolic extract of *Mentha arvensis* L.," *Asian Pacific Journal of Tropical Biomedicine*, vol. 4, no. 10, pp. 792–797, 2014.

[343] B. Adorjan and G. Buchbauer, "Biological properties of essential oils: an updated review," *Flavour and Fragrance Journal*, vol. 25, no. 6, pp. 407–426, 2010.

[344] M. Nicolai, P. Pereira, R. F. Vitor, C. P. Reis, A. Roberto, and P. Rijo, "Antioxidant activity and rosmarinic acid content of ultrasound-assisted ethanolic extracts of medicinal plants," *Measurement*, vol. 89, pp. 328–332, 2016.

[345] S. C. Duda, L. A. Mărghitaş, D. Dezmirean, M. Duda, R. Mărgăoan, and O. Bobiş, "Changes in major bioactive compounds with antioxidant activity of *Agastache foeniculum, Lavandula angustifolia, Melissa officinalis* and *Nepeta cataria* : effect of harvest time and plant species," *Industrial Crops and Products*, vol. 77, pp. 499–507, 2015.

[346] Z. Rabiei, M. Rafieian-Kopaei, S. Mokhtari, Z. Alibabaei, and M. Shahrani, "The effect of pretreatment with different doses of *Lavandula officinalis* ethanolic extract on memory, learning and nociception," *Biomedicine and Aging Pathology*, vol. 4, no. 1, pp. 71–76, 2014.

[347] S. B. Waller, M. B. Cleff, E. F. Serra et al., "Plants from Lamiaceae family as source of antifungal molecules in humane and veterinary medicine," *Microbial Pathogenesis*, vol. 104, pp. 232–237, 2017.

[348] Z. Xiao, Q. Li, Y. Niu et al., "Odor-active compounds of different lavender essential oils and their correlation with sensory attributes," *Industrial Crops and Products*, vol. 108, pp. 748–755, 2017.

[349] V. Hajhashemi, A. Ghannadi, and B. Sharif, "Anti-inflammatory and analgesic properties of the leaf extracts and essential oil of *Lavandula angustifolia* Mill.," *Journal of Ethnopharmacology*, vol. 89, pp. 67–71, 2003.

[350] Z. Rabiei and M. Rafieian-Kopaei, "Neuroprotective effect of pretreatment with *Lavandula officinalis* ethanolic extract on blood-brain barrier permeability in a rat stroke model," *Asian Pacific Journal of Tropical Medicine*, vol. 7, pp. S421–S426, 2014.

[351] L. Pistelli, B. Najar, S. Giovanelli, L. Lorenzini, S. Tavarini, and L. G. Angelini, "Agronomic and phytochemical evaluation of lavandin and lavender cultivars cultivated in the Tyrrhenian area of Tuscany (Italy)," *Industrial Crops and Products*, vol. 109, pp. 37–44, 2017.

[352] A. Chrysargyris, C. Panayiotou, and N. Tzortzakis, "Nitrogen and phosphorus levels affected plant growth, essential oil composition and antioxidant status of lavender plant (*Lavandula angustifolia* Mill.)," *Industrial Crops and Products*, vol. 83, pp. 577–586, 2016.

[353] E. Barocelli, F. Calcina, M. Chiavarini et al., "Antinociceptive and gastroprotective effects of inhaled and orally administered *Lavandula hybrida* Reverchon "grosso" essential oil," *Life Sciences*, vol. 76, no. 2, pp. 213–223, 2004.

[354] Y. Husseini, H. Sahraei, G. H. Meftahi et al., "Analgesic and anti-inflammatory activities of hydro-alcoholic extract of Lavandula officinalis in mice: possible involvement of the cyclooxygenase type 1 and 2 enzymes," *Revista Brasileira de Farmacognosia*, vol. 26, pp. 102–108, 2016.

[355] M. R. Serafini, M. Campos, K. Rabelo et al., "Determination of chemical and physical properties of *Hyptis pectinata* essential oil and their redox active profile," *Free Radical Biology and Medicine*, vol. 3, pp. 1–9, 2012.

[356] S. Gavanji, E. Mohammadi, B. Larki, and A. Bakhtari, "Antimicrobial and cytotoxic evaluation of some herbal essential oils in comparison with common antibiotics in bioassay condition," *Integrative Medicine Research*, vol. 3, no. 3, pp. 142–152, 2014.

[357] G. Flamini, P. L. Cioni, and I. Morelli, "Composition of the essential oils and in vivo emission of volatiles of four *Lamium* species from Italy: *L. purpureum*, *L. hybridum*, *L. bifidum* and *L. amplexicaule*," *Food Chemistry*, vol. 91, no. 1, pp. 63–68, 2005.

[358] Y. El Ouadi, M. Manssouri, A. Bouyanzer et al., "Essential oil composition and antifungal activity of *Melissa officinalis* originating from north-east Morocco, against postharvest phytopathogenic fungi in apples," *Microbial Pathogenesis*, vol. 107, pp. 321–326, 2017.

[359] C. Mogosan, O. Vostinaru, R. Oprean et al., "A comparative analysis of the chemical composition, anti-inflammatory, and antinociceptive effects of the essential oils from three species of Mentha cultivated in Romania," *Molecules*, vol. 22, no. 2, p. 263, 2017.

[360] A. Kadri, Z. Zarai, A. Békir, N. Gharsallah, and M. Damak, "Chemical composition and antioxidant activity of *Marrubium vulgare* L. essential oil from Tunisia," *African Journal of Biotechnology*, vol. 10, no. 19, pp. 3908–3914, 2011.

[361] G. De Mastro, W. Tarraf, L. Verdini, G. Brunetti, and C. Ruta, "Essential oil diversity of *Origanum vulgare* L. populations from Southern Italy," *Food Chemistry*, vol. 235, pp. 1–6, 2017.

[362] D. Benedec, I. Oniga, R. Oprean, and M. Tamas, "Chemical composition of the essential oils of *Ocimum basilicum* L. cultivated in Romania," *Farmacia*, vol. 57, pp. 625–629, 2009.

[363] A. L. Martínez, M. E. González-Trujano, F. Pellicer, F. J. López-Muñoz, and A. Navarrete, "Antinociceptive effect and GC/MS analysis of *Rosmarinus officinalis* L. essential oil from its aerial parts," *Planta Medica*, vol. 75, no. 5, pp. 508–511, 2009.

[364] L. De Martino, V. De Feo, and F. Nazzaro, "Chemical composition and in vitro antimicrobial and mutagenic activities of seven Lamiaceae essential oils," *Molecules*, vol. 14, no. 10, pp. 4213–4230, 2009.

[365] M. Moosavi-Nasab, M. J. Saharkhiz, E. Ziaee, F. Moayedi, R. Koshani, and R. Azizi, "Chemical compositions and antibacterial activities of five selected aromatic plants essential oils against food-borne pathogens and spoilage bacteria," *Journal of Essential Oil Research*, vol. 28, no. 3, pp. 241–251, 2016.

[366] F. N. Yalçin, D. Kaya, I. Çaliş, T. Ersöz, and E. Palaska, "Determination of iridoid glycosides from four Turkish *Lamium* species by HPLC-ESI/MS," *Turkish Journal of Chemistry*, vol. 32, no. 4, pp. 457–467, 2008.

[367] M. Carocho, L. Barros, R. C. Calhelha et al., "*Melissa officinalis* L. decoctions as functional beverages: a bioactive approach and chemical characterization," *Food and Function*, vol. 6, pp. 2240–2248, 2015.

[368] M. Cirlini, P. Mena, M. Tassotti et al., "Phenolic and volatile composition of a dry spearmint (*Mentha spicata* L.) extract," *Molecules*, vol. 21, pp. 1–15, 2016.

[369] N. Amessis-Ouchemoukh, I. M. Abu-Reidah, R. Quirantes-Piné, K. Madani, and A. Segura-Carretero, "Phytochemical profiling, *in vitro* evaluation of total phenolic contents and antioxidant properties of *Marrubium vulgare* (horehound) leaves of plants growing in Algeria," *Industrial Crops and Products*, vol. 61, pp. 120–129, 2014.

[370] A. Vallverdú-Queralt, J. Regueiro, M. Martínez-Huélamo, J. F. Rinaldi Alvarenga, L. N. Leal, and R. M. Lamuela-Raventos, "A comprehensive study on the phenolic profile of widely used culinary herbs and spices: rosemary, thyme, oregano, cinnamon, cumin and bay," *Food Chemistry*, vol. 154, pp. 299–307, 2014.

[371] R. Pandey and B. Kumar, "HPLC-QTOF-MS/MS-based rapid screening of phenolics and triterpenic acids in leaf extracts of *Ocimum* species and their interspecies variation," *Journal of Liquid Chromatography and Related Technologies*, vol. 39, no. 4, pp. 225–238, 2016.

[372] P. Mena, M. Cirlini, M. Tassotti, K. A. Herrlinger, C. Dall'Asta, and D. Del Rio, "Phytochemical profiling of flavonoids, phenolic acids, terpenoids, and volatile fraction of a rosemary (*Rosmarinus officinalis* L.) extract," *Molecules*, vol. 21, no. 11, pp. 1–15, 2016.

[373] B. F. Zimmermann, S. G. Walch, L. N. Tinzoh, W. Stühlinger, and D. W. Lachenmeier, "Rapid UHPLC determination of polyphenols in aqueous infusions of *Salvia officinalis* L. (sage tea)," *Journal of Chromatography B*, vol. 879, no. 24, pp. 2459–2464, 2011.

[374] M. Marrelli, F. Conforti, D. Rigano et al., "Cytotoxic properties of *Marrubium globosum* ssp. *libanoticum* and its bioactive components," *Natural Product Communications*, vol. 8, no. 5, pp. 567–569, 2013.

[375] N. Mnonopi, R. Levendal, M. T. Davies-Coleman, and C. L. Frosta, "The cardioprotective effects of marrubiin, a diterpenoid found in *Leonotis leonurus* extracts," *Journal of Ethnopharmacology*, vol. 138, no. 1, pp. 67–75, 2011.

[376] N. Zaabat, A.-E. Hay, S. Michalet et al., "Antioxidant and antigenotoxic properties of compounds isolated from *Marrubium deserti* de Noé," *Food and Chemical Toxicology*, vol. 49, no. 12, pp. 3328–3335, 2011.

[377] A. Paula de Oliveira, J. R. Santin, M. Lemos et al., "Gastroprotective activity of methanol extract and marrubiin obtained from leaves of *Marrubium vulgare* L. (Lamiaceae)," *Journal of Pharmacy and Pharmacology*, vol. 63, no. 9, pp. 1230–1237, 2011.

[378] N. Mnonopi, R.-A. Levendal, M. T. Davies-Coleman, and C. L. Frost, "The cardioprotective effects of marrubiin, a diterpenoid found in *Leonotis leonurus* extracts," *Journal of Ethnopharmacology*, vol. 138, no. 1, pp. 67–75, 2011.

[379] R. Lucarini, W. A. Bernardes, D. S. Ferreira et al., "In vivo analgesic and anti-inflammatory activities of *Rosmarinus officinalis* aqueous extracts, rosmarinic acid and its acetyl ester derivative," *Pharmaceutical Biology*, vol. 51, no. 9, pp. 1087–1090, 2013.

[380] H. Hosseinzadeh and M. Nourbakhsh, "Effect of *Rosmarinus offcinalis* L. aerial parts extract on morphine withdrawal syndrome in mice," *Phytotherapy Research*, vol. 17, no. 8, pp. 938–941, 2003.

[381] C. Chen, H. Chen, C. Hsieh, Y. Yang, and B. Wung, "Upregulation of NF-E2-related factor-2-dependent glutathione by carnosol provokes a cytoprotective response and enhances cell survival," *Acta Pharmacologica Sinica*, vol. 32, no. 1, pp. 62–69, 2011.

[382] C.-F. Kuo, J.-D. Su, C.-H. Chiu et al., "Anti-inflammatory effects of supercritical carbon dioxide extract and its isolated carnosic acid from *Rosmarinus officinalis* leaves," *Journal of Agricultural and Food Chemistry*, vol. 59, no. 8, pp. 3674–3685, 2011.

[383] Y. Shingai, A. Fujimoto, M. Nakamura, and T. Masuda, "Structure and function of the oxidation products of polyphenols and identification of potent lipoxygenase inhibitors from fe-catalyzed oxidation of resveratrol," *Journal of Agricultural and Food Chemistry*, vol. 59, no. 15, pp. 8180–8186, 2011.

[384] E. S. Mengoni, G. Vichera, L. A. Rigano et al., "Suppression of COX-2, IL-1β and TNF-α expression and leukocyte infiltration in inflamed skin by bioactive compounds from *Rosmarinus officinalis* L.," *Fitoterapia*, vol. 82, no. 3, pp. 414–421, 2011.

[385] L. D. C. Mannelli, L. Micheli, M. Maresca et al., "Anti-neuropathic effects of *Rosmarinus officinalis* L. terpenoid fraction: relevance of nicotinic receptors," *Scientific Reports*, vol. 6, pp. 1–15, 2016.

[386] M. V. Ivan, A. Zala, A. Agop et al., "Several aspects about fractalitaty role in the dynamics of complex systems," *UPB Scientific Bulletin, Series A: Applied Mathematics and Physics*, vol. 79, no. 3, pp. 235–246, 2017.

[387] A. T. Peana, P. S. D'Aquila, F. Panin, G. Serra, P. Pippia, and M. D. L. Moretti, "Anti-inflammatory activity of linalool and linalyl acetate constituents of essential oils," *Phytomedicine*, vol. 9, no. 8, pp. 721–726, 2002.

[388] A. T. Peana, P. S. D'Aquila, M. L. Chessa, M. D. L. Moretti, G. Serra, and P. Pippia, "(−)-Linalool produces antinociception in two experimental models of pain," *European Journal of Pharmacology*, vol. 460, no. 1, pp. 37–41, 2003.

[389] V. S. Rao, A. M. Menezes, and G. S. Viana, "Effect of myrcene on nociception in mice," *Journal of Pharmacy and Pharmacology*, vol. 42, pp. 877-878, 1990.

[390] P. J. C. Sousa, C. F. B. M. Linard, D. Azevedo-Batista, A. C. Oliveira, A. N. Coelho-de-Souza, and J. H. Leal-

Cardoso, "Antinociceptive effects of the essential oil of *Mentha x villosa* leaf and its major constituent piperitenone oxide in mice," *Brazilian Journal of Medical and Biological Research*, vol. 42, no. 7, pp. 655–659, 2009.

[391] D. Le Bars, M. Gozariu, and S. W. Cadden, "Animal Models of Nociception," *Pharmacological Reviews*, vol. 53, no. 4, pp. 597–652, 2001.

[392] E. Williamson, D. Okpako, and F. Evans, *Selection, Preparation and Pharmacological Evaluation of Plant Material*, John Wiley & Sons, Hoboken, NJ, USA, 1996.

[393] A. W. Bannon and A. B. Malmberg, *Models of Nociception: Hot-Plate, Tail-Flick, and Formalin Tests in Rodents, in: Curr. Protoc. Neurosci.*, John Wiley & Sons, Inc., Hoboken, NJ, USA, 2007.

Permissions

All chapters in this book were first published in PRM, by Hindawi Publishing Corporation; hereby published with permission under the Creative Commons Attribution License or equivalent. Every chapter published in this book has been scrutinized by our experts. Their significance has been extensively debated. The topics covered herein carry significant findings which will fuel the growth of the discipline. They may even be implemented as practical applications or may be referred to as a beginning point for another development.

The contributors of this book come from diverse backgrounds, making this book a truly international effort. This book will bring forth new frontiers with its revolutionizing research information and detailed analysis of the nascent developments around the world.

We would like to thank all the contributing authors for lending their expertise to make the book truly unique. They have played a crucial role in the development of this book. Without their invaluable contributions this book wouldn't have been possible. They have made vital efforts to compile up to date information on the varied aspects of this subject to make this book a valuable addition to the collection of many professionals and students.

This book was conceptualized with the vision of imparting up-to-date information and advanced data in this field. To ensure the same, a matchless editorial board was set up. Every individual on the board went through rigorous rounds of assessment to prove their worth. After which they invested a large part of their time researching and compiling the most relevant data for our readers.

The editorial board has been involved in producing this book since its inception. They have spent rigorous hours researching and exploring the diverse topics which have resulted in the successful publishing of this book. They have passed on their knowledge of decades through this book. To expedite this challenging task, the publisher supported the team at every step. A small team of assistant editors was also appointed to further simplify the editing procedure and attain best results for the readers.

Apart from the editorial board, the designing team has also invested a significant amount of their time in understanding the subject and creating the most relevant covers. They scrutinized every image to scout for the most suitable representation of the subject and create an appropriate cover for the book.

The publishing team has been an ardent support to the editorial, designing and production team. Their endless efforts to recruit the best for this project, has resulted in the accomplishment of this book. They are a veteran in the field of academics and their pool of knowledge is as vast as their experience in printing. Their expertise and guidance has proved useful at every step. Their uncompromising quality standards have made this book an exceptional effort. Their encouragement from time to time has been an inspiration for everyone.

The publisher and the editorial board hope that this book will prove to be a valuable piece of knowledge for researchers, students, practitioners and scholars across the globe.

List of Contributors

Michael Brinkers, Moritz Kretzschmar and Giselher Pfau
Department of Anaesthesiology and Intensive Care Medicine, Otto-von-Guericke-University Magdeburg, Magdeburg, Germany

Paulina Rumpelt
Department of Diagnostic and Interventional Radiology, Oberlausitz-Kliniken, Bautzen, Germany

Anke Lux
Department for Biometrics and Medical Informatics, Otto-von-Guericke-University Magdeburg, Magdeburg, Germany

Roberta Maria Drumond Furtado Bossi Fonseca
Programa de Pós-Graduação em Patologia, Faculdade de Medicina, Universidade Federal de Minas Gerais (UFMG), Belo Horizonte, MG, Brazil

Eduardo Januzzi
Faculdade Ciodonto, Sete Lagoas, MG, Brazil

Antonio Carlos Pires Carvalho
Departamento de Radiologia, Faculdade de Medicina, Universidade Federal do Rio de Janeiro, Rio de Janeiro, RJ, Brazil

Luciano Ambrosio Ferreira
Departamento de Radiologia, Faculdade de Medicina, Universidade Federal do Rio de Janeiro, Rio de Janeiro, RJ, Brazil
Hospital Maternidade, erezinha de Jesus-HMTJ/JF, Suprema-Faculdade de CiênciasMédicas e da Saúde, Juiz de Fora, Brazil

Eduardo Grossmann
Departamento de Ciências Morfológicas, Instituto de Ciências Básicas da Saúde, Universidade Federal do Rio Grande do Sul, Porto Alegre, RS, Brazil

Pedro Gonçalves de Oliveira
Faculdade de Farmácia, Universidade Anhembi Morumbi, São Paulo, SP, Brazil

Érica Leandro Marciano Vieira
Departamento de Clínica Médica, Faculdade de Medicina, UFMG, Belo Horizonte, MG, Brazil

Antônio Lúcio Teixeira
Departamento de Clínica Médica, Faculdade de Medicina, UFMG, Belo Horizonte, MG, Brazil
Department of Psychiatry and Behavioral Sciences, The University of Texas, Houston, TX, USA

Camila Megale Almeida-Leite
Programa de Pós-Graduação em Patologia, Faculdade de Medicina, Universidade Federal de Minas Gerais (UFMG), Belo Horizonte, MG, Brazil
Departamento de Morfologia, Instituto de Ciências Biológicas, UFMG, Belo Horizonte, MG, Brazil

Humberto Guevara-García, Francisco J. García-Guillén and Ángel Herrera-Gómez
Department of Critical Care Medicine, Instituto Nacional de Cancerología, Mexico City, Mexico

Luis A. Sánchez-Hurtado
Department of Critical Care Medicine, Instituto Nacional de Cancerología, Mexico City, Mexico
Department of Critical Care Medicine, Hospital Especialidades Centro Médico Nacional La Raza, Mexican Institute of Social Security, Mexico City, Mexico

Mario Del Moral-Armengol
Department of Critical Care Medicine, Hospital Especialidades Centro Médico Nacional La Raza, Mexican Institute of Social Security, Mexico City, Mexico

Nancy Hernández-Sánchez
Department of Critical Care Medicine, UMAE Hospital de Traumatologia "Dr. Victor de la Fuente Narvaez", Mexican Institute of Social Security, Mexico City, Mexico

Silvio A. Ñamendys-Silva
Department of Critical Care Medicine, Instituto Nacional de Cancerología, Mexico City, Mexico
Department of Critical Care Medicine, Instituto Nacional de Ciencias Médicas y Nutrición Salvador Zubirán, Mexico City, Mexico
Department of Critical Care Medicine, Medica Sur Clinic and Foundation, Mexico City, Mexico

Ilhem Rjeibi, Anouar Feriani and Najla Hfaiedh
Research Unit of Macromolecular Biochemistry and Genetic, Faculty of Sciences of Gafsa, University of Gafsa, 2112 Gafsa, Tunisia

Jazia Sdayria
Research Unit of Macromolecular Biochemistry and Genetic, Faculty of Sciences of Gafsa, University of Gafsa, 2112 Gafsa, Tunisia

Laboratory of Animal Ecophysiology, Faculty of Science of Sfax, University of Sfax, 3018 Sfax, Tunisia

Abdelfattah Elfeki and Mohamed Salah Allagui
Laboratory of Animal Ecophysiology, Faculty of Science of Sfax, University of Sfax, 3018 Sfax, Tunisia

Sana Ncib and Wided Bouguerra
Common Services Unit for Research, Faculty of Sciences of Gafsa, University of Gafsa, 2112 Gafsa, Tunisia

Xaver Fuchs
Biopsychology and Cognitive Neuroscience, Faculty of Psychology and Sports Science, Bielefeld University, Bielefeld, Germany
Department of Cognitive and Clinical Neuroscience, Central Institute of Mental Health, Medical Faculty Mannheim, Heidelberg University, Mannheim, Germany

Robin Bekrater-Bodmann
Department of Cognitive and Clinical Neuroscience, Central Institute of Mental Health, Medical Faculty Mannheim, Heidelberg University, Mannheim, Germany

Herta Flor
Department of Cognitive and Clinical Neuroscience, Central Institute of Mental Health, Medical Faculty Mannheim, Heidelberg University, Mannheim, Germany
Center for Neuroplasticity and Pain (CNAP), SMI, Department of Health Science and Technology, Aalborg University, Aalborg, Denmark

Hiroshi Nagahisa, Kazumi Ikezaki and Hirofumi Miyata
Biological Sciences, Graduate School of Sciences and Technology for Innovation, Yamaguchi University, Yoshida 1677-1, Yamaguchi 753-8515, Japan

Ryotaro Yamada and Takashi Yamada
Graduate School of Health Sciences, Sapporo Medical University, Sapporo 060-8556, Japan

Monica L. Joustra, Wilma L. Zijlema and Karin A. M. Janssens
University of Groningen, University Medical Center Groningen, Department of Psychiatry, Groningen, Netherlands

Judith G. M. Rosmalen
University of Groningen, University Medical Center Groningen, Department of Psychiatry, Groningen, Netherlands
University of Groningen, University Medical Center Groningen, Department of Internal Medicine, Groningen, Netherlands

Izumi Makino, Yusuke Ohmichi, Shuichi Aono, Makoto Nishihara, Jun Sato and Noboru Hatakeyama
Multidisciplinary Pain Center, Aichi Medical University School of Medicine, Aichi, Japan

Young-Chang Arai, Masayuki Inoue, Tatsunori Ikemoto, Takahiro Ushida and Kazuhiro Shimo
Multidisciplinary Pain Center, Aichi Medical University School of Medicine, Aichi, Japan
Institute of Physical Fitness, Sports Medicine and Rehabilitation, Aichi Medical University

Hiroki Sakurai
Faculty of Health and Medical Sciences, Tokoha University, Shizuoka, Japan

Takako Matsubara
Multidisciplinary Pain Center, Aichi Medical University School of Medicine, Aichi, Japan
Faculty of Health and Medical Sciences, Tokoha University, Shizuoka, Japan

Emilie Paul-Savoie, Patricia Bourgault and Emilie Gosselin
School of Nursing, Faculty of Medicine and Health Sciences, Université de Sherbrooke, Sherbrooke, QC, Canada

Stéphane Potvin
Centre de Recherche de L'Institut Universitaire en Santé Mentale de Montréal, Department of Psychiatry, Faculty of Medicine, Université de Montréal, Montreal, QC, Canada

Sylvie Lafrenaye
Department of Pediatrics, Faculty of Medicine and Health Sciences, Université de Sherbrooke, Sherbrooke, QC, Canada

Paola Di Giacomo, Valeria Ferrara, Ettore Accivile, Giacomo Ferrato, Antonella Polimeni and Carlo Di Paolo
Department of Oral and Maxillofacial Sciences, Sapienza University of Rome, Rome, Italy

Junya Sakamoto, Jiro Nakano and Minoru Okita
Department of Physical Therapy Science, Nagasaki University Graduate School of Biomedical Sciences, Sakamoto 1-7-1, Nagasaki 852-8520, Japan

Yuichiro Honda, Ryo Sasabe and Takuya Fukushima
Department of Physical Therapy Science, Nagasaki University Graduate School of Biomedical Sciences, Sakamoto 1-7-1, Nagasaki 852-8520, Japan
Department of Rehabilitation, Nagasaki University Hospital, Sakamoto 1-7-1, Nagasaki 852-8520, Japan

Natsumi Tanaka
Department of Physical Therapy Science, Nagasaki University Graduate School of Biomedical Sciences, Sakamoto 1-7-1, Nagasaki 852-8520, Japan
Department of Physical Therapy, Niigata University of Health and Welfare, Shimami-cho 1398, Kitaku, Niigata 950-3198, Japan

Yohei Hamaue
Department of Physical Therapy, Niigata University of Health and Welfare, Shimami-cho 1398, Kitaku, Niigata 950-3198, Japan
Institute for Human Movement and Medical Sciences, Niigata University of Health and Welfare, Shimami-cho 1398, Kitaku, Niigata 950-3198, Japan

Hideki Kataoka and Kyo Goto
Department of Physical Therapy Science, Nagasaki University Graduate School of Biomedical Sciences, Sakamoto 1-7-1, Nagasaki 852-8520, Japan
Department of Rehabilitation, Nagasaki Memorial Hospital, Fukahori 1-11-5, Nagasaki 851-0301, Japan

Yasutaka Kondo
Department of Rehabilitation, Japanese Red Cross Nagasaki Atomic Bomb Hospital, Mori 3-15, Nagasaki 852-8104, Japan

Satoshi Oga
Department of Physical Therapy Science, Nagasaki University Graduate School of Biomedical Sciences, Sakamoto 1-7-1, Nagasaki 852-8520, Japan
Department of Rehabilitation, Saiseikai Nagasaki Hospital, Kitafuchi 2-5-1, Nagasaki 850-0003, Japan

Ryo Sasaki
Department of Physical Therapy Science, Nagasaki University Graduate School of Biomedical Sciences, Sakamoto 1-7-1, Nagasaki 852-8520, Japan
Department of Rehabilitation, Juzenkai Hospital, Kago 7-18, Nagasaki 850-0905, Japan

Daisuke Uritani
Department of Physical Therapy, Faculty of Health Science, Kio Univeristy, 4-2-2 Umaminaka, Koryocho, Kitakatsuragigun, Nara 6350832, Japan

Tomoko Nishida
Department of Rehabilitation, Japanese Red Cross Kyoto Daiichi Hospital, 15-749 Honmachi, Higashiyamaku, Kyoto 6050981, Japan

Nanami Sakaguchi
Department of Rehabilitation, Higashiosaka Yamaji Hospital, 1-7-5 Inaba, Higashiosaka, Osaka 5780925, Japan

Tetsuji Kawakami and Tadaaki Kirita
Department of Oral and Maxillofacial Surgery, Nara Medical University, 840 Shijo-Cho, Kashihara, Nara 6348521, Japan

Lester E. Jones
Judith Lumley Centre, La Trobe University, Plenty Road, Bundoora, Melbourne, VIC 3086, Australia

Maarten van Kleef
Department of Anesthesiology and Pain Medicine, Maastricht University Medical Centre, Maastricht, Netherlands

José W. Geurts
Department of Anesthesiology and Pain Medicine, Maastricht University Medical Centre, Maastricht, Netherlands
Department of Anesthesiology and Pain Management, Rijnstate Hospital, Arnhem, Netherlands

Jan-Willem Kallewaard
Department of Anesthesiology and Pain Management, Rijnstate Hospital, Arnhem, Netherlands

Paul C. Willems
Department of Orthopedic Surgery, Maastricht University Medical Centre, Maastricht, Netherlands

Carmen Dirksen
Department of Clinical Epidemiology and Medical Technology, Maastricht University Medical Centre, CAPHRI—Care and Public Health Research Institute, Maastricht, Netherlands

Fushui Liu, Ting Fang, Fanyuan Zhou, Meimei Zhao, Mei Chen, Jianyu You, Yuli Jin and Jinmei Xie
School of Moxibustion, Jiangxi University of Traditional Chinese Medicine, Nanchang, China

Zhongyong Liu
College of Clinical Medicine, Jiangxi University of Traditional Chinese Medicine, Nanchang, China

Willias Masocha
Department of Pharmacology and Therapeutics, Faculty of Pharmacy, Kuwait University, Safat 13110, Kuwait

C. Praz, P. Terrier, P. Vuistiner and B. Léger
Institute for Research in Rehabilitation, Clinique Romande de Réadaptation Suvacare, Avenue Grand-Champsec 90, 1950 Sion, Switzerland

J. Ducki and M. L. Connaissa
Institute of Sports Sciences, University of Lausanne, Géopolis, Campus Dorigny, 1015 Lausanne, Switzerland

F. Luthi
Institute for Research in Rehabilitation, Clinique Romande de R´eadaptation Suvacare, Avenue Grand-Champsec 90, 1950 Sion, Switzerland
Department for Musculoskeletal Rehabilitation, Clinique Romande de R´eadaptation Suvacare, Avenue Grand-Champsec 90, 1950 Sion, Switzerland
Department of Physical Medicine and Rehabilitation, Orthopaedic Hospital, Lausanne University Hospital, Rue du Bugnon 21, 1011 Lausanne, Switzerland

Hyeun Sung Kim, Nitin Adsul, Byapak Paudel, Ki Joon Kim, Sung Ho Choi, Jeong Hoon Kim, Sung Kyun Chung, Jeong-Hoon Choi and Jee-Soo Jang
Department of Neurosurgery, Nanoori Suwon Hospital, Suwon, Republic of Korea

Farid Yudoyono
Department of Neurosurgery, Hasan Sadikin Hospital, College of Medicine, Universitas Padjadjaran, Bandung, Jawa Barat, Indonesia

Il-Tae Jang
Department of Neurosurgery, Nanoori Hospital, Seoul, Republic of Korea

Seong-Hoon Oh
Department of Neurosurgery, Nanoori Incheon Hospital, Incheon, Republic of Korea

Renata Zajączkowska, Jarosław Woroń, Anna Wrzosek and Jerzy Wordliczek
Department of Interdisciplinary Intensive Care, Jagiellonian University Medical College, Kraków, Poland

Wojciech Leppert
Department of Palliative Medicine, Poznan University of Medical Sciences, Poznan, Poland

Joanna Mika
Department of Pain Pharmacology, Institute of Pharmacology, Polish Academy of Sciences, Kraków, Poland

Magdalena Kocot-Kępska
Department of Pain Research and Treatment, Jagiellonian University Medical College, Kraków, Poland

Carlos Suso-Ribera
Department of Basic and Clinical Psychology and Psychobiology, Jaume I University, Castell´on de la Plana, Spain

Michael J. L. Sullivan
Department of Psychology, McGill University, Montreal, Canada

Santiago Suso-Vergara
Department of Traumatology, Clinic Hospital, Barcelona, Spain

Ann-Katrin Stensdotter
Department of Neuromedicine and Movement Science, Faculty of Medicine and Health Sciences, Norwegian University of Science and Technology (NTNU), Trondheim, Norway

Omid Rasouli
Department of Neuromedicine and Movement Science, Faculty of Medicine and Health Sciences, Norwegian University of Science and Technology (NTNU), Trondheim, Norway
Department of Public Health and Nursing, Faculty of Medicine and Health Sciences, Norwegian University of Science and Technology (NTNU), Trondheim, Norway

Egil A. Fors, Ottar Vasseljen, Egil A. Fors and Ottar Vasseljen
Department of Public Health and Nursing, Faculty of Medicine and Health Sciences, Norwegian University of Science and Technology (NTNU), Trondheim, Norway

Yuhua Yin and Dong Woon Kim
Department of Medical Science, Chungnam National University School of Medicine, Daejeon 35015, Republic of Korea
Department of Anatomy and Cell Biology, Brain Research Institute, Chungnam National University School of Medicine, Daejeon 35015, Republic of Korea

Min-Hee Yi
Department of Neurology, Mayo Clinic, Rochester, MN 55905, USA

Marit Slåttelid Skeie
Department of Clinical Dentistry, Pediatric Dentistry, The Faculty of Medicine, University of Bergen, Bergen, Norway

Paula Frid
Department of Otorhinolaryngology, Division of Oral and Maxillofacial Surgery, University Hospital North Norway and Public Dental Service Competence Centre of North Norway and Department of Clinical Medicine, Faculty of Health Sciences, The Arctic University of Norway, Tromsø, Norway

Manal Mustafa
Oral Health Centre of Expertise in Western Norway, Hordaland, Norway

Jörg Aßmus
Centre for Clinical Research, Haukeland University Hospital, 5021 Bergen, Norway

Annika Rosén
Department of Clinical Dentistry, Division of Oral and Maxillofacial Surgery, The Faculty of Medicine, University of Bergen, Bergen, Norway

Regina Schultz and Tania Gardner
Department of Pain Medicine, St Vincent's Hospital, Sydney, NSW, Australia

Jessica Smith and Gavin Andrews
Clinical Research Unit for Anxiety and Depression (CRUfAD), School of Psychiatry, St Vincent's Hospital, University of New South Wales, Sydney, NSW, Australia

Jill M. Newby
Clinical Research Unit for Anxiety and Depression (CRUfAD), School of Psychiatry, St Vincent's Hospital, University of New South Wales, Sydney, NSW, Australia
School of Psychology, University of New South Wales, Sydney, Australia

Christine T. Shiner and Steven G. Faux
Department of Pain Medicine, St Vincent's Hospital, Sydney, NSW, Australia
St Vincent's Clinical School, University of New South Wales, Sydney, Australia

Raúl Ferrer-Peña
Physical Therapy Department and Motion in Brains Research Group, Instituto de Neurociencias y Ciencias del Movimiento (INCIMOV), Centro Superior de Estudios Universitarios La Salle, Universidad Aut´onoma de Madrid, Madrid, Spain Centro de Salud Entrevías, Gerencia de Atención Primaria, Servicio Madrileño de Salud, Madrid, Spain
Escuela Internacional de Doctorado, Department of Physical Therapy, Occupational Therapy, Rehabilitation and Physical Medicine, Universidad Rey Juan Carlos, Alcorcón, Spain

César Calvo-Lobo
Nursing and Physical Therapy Department, Faculty of Health Sciences, Universidad de León, Ponferrada, León, Spain

Ramón Aiguadé
Departamento de enfermería y fisioterapia, Universitat de Lleida, Lleida, Spain

Josué Fernández-Carnero
Department of Physical Therapy, Occupational Therapy, Rehabilitation and Physical Medicine, Universidad Rey Juan Carlos, Alcorcón, Spain

Mefkure Eraslan Sahin and Erdem Sahin
Department of Obstetrics and Gynecology, Health Sciences University Sivas Sarkışla Government Hospital, Sivas, Turkey

Yusuf Madendag, Fatma Özdemir, Gokhan Acmaz and Iptisam Ipek Muderris
Department of Obstetrics and Gynecology, Erciyes University Medicine Faculty, Kayseri, Turkey

Ilknur Col Madendag
Department of Obstetrics and Gynecology, Health Sciences University Kayseri Education and Research Hospital, Kayseri, Turkey

Ahter Tanay Tayyar
Department of Obstetrics and Gynecology, Acibadem Maslak Hospital, Istanbul, Turkey

Malgorzata Pihut and Andrzej Gala
Prosthodontics Department, Consulting Room of Temporomandibular Joint Dysfunction, Jagiellonian University Medical Collage, 4 Montelupich Str., 31-155 Krakow, Poland

Piotr Ceranowicz
Department of Physiology, Faculty of Clinical Physiology, Jagiellonian University Medical College, 16 Grzegorzecka Str., 31-531 Krakow, Poland

Ewa Wozniak, Jolanta E. Loster and Aneta Wieczorek
Department of Dental Prosthetics, Institute of Dentistry at Jagiellonian University, Krakow, Poland

Walid Frigui
Department of Anesthesia and Intensive Care, Sahloul Academic Hospital, Sousse, Tunisia

Mohamed Said Nakhli, Mohamed Kahloul and Walid Naija
Department of Anesthesia and Intensive Care, Sahloul Academic Hospital, Sousse, Tunisia
University of Medicine "Ibn Al Jazzar", Sousse, Tunisia

Chawki Jebali
University of Medicine "Ibn Al Jazzar", Sousse, Tunisia
Emergency Medical Service, Sahloul Academic Hospital, Sousse, Tunisia

Susanna Zanini, Alessandra Voltolini and Emilia Fumagalli
Clinical Psychology Service, ASST Grande Ospedale Metropolitano Niguarda, Piazza Dell'Ospedale Maggiore 3, 20162 Milan, Italy

Gaia Gragnano
Department of Psychology, Università Cattolica del Sacro Cuore, Largo Agostino Gemelli 1, 20123 Milan, Italy

Francesco Pagnini
Department of Psychology, Università Cattolica del Sacro Cuore, Largo Agostino Gemelli 1, 20123 Milan, Italy
Department of Psychology, Harvard University, 33 Kirkland Street, Cambridge, MA 02138, USA

Cristina M. Uritu, Cosmin T. Mihai, Gabriela-Dumitrita Stanciu, Gianina Dodi, Teodora Alexa-Stratulat, Andrei Luca, Maria-Magdalena Leon-Constantin, Raluca Stefanescu, Veronica Bild and Bogdan I. Tamba
"Grigore T. Popa" University of Medicine and Pharmacy, 700115 Iasi, Romania

Silvia Melnic
Institute of Chemistry, Academy of Sciences of Moldova, MD-2028 Chisinau, Moldova

Index